NGE medical b

This b

URGERY ON CALL

d Edition

d by

T. Lefor, MD, MPH, FACS
or, Division of Surgical Oncology
or, Surgical Education and Academic Affairs
rs-Sinai Medical Center
ciate Professor of Clinical Surgery
artment of Surgery
versity of California, Los Angeles
Angeles, California

nard G. Gomella, MD, FACS
Bernard W. Goodwin Jr. Associate Professor
partment of Urology
rson Medical College
mas Jefferson University
adelphia, Pennsylvania

Lange Medical Books/McGraw-Hill
Medical Publishing Division

New York Chicago San Francisco Lisbon London
Madrid Mexico City San Juan
Seoul

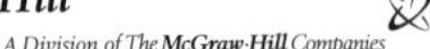

Surgery On Call, Third Edition

1234567890 DOC/DOC 0987654321

ISSN: 1044-4033
ISBN: 0-8385-8817-4 (Domestic)

Notice

Medicine is an ever-changing science. As new research and clinical experience broaden our knowledge, changes in treatment and drug therapy are required. The authors and the publisher of this work have checked with sources believed to be reliable in their efforts to provide information that is complete and generally in accord with the standards accepted at the time of publication. However, in view of the possibility of human error or changes in medical sciences, neither the authors nor the publisher nor any other party who has been involved in the preparation or publication of this work warrants that the information contained herein is in every respect accurate or complete, and they disclaim all responsibility for any errors or omissions or for the results obtained from use of the information contained in this work. Readers are encouraged to confirm the information contained herein with other sources. For example and in particular, readers are advised to check the product information sheet included in the package of each drug they plan to administer to be certain that the information contained in the this work is accurate and changes have not been made in the recommended dose or in the contraindications for administration. This recommendation is of particular importance in connection with new or infrequently used drugs.

The book was set in Helvetica by Pine Tree Composition, Inc.
The editors were Janet Foltin, Isabel Nogueira, and Barbara Holton.
The production supervisor was Phil Galea.
The cover designer was Mary McKean.
The index was prepared by Marianna Wackerman
The art manager was Charissa Baker.

R. R. Donnelley & Sons Company was the printer and binder.

This book is printed on acid-free paper.

INTERNATIONAL EDITION ISBN 0–07–-118219–5

To Sheila and Maarten, and to Tricia, Leonard, Patrick, Andrew, Michael and Aunt Lucy for their gift of time.

Contents

Associate Editors

Eric A. Wiebke, MD, FACS
Associate Professor
Department of Surgery
Indiana University
Indianapolis, Indiana

Douglas L. Fraker, MD, FACS
Associate Professor of Surgery
Head, Division of Surgical Oncology
University of Pennsylvania
Philadelphia, Pennsylvania

Contributors

Dana Balderrama, MD
Chief Resident in Surgery
Department of Surgery
Kern Medical Center
Bakersfield, California

Marianne Billeter, PharmD, BCPS
Associate Professor of Pharmacy Practice
Division of Distance Education
Bernard J. Dunn School of Pharmacy
Shenandoah University
Winchester, Virginia

Pasquale Casale, MD
Resident in Urology
Department of Urology
Thomas Jefferson University
Philadelphia, Pennsylvania

Jeannie G. Chen, PharmD
SICU Clinical Pharmacist
Department of Pharmacy
Cedars-Sinai Medical Center
Los Angeles, California

Marisa Davis, PharmD Candidate
Bernard J. Dunn School of Pharmacy
Shenandoah University
Winchester, Virginia

Vipul Dev, MD
Chief Resident in Surgery
Department of Surgery
Kern Medical Center
Bakersfield, California

Joseph B. Eby, MD
Resident in Surgery
Department of Surgery
Cedars-Sinai Medical Center
Los Angeles, California

Ehab El-Gabry, MD
Fellow, Urologic Oncology
Thomas Jefferson University
Philadelphia, Pennsylvania

Douglas L. Fraker, MD, FACS
Associate Professor of Surgery
Head, Division of Surgical Oncology
University of Pennsylvania
Philadelphia, Pennsylvania

Leonard G. Gomella, MD, FACS
The Bernard W. Goodwin Jr. Associate Professor
Department of Urology
Jefferson Medical College
Thomas Jefferson University
Philadelphia, Pennsylvania

John C. Kairys, MD
Assistant Professor
Program Director, Department of Surgery
Thomas Jefferson University
Philadelphia, Pennsylvania

Andreas Kamlot, MD
Resident in Surgery
Department of Surgery
Cedars-Sinai Medical Center
Los Angeles, California

Scott Karlan, MD
Attending Surgeon
Department of Surgery
Cedars-Sinai Medical Center
Los Angeles, California

Alan T. Lefor, MD, MPH, FACS
Director, Division of Surgical Oncology
Director, Surgical Education and Academic Affairs
Cedars-Sinai Medical Center
Los Angeles, California
Associate Professor of Clinical Surgery
Department of Surgery
University of California, Los Angeles

Carlo Manookian, MD
Administrative Chief Resident
Department of Surgery
Cedars-Sinai Medical Center
Los Angeles, California

Ganesh V. Raj, MD, PhD
Resident in Urology
Division of Urology
Department of Surgery
Duke University Medical Center
Durham, North Carolina

Darshan Shah, MD
Fellow in Plastic Surgery
Department of Surgery, Mayo Clinic
Rochester, Minnesota

Richard Suh, MD
Administrative Chief Resident
Department of Surgery
Cedars-Sinai Medical Center
Los Angeles, California

Eric A. Wiebke, MD, FACS
Associate Professor
Department of Surgery
Indiana University
Indianapolis, Indiana

Alexander Zilberman, MD
Chief Resident in Surgery
Department of Surgery
Kern Medical Center
Bakersfield, California

Preface

We are grateful to be able to bring to you the third edition of *Surgery On Call.* The "On Call" series is based on Dr. Tricia Gomella's concept that first appeared in 1988 in her book *Neonatology: Basic Management, On-call Problems, Diseases, and Drugs.* The idea is a simple one: house officers are not usually presented with a diagnosis when on-call, but with a specific complaint or problem that requires action and ultimately leads to a diagnosis. Most medical books approach diseases from the diagnosis and disease perspective. Medical education requires a careful synthesis of the practicality of dealing with patient issues on a day-to-day basis with the essentials of medicine. We hope that this manual will provide the house officer and student with the tools to provide the patient with well thought out initial care. This initial care should be followed by a more detailed study of the patient's problem available in standard textbooks of surgery.

In general, the problems reflect that of adult patients, with consideration to pediatric surgical issues supplied where appropriate. Contributions of house staff are invaluable in identifying the issues addressed while on call on a given surgical service. We take great pride in the fact that most of the contributors to this book are residents working daily "in the trenches." This book reflects generally accepted practices from major medical centers around the country. All sections of the book have been updated from the previous edition to reflect the ever-changing practice of medicine. All of the clinical problems have been revised and refined to reflect current practices. New medications have been added to the existing comprehensive list to make it a more useful reference.

We would like to acknowledge our contributors for their efforts, McGraw-Hill for their encouragement and patience, and Janet Foltin for her outstanding editorial assistance. Please contact us with any suggestions you may have so that the book will be able to provide our readership with the essential skills needed to make the all important on-call experience one of efficient patient care and a sound educational opportunity.

Alan T. Lefor, MD, MPH, FACS
Leonard G. Gomella, MD, FACS

Los Angeles and Philadelphia
June 2001

I. On-Call Problems

1. ABDOMINAL DISTENTION

I. **Problem.** A 42-year-old female patient is complaining of abdominal bloating.

II. **Immediate Questions**

A. **Was the patient recently operated upon?** Distention is common after abdominal and retroperitoneal surgery and may be related to ileus or gastric distention. Retroperitoneal surgery may also cause an ileus.

B. **Is there a nasogastric tube in place?** Nasogastric tubes can relieve gastric distention, but will be of little use in draining colonic gas. Verify that the tube is functioning (see Problem 55, page 211).

C. **What medication is the patient taking?** Certain medications such as narcotics (eg, codeine, morphine) and anticholinergics (eg, atropine, belladonna) slow intestinal motility. Diuretic-induced hypokalemia may also cause decreased motility.

D. **What previous operations has the patient had?** The patient may have a bowel obstruction causing distention. Remember the mnemonic "HAM" (Hernia, Adhesions, Malignancy) that lists the causes of bowel obstruction in the adult.

E. **What are the vital signs?** Abdominal distention may restrict pulmonary function and cause tachypnea. Fever suggests an infectious process, such as peritonitis or pneumonia, which may cause a reflex ileus. When a patient with a bowel obstruction has a fever or tachycardia, consider ischemia, as the patient may need urgent surgery. In the absence of fever, tachycardia, leukocytosis, fluid sequestration, and localized pain (all 5 symptoms), the risk of ischemia is low.

F. **When was the most recent bowel movement or flatus?** Bowel movements and the passage of flatus are useful indicators of bowel activity. Their absence suggests (mechanical) obstruction or (functional) adynamic ileus. A patient with a partial small- bowel obstruction (SBO) may still be able to pass flatus.

G. **Has the patient been vomiting?** Vomiting is often a sign of obstruction. The characteristics of the material may aid in diagnosing the site of obstruction. In gastric outlet obstruction, vomitus tends to be clear with little or no bile; in distal SBO, vomitus tends to be bilious or feculent.

III. Differential Diagnosis

A. Gastrointestinal Tract Obstruction

1. **Stomach.** Gastric outlet obstruction by tumor, ulcer or gastric atony secondary to surgery or diabetes can lead to gastric dilatation and a sensation of bloating. This is common in pediatric patients who tend to swallow large amounts of air while crying. Hiccups, from diaphragmatic irritation, can be an early sign of gastric distention.
2. **Small intestine.** Adhesions from previous surgery and other mechanical causes, such as intraluminal obstruction (foreign body, gallstone, etc) and extraluminal obstruction from tumors, commonly cause small-bowel obstruction. Internal hernias or strangulated/incarcerated external hernias can also cause small-bowel obstruction. A "gallstone ileus" is actually a small-bowel obstruction caused by a gallstone impacted at the ileocecal valve. This is usually seen in an elderly patient who has had a previous attack of acute cholecystitis that has led to a cholecystoduodenal fistula.

   Intussusception is the telescoping of one piece of bowel into another. It most often occurs in the pediatric population, usually at the ileocecal valve. When intussusception occurs in adults, there is usually a tumor or polyp acting as a lead point.
3. **Large intestine.** Obstruction may be from tumors, volvulus, foreign bodies, and fecal impaction (particularly in elderly, bedridden patients). Pseudoobstruction of the colon (Ogilvie's syndrome) should also be included in the differential.
4. **Nongastrointestinal tract.** Rarely, gynecologic tumors, retroperitoneal sarcomas, lymphomas or genitourinary tumors (as well as others) may cause obstruction. Pneumonia can cause a reflex ileus below the diaphragm.

B. Intestinal Ischemia.
This diagnosis is based on "pain out of proportion to physical findings." The patient will eventually develop an elevated WBC and acidosis. An elevated amylase and lactic acid level may also aid in the diagnosis.

C. Paralytic Ileus (adynamic ileus).
This can be secondary to intra-abdominal infection (peritonitis), or inflammation (pancreatitis, cholecystitis), or can be caused by systemic disease (sepsis). It occurs commonly after abdominal or retroperitoneal surgery, after blunt abdominal trauma, and

as a result of medications (see page 1). "Reflex" ileus can be the result of pneumonia or urinary tract infection (pyelonephritis). Some electrolyte abnormalities (K^+, Ca^{2+}, Mg^{2+}) cause an ileus.

D. **Organomegaly.** Massive hepatomegaly and splenomegaly may be confused with distention.

E. **Intra-abdominal Mass.** A variety of lesions, such as cysts (mesenteric, ovarian, renal), tumors, aneurysms, or even an unrecognized pregnancy can lead to complaints of distention.

F. **Bladder Distention.** Bladder outlet obstruction may cause massive bladder distention. Prostatic enlargement and neurogenic bladder (spinal cord injury, diabetic) are often responsible. Placement of a Foley catheter can immediately diagnose and manage this problem.

G. **Abdominal Wall or Groin Hernia.** These may allow incarceration (with obstruction) or strangulation (with ischemia) of a loop of bowel.

H. **Hirschsprung's Disease.** Also known as aganglionic megacolon, this is usually diagnosed early in life and causes intermittent constipation with bloating and vomiting.

I. **Ascites.** This is usually a chronic condition related to liver diseases (alcoholic cirrhosis) or carcinoma (malignant ascites). Inquire about a history of alcohol abuse.

IV. Database

A. Physical Exam Key Points

1. **Vital signs.** Fever suggests an inflammatory process, and tachypnea may represent respiratory compromise. Tachycardia and hypotension are usually present with more serious causes of obstruction.
2. **Heart.** Check for atrial fibrillation, which can lead to arterial embolization and intestinal ischemia.
3. **Lungs.** Auscultation may reveal evidence of pneumonia.
4. **Abdomen.** Perform auscultation, percussion, inspection, and palpation. Direct special attention to the left upper quadrant for evidence of gastric distention (such as tympany). Evaluate for the presence of bowel sounds (usually absent with peritonitis and severe ileus, increased and high pitched with SBO). Note any surgical scars and palpate for any tenderness to suggest peritoneal irritation (generalized with peritonitis, or localized with other causes of an acute abdomen such as cholecystitis, see Problem 2, page 6). Abdom-

inal wall hernias may be present. Costovertebral angle tenderness suggests an inflammatory process involving the kidney, diaphragm, liver, or spleen. A fluid wave is seen in ascites. Check for organomegaly.

5. **Rectal exam.** Digital exam may reveal fecal impaction, a foreign body, or rectal tenderness. Test for the presence of occult blood on a fecal sample.
6. **Inguinal.** Check for hernias in the inguinal and femoral areas.
7. **Skin.** There may be changes typical of alcohol abuse, such as spider angiomata, palmar erythema, and caput medusae.
8. **Peripheral vascular.** Signs of peripheral embolization may be the best clue to intestinal embolization and ischemia (eg, absent pulses or ischemic fingers and toes).
9. **Pelvic exam.** A tender adnexal mass suggests pelvic inflammatory disease. Ovarian cancer is likely if the patient has a pelvic mass with ascites.
10. **Intake/ Output:** Check for fluid sequestration, a sign of possible ischemia.

B. Laboratory Data

1. **CBC.** Leukocytosis and left shift suggest an infectious process or ischemic bowel.
2. **Serum electrolytes.** Severe hypokalemia may cause an ileus. Third spacing of fluid with an obstruction may cause a number of electrolyte imbalances.
3. **Liver function tests.** The bilirubin, alkaline phosphatase, ALT, and AST are useful to identify liver and biliary disease.
4. **Urinalysis.** White cells and a positive leukocyte esterase suggest a urinary tract infection.
5. **Serum amylase and lipase.** These are typically elevated with pancreatitis. The amylase may also be elevated with a perforated viscus, an intestinal obstruction or mesenteric ischemia.
6. **Arterial blood gas.** Acidosis can be present with bowel ischemia.
7. **Lactic acid level.** Can be elevated with bowel ischemia.

C. Radiographic and Other Studies

1. **Abdominal radiographs.** Supine and upright abdominal radiographs should be ordered. **Note:** An upright chest radiograph should also always be included in the evaluation; see below). Distended loops of bowel or air fluid levels on the upright film can be seen with an ileus or obstruction, and a large gastric bubble may suggest

acute gastric dilatation (from postoperative gastric atony) or gastric outlet obstruction. When the cecum is markedly dilated (10–12 cm across), emergent intervention is needed to prevent cecal perforation. A "ground-glass" appearance is seen with ascites. Also look for air in the colon, signs of volvulus, colicked springs (intussusception), and a sentinel loop (pancreatitis).

2. **Chest radiograph.** An upright chest radiograph is often the best film to detect free air under the diaphragm. Free air may be normal for a few days after a laparotomy; at other times, this suggests a perforation. Pneumonia may also be diagnosed. Pleural effusion is usually caused by and directs attention to a subdiaphragmatic inflammatory process.
3. **Barium studies.** Do not order these studies when you suspect perforation. If you suspect obstruction, use very careful consideration. Barium that extravasates through a perforation causes severe peritonitis and increases the risk of subsequent infection. Barium studies can also be problematic if a patient is obstructed. Barium given proximal to a partial obstruction can harden and lead to a full obstruction. Water- soluble contrast media (eg, meglumine diatrizoate [Gastrogafin]) are a good alternative when there is any chance of perforation. In an infant with intussusception, however, a barium enema may be both diagnostic and therapeutic.
4. **Ultrasound and CT scan.** This can help establish the diagnosis, especially if a tumor, ascites, or organomegaly is suspected. Cholelithiasis and cholecystitis may be detected on CT, although ultrasound is more sensitive.
5. **Endoscopy.** This technique should be used in select circumstances. EGD is invaluable in assessing gastroduodenal obstruction. Colonoscopy is helpful in evaluating colon masses and colon distension. Be very careful not to sedate a patient for endoscopy when the patient has a full or distended stomach, unless you protect the patient from aspiration.

V. **Plan.** Relieve the distention first and then identify and treat the underlying cause.

A. **Initial Management.** In most cases, keeping the patient NPO with adequate intravenous hydration is acceptable initial therapy while the workup is in progress (see Section IV, page 381).

B. **Nasogastric Intubation.** For most patients with gastrointestinal obstruction and for all patients vomiting, a function-

.g nasogastric tube (NGT) is essential. In the absence of gastric distention, an NGT may be less useful at relieving distention, but should be tried empirically (see Section III, page 352).

C. **Fluid Balance.** Carefully monitor fluid intake and output, especially if an NGT is in place. Replacement of NGT aspirate may be indicated if large volumes are being evacuated.

D. **Specific Treatment Plans.** The underlying cause must be clearly identified and appropriately treated. Common treatment plans include

1. Correct any electrolyte abnormalities, especially hypokalemia. Use IV potassium chloride in divided doses (see page 177).
2. Review the patient's medications for agents that may slow intestinal motility, and adjust accordingly.
3. Fecal impaction should be cleared with gentle digital extraction or enemas.
4. Ascites is usually managed medically (sodium restriction, spironolactone), although therapeutic paracentesis may be needed when there is respiratory compromise.
5. Postoperative ileus usually clears spontaneously, unless complications such as infection intervene.
6. Operative intervention is indicated in most cases of bowel ischemia, incarcerated hernias, and intestinal perforation, and in many cases of mechanical obstruction. Sometimes, surgery is necessary to rule out these possibilities when no other diagnosis is apparent preoperatively.
7. Colonoscopy can be used to treat volvulus and pseudo-obstruction. Newer techniques of GI stenting may also prove valuable.
8. Neostigmine can be used to treat pseudo-obstruction.

2. ABDOMINAL PAIN

I. **Problem.** Seven days after a 40% burn, the patient, a 60-year-old man, complains of pain in the right upper quadrant.

II. **Immediate Questions**

A. **What are the vital signs?** Fever indicates an inflammatory process. Hypotension and tachycardia may indicate shock owing to sepsis or hemorrhage. Fever may be absent in the elderly or in those patients receiving immunosuppressive or antipyretic medications.

B. **Where is the pain located?** This is only a general guide to the diagnosis of abdominal pain, since early in the course of the illness, pain may be "shifted" away from the actual site of pathology, and late in the course, pain may become generalized. The classic example is appendicitis, where the discomfort is initially periumbilical or epigastric and later localized in the right lower quadrant. When the process goes unchecked, the appendix perforates, and the patient develops generalized abdominal pain. Referred pain to the groin can be seen with ureteral colic. Referred back pain suggests pancreatitis or a ruptured abdominal aneurysm (Figures I–1 and I–2).

C. **When did it start?** Sudden, explosive pain is typical of a perforated viscus or rupture of an aneurysm or abscess or ectopic pregnancy. Pain intensifying over 1–2 h is typical of acute cholecystitis, acute pancreatitis, strangulated bowel, mesenteric thrombosis, proximal small bowel obstruction or renal or ureteral colic. Vague pain that increases over several hours is most often seen with acute appendicitis, distal small bowel and large bowel obstructions, uncomplicated peptic ulcer disease, and various gynecologic and genitourinary conditions (Figure I–2).

D. **What is the pain like (dull, sharp, intermittent, constant, worst in life, burning)?** Classically described patterns include "burning" (eg, peptic ulcer disease), "searing" (eg, ruptured aortic aneurysm), "intermittent" (eg, renal or ureteral colic) (Figure I–2). Have the person rate the severity of the pain on a scale from 1 (least painful) to 10 (most painful). This allows you to follow the course more objectively.

E. **What makes the pain better or worse?** Pain that increases with deep inspiration is associated with diaphragmatic irritation (eg, pleurisy or inflammatory lesions of upper abdomen). Food often relieves the pain of peptic ulcer disease. Narcotics relieve colic, but are less effective when pain is from strangulated bowel or mesenteric thrombosis. Bending forward often relieves the pain of pancreatitis.

F. **What are the associated symptoms, if any?** Vomiting with the onset of pain is seen with perforation of a hollow viscus, Boerhaave's syndrome, acute gastritis, pancreatitis, and in many cases of peritoneal irritation. In distal small bowel or large bowel obstruction, nausea is usually present long before vomiting begins. Hematemesis suggests upper GI bleeding (ulcer disease, Mallory-Weiss syndrome). Diarrhea, if severe and associated with abdominal

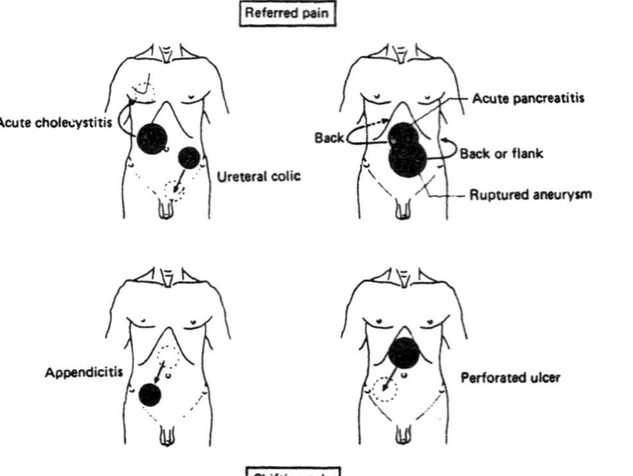

Figure I–1. Referred and shifting pain in the acute abdomen. Solid circles indicate the site of maximum pain, and dashed circles show the sites of lesser pain. *(Reproduced, with permission, from Boey JH: Acute Abdomen. In Way LW (editor):* Current Surgical Diagnosis & Treatment, *10th ed. Originally published by Appleton & Lange. Copyright © 1994 by The McGraw-Hill Companies, Inc.)*

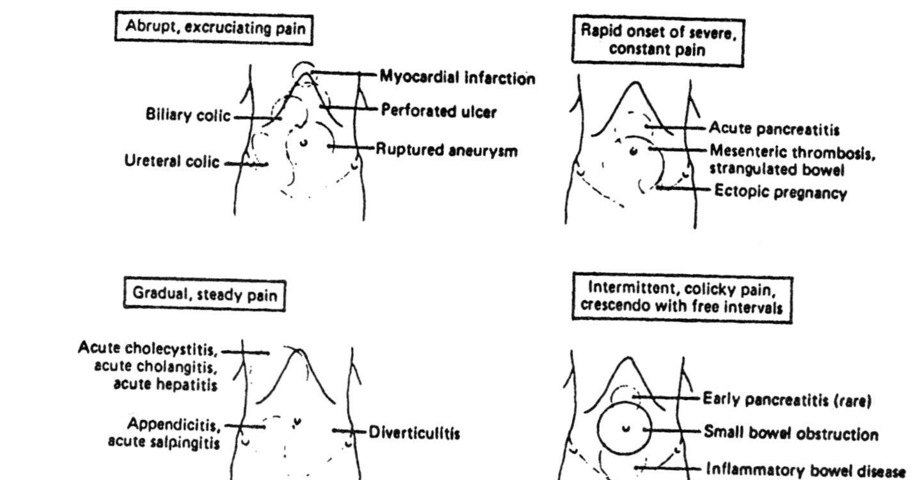

Figure I–2. The location and character of the pain are useful in the differential diagnosis of the acute abdomen. *(Reproduced, with permission, from Boey JH: Acute Abdomen. In Way LW (editor):* Current Surgical Diagnosis & Treatment, *10th ed. Originally published by Appleton & Lange. Copyright © 1994 by The McGraw-Hill Companies, Inc.)*

pain, suggests infectious gastroenteritis, and if bloody, may represent ischemic colitis, ulcerative colitis, Crohn's disease or amebic dysentery. Constipation alternating with diarrhea may be seen with diverticular disease. Although constipation is often nonspecific, obstipation (absence of passage of both stool and flatus) is strongly suggestive of mechanical bowel obstruction. Hematuria suggests a genitourinary cause.

G. **What are the characteristics of the vomitus?** (see Problem 53, page 205).

H. **When did the patient eat last?** This allows an assessment of the time course of the illness and is particularly important if anesthesia is planned.

I. **What is a female patient's menstrual history?** Missed or late period may suggest an ectopic pregnancy. Mittelschmerz (mid-cycle pain) is due to a ruptured ovarian follicle.

J. **What is the patient's medical and surgical history?** Knowledge of a history of ulcers, gallstones, alcohol abuse, or previous operations along with a list of current medications aids in establishing the diagnosis. A history of recent blunt abdominal trauma (1–3 d before the onset of the pain) may signify subcapsular hemorrhage of the liver, spleen, or kidney, or delayed perforation of an injured viscus.

III. **Differential Diagnosis.** Abdominal pain has both intra-abdominal and extra-abdominal sources and can be associated with both medical and surgical diseases. The list is too long to reproduce in its entirety here, but some of the more frequently encountered causes follow.

A. **Intra-abdominal**

1. **Hollow viscera.** Hollow viscera can perforate in the face of obstruction; this represents an acute surgical emergency.
   a. **Upper abdominal:** esophagitis, gastritis, peptic ulcer disease, cholecystitis.
   b. **Mid gut:** small bowel obstruction or infarction. Obstruction may be a result of adhesions (benign and malignant), hernias (internal and external), or volvulus.
   c. **Lower abdominal:** inflammatory bowel disease, appendicitis, mesenteric lymphadenitis, obstruction.
   d. **Gastroenteritis, colitis.**
2. **Solid organs.**
   a. **Liver:** Hepatitis.
   b. **Pancreas:** Pancreatitis.

c. **Spleen:** Splenic infarction.
d. **Kidney:** Stones, pyelonephritis, abscess.

3. **Pelvic.**
   a. Pelvic inflammatory disease.
   b. Ectopic pregnancy (rupture is a surgical emergency).
   c. **Other:** Fibroid torsion, cysts, endometriosis.
4. **Vascular.** Vascular catastrophes are surgical emergencies.
   a. Ruptured aneurysm.
   b. Aortic dissection.
   c. Mesenteric thrombosis or embolism.
   d. Splenic or hepatic rupture (usually posttraumatic).

B. **Extra-abdominal.** Pathology in extra-abdominal diseases may rarely present as referred abdominal pain. The most important to remember are sickle cell crisis, pneumonia (especially lower lobe), myocardial infarction, and rarely, diabetic ketoacidosis.

C. **Other**
1. **Trauma patients.** Blunt trauma may cause injuries to solid viscera (spleen, liver, kidney, pancreas) or to fixed structures such as the duodenum. Penetrating trauma may injure any intra-abdominal structure.
2. **Postoperative patients.** Postoperative abdominal pain usually improves significantly during the first 2–3 postoperative days. Persistent pain may indicate a complication, such as a wound infection, an intestinal obstruction, or abscess. Postoperative pain is derived from both visceral afferent fibers (because of surgical injury to peritoneal linings) and from somatic fibers (innervating the abdominal wall).
3. **Critically ill patients.** Patients with serious injuries (multiple trauma or burns) or sepsis are at risk for potentially life-threatening intra-abdominal events.
   a. Acute stress gastritis (usually manifested as massive upper GI bleeding).
   b. Curling's ulcer with or without perforation (after burns).
   c. Acalculous cholecystitis and cholestasis from the prolonged use of total parenteral nutrition.

IV. Database

A. Physical Exam Key Points

1. **Overall appearance.** Patients writhe in agony when they have colic and stay motionless when they have peritoneal irritation.

2. **Lungs.** Listen for basilar rales or rhonchi indicating possible pneumonia. Dullness to percussion may represent pleural effusion or consolidation.
3. **Heart.** Look for evidence of cardiac decompensation (distended neck veins, S3 gallop, peripheral edema), especially in the patient with preexisting coronary disease. This may direct attention toward an acute myocardial infarction or new-onset atrial fibrillation, which can be sources for intestinal emboli.
4. **Abdomen.**
   a. **Inspection:** Is the abdomen distended (obstruction, ileus, ascites), or scaphoid (perforated ulcer)? Are there flank ecchymoses (hemorrhagic pancreatitis), caput medusae (portal hypertension), or surgical scars (adhesions, tumor)?
   b. **Auscultation:** Listen for bowel sounds (absent or occasional tinkles with obstruction or ileus; hyperperistaltic with gastroenteritis; rushes with small bowel obstruction).
   c. **Percussion:** Tympany is associated with distended loops of bowel; dullness and a fluid wave with ascites; loss of liver dullness with free air.
   d. **Palpation:** Guarding, rigidity, tenderness to percussion, and rebound tenderness are hallmarks of peritonitis. Localized tenderness is often seen with cholecystitis, appendicitis, salpingitis, and diverticulitis. Costovertebral angle tenderness is common with pyelonephritis. Murphy's sign suggests acute cholecystitis. Patients with Murphy's sign are unable to take a deep breath when you press deeply in the right upper quadrant (they inspire to a point, then abruptly stop). Pain with active hip flexion (psoas sign) can represent a retrocecal appendix or psoas abscess. The obturator sign (pain on internal and external rotation of the flexed thigh) can be found with a retrocecal appendix or an obturator hernia. Palpation may also reveal masses.
5. **Rectal exam.** There is usually a mass with rectal carcinoma; a fistula or fissure may indicate Crohn's disease, right-sided rectal tenderness suggests appendicitis (usually retrocecal) or an abscess. If stool is present, test for occult blood (see page 324).
6. **Pelvic exam.** Cervical motion tenderness and purulent cervical discharge suggest pelvic inflammatory disease (salpingitis, tuboovarian abscess). Masses may also be felt (ectopic pregnancy, ovarian cyst, or neoplasm).
7. **Extremities.** Asymmetric pedal pulses, pain, pallor, and paresthesia are evidence of peripheral ischemia that may be associated with systemic emboli.

8. **Skin.** Look for jaundice and spider angiomata as a sign of liver disease. Cool and clammy skin (from peripheral vasoconstriction) is a sign of shock.

B. Laboratory Data

1. **CBC.** Anemia may indicate hemorrhage from an ulcer, colon cancer, or leaking aneurysm. Leukocytosis indicates inflammation. Patients with viral infections, such as gastroenteritis or mesenteric adenitis, usually have a normal white count.
2. **Serum electrolytes, BUN, creatinine.** Bowel obstruction with vomiting can cause hypokalemia, dehydration, or both (BUN/creatinine ratio > 20:1).
3. **Bilirubin, AST, ALT, alkaline phosphatase.** Hepatitis, cholecystitis and other liver diseases may be diagnosed.
4. **Amylase.** Markedly elevated levels are associated with acute pancreatitis. Mild elevations occur with perforated ulcers and small bowel obstruction. Patients with chronic pancreatitis, hemorrhagic pancreatitis, and pseudocysts occasionally have a normal amylase level.
5. **Arterial blood gases.** Hypoxia is often an early sign of sepsis (from pulmonary shunting). When you suspect a pulmonary embolus, also consider sepsis. Acidosis may be present in ischemic bowel.
6. **Pregnancy test.** Premenopausal women should be tested (Urinary hCG-β) to rule out ectopic pregnancy, whether they use birth control or not.
7. **Urinalysis.** Hematuria may indicate urolithiasis or cancer; pyuria (occasionally with hematuria) suggests a urinary tract infection, can be is rarely seen in appendicitis.
8. **Cervical culture.** Send a specimen specifically for gonorrhea (in GC media) when pelvic inflammatory disease is suspected.

C. Radiographic and Other Studies

1. **Flat and upright abdominal films.** If the patient is debilitated, a left lateral decubitus film may be substituted for the upright. Observe for the following key elements: gas pattern, bowel dilatation, air-fluid levels, presence of air in rectum, pancreatic calcifications, loss of psoas margin, displacement of hollow viscera, gallstones and renal stones, portal vein air, and aortic calcifications. On a left lateral decubitus film, free air makes the liver stand out.
2. **Chest film.** This may reveal pneumonia, a widened mediastinum (dissecting aneurysm), a pleural effusion, or elevation of a hemidiaphragm (subdiaphragmatic inflammatory process). Free air under the diaphragm

suggests a perforation and is most often seen on the upright chest radiograph.

3. **Ultrasound.** May reveal gallstones, ectopic pregnancy, or other diseases.
4. **Electrocardiogram.** Rule out myocardial infarction as a cause of upper abdominal pain and nausea.
5. **Other studies as clinically indicated:**
   a. IVP (an excretory urogram is helpful in the workup of urolithiasis).
   b. Abdominal CT scan.
   c. Biliary scintigraphy.
   d. Contrast bowel studies: Swallowing studies, upper GI series, small-bowel series, and enemas (barium, dilute barium, Gastrografin).
   e. Endoscopic studies: Esophagogastroduodenoscopy (EGD), colonoscopy, endoscopic retrogradcholangiopancreatography (ERCP).
   f. Arteriography.
   g. Peritoneal lavage (page 366) or paracentesis (page 363).

V. Plan. Abdominal pain in any patient can present a diagnostic dilemma, but even more so in patients at the extremes of age or in those unable to communicate. The surgeon's primary goal is to determine whether the abdominal pain requires surgical treatment to prevent further morbidity. Entire books have been written on the proper management of a patient with an acute abdomen. In rough terms, pain that has been present for 6 or more hours is likely to have a cause requiring surgical intervention. In many cases of abdominal pain, patients are taken to surgery without a definite diagnosis before laparotomy. A brief period of observation may ultimately point to the cause, but operation is safer in most cases. The use of analgesics remains controversial, but most clinicians now believe that limited doses of pain medicine will not mask symptoms enough to impede diagnosis and will make patients much more comfortable during their workup. There are too many specific types of therapy and operations to describe them here, although information is available in surgical and medical textbooks. It is essential to recognize that certain conditions are life threatening and most of these require urgent operation (Table I–1).

A. Observation. With the exception of catastrophes that require urgent surgical exploration (Table I–1), most cases of abdominal pain require close observation, medical management, and occasionally analgesics. In the case of postoperative abdominal pain, analgesics are usually necessary.

1. Keep the patient NPO and consider nasogastric suction, especially if the patient is vomiting.

TABLE I–1. INDICATIONS FOR URGENT OPERATION IN PATIENTS WITH ACUTE ADOMEN.

Physical findings

Involuntary guarding or rigidity, especially if spreading
Increasing or severe localized tenderness
Tense or progressive distention
Tender abdominal or rectal mass with high fever or hypotension
Rectal bleeding with shock or acidosis
Equivocal abdominal findings along with—
- Septicemia (high fever, marked or rising leukocytosis, mental changes, or increasing glucose intolerance in a diabetic patient)
- Bleeding (unexplained shock or acidosis, falling hematocrit)
- Suspected ischemia (acidosis, fever, tachycardia)
- Deterioration on conservative treatment

Radiologic findings

Pneumoperitoneum
Gross or progressive bowel distention
Free extravasation of contrast material
Space-occupying lesion on scan, with fever
Mesenteric occlusion on angiography

Endoscopic findings

Perforated or uncontrollably bleeding lesion

Paracentesis findings

Blood, bile, pus, bowel contents, or urine.

(Reproduced, with permission, from Boey JH: Acute Abdomen. In: Current Surgical Diagnosis and Treatment, *10/e. LW Way (editor). Appleton & Lange, 1994).*

2. Start intravenous hydration (see Section IV, page 381) with careful attention to intake and output.
3. Parenteral analgesics are used sparingly to avoid masking pathologic processes.
4. Serial physical exams by the same examiner are useful in determining the progression of symptoms, which will aid in securing the diagnosis and managing the patient.

B. Surgery. Vascular catastrophes, perforated viscus, most causes of bowel obstruction, many splenic and hepatic injuries, ruptured ectopic pregnancies, and appendicitis require emergency surgery. Indications for urgent operation without a precise preoperative diagnosis are outlined in Table I–1.

3. ACIDOSIS

(See also Section II, page 278)

I. Problem. A patient with fulminant acute pancreatitis and accompanying ARDS requires intubation and mechanical ventilation. The initial arterial blood gas following intubation reveals a pH of 7.14.

II. Immediate Questions

A. **Is the acidosis respiratory, metabolic, or a combination of both?** The blood gas report will often list the calculated base excess/deficit at the end of the report (eg, Po_2/Pco_2/pH/bicarbonate/base excess). If the base excess is negative (or a positive deficit), the acidosis is at least partially metabolic. If the base excess is not reported with the results of the ABG, the differentiation between metabolic and respiratory causes can still be quickly made. If the $Pco_2 < 40$, then the acidosis is metabolic, possibly with respiratory compensation. If the $Pco_2 > 40$, the acidosis is at least partially respiratory. Every 10 torr that the Pco_2 is greater than 40, the pH will be lowered by 0.08 in normal circumstances. For example, if the Pco_2 is 60, one would expect a pH of 7.24; any additional acidosis should be attributed to metabolic causes. Respiratory compensation for acute metabolic acidosis disturbances can be estimated as follows:

$$Pco_2 = 1.5\ (\text{serum } HCO_3) + 8\ (\pm 2)$$

B. **Is the patient hypovolemic?** Lactic acidosis, a common cause of metabolic acidosis in the acute setting, is caused by poor tissue perfusion. Examine the patient, look at the recent urine output and the cardiac filling pressures (if available) to determine whether the patient is hypovolemic. Diuretic-induced volume contraction without hypoperfusion is often associated with alkalosis.

C. **Is there any problem with the ventilator circuit?** A nonintubated patient with a respiratory acidosis usually has some apparent difficulty with breathing. In a sedated or obtunded patient on a ventilator, respiratory acidosis may not be clinically apparent. Check the ventilator circuit, the exhaled volume, and the settings on the ventilator to make certain there is no technical explanation for the acidosis. Verify the position of the endotracheal tube on chest radiograph to make sure it has not slipped distally into the right mainstem bronchus.

D. **Are there any arrhythmias or ectopy?** With a profound acidosis of any cause, there may be atrial or ventricular arrhythmias. Obtain an ECG and monitor the patient.

III. **Differential Diagnosis.** As previously mentioned, the most important distinction to make in diagnosing the cause of acidosis is apportioning respiratory and metabolic contributions. In the acutely ill surgical patient, both causes may be present as in the example above.

A. Respiratory Acidosis. By definition, this is alveolar hypoventilation. There are two main categories: acute and chronic, and these have relative compensatory adjustments, depending on their chronicity. Acute is < 24 h, and the expected pH = 0.008 X change in Pco_2. Chronic is > 24 h, and the expected pH = 0.003 x change in Pco_2.

1. **Pulmonary conditions**
   a. **Asthma:** If an asthmatic has progressed to a respiratory acidosis, they have very severe disease and usually require prompt intubation.
   b. **Mechanical upper airway obstruction:** A foreign body or laryngospasm may be the cause.
   c. **Space-occupying lesions:** Pneumothorax, pleural effusion, or hemothorax may result in respiratory compromise.
   d. **Severe pulmonary edema:** As in congestive heart failure.
   e. **Pneumonia:** Usually with baseline respiratory compromise (COPD).
2. **Drugs/toxins**
   a. Alcohol ingestion.
   b. Narcotics/sedative overdose.
   c. Neuromuscular blocking agents (eg, curare).
3. **Neuromuscular conditions**
   a. Myasthenia gravis
   b. Pickwickian syndrome
   c. Cerebrovascular accident
   d. Guillain-Barré syndrome

B. Metabolic Acidosis. This can be subdivided into conditions with a normal anion gap and those with an increased anion gap (implying an elevated unmeasured anion). The anion gap is calculated by Na + Cl – HCO_3. The normal range is 8–12 mEq/L.

1. **Normal anion gap**
   a. Loss of bicarbonate: Losses are usually from the GI tract with diarrhea, a small bowel fistula, a pancreatic-cutaneous fistula, or a large amount of external biliary drainage.
   b. Renal tubular acidosis. When the patient has a normal anion gap and a loss of bicarbonate is evident, it may help to calculate a urinary cation gap (urine Na + urine K) – urine Cl. A positive value indicates renal tubular acidosis, whereas a negative value indicates GI losses.

2. **Elevated anion gap**
   a. Lactic acidosis: Poor perfusion prevents normal oxidative metabolism.
   b. Diabetic ketoacidosis
   c. Alcoholic ketoacidosis
   d. Chronic renal insufficiency: The elevated unmeasured anions include sulfates and phosphates.
   e. Drugs and poisoning: Overdosage of aspirin or ingestion of methanol, ethylene glycol, or paraldehyde.

IV. Database

A. Physical Exam Key Points

1. **Vital signs.** Look for evidence of hypoventilation, hypotension, tachycardia, or fever. Sepsis can cause shock—a common cause of acidosis.
2. **Skin.** Look for cool, clammy, and mottled skin as in shock, with clamped-down peripheral perfusion.
3. **HEENT.** Ketosis or a fruity odor on the breath suggests diabetic ketoacidosis. Look for tracheal shift (from a space-occupying lesion) or jugular venous distention (from CHF, cardiac tamponade, or tension pneumothorax).
4. **Pulmonary.** Listen for absent or decreased breath sounds, stridor (in upper airway obstruction), wheezes, rales, or evidence of accessory muscle use (sternocleidomastoid, rectus).
5. **Abdomen.** Peritoneal signs indicate an acute abdomen, and marked distention may inhibit respiration. There may also be evidence of paradoxical motion (abdominal breathing).
6. **Neuromuscular.** Generalized weakness or focal neurologic signs, a depressed level of consciousness, obtundation, or coma should be noted.

B. Laboratory Data

1. **CBC.** Leukocytosis is seen with sepsis. Anemia is common with chronic renal insufficiency.
2. **Electrolytes, BUN and creatinine.** There should be an elevated serum chloride in non-anion gap metabolic acidosis. Calculate the anion gap from the electrolytes (see page 17). Renal insufficiency may be present.
3. **Blood glucose, ketone levels.** Elevations are associated with diabetic ketoacidosis.
4. **Lactate levels.** Levels are elevated with sepsis and poor perfusion.
5. **Arterial blood gas.** Repeat the ABG to follow therapeutic interventions.

C. **Other Studies**

1. **Chest radiograph.** To evaluate for infiltrates, pulmonary edema, effusions, and endotracheal tube positioning (the ideal position is approximately 2 cm above the carina).
2. **ECG with rhythm strip.** To identify arrhythmias, heart failure, or myocardial infarction. Cardiac enzymes (creatine kinase and troponin I) will confirm the diagnosis of myocardial infarction.
3. **EMG.** This and other specialized neurology tests may be needed to diagnose primary neurologic conditions.

V. **Plan.** In general for both respiratory and metabolic acidosis, the primary goal is to identify and treat the underlying cause of the acidosis. In emergent situations, treat the acidosis first by hyperventilating the patient and administering sodium bicarbonate intravenously (reserved for severe acidemia, ie, pH < 7.2). Be sure to check serial pH values to monitor the progress of therapy.

A. **Metabolic Acidosis**

1. **Bicarbonate therapy.** In general, administer IV bicarbonate if the pH < 7.20.
   a. Calculate the total body bicarbonate need:

Patient's body weight (in kg) $\times$ 0.40 $\times$ (24 – [HCO_3]) = Total number of mEq of HCO_3 needed

   b. Give 50% of this amount over the first 12 h as a mixture of bicarbonate with D5W.
   c. Complications of bicarbonate therapy include
      i. Hypernatremia
      ii. Volume overload
      iii. Hypokalemia: Caused by intracellular shifts of potassium as the pH increases.
      iv. Intracellular hypercarbia with myocardial depression.
2. **Treat the underlying causes**
   a. Volume resuscitate the patient in sepsis, hemorrhagic shock and other causes of lactic acidosis.
   b. Administer insulin and saline for diabetic ketoacidosis (see page 496).
   c. Dialyze patients as needed for renal failure.

B. **Respiratory Acidosis.** The main goal is to treat the underlying cause.

1. If necessary, intubate the patient and start mechanical ventilation. If a patient is already intubated and has a significant respiratory acidosis, then increase the alveo-

lar ventilation by either increasing the tidal volume (up to 10–15 mL/kg) while following peak inspiratory pressures or by increasing the respiratory rate.

2. In an emergent situation, disconnect the patient from the ventilator and hyperventilate by hand using the bag device. The importance of good pulmonary toilet, ie, suctioning of secretions, cannot be overemphasized. Sedation is often a necessary adjunct to mechanical ventilation (see page 414).

4. ALKALOSIS

(See also Section II, page 278)

I. **Problem.** A 47-year-old female is in the ICU and has a pH of 7.56 one day after thoracotomy for a Belsey antireflux procedure.

II. **Immediate Questions**

A. **Is the patient on a ventilator and if so, what is the respiratory rate and tidal volume?** Alkalosis may be a result of over ventilation ("blowing off CO_2"). The minute ventilation is what matters. Thus, both rate (IMV or Assist Control) and volume for each delivered breath (tidal volume) are important. The tidal volume should be set at 10–15 mL/kg. Minute ventilation = rate X tidal volume, so a change in either parameter will affect the minute ventilation.

B. **What medications is the patient receiving?** Thiazide diuretics can result in a "contraction" alkalosis, and excess bicarbonate and bicarbonate precursors (such as acetate in hyperalimentation solutions) can cause a metabolic alkalosis.

C. **What is the composition of IV fluids?** Be sure there is no added bicarbonate (avoid Ringer's lactate) and make sure the patient is receiving sufficient chloride (80–100 mEq/d as NaCl, plus excess losses).

D. **Does the patient have a nasogastric tube, or is the patient vomiting?** Nasogastric drainage of the GI tract is a common cause of alkalosis in surgical patients. Most patients develop a hypokalemic hypochloremic metabolic alkalosis. The alkalosis is a result of renal exchange of K^+ for H^+, and is **not** from the loss of HCl from the stomach. These patients are alkalotic, yet have aciduria ("paradoxical aciduria"). As K^+ is removed by the NGT, the kidney attempts to hold onto K^+, so it exchanges K^+ with H^+, leaving the patient alkalotic. Thus, therapy should be directed at volume repletion and K^+ repletion.

III. Differential Diagnosis. Just as with acidosis, the key point here is to determine whether the alkalosis is primarily metabolic or respiratory.

A. Metabolic Alkalosis. There is an elevated serum bicarbonate with compensation by hypoventilation and increased renal excretion of bicarbonate. Patients have an increased pH with a normal or increased arterial P_{CO_2}. Chloride deficit and hydrogen deficit can be calculated by the following two equations

$$\text{Chloride deficit} = 0.5\ (\text{body wt in kg}) \times (103 - \text{measured Cl})\ \text{mEq}$$

$$\text{Hydrogen deficit} = 0.5\ (\text{wt in kg}) \times (\text{measured } HCO_3 - 24)\ \text{mEq}$$

1. Loss of HCl (chloride responsive) urine Cl < 10 meq/L
   - **a.** Nasogastric suction, vomiting
   - **b.** Villous adenoma (potassium wasting)
   - **c.** Diuretics (especially thiazides)
   - **d.** Posthypercapnia
   - **e.** Cystic fibrosis
2. Chloride resistant (chloride unresponsive) urine Cl > 10 meq/L
   - **a.** Bicarbonate administration (oral and parenteral)
   - **b.** Chronic hypokalemia
   - **c.** Primary hyperaldosteronism
   - **d.** Cushing's syndrome, exogenous steroids
   - **e.** Bartter's syndrome
   - **f.** Hypercalcemia and hypoparathyroidism

B. Respiratory Alkalosis. Hyperventilation results in a decreased P_{CO_2} and the compensatory mechanism is through increased renal bicarbonate excretion.

1. Anxiety.
2. Hypermetabolic states (eg, fever, early sepsis).
3. Iatrogenic. The ventilator rate is set for too many breaths, or the tidal volume is set too high.
4. Pregnancy.
5. Cirrhosis.
6. Cardiac disease (refer to Problem 12, page 54).
7. Pulmonary disease (refer to Problem 26, page 113).
8. Brain stem lesion (refer to Problem 14, page 70).
9. Salicylate intoxication (alkalosis early, with metabolic acidosis later).

IV. Database

A. Physical Exam Key Points

1. **Vital signs.** Pay particular attention to the respiratory rate. Tachypnea may signify a respiratory cause.

2. **Lungs.** Check for signs of pulmonary edema (rales).
3. **Skin.** Look for changes associated with alcohol abuse such as palmar erythema, spider angiomata, etc. Signs of sepsis or decreased perfusion may be present.

B. Laboratory Data. Simultaneously obtain an arterial blood gas and electrolytes.

1. **Arterial blood gases.** As noted above.
2. **Serum electrolytes.** Pay particular attention to hypokalemia, which may accompany alkalosis. (Low serum H^+ balanced by exchange of K^+ in the kidney).
3. **Serum salicylate levels.** If aspirin intoxication is suspected.
4. **Spot urine electrolytes for chloride.** This is most helpful in the diagnosis and treatment of metabolic alkalosis. If the urine chloride is < 10 mEq/L, the patient has a "chloride responsive" alkalosis (caused by diuretics or GI tract losses) that can often be corrected by the administration of chloride-containing IV fluids. If the urine chloride is > 10 mEq/L, this represents a "chloride resistant" alkalosis (caused by adrenal diseases, exogenous steroid use) and usually cannot be corrected by chloride infusion.

V. Plan. It is essential to identify the cause of alkalosis and treat it.

A. Discontinue Exogenous Bicarbonate. Is the patient receiving bicarbonate precursors, such as the acetate salts (amino acids) found in hyperalimentation solutions? When hyperalimentation is essential, attempt to increase the chloride salts in the solution. You may also need to reduce the amino acid content.

B. IV Replacement. For alkalosis resulting from the loss of HCl, give NaCl as normal saline IV. For alkalosis that is chloride resistant, give KCl IV.

C. Sedation. Sedate ventilated patients when anxiety is contributing to respiratory alkalosis. Use agents such as diazepam, lorazepam, or midazolam.

D. Increase F_ICO_2. Use a rebreathing mask for the nonintubated patient with respiratory alkalosis. For an intubated patient, decrease the minute ventilation by decreasing the rate or the tidal volume. Aim for a tidal volume of 10–15 mL/kg.

E. Treat Hypokalemia. Use KCl supplementation.

F. Replace Volume Losses. Replace fluid volume lost through the nasogastric tube or vomiting, using D5 1/2 NS with 20 mEq KCl/L.

5. ANAPHYLAXIS (DRUG REACTION)

Immediate Actions

1. Stop administering the allergen (eg, blood, medication, IV contrast).
2. Assess the patient's airway, and intubate if necessary (this may be difficult secondary to laryngeal edema or laryngospasm and may require the use of a smaller endotracheal tube or a cricothyrotomy).
3. Check breathing, administer oxygen.
4. Ensure adequate IV access (14- or 16-gauge IV) and begin fluids (LR 500-ml bolus)
5. Use continuous electrocardiogram monitoring and pulse oximetry.
6. Treat patients having drug reactions with epinephrine, diphenhydramine, and steroids (see following section, "Plan").

I. **Problem.** A postoperative patient has developed severe dyspnea and a generalized rash after receiving intravenous penicillin.

II. **Immediate Questions.**

A. **What are the patient's vital signs?** Tachycardia is a common finding and could represent a response to hypoxia, fear, hypotension, or an arrhythmia. Respiratory distress and hypotension can be life-threatening, and patients with such conditions should be treated immediately. Treat the patient with IV crystalloid, epinephrine, and diphenhydramine as soon as available.

B. **Can the patient communicate appropriately?** An appropriate answer to simple questions indicates that cerebral oxygenation is adequate. Inability to speak suggests severe respiratory deterioration with hypoxia, upper airway obstruction from laryngospasm, or laryngeal edema.

C. **What medications is the patient receiving?** Many medications can cause anaphylaxis, but the most common in this setting are penicillins, cephalosporins (which have a low rate of allergic reactions but a very high rate of use), and intravenous contrast. Aspirin and other nonsteroidal anti-inflammatory drugs (NSAIDs) may cause reactions in sensitive patients. Transfusion reactions are discussed in Problem 68, page 247. Insect stings are another cause managed the same way.

III. Differential Diagnosis. Anaphylaxis technically refers to the signs and symptoms caused by an antigen-mediated release of IgE-induced mediators. It can be localized (as in allergic rhinitis) or can be systemic and life-threatening.

A. Acute Allergic Reaction (Anaphylaxis). In the hospital setting, this is most often caused by the medications noted in Section II-C above. Less frequently, anaphylaxis may be caused by food, environmental agents (dust, pollen) or insects.

B. Upper Airway Obstruction. May be caused by a foreign body or laryngeal edema and classically presents as stridor.

C. Acute Asthmatic Attack. Patients usually wheeze and have a history of asthma.

D. Pulmonary Embolus. This should be considered in all patients acutely short of breath, especially in the postoperative setting.

E. Tachypnea and Dyspnea. These conditions can be caused by sepsis. Streptococcal and other bacterial infections occasionally cause a rash.

F. Pulmonary Edema. This may be caused by postoperative fluid shifts and should be suspected in elderly patients and in patients with cardiac disease. Symptoms can appear as dyspnea, "cardiac" wheezes, and sometimes hypotension. A chest radiograph confirms the diagnosis.

G. Others. Other causes for this constellation of symptoms are discussed in other sections: Dyspnea (Problem 26, page 113), Hypotension (Problem 47, page 184), Pruritus (Problem 60, page 224) and Wheezing (Problem 75, page 268).

IV. Database. Knowledge of the patient's allergies and current medications is essential. The relationship of medication administration to the onset of symptoms is also important, because anaphylaxis usually occurs within minutes of medication administration.

A. Physical Exam Key Points

1. **Vital signs.** Tachycardia is an early sign. Hypotension must be recognized early and may appear as syncope
2. **Lungs.** Listen for wheezing (suggests bronchospasm), stridor (suggests laryngospasm), and adequacy of air movement.
3. **Skin.** Generalized rash, urticaria, and pruritus are the most common signs seen in an anaphylactic reaction.
4. **Extremities.** Look for evidence of cyanosis. A Medic-Alert bracelet may document prior allergic reactions.

5. **Mental status.** Somnolence in this setting is indicative of severe hypercapnia and warrants immediate respiratory support.
6. **Gastrointestinal.** Nausea, vomiting, abdominal pain, tenesmus or diarrhea may accompany anaphylaxis.

B. Laboratory Data

1. **Arterial blood gas.** Usually has no role in the immediate management of the patient with acute respiratory distress. This should be obtained after the "ABCs" are managed.

C. Radiographic and Other Studies

1. **Chest radiograph.** When time permits, a chest radiograph will rule out other causes of respiratory distress (CHF, pneumonia, etc).
2. **Electrocardiogram.** An acute myocardial infarction can present as pulmonary edema with severe dyspnea. Right ventricular strain can be seen in a pulmonary embolus.

V. Plan. Treatment should be initiated quickly on the basis of clinical findings and before performing other studies and lab exams. Treatment is dictated by the severity of the reaction. Be prepared to initiate cardiopulmonary resuscitation.

A. Laryngeal edema. Start oxygen by face mask for moderate dyspnea. Intubation (or surgical airway) may be required if the patient is in severe respiratory distress (stridor), is somnolent, or desaturating. Sedation and paralysis are contraindicated. Racemic epinephrine in a nebulizer may temporize laryngeal edema. Consider steroids (methylprednisolone 125–250 mg IV every 6 h) for protracted mild-to-moderate laryngeal edema. Epinephrine (as outlined in section V.C. below) and diphenhydramine (Benadryl)—25–50 mg PO/IM for mild reactions, 50–100 mg IV for severe reactions—should be given immediately.

B. Bronchospasm. In addition to oxygen, give diphenhydramine, epinephrine, and, in consideration of intubation, albuterol by inhalation. Also consider the use of aminophylline, ipratropium bromide, and steroids (as outlined above).

C. Hypotension. Epinephrine 1:1,000 solution 0.3–0.5 mL (0.01 mL/kg for children) subcutaneously or intramuscularly (for improved absorption with generalized urticaria) should be given immediately for moderate to severe anaphylaxis (laryngospasm, bronchospasm, or hypotension). Improvement is often dramatic. Repeat the dose in 5–10 min as needed. The epinephrine used for CPR is a 1:10,000 solution and should **not** be used in this situation. Use epinephrine with caution in patients over age 40 (there is a risk of arrhythmias and cardiac ischemia). In severe hypotension, acute respiratory failure from bronchospasm or upper airway obstruction, epinephrine is administered intravenously, (5–10 mL of a 1:10,000 solution). Volume repletion should start immediately with crystalloid. In refractory hypotension, consider vasopressors (dopamine, isoproterenol or norepinephrine), Glucagon (1 mg IV), or steroids (as above).

D. **Other considerations.** Consider activated charcoal for ingested antigens. Cimetidine (300 mg IV every 6 h) should be given for persistent anaphylaxis.

E. **Monitoring.** Resolution of the respiratory distress associated with anaphylaxis is usually so dramatic that ICU monitoring after the episode is often unnecessary. However, clinical judgment is needed, and exceptions include elderly or severely ill patients and patients who experience arrhythmias or appear near to respiratory arrest before treatment. Patients given epinephrine need cardiac monitoring for at least 30 min. Benadryl should be continued for the next 48 h, and steroids should be tapered in cases of persistent bronchospasm or hypotension.

F. **Prophylaxis.** Patients known to have an allergy to IV contrast should be premedicated with prednisone (50 mg given 13 h, 7 h, and 1 h before the procedure), Benadryl (given 50 mg IM 1 h before procedure), and should receive low-osmolality dye.

6. ANEMIA

I. **Problem.** A patient admitted for a varicose vein stripping has a hematocrit of 19% on preoperative laboratory evaluation.

II. **Immediate Questions**

A. **Is the patient hemodynamically stable?** A patient with a chronic anemia has usually already compensated for volume loss. The evaluation and treatment of these patients can proceed in an orderly fashion. Patients with a low hematocrit secondary to an acute bleed may need urgent volume resuscitation. However, those patients almost always present with clinically apparent bleeding as opposed to being diagnosed on a routine lab study. Tachycardia and postural hypotension are important signs of hypovolemia.

B. **Is the patient's stool positive for occult blood?** On a surgical service, a patient with an unexpected drop in hematocrit should be assumed to have GI bleeding until proven otherwise. Check the indices (MCV, MCH, MCHC) on the CBC, and if they show a microcytic, hypochromic anemia (see Section II, page 278), chances are even greater that the cause is chronic GI blood loss. Ask about melena (tarry stools) or a change in bowel habits. Even if the stool is negative on the first check, obtain 2–3 more specimens at different times, because GI bleeding tends to be intermittent.

C. **Does the patient have a history of anemia?** Review the chart or clinic records to find the most recent hematocrit. Ask the patient whether they have had a history of anemia or whether there is a family history of anemia.

D. **Is the low hematocrit correct?** If the lab result is unexpected or if it does not correlate with the clinical appearance of the patient, question the validity of the test. Sources of lab error causing a low hematocrit include (1) the sample is from a different patient; (2) there is a technical problem with the machine; or (3) blood is drawn proximal to an open IV line. Incorrect laboratory results are unusual, but it is worth repeating the test before embarking on an extensive workup.

E. **Is there blood available in the blood bank?** If there is any possibility that an emergency transfusion will be needed, call the blood bank to determine whether blood is already set up for the patient. If not, obtain the specimens needed to type and cross-match blood. Do not transfuse the patient unless clinically indicated (hemodynamically unstable, etc) or before completing the initial evaluation, confirming the validity of the result, and drawing blood specimens for the laboratory tests discussed below.

III. **Differential Diagnosis.** Anemia is present in many disease states. Chronic anemia can be categorized as either microcytic or macrocytic. Microcytic anemias are easy to remember by the acronym **TAILS,** which is Thalassemia, Anemia of chronic disease, Iron deficiency, Lead poisoning, or Sideroblastic. Macrocytic anemias are usually due to B_{12} or folate deficiencies (usually seen in alcoholic patients) or in patients after extensive ileal resection. Acute anemia due to blood loss can be from many different sources, and must be dealt with in a timely fashion.

IV. **Database**

A. **Physical Exam Key Points**

1. **Vital signs.** Orthostatic hypotension and tachycardia indicate hemodynamically significant anemia.
2. **Skin.** Pallor, pale conjunctiva and nail beds correlate with the degree of anemia reported by the lab.
3. **Abdomen.** Splenomegaly is present in hemolytic anemias, in disorders with intracorpuscular defects leading

to RBC destruction, and in myeloid metaplasia. A mass may be palpable with malignancies.

4. **Rectal exam.** Pay close attention to any mass and test for the presence of occult blood.
5. **Dressings, drains, and surgical sites should be inspected.** An NGT can be used to rule out an upper GI source of bleeding (ulcer, varices, etc.)

B. **Laboratory Data (see Section II, page 278 for more details)**

1. **CBC.** Aside from the hematocrit, look at the white blood count and platelet count for evidence of general bone marrow depression or leukemia.
2. **Red blood cell indices.** MCV and MCHC allow a classification of anemia according to RBC size (microcytic, normocytic, or macrocytic) and hemoglobin content (hypochromic or normochromic). Iron deficiency anemia is microcytic and hypochromic, whereas megaloblastic anemia is typically macrocytic.
3. **Peripheral blood smear.** This can also be used to look at the actual size of red cells, as the indices may be occasionally misleading. For example, if a microcytic and a macrocytic process were occurring together, the MCV may be normal owing to a mixed population of red cells. Examining the shape of the cells (spherocytosis, elliptocytosis, RBC fragments) may lead to several diagnoses. An RDW (red cell distribution width) can help identify a mixed population of macro- and microcytic cells and is available in some centers.
4. **Reticulocyte count.** This reflects the rate of production of red cells. A low reticulocyte count suggests inadequate production of red cells (anemia of chronic disease, vitamin deficiencies, bone marrow suppression), whereas an increased count is associated with chronic blood loss (GI bleeding) or increased destruction of red cells.
5. **Serum chemistries, BUN, and creatinine.** GI bleeding increases the BUN. The levels of potassium and creatinine are elevated in renal failure, as is the level of indirect bilirubin in hemolytic anemias.
6. **Iron, total iron-binding capacity (TIBC).** In iron deficiency, serum iron is decreased and TIBC is increased. In anemia of chronic disease, serum iron is decreased or normal and TIBC is decreased.
7. **Haptoglobin.** Often decreased in hemolytic anemia.
8. **Folate, Vitamin B_{12} levels.** These measure deficiencies of specific metabolites.
9. **Coombs' test.** This measures IgM and IgG antibodies in hemolytic anemias.

C. **Radiographic and Other Studies**
   1. **Bone marrow biopsy.** When the reticulocyte count is low, this assesses erythrocyte precursors, iron stores, and bone marrow replacement by infiltrative disease processes.
   2. **GI workup.** May include an upper GI series, barium enema, upper GI endoscopy, colonoscopy, angiography, or tagged red blood cell nuclear scan when the workup suggests GI bleeding.
   3. **Ultrasound and CT scans.** May help identify a tumor.

V. **Plan.** Notify the senior staff because an elective operation may need to be postponed when anemia is identified.

A. **Acute Management.** When hemodynamically significant anemia is present, start a large bore IV (16 gauge or larger), draw necessary blood samples for the lab and blood bank, and begin fluid resuscitation. Check stools for occult blood. If heme-positive, consider passing a nasogastric tube as an initial diagnostic maneuver to check for an upper GI source of bleeding. Blood transfusions should be initiated when indicated.

B. **Evaluation.** Continue with GI workup as described above. When the anemia is due to causes other than acute blood loss, gather laboratory data as discussed above, and obtain a hematology consultation.

C. **Specific Treatments**
   1. **Iron deficiency.** Ferrous sulfate or gluconate 325 mg three times a day for several weeks (iron absorption is poor). Also give a stool softener (eg, Colace), because iron pills cause constipation. Inform patients that their stools may turn black from the iron.
   2. **Folate deficiency.** Folic acid 1 mg PO or mixed with IV every day.
   3. **Vitamin B_{12} deficiency.** 1000 mg IM daily for 14 d, then 1000 mg IM monthly.
   4. **Hemolytic anemia.** Often treated with glucocorticoids such as prednisone 60–100 mg/d and may require splenectomy.
   5. **Intracorpuscular red blood cell defect.** Splenectomy will often help to reduce RBC destruction.
   6. Transfuse as needed.
   7. Urgent surgery may be needed for GI bleeding; elective surgery (splenectomy) for hematologic disorders.
   8. Order H_2-receptor blockers (eg, Tagamet or Zantac) and antacids for ulcer disease.

7. ARTERIAL LINE PROBLEMS

(The technique for arterial line placement is discussed in Section III, page 335).

I. **Problem.** The arterial line is not functioning in a 65-year-old patient on the first postoperative day after pulmonary lobectomy.

II. **Immediate Questions**

A. **What is the appearance of the tracing?** An absent tracing may indicate clotting of the catheter. A normal tracing suggests that there is adequate arterial flow in the catheter. A dampened tracing usually indicates air or a clot in the system. When this is noted, flush the tubing that originates from the pressure bag after disconnecting it from the arterial line.

B. **Is the extremity distal to the line compromised?** Be sure that the fingers (or toes) are not ischemic. A pulse oximeter may be helpful in assessing this. When there is any question, remove the line and replace it elsewhere (if still indicated).

C. **Can blood be drawn back through the catheter?** Even if the catheter cannot be used to draw blood, it can often function as a blood pressure monitor.

D. **Does the arterial pressure measured correlate with a cuff pressure?** Find out how well arterial pressure was measured when the catheter did work. In general, cuff measurements should be within 10–15 mm Hg of the arterial line reading.

III. **Differential Diagnosis**

A. **Mechanical**

1. **Kinked catheter.** This can lead to a dampened inaccurate tracing or no tracing with an inability to draw blood. The catheter and tubing should be properly connected and secured with smooth curves (no kinks).
2. **Clotted catheter.** Often caused by insufficient heparin in the flush solution.
3. **Faulty monitor or transducer.** The ICU staff will be helpful in solving this problem. There may be a connector, an electrical, or a transducer malfunction or air in the system.
4. **Cracked catheter.** Bleeding, air on drawing back through the line, or lack of a tracing may be present. Replacing the line over a guidewire is often successful.

5. **Positional catheter.** This is often a problem with the way the catheter was sutured in place or the positioning of the wrist on the armboard. If the line is truly positional, it is prudent to remove the line and establish a proper functioning line.

B. Vascular

1. **Thrombosed vessel.** Check the pulse proximally, using a Doppler probe if necessary. Risk factors include (1) hypotension, (2) mechanical pressure to control bleeding at the site, (3) the use of a catheter too large for the vessel, (4) prolonged use of a catheter, (5) an underlying hypercoagulable state, and (6) an existing coagulopathy.
2. **Bleeding around the catheter from a torn artery.** This occurs most often after a problematic cut-down. The application of pressure, as with any bleeding, should control the problem. Failure to prevent a large periarterial hematoma may result in a pseudoaneurysm later.

IV. Database

A. Physical Exam Key Points

1. Examine the insertion site for signs of infection or bleeding. Check the suture securing the catheter. Obtain a cuff pressure and compare it to the arterial line measurement.
2. The distal extremity (hand or foot) should be examined for evidence of ischemia. Place a pulse oximeter on a digit of the extremity in question.
3. The entire tubing, transducer, and monitoring system should be checked for problems like kinking, disconnections, air in the system, and insufficient pressure in the pressure infusion bag.

B. Laboratory Data. Laboratory data is only useful when there is bleeding from the site. Check the PT/PTT, platelets, and fibrin split products are helpful if diffuse bleeding is present. A hematocrit is essential if bleeding has been excessive.

V. Plan. Check the pressure tracing against a standard blood pressure cuff measurement. Verify the acceptable withdrawal of arterial blood. Occasionally, a catheter may be used to withdraw arterial blood but not to provide reliable pressure monitoring and vice-versa. A highly subjective decision must often be made whether to remove or change the site, and this decision is based on the physician's preference and the patient's condition.

A. **Bleeding**
   1. Apply direct pressure or a pressure dressing when bleeding from the site is a problem. Bleeding from other sites may signify disseminated intravascular coagulation.
   2. After a catheter is removed, pressure should be applied to the site for at least 10 min to prevent bleeding with resultant hematoma and later pseudoaneurysm formation.

B. **Mechanical Problems**
   1. The use of an armboard will help prevent many of the mechanical problems with arterial lines. If a catheter is positional, try an armboard or resuture the catheter. If possible, avoid placing arterial lines across joints (such as the antecubital region).
   2. Kinked or clotted catheters usually must be replaced.
      a. If a catheter clots, verify that there is sufficient heparin in the flush bag (usually 2–4 U heparin/mL).
      b. Continuous flushing systems are preferred over intermittent flush systems.
      c. If the vessel appears undamaged, consider changing the catheter over a guidewire using sterile technique. Be sure to carefully suture it in place to avoid kinking and movement of the catheter.
   3. A dampened wave form usually indicates air in the transducer system or a clot in the catheter. Air bubbles can usually be flushed clear.
   4. Line leaks or connection problems can usually be solved by the ICU nursing staff.

C. **Reading Errors.** As previously mentioned, the difference between the cuff and arterial line pressure should be less than 10–15 mm Hg. Using an appropriate sized BP cuff, keeping tubing lengths as short as possible, verifying that the transducer is properly "zeroed", and checking that no air is in the system should minimize the differences.

D. **Thrombosis.** Usually requires removal of the catheter and observation for ischemic changes. Because ischemic changes can progress, careful follow-up is important to monitor an ischemic limb.

8. ASPIRATION

I. **Problem.** An obtunded trauma patient in the emergency room vomits and develops acute respiratory distress.

II. **Immediate Questions**

A. **What are the vital signs?** Significant respiratory distress (tachypnea and tachycardia) may indicate airway obstruction or aspiration of gastric contents. A decrease in oxygen saturation should alert the physician to respiratory decompensation. Fever may indicate infection, and signs of septic shock may eventually ensue.

B. **Is the airway protected?** If the patient's airway cannot be protected, then intubation is indicated. Check the patient's Glasgow Coma Scale. Any number less than 8 is an indication for emergent intubation. Also, check for a gag reflex and check the neck and oral cavity for signs of trauma.

C. **Is the patient cyanotic?** If the patient is hypoxic to the point of cyanosis, intubation is indicated.

D. **What is the patient's neurologic status?** Patients who are unconscious or obtunded are at higher risk for aspiration.

III. Differential Diagnosis

A. **Aspiration Pneumonitis.** Risk factors include (1) altered mental status (due to head injury, drugs or alcohol), (2) reflux disease, (3) nasogastric tube placement, (4) tracheostomy, and (5) vomiting. Emergency intubation has a high incidence of aspiration. Emergent intubation for pregnant patients, patients who recently ate, or patients with bowel obstruction requires rapid sequence induction with cricoid pressure to reduce the aspiration risk. Aspiration of acidic gastric contents causes bronchospasm and respiratory distress; large food particles may cause obstruction; smaller particles may lead to pneumonia or lung abscess formation.

B. **Asthma.** Wheezing from aspiration, especially chronic aspiration, can mimic asthma. Aspiration can be especially dangerous in a patient with a history of asthma.

C. **Pneumonia.** May precede aspiration or be caused by aspiration.

D. **Pulmonary Embolus and Infarction.** Acute dyspnea and tachypnea (with associated respiratory alkalosis) are the most common symptoms from a pulmonary embolus. Hypoxia, hypotension, and pulmonary infarction occur with larger emboli (refer to Problem 26, page [113]).

E. **Foreign Body Aspiration.** A problem mostly in children. Older patients with poor dentition may aspirate loose teeth.

F. **Pneumothorax.** This can also mimic aspiration, especially in a trauma patient.

IV. Database. Check for a history of asthma. Consider the risk factors for pulmonary embolus (birth control pills, recent surgery, prolonged bedrest, cancer, obesity, previous deep venous thrombosis).

A. Physical Exam Key Points

1. **Vital signs.** Pay close attention to the respiratory rate and oxygen saturation.
2. **HEENT.** Check dentition for loose or missing teeth. Look for oral foreign bodies or vomitus. If a nasogastric (NG) or feeding tube is present, check its position.
3. **Neck.** Make note of head and neck tumors, radiation, and surgery (eg, tracheostomy). Also, check for jugular venous distention (JVD), which may indicate a tension pneumothorax or cardiac tamponade.
4. **Lungs.** Decreased breath sounds can occur with foreign body aspiration and pneumothorax. Aspiration can cause wheezing (by irritating the airways). Rales can also be present when a large volume of aspiration has occurred.
5. **Skin.** Look for cyanosis to suggest hypoxia.
6. **Extremities.** Look for evidence of deep vein thrombosis (DVT)(eg, swelling, pain).
7. **Neurologic exam.** It is important to carefully evaluate the patient's mental status and gag reflex. Determine the patient's Glasgow Coma Scale level.

B. Laboratory Data

1. **Arterial blood gas.** This is key to assessing the degree of respiratory distress. Intubate the patient when you cannot maintain adequate oxygenation.
2. **CBC.** Pay particular attention to the white count.
3. **Sputum Gram's stain and culture.** Pathogenic organisms may grow in acute or chronic aspiration.
4. **Glucose test of tracheal aspirate.** A glucose level of > 20 mg/dL indicates aspiration of feeding formulas.

C. Radiographic and Other Studies

1. The chest radiograph may show
   - **a.** Air trapping ("hyperaeration") on side of foreign body aspiration.
   - **b.** Infiltrates that vary with the position of the patient at the time of aspiration. The right superior basal segment is most often involved (right mid-lung field on chest radiograph), particularly when the patient is supine. (Aspirated gastric contents tend to flow downward and posterior because of gravity.) Aspiration can result in infiltrates in any portion of either lung or none at all, depending on quantity and quality of the material aspirated. Infiltrates may not be seen for 24h after aspiration.

c. A wedge-shaped infarct in some cases of pulmonary embolus.
d. Air outside the border of the lung in a pneumothorax.
e. Clear fields and a flattened diaphragm in uncomplicated asthma or COPD.
f. A cavity with air-fluid levels with lung abscess formation. This is usually a late finding or is associated with chronic aspiration.

2. **Other Studies.** Ventilation/perfusion scans, spiral CT scans of the chest, and pulmonary angiograms all help to diagnose pulmonary emboli. A barium swallow can be done at a later time to look for reflux. It is important that Gastrografin not be used because of its severe pulmonary toxicity when aspirated.

V. **Plan.** Aspiration should be suspected in patients who (1) may be unable to protect their airway because of neurologic or oncologic disease affecting swallowing and coughing; (2) have an altered mental status (sedated, confused, obtunded), particularly with abdominal distention; (3) have no gag reflex (eg, head trauma or alcohol intoxication), or (4) have required intubation on a full stomach. Patients undergoing gavage feedings are also at increased risk. The goal should be to recognize the at-risk population and prevent aspiration.

A. **Prevention**

1. For emergent intubation, use a rapid sequence induction with cricoid pressure.
2. For patients being gavage fed, confirm gastric emptying by checking residuals every 4 h, and elevate the head of the bed.
3. Unconscious patients should be placed in a lateral, slightly head down position (whenever possible) and monitored closely.
4. If in place, NG tubes should be placed to suction.

B. **Oxygenation.** Supplemental oxygen is usually given by mask initially. Carefully monitor oxygenation with a pulse oximeter or repeat arterial blood gases.

C. **Intubation and Pulmonary Toilet.** When oxygenation is poor or when a patient is obtunded, intubate the patient to provide adequate oxygenation and to protect the airway from further aspiration.

D. **Remove the Nasogastric Tube.** If the patient does not need the tube, remove it because gastric contents can "wick" up the tube and enter the trachea. The tube also irritates the oropharynx and interferes with effective coughing.

E. **Replace a Metal Tracheostomy.** Use a plastic nonfenestrated cuffed tracheostomy tube. Metal tubes are used rarely now, but may be found in patients with old tracheostomies. Most outpatient tracheostomy tubes are fenestrated and noncuffed.

F. **Medications**
   1. Corticosteroids are not generally indicated in the acute management of aspiration, but there is some debate about this. Some clinicians feel hydrocortisone 30 mg/kg/d IV should be given for 3 d.
   2. Start antibiotics on the basis of culture results when there is evidence of an established pneumonia. Acute aspiration pneumonia may have an aerobic or mixed anaerobic-aerobic flora.
   3. Anaerobic organisms are more likely with poor dentition. If empiric antibiotic therapy is chosen for an out-of-the hospital aspiration, penicillin G (2–6 million U/d) is recommended; for hospitalized patients, tobramycin with ticarcillin is a reasonable initial choice, pending culture results.

G. **Bronchoscopy.** Performed when foreign body aspiration is suspected or for those patients who aspirate particulate gastric material that cannot be adequately suctioned. This procedure should be performed as early as possible, as it is the best way to ensure clearance of the airway.

H. **Chest Tube or CT-guided aspiration.** May be needed later for drainage of an empyema. Chronic aspiration pneumonia may be necrotizing with formation of a lung abscess or progression to empyema.

I. **Respiratory therapy.** This is the most important aspect of treatment. Every 2- to 4-h albuterol treatments should be administered to treat bronchospasm. This should be accompanied by frequent tracheal suctioning and bicarbonate lavages. Postural drainage should also be done as frequently as possible.

9. BRADYCARDIA

I. **Problem.** A postoperative hernia patient is found to have a heart rate of 42 on a routine vital signs check.

II. **Immediate Questions**

A. **What is the patient's blood pressure, and is the patient alert and oriented?** The initial questions define the severity of the problem. Because the clinical consequence of a significant bradycardia is reduced perfusion, the rapid assessment of perfusion—the blood pressure and the mental status—should be performed.

B. **What is the patient's normal resting heart rate?** The range of normal heart rates is wide and a resting pulse of 42 bpm may not be abnormal in a highly conditioned athlete.

C. **Are there any associated symptoms of chest pain or pressure, dyspnea, diaphoresis, or nausea?** Bradycardia is a common manifestation of an acute inferior wall myocardial infarction. Question the patient about any concurrent symptoms.

D. **Has the patient felt dizzy or lightheaded in the recent past?** The clinical presentation of sinus node dysfunction may be episodic syncope or near-syncope.

E. **What medication is the patient taking, and does the patient have a pacemaker?** Certain medications, such as β-blockers (propranolol, etc), verapamil, digitalis, and others can lead to bradycardia. A patient with a pacemaker may be suffering from pacer malfunction.

F. **Does the patient have a history of cardiovascular disease?** This may further clarify the nature of the slow heart rate.

III. **Differential Diagnosis.** Disturbances in the cardiac conduction pathway leading to bradydysrhythmias are due to dysfunction at the level of the sinus node or at the level of the atrioventricular (AV) node/His Purkinje system. Within these two categories, a variety of conditions exist defined by characteristic ECG patterns and associated with particular clinical conditions.

A. **Sinus Node Disease**
   1. **Sinus bradycardia**
      a. **Vasovagal syncope**
      b. **High vagal tone:** More common in conditioned athletes and in the elderly.
      c. **Increased intracranial pressure:** Cushing's reflex results in bradycardia and hypertension.
   2. **Sinus node dysfunction.** Sick sinus syndrome and tachycardia-bradycardia syndrome are variants of sinus node disease characterized by intermittent sinus pauses.
      a. Ischemic cardiomyopathy
      b. Hypertensive cardiomyopathy
      c. Hypothyroidism
      d. Hypothermia

e. Infiltrative diseases (amyloidosis, etc)

B. **Atrioventricular Node Disease**
1. **First-degree AV block.** PR interval > 0.2 s.
2. **Second-degree AV block Mobitz type 1 (Wenckebach).** Successive prolongation of the PR interval with eventual dropped ventricular beat.
   a. **Inferior myocardial infarction**
   b. **Drug toxicity:** Frequently implicated drugs include digoxin, β-blockers (propranolol), and calcium-channel blockers (verapamil).
3. **Second-degree AV block Mobitz type II.** Intermittent missed ventricular beats. Associated conditions are the same as for third-degree AV block, and this condition may progress to third-degree AV block.
4. **Third-degree AV block.** Also called "AV dissociation."
   a. **Myocardial infarction:** Most common sites are anteroseptal or inferior.
   b. Primary degenerative disease of the conducting system.
   c. **Infiltrative conditions:** Sarcoidosis, amyloidosis, neoplasms.
   d. **Infectious diseases:** Viral myocarditis, acute rheumatic fever, Lyme disease.

IV. **Database.** The primary test to diagnose a bradycardia is a 12-lead ECG and rhythm strip, which should be obtained concurrently with the initial history and physical exam.

A. **Physical Exam Key Points**
1. **Vital signs.** Note the heart rate, blood pressure, and respiratory rate. Hypotension < 90 mm Hg requires emergent treatment.
2. **Lungs.** Listen for evidence of congestive heart failure (crackles).
3. **Cardiac.** Note any new murmurs or gallops. Is the rhythm regular or irregular?
4. **Skin.** Pallor, cool, moist skin is evidence of poor perfusion or increased vagal tone.
5. **Neurologic.** Look for evidence of elevated intracranial pressure (papilledema). Decreased mental status may be a sign of inadequate cerebral perfusion pressure.

B. **Laboratory Data**
1. **Electrolytes, calcium.** Hypokalemia can potentiate digoxin toxicity and hypocalcemia can result in a prolonged QT interval and bradycardia.
2. **Troponin-I/CPK with isoenzymes.** Defines myocardial injury (see Section II, page 327).

3. **Digoxin level if indicated.** Toxicity is often manifested as bradycardia. Toxic levels usually > 2.5 ng/mL.
4. **Thyroid hormone levels.** Hypothyroidism can cause bradycardia.
5. Arterial blood gases if indicated by respiratory distress or dyspnea.

C. Radiographic and Other Studies

1. **ECG.** This should be analyzed systematically looking for the atrial rate (lead II is good), ventricular rate, PR interval, relation of P waves to QRS complexes, and for evidence of ischemia (inverted T waves, ST segment depression).
2. **Chest radiograph.** A change in cardiac silhouette and lung fields may be associated with myocardial dysfunction.
3. Specialized tests conducted by cardiologists include electrophysiologic mapping (to define the precise location of blocks) and complete autonomic blockade using atropine and propranolol (to determine the intrinsic heart rate and document the contribution of vagal tone to the bradycardia).

V. Plan. The treatment will be dictated by the type and degree of bradycardia and any underlying clinical condition. Remember that not all bradycardia is clinically significant. Use extreme caution when treating bradycardia, especially in elderly patients. In urgent situations, treat with IV fluids, IV atropine, apply oxygen, and obtain an ECG as soon as possible.

Critical management can be found in the advanced cardiac life support (ACLS) algorithm for bradycardia (see Figure I–3, below).

A. Critical Symptomatic Bradycardia. Should be used in cases of acute, clinically significant bradycardia usually associated with hypotension in the following sequence:

1. Atropine 0.5–1.0 mg IV (0.01 mg/kg). May be repeated every 5–10 min to a total dose of 2 mg.
2. Transcutaneous pacing if available.
3. Dopamine 5–20 mg/kg/min IV.
4. Epinephrine 2–10 mg/min IV.
5. Isoproterenol (Isuprel) 1–3 mg/min IV continuous infusion (low dose).
6. Consider giving an IV fluid bolus to ensure adequate preload when a patient does not appear to be in pulmonary edema.

B. Treat the Underlying Condition

1. **Myocardial ischemia.** Should be treated with nitrates (such as sublingual nitroglycerin) and oxygen.

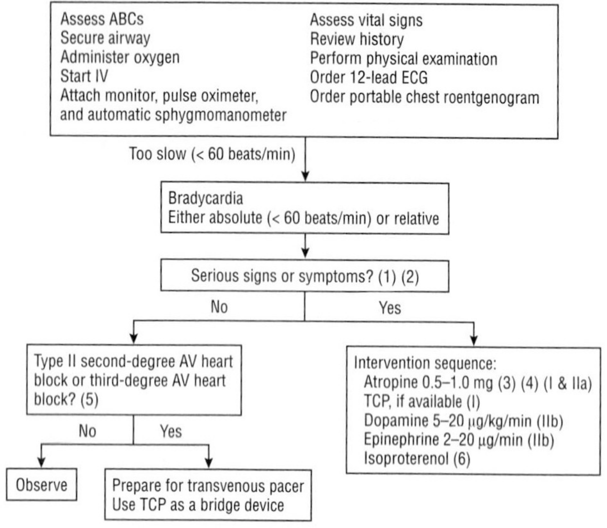

Footnotes

(1) Serious signs or symptoms must be related to the slow rate.
Clinical manifestations include:
Symptoms (chest pain, shortness of breath, decreased level of consciousness) and signs (low BP, shock, pulmonary congestions, CHF, acute MI).

(2) Do not delay TCP while awaiting IV access or for atropine to take effect if patient is symptomatic.

(3) Denervated transplanted hearts will not respond to atropine. Go at once to pacing, catecholamine infusion, or both.

(4) Atropine should be given in repeat doses in 3–5 min up to a total of 0.04 mg/kg. Consider shorter dosing intervals in severe clinical conditions. It has been suggested that atropine should be used with caution in atrioventricular (AV) block at the His-Purkinje level (type II AV block and new third degree block with wide QRS complexes) (class IIb).

(5) Never treat third-degree heart block plus ventricular escape beats with Lidocaine.

(6) Isoproterenol should be used, if at all, with extreme caution. At low doses it is class IIb (possibly helpful); at higher doses it is class III (harmful).

(7) Verify patient tolerance and mechanical capture. Use analgesia and sedation as needed.

Figure I–3. Bradycardia algorithm (patient not in cardiac arrest). *(Reproduced, with permission, from Adult Advanced Cardiac Life Support.* JAMA *1992;268:16.) (Updated according to American Heart Assn. Guidelines, 2000).*

2. **Increased intracranial pressure.** Maneuvers to decrease pressure include mannitol diuresis, elevating the head of the bed, intubation, and hyperventilation.

C. **Pacemaker Therapy.** When the bradydysrhythmia does not respond to medical therapy or in certain critical situations as listed below, ventricular pacing should be used. External pacer pads are the quickest method of pacing the heart but do not "capture" consistently. Transvenous pacers (eg, pacing using a Swan-Ganz catheter designed for pacing) should be used for more prolonged pacing. If this option is needed, contact the cardiology consultant.

1. Indications for a temporary pacemaker:
   a. Transient second-degree AV block with an inferior myocardial infarction.
   b. AV block as a result of drug toxicity.
   c. As temporizing measure before permanent pacemaker insertion.
2. Indications for a permanent pacemaker:
   a. **Sinus node dysfunction.** When symptomatic.
   b. Second- or third-degree AV block associated with an acute myocardial infarction.
   c. Symptomatic Mobitz type II and third degree AV block.
   d. **Digoxin Toxicity.** Check the level, hold further doses, and consider digoxin antibody (Digibind) 60 mg per 1-mg digoxin, IV.

10. BRIGHT RED BLOOD PER RECTUM (HEMATOCHEZIA)

I. **Problem.** You are called to see a 60-year-old female patient who is passing red blood per rectum 3 d after undergoing a modified radical mastectomy.

II. **Immediate Questions**

A. **What are the vital signs?** Look for signs of hemodynamically significant blood loss, such as tachycardia and hypotension.

B. **How much blood has been passed and over what time period?** The volume of blood may help assess the significance of the bleed, as the hematocrit may not decrease until later. Inquiring when blood was last passed may tell you if this is an ongoing process (blood passes quickly through the GI tract).

C. **What was the most recent hematocrit?** A baseline value is needed to assess the amount of bleeding.

D. **What is the nature of the stool?** Coating of the stool often indicates an anal process such as hemorrhoids but may also suggest a colonic tumor. Bright red blood is more likely to be from the distal left colon. Melena usually signifies bleeding proximal to the right colon. Because the color of the stool is primarily determined by the length of time the blood has been in the bowel, bright red rectal blood occasionally can be a result of an upper GI source and a rapid transit through the bowel.

E. **What medications is the patient taking, and is there any history of alcohol abuse?** A history of alcoholism suggests varices; aspirin and other nonsteroidal anti-inflammatory agents commonly cause ulcers; overuse of warfarin (Coumadin) may cause GI tract bleeding.

F. **Has the patient had recent GI tract surgery?** It is common to have some blood in the bowel movements immediately after GI tract surgery.

G. **Are there any associated symptoms?** Crampy abdominal pain or fever suggests an infectious cause, inflammatory bowel disease, or diverticulitis. A change in bowel habits or decreased caliber of stools may indicate a neoplasm, whereas polyps and angiodysplasia are usually free of other symptoms.

III. Differential Diagnosis

A. **Diverticular Disease.** A common cause of massive lower gastrointestinal bleeding, most often from the left colon.

B. **Angiodysplasia.** These are usually right-sided lesions and thus most often associated with melena. They are more frequent in elderly patients. The natural history of bleeding from angiodysplasia usually includes rebleeding. This is usually venous or capillary bleeding as contrasted with the arterial bleeding associated with diverticula.

C. **Polyps.** The larger the polyp, the greater the chance it contains cancer. Villous adenomas can also cause potassium loss.

D. **Carcinoma.** Usually adenocarcinoma of the colon.

E. **Inflammatory Bowel Disease.** Ulcerative colitis is more frequently associated with bloody diarrhea than Crohn's disease. Look for a history of chronic diarrhea.

F. **Hemorrhoids.** Although hemorrhoids are commonly present, this does not preclude the presence of a simultaneous tumor or angiodysplasia. Bleeding from cancer is commonly attributed to hemorrhoids.

G. **Mesenteric Thrombosis.** This may lead to bowel infarction or ischemic colitis. Remember that "abdominal pain out of proportion to findings on exam" is the key indicator of bowel ischemia.

H. **Meckel's Diverticulitis.** A Meckel's scan is usually diagnostic in this setting, because Meckel's diverticula generally do not bleed unless they contain ectopic gastric mucosa.

I. **Anal Fissures.** Patients usually have severe anal pain, particularly with bowel movements.

J. **Excessive Anticoagulation.** Be sure to review the medications the patient is taking. Check clotting studies as needed.

K. **Massive Upper GI Bleed.** Results in rapid intestinal transit and resulting hematochezia (see Problem 34, page 137). Blood is an excellent cathartic. Remember that lower GI bleeding (bright red blood) can originate anywhere in the GI tract.

L. **Infectious Colitis.** *Shigella*, *Yersinia*, entero-invasive *Escherichia coli*, and *Salmonella* infections often cause bloody diarrhea. Order stool cultures in a patient with a history of chronic diarrhea or travel.

IV. Database

A. Physical Exam Key Points

1. **Vital Signs.** Look for evidence of hypovolemia (tachycardia and hypotension). Fever may represent inflammatory bowel disease or an infectious gastroenteritis.
2. **Abdomen.** Palpation for masses or tenderness. A left lower quadrant mass may be associated with diverticulitis; a right lower quadrant mass may be from Crohn's disease; any mass may represent cancer. Bowel sounds may be hyperactive, because blood is a cathartic.
3. **Rectal.** Hemorrhoids, fissures, or masses may be detected.
4. Is bleeding present at other sites to suggest a systemic cause?
5. Check for signs of cirrhosis (palmar erythema, caput medusae) to suggest a possible upper GI source.

B. Laboratory Studies

1. **CBC.** Serial hematocrits are helpful because rapid bleeding may not reflect itself as a change in hematocrit for some time. Microcytic and hypochromic indices are indicative of chronic blood loss.
2. **Clotting studies.** The PT/PTT and platelet count may reveal a coagulation disorder.

3. **Blood bank.** Obtain a type and crossmatch.

C. **Radiographic and Other Studies**

1. **Nasogastric tube.** Pass a nasogastric tube to rule out upper GI bleeding.
2. **Colonoscopy.** Should be done as soon as possible to evaluate the cause (cancer, IBD, ischemic colitis) and location of bleeding and possibly to treat lesions, such as polyps or angiodysplasia. A quick rigid sigmoidoscopy may be helpful.
3. **Angiography.** Is indicated for the diagnosis of lower GI bleeding in any patient who requires more than 2 units of blood to maintain their hematocrit or becomes hypotensive. Remember that angiography is impossible with barium in the gut. For this reason, endoscopy, nuclear studies, and angiography are preferred for the initial workup of a patient with GI bleeding, rather than contrast studies. For angiography to be helpful, bleeding must usually be > 0.5–1.0 mL/min. Selective embolization or vasopressin infusion may be possible to control bleeding.
4. **Radiolabeled red cell study (Usually ^{99m}Tc.** This can sometimes localize lesions in the GI tract, especially with slower rates of bleeding than needed for angiography (0.2 mL/min). These are less reliable than angiography (a hot spot in the left upper quadrant may indicate bleeding from the stomach, small bowel, or splenic flexure of the colon).
5. **Upper GI Endoscopy (esophagogastroduodenoscopy [EGD]).** Although a nasogastric tube can usually rule out upper GI sources of bleeding, an inconclusive workup for lower GI bleeding necessitates a definitive look at the upper GI tract.

V. **Plan.** Approximately 80% of patients with lower GI bleeding stop bleeding spontaneously. Acute, severe hemorrhage is potentially life-threatening and should be treated emergently.

A. **Acute Intervention.** Large-bore IVs (16 gauge) should be placed for volume resuscitation. Use crystalloid or blood if there is a low hematocrit. Attempt to keep the hematocrit > 30%. A Foley catheter will allow more accurate assessment of volume status. Consider a central venous pressure (CVP) line when there is any instability and when the patient is elderly. The philosophy should be to treat these people like trauma patients (ABCs, etc.).

B. **Diagnosis and Treatment.** A suggested algorithm for the diagnosis and treatment of acute lower GI bleeding is outlined in Figure I–4. (page 46).

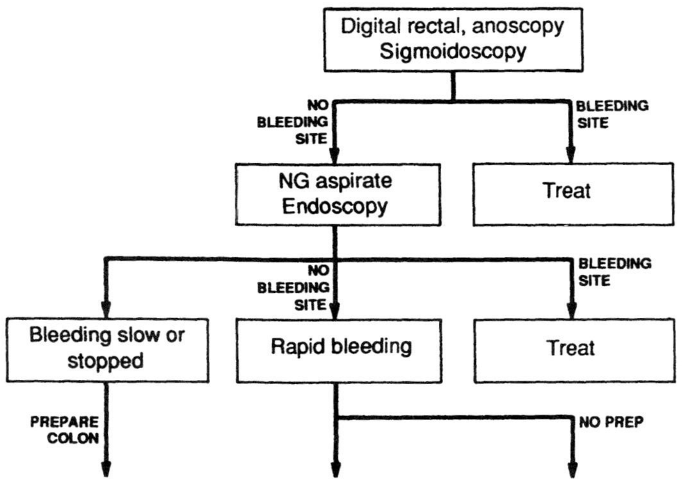

Digital rectal, anoscopy
Sigmoidoscopy
NO BLEEDING SITE
BLEEDING SITE
NG aspirate
Endoscopy
Treat
NO BLEEDING SITE
BLEEDING SITE
Bleeding slow or stopped
Rapid bleeding
Treat
PREPARE COLON
NO PREP

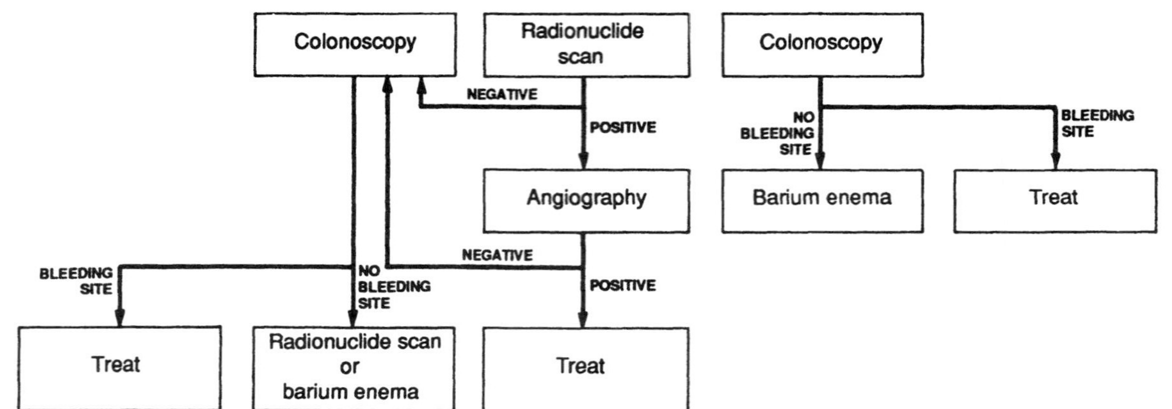

Figure I–4. Suggested scheme for the management of lower gastrointestinal hemorrhage. NG = nasogastric tube. *(Reproduced, with permission, from Schrock TR: Large intestine. In Way LW (editor):* Current Surgical Diagnosis & Treatment, *10th ed. Originally published by Appleton & Lange. Copyright © 1994 by The McGraw-Hill Companies, Inc.)*

1. Treatment is directed at the cause.
2. The combined approach of angiography and colonoscopy can usually localize the bleeding site. In those extreme cases where the site cannot be identified, subtotal colectomy may be necessary.
3. Surgery may eventually be needed to treat lesions such as carcinoma, polyps, hemorrhoids, and the consequences of inflammatory bowel disease.
4. Local care for hemorrhoids includes sitz baths, stool softeners, and topical hydrocortisone (Anusol-HC, etc). Dietary fiber reduces the incidence of recurrence. Chronic anal fissures are treated with topical creams (nitroglycerine, tetracaine), botox injections, or surgery (lateral sphincterotomy).

11. CARDIOPULMONARY ARREST

Immediate Actions

1. Assess responsiveness.
2. If unresponsive, follow algorithm in Figure I–5. (page 48)

I. **Problem.** One week after an above-the-knee amputation, a patient is found unresponsive and pulseless in bed.

II. **Immediate Questions**

A. **Is the patient responsive?** Basic cardiopulmonary resuscitation (CPR) begins with a vigorous attempt to arouse the patient. The patient should be called and shaken by the shoulders. Always be certain that you are not alone; always get help.

B. **Is the airway obstructed?** Finger sweep or suction out the patient's mouth. Listen for air movement.

C. **Are there vital signs?** Check for carotid pulse and blood pressure. If the patient is not breathing, begin mouth-to-mouth or, preferably, ventilation with 100% oxygen by bag and mask. If the patient has no pulse, begin chest compressions. The following questions are then asked as ACLS is started.

D. **What medications is the patient taking?** Cardiac medications are particularly important, especially antiarrhythmics and digoxin. An adverse reaction to a recently administered medication may be identified. Have someone obtain the patient's most recent medication list.

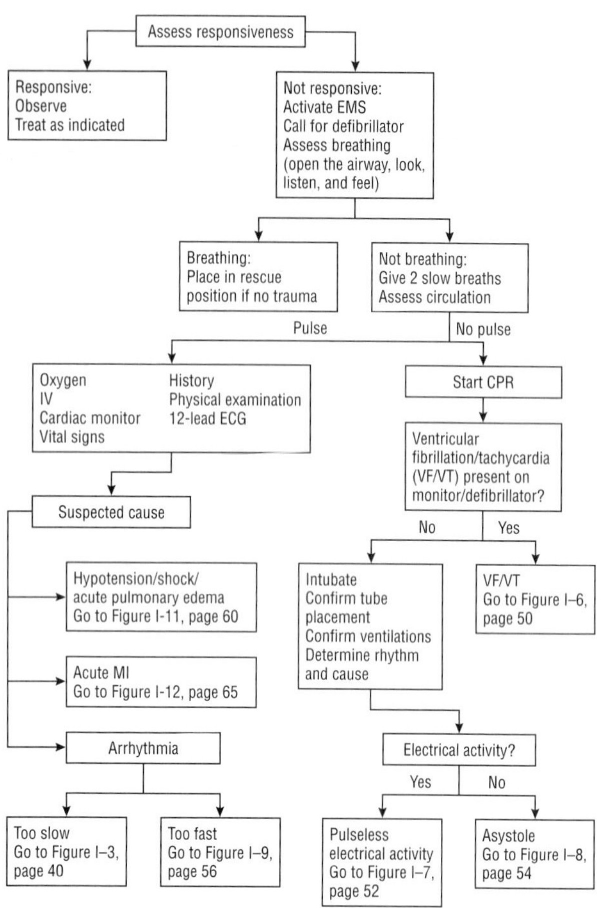

Figure I–5. Universal algorithm for adult emergency cardiac care (ECC). *(Reproduced, with permission, from Adult Advanced Cardiac Life Support.* JAMA *1992;268:16.) (Updated according to American Heart Assn. Guidelines, 2000).*

E. **Are there any recent lab values, particularly the potassium or hematocrit?** Hyperkalemia (usually > 7 mEq/L) and hypercalcemia (> 11 mEq/dL) may cause cardiac arrest. Acute anemia may cause cardiac arrest, but this is usually from hypovolemia (related to bleeding) rather than a lack of hemoglobin.

F. **What are the patient's major medical problems?** Ask about coronary artery disease, previous myocardial infarction, hypertension, previous pulmonary embolus, and recent surgery.

III. Differential Diagnosis.

III. Differential Diagnosis. Arrest rhythms include ventricular fibrillation and tachycardia, asystole, bradycardia, and electromechanical dissociation (EMD). Causes of cardiopulmonary arrest may include:

A. Cardiac

1. Myocardial infarction.
2. Congestive heart failure.
3. Ventricular arrhythmias.
4. Cardiac tamponade. Usually posttraumatic.

B. Pulmonary

1. Pulmonary embolus.
2. Acute respiratory failure.
3. Aspiration.
4. Tension pneumothorax.

C. **Hemorrhagic.** Unrecognized bleeding can result in a cardiac arrest, (as in a ruptured aortic aneurysm).

D. Metabolic

1. **Hypokalemia, hyperkalemia.** These may induce arrhythmias.
2. **Acidosis.** Severe acidosis may suppress myocardial function.
3. **Warming from hypothermia.** Arrhythmias are common.

IV. Database

A. **Physical Exam Key Points.** As described, check responsiveness and vital signs. Resuscitation should always be initiated before a detailed physical exam is performed. Always remember the ABCs.

1. Check ventilation and perform airway opening maneuvers (jaw thrust or chin lift) as needed.
2. Look for tracheal deviation as evidence of a tension pneumothorax.
3. Distended neck veins may indicate pericardial tamponade or tension pneumothorax.

B. Laboratory Data. These should be obtained as soon as possible but should not delay the start of therapy.

1. Arterial blood gas.
2. Serum electrolytes, with special attention to the potassium.
3. **CBC.** Especially the hematocrit.

C. Radiographic and Other Studies

1. Continuous cardiac monitoring, frequently checking lead placement.

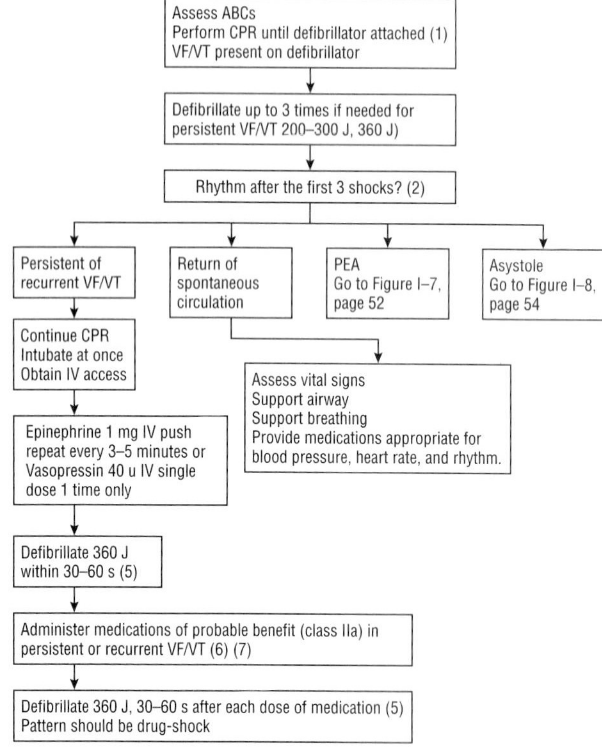

Figure I–6. Algorithm for ventricular fibrillation and pulseless ventricular tachycardia (VF/VT). *(Reproduced, with permission, from Adult Advanced Cardiac Life Support.* JAMA *1992;268:16.) (Updated according to American Heart Assn. Guidelines, 2000).*

2. Other studies may be performed after the patient has been resuscitated. A chest radiograph may be the single most important immediate study. This will help diagnose a pneumothorax, hemothorax, or pericardial effusion.

V. Plan. Therapy for cardiac arrest is based on specific algorithms outlined by the American Heart Association (AHA). Specific AHA algorithms for bradycardia, ventricular fibrillation, electromechanical dissociation, asystole treatment, and tachycardia are shown in Figure I–3 (page 40) and Figure I–6 (page 50) through Figure I–9 (page 56) respectively. Frequently used resuscitation medications are located inside the back cover of this book. Every physician should have these memorized.

In addition, successful resuscitation is based on a team approach with one leader monitoring the rhythm and ordering therapy, according to the appropriate algorithm. Everyone must remain calm and must be assigned to a specific job.

Resuscitation begins with the **ABC**s: **A**irway (intubate whenever possible), **B**reathing (ventilate), and **C**irculation

Footnotes to Figure I–6

Class I: Definitely helpful.
Class IIa: Acceptable, probably helpful.
Class IIb: Acceptable, possibly helpful.
Class III: Not indicated, may be harmful.

(1) Precordial thump is a class IIb action in witnessed arrest, no pulse, and no defibrillator available.
(2) Hypothermic cardiac arrest is treated differently after this point. See section on hypothermia.
(3) Multiple sequenced shocks (200 J, 200–300 J, 360 J) are acceptable here (class I), especially when medications are delayed.
(4) Lidocaine 1.5 mg/kg IV push. Repeat in 3–5 min to total loading dose of 3 mg/kg; then use:
    Bretylium 5 mg/kg IV push. Repeat in 5 min at 10 mg/kg.
    Magnesium sulfate 1–2 g IV in torsades de pointes or suspected hypomagnesemic state or severe refractory VF.
    Procainamide 30 mg/min in refractory VF (maximum total 17 mg/kg).
(5) Sodium bicarbonate (1 mEq/kg IV):
    Class IIa
        If known preexisting bicarbonate-responsive acidosis.
        If overdose with tricyclic antidepressants.
        To alkalinize the urine in drug overdoses.
    Class IIb
        If intubated and continued long arrest interval.
        Upon return of spontaneous circulation after long arrest interval.
    Class III
        Hypoxic lactic acids.

PEA includes:
- Electromechanical dissociation (EMD)
- Pseudo-EMD
- Idioventricular rhythms
- Ventricular escape rhythms
- Bradyasystolic rhythms
- Postdefibrillation idioventricular rhythms

Continue CPR	Obtain IV access
Intubate at once	Assess blood flow using Doppler ultrasound

↓

Consider possible causes:
Hypovolemia (volume infusion)
Hypoxia (ventilation)
Cardiac tamponade (pericardiocentesis)
Tension pneumothorax (needle decompression)
Hypothermia (see Hypothermia, page 83)
Massive pulmonary embolism (surgery thrombolytics)
Drug overdoses such as tricyclics, digitalis, β-blockers, calcium channel blockers
Hyperkalemia [1]
Acidosis [2]
Massive acute myocardial infarction (go to Figure I–12, page 65)

↓

Epinephrine 1 mg IV push [1] [3] repeat every 3–5 minutes

↓

If absolute bradycardia (< 60 beats/min) or relative bradycardia, give atropine 1 mg IV.
Repeat every 3–5 min to a total of 0.04 mg/kg [4].

Figure I–7. Algorithm for pulseless electrical activity (PEA) (electromechanical dissociation [EMD]). *(Reproduced, with permission, from Adult Advanced Cardiac Life Support.* JAMA *1992;268:16.) (Updated according to American Heart Assn. Guidelines, 2000).*

(chest compression). For adults, the ratio of 5 compressions to 1 breath is used in two-person CPR.

A. Ventricular Fibrillation and Pulseless Tachycardia. See Figure I–6 (pages 50–51). Torsade de pointes, a rare ventricular arrhythmia, is treated with a temporary pacemaker, rarely bretylium, but never lidocaine. This is most often congenital or drug induced and is characterized by "twisting" or direction changes of the QRS complex around the isoelectric line.

B. Electromechanical Dissociation. See Figure I–7 (page 52). In surgical patients, always consider pulmonary em-

Footnotes to Figure I–7
Class I: Definitely helpful.
Class IIa: Acceptable, probably helpful.
Class IIb: Acceptable, possibly helpful.
Class III: Not indicated, may be harmful.

[1] Sodium bicarbonate 1 mEq/kg is class I if patient has known preexisting hyperkalemia.
[2] Sodium bicarbonate 1 mEq/kg:
Class IIa
If known preexisting bicarbonate-responsive acidosis.
If overdose with tricyclic antidepressants.
To alkalinize the urine in drug overdoses.
Class IIb
If intubated and continued long arrest interval.
Upon return of spontaneous circulation after long arrest interval.
Class III
Hypoxic lactic acids.
[3] The recommended dose of epinephrine is 1 mg IV push every 3–5 min. If this approach fails, several class IIb dosing regimens can be considered:
Intermediate: epinephrine 2–5 mg IV push, every 3–5 min.
Escalating: epinephrine 1 mg–3 mg–5 mg IV push (3 min apart).
High: epinephrine 0.1 mg/kg IV push, every 3–5 min.
[4] Shorter atropine dosing intervals are possibly helpful in cardiac arrest (class IIb).

bolism, especially in high-risk patients (obese, prolonged bed rest, history of cancer, previous embolism, certain pelvic and orthopedic cases), and hypovolemia as causes of EMD. In trauma patients, consider tension pneumothorax and cardiac tamponade. Treat hypovolemia with aggressive fluid resuscitation, tension pneumothorax with tube thoracostomy, and pericardial tamponade with pericardiocentesis. Tamponade should be treated with volume while setting up for paracentesis.

C. **Asystole.** See algorithm in Figure I–8 (page 54). The prognosis is very poor in cases of asystole. Defibrillate if there is any question about the rhythm being fine ventricular tachycardia.

D. **Tachycardia.** See Figure I–9 (page 56) and Problem 67, page 244.

E. **Bradycardia.** See Figure I–3 (page 40) and Problem 9, page 36. Emergency cardioversion is reviewed in Figure I–10 (page 58).

F. **Hypotension, shock, and acute pulmonary edema.** May arise independently or associated with a cardiac event. See Figure I–11 and Problem 47, page 184

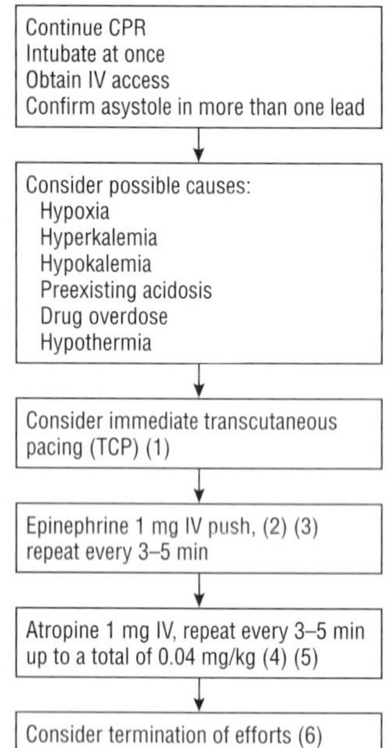

Figure I–8. Asystole treatment algorithm. *(Reproduced, with permission, from Adult Advance Cardiac Life Support.* JAMA *1992; 268:16.) (Updated according to American Heart Assn. Guidelines, 2000).*

REFERENCE

Adult Advanced Cardiac Life Support. *JAMA* 1992;268:2199.

12. CHEST PAIN

I. **Problem.** Four days following a radical nephrectomy a 62-year-old patient tells the nurse of an ongoing episode of chest pain that has lasted for 10 min.

II. **Immediate Questions.** The conditions that lead a patient to complain of "chest pain" range from inconsequential to life-threatening. The purpose of the immediate questions is to determine the urgency of response and, in particular, to ascertain if ischemic heart disease is the cause of the pain.

   A. **Does the patient have a history of coronary artery disease?** If so, does the current pain resemble previous episodes of angina pectoris? In patients with documented cardiac disease, particularly if the current episode resem-

Footnotes to Figure I–8
Class I: Definitely helpful.
Class IIa: Acceptable, probably helpful.
Class IIb: Acceptable, possibly helpful.
Class III: Not indicated, may be harmful.

(1) TCP is a class IIb intervention. Lack of success may be due to delays in pacing. To be effective TCP must be performed early, simultaneously with drugs. Evidence does not support routine use of TCP for asystole.
(2) The recommended dose of epinephrine is 1 mg IV push every 3–5 min. If this approach fails, several class IIb dosing regimens can be considered:
Intermediate: epinephrine 2–5 mg IV push, every 3–5 min.
Escalating: epinephrine 1 mg–3 mg–5 mg IV push (3 min apart).
High: epinephrine 0.1 mg/kg IV push, every 3–5 min.
(3) Sodium bicarbonate 1 mEq/kg is class I if patient has known preexisting hyperkalemia.
(4) Shorter atropine dosing intervals are class IIb in asystolic arrest.
(5) Sodium bicarbonate 1 mEq/kg IV:
Class IIa
If known preexisting bicarbonate-responsive acidosis.
If overdose with tricyclic antidepressants.
To alkalinize the urine in drug overdoses.
Class IIb
If intubated and continued long arrest interval.
Upon return of spontaneous circulation after long arrest interval.
Class III
Hypoxic lactic acids.
(6) If patient remains in asystole or other agonal rhythms after successful intubation and initial medications and no reversible causes are identified, consider termination of resuscitative efforts by a physician.
Consider interval since arrest.

bles previous known anginal attacks, the pain should be treated as myocardial ischemia with sublingual nitroglycerin (0.4 mg typical initial dose) and oxygen without delay. The patient should be transferred immediately to at least a telemetry unit, and a cardiology consultation should be obtained.

B. **What is the location, nature, and severity of the pain?** The location of the pain (substernal, epigastric), radiation of the pain to other areas (jaw, arms, flank, abdomen), the nature of the pain (burning, crushing, tearing, stabbing), and the severity of the pain (mild, moderate, severe) can help define patterns of chest pain that fit certain diagnostic categories. However, chest pain cannot be defined by clinical criteria alone, because there is considerable overlap in pain from varied causes as the thoracic viscera share common neural pathways. Classic angina is a retrosternal crushing pain ("an elephant sitting on my chest") and may radiate to

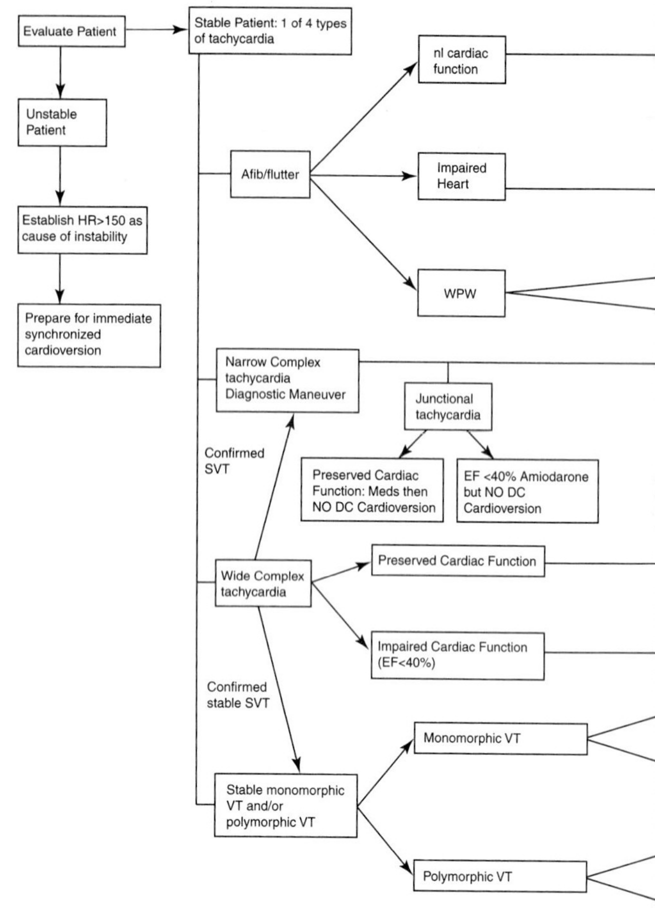

Figure I–9. Tachycardia algorithm. *(Modified with permission from American Heart Assn 2000 Handbook of Emerg Cardiovasc Care.)*

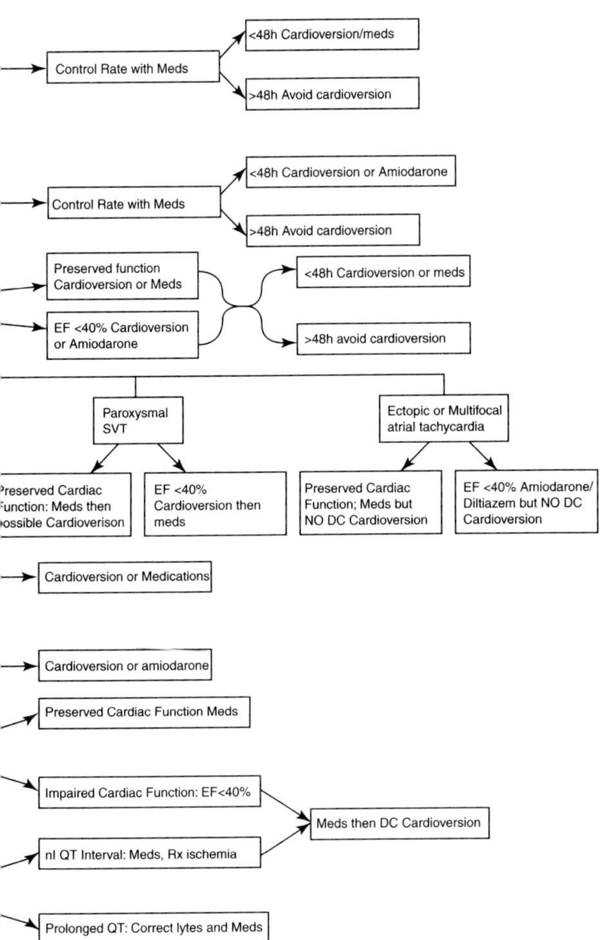
Control Rate with Meds
<48h Cardioversion/meds
>48h Avoid cardioversion
Control Rate with Meds
<48h Cardioversion or Amiodarone
>48h Avoid cardioversion
Preserved function Cardioversion or Meds
EF <40% Cardioversion or Amiodarone
<48h Cardioversion or meds
>48h avoid cardioversion
Paroxysmal SVT
Ectopic or Multifocal atrial tachycardia
Preserved Cardiac Function: Meds then possible Cardioverison
EF <40% Cardioversion then meds
Preserved Cardiac Function; Meds but NO DC Cardioversion
EF <40% Amiodarone/ Diltiazem but NO DC Cardioversion
Cardioversion or Medications
Cardioversion or amiodarone
Preserved Cardiac Function Meds
Impaired Cardiac Function: EF<40%
nl QT Interval: Meds, Rx ischemia
Meds then DC Cardioversion
Prolonged QT: Correct lytes and Meds

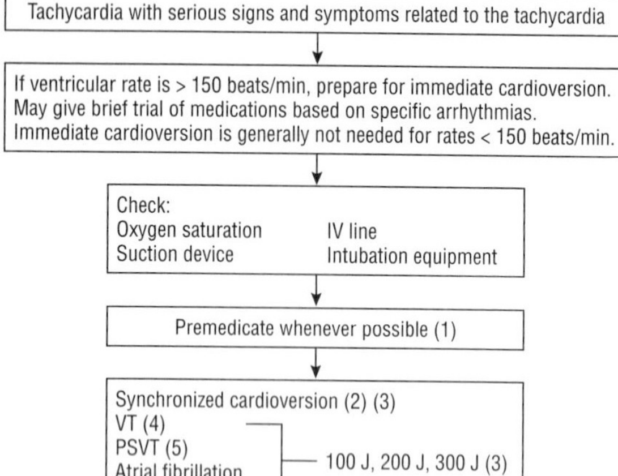

Footnotes

(1) Effective regimens have included a sedative (eg, diazepam, midazolam, barbituates, etomidate, ketamine, methohexital) with or without an analgesic agent (eg, fentanyl, morphine, meperidine).
Many experts recommend anesthesia if service is readily available.

(2) Note possible need to resynchronize after each cardioversion.

(3) If delays in synchronization occur and clinical conditions are critical, go to immediate unsynchronized shocks.

(4) Treat polymorphic VT (irregular form and rate) like VF:
200 J, 200–300 J, 260 J.

(5) PSVT and atrial flutter often respond to lower energy levels (start with 50 J).

Figure I–10. Electrical cardioversion algorithm (patient not in cardiac arrest). *(Reproduced, with permission, from Adult Advanced Cardiac Life Support.* JAMA *1992; 268:16.) (Updated according to American Heart Assn. Guidelines, 2000).*

the left arm or jaw. Thoracic aortic dissection is usually described as tearing or ripping. Peptic ulcer disease and esophageal reflux (GERD) are often burning or gnawing.

C. **What was the patient doing when the pain began?** The inciting activity (or factors that alleviate pain) at the onset of an episode of chest pain is helpful in defining the diagnosis. Classic angina is brought on by exertion, pleuritic pain is exacerbated by coughing, and esophagitis is often exacerbated by recumbency.

D. **Are there any symptoms associated with the episode of chest pain?** Inquire specifically about nausea, dyspnea, diaphoresis, dizziness, syncope, abdominal pain, pleuritic pain, palpitations, and the presence of an acid taste in the mouth.

III. Differential Diagnosis.

A. Cardiac/Vascular

1. **Acute myocardial infarction.** Patients typically have crushing retrosternal chest pain lasting longer than 1 h and unrelieved by nitroglycerin. An MI is usually associated with ECG changes and may be associated with hypotension or signs of CHF.
2. **Angina pectoris.** Angina is typically described as crushing, substernal chest pain, often with radiation to the left arm or jaw. There may be associated nausea, diaphoresis, dyspnea, or palpitations, and pain is usually relieved by nitroglycerin. Angina is caused by coronary artery narrowing or blockage (atherosclerosis) or spasm (Prinzmetal's angina).
3. **Aortic dissection.** The pain is tearing in nature and radiates to the back. It is usually associated with hypertension.
4. **Acute pericarditis.** A friction rub may be present and an effusion seen on an echocardiogram.
   a. **Infectious:** Most commonly viral, rarely from tuberculosis.
   b. **Myocardial infarction (MI):** There can be early pericarditis (within a few days of the MI) or Dressler's syndrome (pericarditis 1–4 wk post MI).
   c. **Uremia.**
   d. **Malignant neoplasm:** Most often breast or bronchogenic.
   e. **Connective tissue diseases.**
5. **Primary pulmonary hypertension:** The pain is mild, and dyspnea on exertion is a prominent symptom.

B. Pulmonary

1. **Pulmonary embolus/infarction.**
2. **Pneumothorax.** Acute onset, often with dyspnea; usually seen in young patients or those with COPD.
3. **Pleurodynia.** Bornholm disease is caused by the Coxsackie virus.
4. **Pneumonia/pleuritis.** This pain is typically pleuritic (made worse on deep inspiration).

C. Gastrointestinal

1. **Gastroesophageal reflux.** The patient often describes an acid taste in their mouth, associated with recumbency. Give the patient an oral antacid, which should immediately relieve the pain.

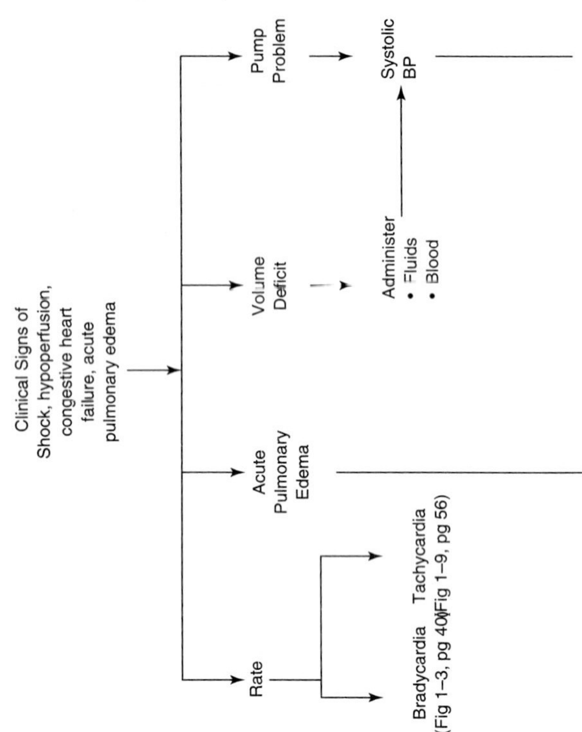
Clinical Signs of Shock, hypoperfusion, congestive heart failure, acute pulmonary edema
Rate
Acute Pulmonary Edema
Volume Deficit
Pump Problem
Bradycardia (Fig 1–3, pg 40)
Tachycardia (Fig 1–9, pg 56)
Administer
• Fluids
• Blood
Systolic BP

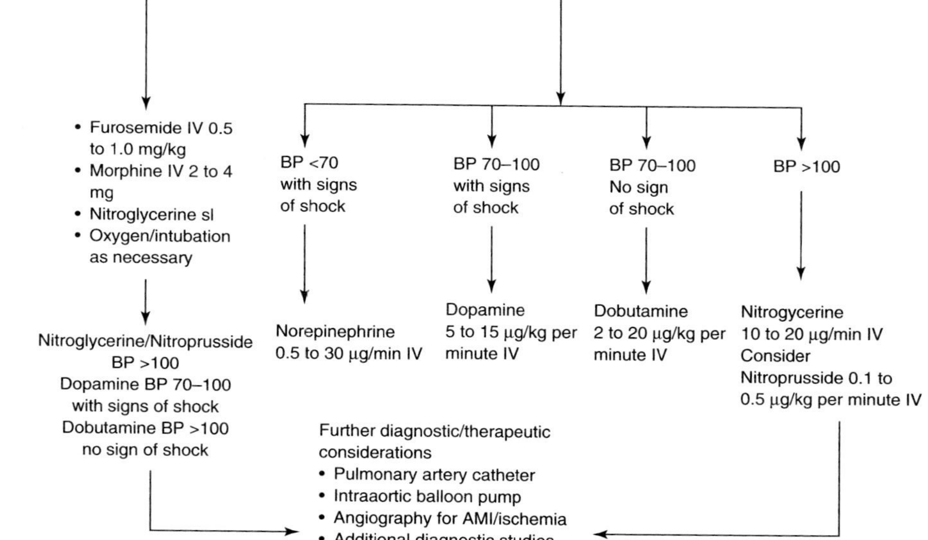

Figure I–11. Algorithm for hypotension, shock, and acute pulmonary edema. *(Modified, with permission from American Heart Assn Guidelines 2000)*

2. **Esophageal spasm.** Easily confused with angina pectoris as it may cause substernal pain relieved by nitrates.
3. **Gastritis.** Caused by alcoholism or an overuse of medications, such as NSAIDs.
4. **Peptic ulcer disease.** Patients commonly describe epigastric pain relieved for an hour or two by eating.
5. **Biliary colic.** Usually associated with eating, especially fatty foods, and located in the epigastrium or right upper quadrant.
6. **Pancreatitis.** Usually caused by gallstones or alcohol; may be relieved by sitting forward.

D. **Musculoskeletal.** Pain is reproduced by palpation of the chest wall.
1. **Costochondritis.** Point tenderness over the costochondral junction.
2. **Muscle strain/spasm.** There is often a history of exercise or exertion.
3. **Rib fractures after trauma.**

IV. Database

A. Physical Exam Key Points

1. **Vital signs.** Hypotension is an ominous sign and may represent cardiovascular collapse (extensive MI, dissecting aneurysm, pulmonary embolus, or tension pneumothorax). Hypertension in the face of a myocardial infarction or aortic dissection requires emergency therapy to reduce the pressure. Fever (usually low grade) may represent an inflammatory process (eg, pneumonia, pleurisy, or pericarditis). Tachycardia may require urgent cardioversion (when a primary arrhythmia causes chest pain or hypotension) or may be secondary to hypovolemia. Tachypnea may be due to pleural effusions, CHF, or pulmonary embolism.
2. **HEENT.** Thrush (especially in immunosuppressed patients) may represent *Candida* esophagitis.
3. **Neck.** Venous distention is seen with CHF, pneumothorax, or tamponade.
4. **Chest.** There is chest wall tenderness or ecchymoses with rib fractures; point costochondral tenderness with costochondritis. Sternal instability after median sternotomy may indicate infection.
5. **Lungs.** Rales occur with CHF, dullness to percussion with fluid or pneumonic consolidation, a friction rub with pleural inflammation, and decreased breath sounds with fluid or pneumothorax.
6. **Heart.** A murmur can be heard with valvular disease, a friction rub with pericarditis (a "normal finding" immedi-

ately after open heart surgery), and a displaced PMI with CHF.

7. **Abdomen.** Determine presence or absence of bowel sounds, distention tympany, tenderness, and other signs of intra-abdominal disease. If you press below the patient's liver and the patient experiences RUQ pain with deep inspiration (Murphy's sign), the patient probably has biliary colic or acute cholecystitis. Hepatomegaly may be due to CHF.
8. **Neurologic.** Aortic dissection may cause a characteristic hemiplegia.
9. **Extremities.** Edema with CHF or asymmetric swelling with venous thrombosis. Aortic dissection may lead to asymmetric pulses.

B. Laboratory Studies

1. **CBC.** Look for a leukocytosis with infections, particularly a lymphocytosis in viral conditions.
2. **CPK and Troponin I** every 6 h to evaluate myocardial injury.
3. **ABG** in most cases and always when there is dyspnea.

C. Radiographic and Other Studies

1. **ECG.** Obtain a baseline study. Evaluate systematically and compare to prior ECGs. Document the presence and degree of pain at the time of the ECG. Look for arrhythmias. ECG findings of an MI may include Q waves, ST-wave changes (depression or elevation) or T-wave inversions. Q waves may not be present with a subendocardial infarction. Note the leads in which changes are present. Changes in leads II, III, and aVF indicate an inferior wall MI, whereas V1–V6 indicate an anterior MI.
2. **Chest radiograph.** If there is any possibility of myocardial ischemia, obtain a portable chest radiograph instead of sending the patient to the radiology department. Look for a pneumothorax, effusions, infiltrates, a globular heart shadow (pericardial effusion), and the silhouette of the thoracic aorta and mediastinum (widened with aneurysm or dissection).
3. **Echocardiogram.** This evaluates the patient for pericardial effusion, cardiac wall motion abnormalities, valvular disease, and aortic dissection.
4. **Aortogram/contrast spiral CT scan.** To diagnose aortic dissection.
5. **Bilateral lower-extremity Doppler study, ventilation/perfusion scan, pulmonary angiogram.** To diagnose pulmonary emboli. A negative $\dot{V}/\dot{Q}$ scan essentially rules out a PE. However, an "indeterminate" scan requires confirmation with pulmonary arteriography. A spiral CT

scan is not as sensitive as an angiogram but is very specific (good at detecting large clots in the main pulmonary arteries).

V. Plan. The treatment plan is dictated by establishing the correct diagnosis. Of the conditions previously listed, myocardial ischemia, aortic dissection, tension pneumothorax, and pulmonary embolism are immediately life threatening but treatable. When you suspect that myocardial ischemia is the source of pain, do not hesitate to treat the patient accordingly (see Figure I–12), page 65.

A. Emergency Management

1. Treat with oxygen therapy by mask or nasal cannula.
2. Obtain an ECG and leave the leads in place to monitor the patient and to repeat the ECG if pain recurs or increases.
3. Request an immediate portable chest radiograph and a room air blood gas.
4. If myocardial ischemia is a possibility, treat with sublingual nitroglycerin as a diagnostic and therapeutic intervention.

B. Myocardial Ischemia

1. **Nitrates.** A typical starting dose of sublingual nitroglycerin is 0.4 mg (1/150 grain). Monitor symptomatic relief and blood pressure. Repeat every 5–10 min up to 3 doses. If nitroglycerin is effective but pain recurs, establish a nitroglycerin drip at 10–20 mg/min and titrate to pain relief. Keep the systolic BP above 90 mm Hg.
2. **Morphine.** If pain is not relieved by nitroglycerin or if the patient cannot tolerate nitrates, treat with 1–3 mg morphine IV.
3. **Oxygen.** Give 4 L by nasal prongs (approximately equal to 35% mask).
4. **Lidocaine.** If the patient has ventricular ectopy, treat with a 75–100 mg bolus IV, then begin a continuous IV infusion at 2 mg/min.
5. Continue monitoring and make arrangement to admit to the CCU/ICU.
6. Coronary thrombolysis or emergent coronary angiography may be indicated and is coordinated by the cardiologist.

C. Aortic Dissection or Rupture. Initial treatment attempts to eliminate pain and reduce systolic blood pressure. Surgical correction is indicated for all symptomatic aneurysms.

1. **Nitroprusside (Nipride).** A continuous infusion of 0.5–1.0 mg/kg/min titrated up to control blood pressure.

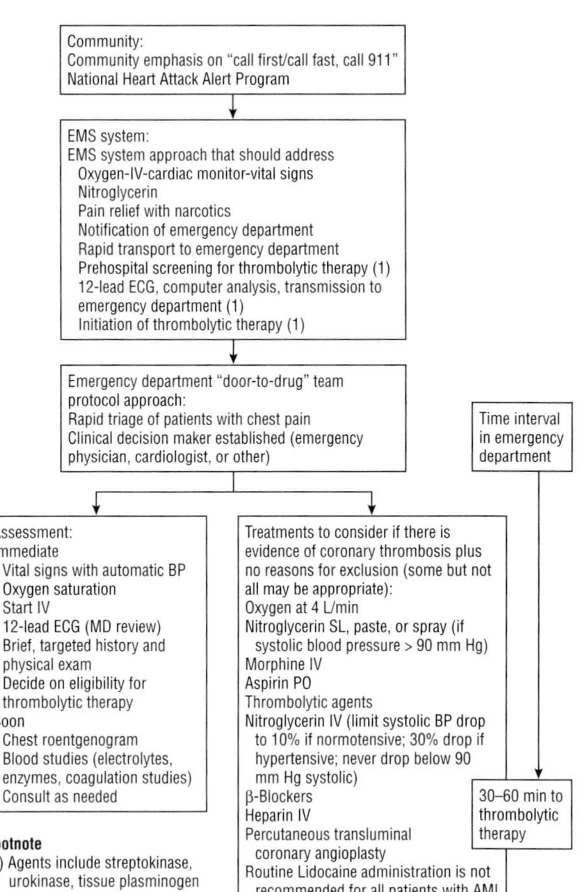

Figure I–12. Acute myocardial infarction (AMI) algorithm. Recommendations for early treatment of patients with chest pain and possible AMI. *(Reproduced, with permission, from Adult Advanced Cardiac Life Support.* JAMA *1992;268:16.)*

Keeping the systolic blood pressure under 120 mm Hg is very important to prevent further dissection.

2. **Esmolol.** Five mg/min IV push in a monitored patient until the systolic blood pressure is less than 120, then 20 μg/min, titrated to effect. As a β-blocker, this not only

lowers the blood pressure, but also the rate of rise and force of cardiac contraction.

3. **Morphine.** Use 1–3 mg IV prn to relieve pain.

D. **Pulmonary Embolus**
   1. Check baseline coagulation parameters (PT/PTT).
   2. Give a bolus of heparin IV (either 10,000 U or 100 U/kg), then begin a continuous IV infusion of 10 U/kg/h. Check the PTT in 3–4 h and adjust the heparin drip to keep the PTT approximately twice normal. Low molecular weight heparin (Lovenox) may also be considered. Even if the patient already has a vena caval filter, you may still want to start anticoagulation to minimize the risk of long-term venous stasis disease from lower-extremity deep vein thrombosis.
   3. If anticoagulation is contraindicated, then Greenfield filter placement is indicated. Filters are also indicated for patients with recurrent emboli despite adequate anticoagulation.

E. **Pneumothorax.** Treated with a chest tube, although a needle thoracostomy may be needed in emergencies (tension pneumothorax).

F. **Pericarditis.** Monitor for tamponade. Administer indomethacin or other anti-inflammatory agents. Needle aspiration may be indicated.

G. **Gastritis/Esophagitis**
   a. Antacids
   b. IV H_2-receptor blockers (cimetidine, ranitidine).

H. **Costochondritis.** Treat with nonsteroidal anti-inflammatory drugs (ibuprofen, etc).

13. CHEST TUBE PROBLEMS

(Chest tube placement is discussed in Section III, Bedside Procedures)

Immediate Actions

When you suspect a tension pneumothorax (on the basis of tachycardia, hypotension, jugular venous distension, and absent or diminished breath sounds) in a patient with a chest tube already in place, immediately insert a large-bore needle (14 gauge) at the anterior axillary line to allow egress of the air. Do not waste time obtaining a chest radiograph. Any patient who has a needle thoracostomy needs a functioning chest tube afterward.

I. **Problem.** The chest tube in a 20-year-old male admitted for spontaneous pneumothorax is malfunctioning.

II. Immediate Questions

A. What are the vital signs? Tachycardia, tachypnea, and hypotension may indicate tension pneumothorax in a patient with a malfunctioning chest tube.

B. What is the problem? Problems may include changes in drainage quality or quantity, persistent air leak, drainage around the tube dressing, increasing subcutaneous emphysema, or persistent complaints of discomfort.

C. When and why was the tube inserted? Tube problems are approached differently, depending on whether the tube was put in during an operation, to drain an effusion, to evacuate air from a spontaneous pneumothorax, or for trauma.

D. When was the last radiograph obtained? If recently, immediately go check the film; if not, obtain a current one.

E. Is the chest tube plugged? Sometimes an obvious clot can be seen in the chest tube. This can be removed by "stripping" the chest tube tubing.

III. Differential Diagnosis

A. Faulty Drainage System. Collection containers may be full, tubing may be kinked, or the wall suction may not be adequate. (You should hear bubbling in the pressure regulator chamber of the chest tube drainage system.)

B. Continuous Air Leak. Indicated by persistent bubbling in the water seal chamber of the chest tube drainage system.

1. These are mechanical problems (cracked tube, tape not air tight, loose connection).
2. The last hole (hole closest to the drainage system) is outside the pleural space.
3. There is a lung parenchymal injury with a persistent air leak (bronchopleural fistula). The injury may be posttraumatic (penetrating injury) or iatrogenic during tube placement.

C. Bloody Drainage

1. **Intercostal vessel injury.** Avoided by placing the tube over the top of the rib and directly abutting the bone.
2. **Bloody effusion.** Malignant effusions are often bloody.
3. **Pulmonary artery injury.** A rare problem.
4. **Posttraumatic.** Most traumatic pneumothoraces are associated with some degree of bleeding. Make sure the tube is large enough to handle this.
5. **Parenchymal lung injury.** Possibly at the time of tube placement. It is also possible to injure the liver or spleen.

D. Decreased Drainage

1. Clotted tube.
2. Resolution of the problem that led to tube placement.

E. Subcutaneous Emphysema

1. Migration of the last hole outside the pleural space but under the skin.
2. Improper placement (subcutaneous tube).
3. A significant air leak, which should be treated by placing a second chest tube.
4. Tension pneumothorax.

IV. Database

A. Physical Exam Key Points

1. **Vital signs.** Tachypnea and decreased oxygen saturation may indicate a pneumothorax or respiratory compromise. When a patient with a pneumothorax is hypotensive, the pneumothorax is under tension (which shifts the mediastinum and interferes with venous return), or the patient has a second life-threatening problem.
2. **Neck.** Tracheal deviation may indicate a tension pneumothorax. (The trachea deviates away from the side of the tension pneumothorax). JVD can also be caused by a tension pneumothorax.
3. **Lungs.** Check for symmetric breath sounds. Hyperresonance may signify a pneumothorax, whereas dullness may suggest an effusion or hemothorax.
4. **Chest wall.** Determine if there is crepitance that signifies subcutaneous emphysema. Examine the insertion site for signs of tube migration, infection, or skin bleeding. Watch for unequal chest rise.

B. Laboratory Data

1. **Arterial blood gases.** Are usually not necessary.
2. **Coagulation studies.** (PT/PTT/platelets) are appropriate in cases of severe bleeding.

C. CBC and serial hematocrits. For hemothorax.

D. Radiographic and Other Studies

1. **Obtain a chest radiograph.** This is probably the most important diagnostic maneuver. Check the tube position, see where the last hole of the tube is located, and note if there is any effusion (either new or recurrent) or any residual pneumothorax.

V. Plan.

A. Air Leak

1. Be sure that the last hole is in the chest cavity (on chest radiograph). A rush of air at the site clinically indicates

that the last hole may be outside the chest. If the last hole is outside the chest, replace the tube. Pushing the tube in is associated with a significant risk of empyema and is strongly contraindicated.

2. To differentiate tube problems from system problems, try clamping the tube briefly at the entry site. A persistent air leak indicates a problem in the drainage system, not the patient or tube. Remember to unclamp the chest tube once you are done.

B. Drainage Around the Tube. Leakage is treated simply by reinforcing the dressing. Be sure the last hole is in the chest. Tight closure of skin around the tube at the entry site may cause subcutaneous dissection of fluid or air.

C. Change in Drainage Quality

1. The sudden appearance of bloody drainage after inserting a tube may indicate damage to an intercostal vessel or, more significantly, may indicate damage to the lung parenchyma. Occasionally, bleeding results from repeated attempts to place an ipsilateral subclavian line.
2. Bleeding from an intercostal vessel may stop on its own, but requires operative exposure and ligation when persistent.
3. Blood tingeing of a previously straw-colored effusion is usually of little significance.
4. Generally, after initial chest tube placement for hemothorax, greater than 1500 cc of blood immediately draining or greater than 200 cc/h for 2 h is an indication for emergent thoracotomy.

D. Change in Drainage Quantity. A sudden increase in drainage is rare, unless the drainage becomes bloody and is related to a vascular mishap. Order a new chest radiograph and compare this with the last film. Is there a new effusion on that side? A sudden decrease in drainage with appearance of a new effusion usually warrants placement of a new tube, with or without removal of the old tube.

E. Subcutaneous Emphysema. A pneumothorax is often associated with subcutaneous air, and some air may persist after placement of the tube. However, new subcutaneous emphysema, especially after a tube has been in for a while, may indicate migration of the tube, such that the last hole is now out of the chest. Even if the tube is properly positioned, subcutaneous emphysema usually indicates a poorly functioning tube and necessitates replacement. The appearance of a great deal of subcutaneous air right after tube placement may be alleviated by enlarging the skin entrance site, to allow egress of the air rather than forcing the air (from a pneumothorax) to track subcutaneously. Large air leaks may require a second tube. Also, check for a concomitant contralateral pneumothorax.

F. **Patient Discomfort.** There is always some pleuritic pain after placement of a tube, especially at the entrance site. Such pain must be differentiated from chest pain of other causes. Sudden onset of a new pain must be investigated, looking at the position of the end of the tube, the skin entrance site, and the lung markings on chest radiograph (look for a persistent pneumothorax, hemothorax, or contusion). Most patients require some narcotics. A patient-controlled analgesia (PCA) machine is often a good choice for patients with chest tubes.

14. CHANGING NEUROLOGIC STATUS

I. **Problem.** You are called to evaluate a 34-year-old woman for somnolence 2 d after a modified radical mastectomy.

II. **Immediate Questions**

A. **What are the vital signs?** Hypotension can cause poor cerebral perfusion and an altered mental status. A changing respiratory pattern may indicate increased intracranial pressure, with an initial slowing followed later by a rapid respiratory rate. Tachycardia or fever may represent sepsis.

B. **Was the patient fully awake at any time since surgery?** Get an idea of the time course for the change in neurologic status.

C. **What medications is the patient taking?** Look at the medication records to see how much pain medicine and sedation the patient has received, not just how much has been ordered.

D. **Is the patient a diabetic?** Either hypoglycemia or hyperglycemia may cause an altered mental status.

E. **Was there a traumatic event?** Did the patient fall out of bed? Trauma patients may have a closed head injury or long-bone fractures causing fat embolism syndrome.

III. **Differential Diagnosis**

A. **Trauma**

1. **Subdural hematoma.** The most common intracranial mass lesion resulting from head injury.
2. **Epidural hematoma.** Usually associated with a skull fracture and a lacerated meningeal vessel.
3. **Concussion.** A clinical diagnosis of cerebral dysfunction that clears within 24 h of the injury.

4. **Contusion.** Usually associated with neurologic deficits that persist for longer than 24 h. The CT scan usually demonstrates small hemorrhages in the cerebral parenchyma.
5. **Fat embolus syndrome.** Look for a petechial rash after a long bone fracture.

B. Metabolic Causes

1. **Exogenous.** Alcohol (including withdrawal "delirium tremens"), drugs (including drug withdrawal), narcotics, anesthetic agents (delayed clearance postop), poisoning.
2. **Endogenous**
   a. **Endocrine**
      i. **Pancreas**—Insulin, hypo- and hyperglycemia
      ii. **Pituitary**—Hyper- and hypopituitarism
      iii. **Thyroid**—Hyper- and hypothyroid
      iv. **Adrenal insufficiency**
      v. **Parathyroid** (hyper- or hypocalcemia)
   b. **Fluids/electrolytes**
      i. **Sodium**—Hypo- and hypernatremia may cause confusion.
      ii. Hypo- and hyperkalemia
      iii. Hypo- and hypercalcemia
      iv. Hypo- and hypermagnesemia
      v. Acidosis (especially respiratory) or alkalosis
      vi. Osmolarity disturbances (hyperosmolar coma)
   c. **Organ Failure:** Including renal, hepatic, or pulmonary (hypoxia, hypercarbia, fat embolism syndrome

C. Infection

1. Central nervous system infections (meningitis, encephalitis).
2. Systemic sepsis.

D. Tumors

1. Primary or metastatic to CNS.
2. Paraneoplastic syndromes.

E. Psychiatric Causes. In psychogenic coma, the neurologic and laboratory profile is completely normal. Depression may cause dementia especially in elderly patients. ICU psychosis and postcardiotomy delirium are seen frequently in elderly patients and can be brought on by sleep deprivation or medications.

F. Miscellaneous

1. **Seizures.** Including postictal states.
2. **Cerebrovascular disease.** Infarction or hemorrhage, arteriovenous malformation (AVM), hypertensive encephalopathy.

3. **Syncope.** (see Problem 66, page 241).
4. **Decreased cardiac output** (shock).
5. **Other CNS diseases.** These are usually chronic and include Alzheimer's disease, normal pressure hydrocephalus, and Wernicke's encephalopathy (thiamine deficiency).

IV. **Database.** If the event occurs during the postoperative period, determine the nature, onset, and duration of the event. Furthermore, ascertain the anesthetics used, medications given, and IV fluids administered.

A. **Physical Exam Key Points**

1. **Vital signs.** Hyper- or hypotension, tachy- or bradycardia, temperature, and respiratory rate may be a clue to the diagnosis.
2. **HEENT.** Look for papilledema (increased intracranial pressure from a mass or hypertensive encephalopathy), meningeal signs such as nuchal rigidity (meningitis), and pupillary reaction (pinpoint with narcotics, unilaterally fixed and dilated with herniation, bilaterally dilated and fixed with anoxia). Conjunctival and fundal petechiae suggest fat embolism. Fruity breath is associated with ketoacidosis. Hemiplegia or aphasia may indicate a stroke. Look for evidence of head trauma.
3. **Skin.** Jaundice, spider angiomata, and palmar erythema occur with liver disease. Look for petechiae in the neck and upper chest.
4. **Neurologic exam.** Evaluate the patient for spontaneous movements, their response to pain, and their cranial nerve function. (See Appendix for Glasgow Coma Scale).

B. **Laboratory Data**

1. **CBC, platelet count.** To identify infection or anemia.
2. **Complete blood chemistry.** Includes electrolytes, BUN, creatinine, calcium, magnesium, and osmolality. Glucose can be rapidly checked with a "finger-stick" glucometer available on most nursing units.
3. **Arterial blood gases.** There may be a respiratory or metabolic cause, hypoxia or hypercarbia (which may also cause delirium). Check the patient's oxygen saturation with a pulse oximeter.
4. **Serum ammonia.** Elevation indicative of hepatic encephalopathy.
5. Urine and serum toxicology screening if indicated.
6. Cultures for sepsis, if indicated.

C. Radiographic and Other Studies

1. **Chest radiograph.** When an infectious or pulmonary source is possible.
2. **CT of the head.** When there is any indication of a CNS cause of coma, especially focal neurologic signs or the presence of papilledema.
3. **Lumbar puncture** (see page 360).
4. **Electrocardiogram.** Will identify myocardial infarction or atrial fibrillation (mural thrombi with emboli).
5. **Electroencephalogram.**

V. Plan. Although the treatment of a patient with changing neurologic status must be directed at the underlying cause, certain initial steps should be taken immediately. Ensure that there is an adequate airway, breathing, and circulation. Intubation may be necessary to protect the airway.

A. Metabolic Causes. Treat any relevant abnormality on lab studies. Refer to specific abnormalities in the Index. Give a single ampule of 50% dextrose when there is any suspicion of hypoglycemia. The effect on a patient in diabetic ketoacidosis is minimal, so it is always safer to give the dextrose than to wait for lab results to confirm hypoglycemia.

B. Exogenous Causes. If you suspect narcotic-induced somnolence, treat with naloxone, 0.4–0.8 mg IV push. Naloxone has a short half-life, so repeated dosing may be necessary (up to 4–5 ampules are commonly given in this situation). A few cases of flash pulmonary edema have been reported after naloxone administration.

C. Tumor. Somnolence in the presence of metastatic or primary CNS tumors is an emergency usually treated by radiotherapy. Give dexamethasone bolus 0.1–0.2 mg/kg.

D. Infection. Treat with high-dose antibiotics on the basis initially of the Gram's stain.

E. Cardiac syncope or low cardiac output. Treat the underlying cardiac problem.

F. Vascular. Intracranial bleeding is usually treated like other causes of increased intracranial pressure. Contact the neurosurgeon. Increased intracranial pressure should be emergently treated because herniation may occur. Intubation with hyperventilation (Pco_2 28–34 mm Hg) is the key; osmotic diuresis with mannitol (1–1.5 gm/kg over 20 min) may be helpful.

G. ICU psychosis. This is a diagnosis of exclusion and is based on clinical suspicion. Provide the patient with a companion and use restraints as a last resort. Haloperidol (Haldol) usually helps, although there is a risk of ventricular dysrhythmias. Avoid benzodiazepines as they may have a paradoxical effect.

15. COAGULOPATHY

I. **Problem.** Following placement of a LeVeen shunt, a patient has bleeding from both peritoneal and neck incisions as well as oozing from an intravenous site.

II. **Immediate Questions**

A. **What is the patient's blood pressure?** Determine if the bleeding episode is extensive enough to cause hypovolemia and shock. Assess the volume status by checking the blood pressure, heart rate, urine output, and central venous pressure. If central lines must be placed, work up and attempt to correct the coagulopathy before inserting needles into major vessels.

B. **How much external bleeding is there?** One of the most frequent calls on a surgical service is for bleeding or blood on a dressing after surgery. One way to separate the clinically significant bleeding episodes from the insignificant ones is to quantify the bleeding. Look at the wound to see if there is active bleeding and ask to have any old dressings saved so that you can see the amount and the nature of the wound drainage. You can also draw the perimeter of a blood stain on a dressing so that additional bleeding can be readily observed.

C. **Do factors exist which increase the likelihood of generalized bleeding?** In the example given, the patient could be expected to have disseminated intravascular coagulation. In general, when confronted with a bleeding or oozing wound, ask patients whether they have a history of bleeding after other surgical or dental procedures. Also ask about liver disease, relatives with bleeding disorders, and use of medications, such as aspirin, NSAIDs, or anticoagulants. Look for bruises or petechia. Posttrauma patients may also be coagulopathic from extensive blood loss (a consumptive coagulopathy).

D. **Could the hematoma compress a major anatomic structure?** This is an important question to ask for neck wounds, where a wound hematoma can compress the trachea, and mediastinal wounds, where blood can cause pericardial tamponade. In both cases, be prepared to open the wound quickly if the patient becomes symptomatic from compression.

III. Differential Diagnosis

A. **Inadequate Surgical Hemostasis.** This is the most common cause of localized bleeding in the postoperative patient.

B. **Platelet Disorders**

1. **Thrombocytopenia**
   a. **Decreased production:** Often secondary to chemotherapy or bone marrow replacement by fibrosis or neoplasia.
   b. **Sequestration:** Caused by splenic enlargement due to portal hypertension, neoplasia, or storage diseases.
   c. **Destruction:** Idiopathic thrombocytopenic purpura, thrombotic thrombocytopenic purpura (TTP), and drug reactions (eg, heparin) can cause platelet destruction.
2. **Qualitative platelet disorders**
   a. **von Willebrand's disease:** An autosomal dominant disease with decreased platelet adhesion. von Willebrand's factor is a factor VIII cofactor.
   b. **Platelet release defects:** Aspirin and NSAIDS interfere with cyclooxygenase metabolism.
   c. **Glanzmann's disease.**
   d. **Bernard-Soulier syndrome.**

C. **Coagulation Defects**

1. **Congenital**
   a. **Hemophilia A:** A factor VIII deficiency, X-linked, with an incidence of 1/10,000 male births.
   b. **Hemophilia B:** A factor IX deficiency, X-linked, with an incidence of 1/100,000 male births.
2. **Acquired**
   a. **Disseminated intravascular coagulation (DIC):** Associated with sepsis, trauma, burns, disseminated malignancy, obstetric catastrophes, and placement of peritoneovenous (LeVeen) shunts (due to proteinaceous material entering the venous system). DIC is a consumptive coagulopathy in which the clotting system is activated, and clotting factors are depleted.
   b. **Vitamin K deficiency:** Vitamin K is needed for synthesis of coagulation factors II, VII, IX, and X.
   c. **Hepatic failure:** Affects not only the vitamin K-dependent factors but factors I, V, and XI (which are also synthesized by the liver).

IV. Database. The keystone in diagnosing a coagulopathy is understanding and using the appropriate laboratory tests. It is important to draw blood for needed tests before instituting therapy or transfusions.

A. Physical Exam Key Points

1. **Vital signs.** Tachycardia and orthostatic hypotension occur with significant blood loss (more than 50% of blood volume or about 750 cc).
2. **Skin.** Petechia, purpura, easy bruising, and oozing from IV sites suggest a systemic rather than a local cause. The skin will be pale with significant blood loss.
3. **Incision.** Examine the incision for hematoma or active bleeding.
4. **Abdomen.** Splenomegaly, hepatomegaly, or ascites may suggest a diagnosis.
5. **Extremity.** Hemarthrosis may be seen with hemophilia.
6. **Neurologic exam.** Needed as a baseline and to identify further CNS bleeding if present.

B. Laboratory Data

1. **CBC.** Follow serial hematocrits to quantify ongoing bleeding.
2. **Platelet count.** Adequate platelet counts do not imply adequate platelet function.
3. **PT and PTT.** The PT is elevated if there is a deficiency of factors I, II, V, VII, or X. The PTT assesses all coagulation proteins except factors VII and XIII. Factor VII has the shortest half-life and is the usual cause of an elevated PT in systemic illnesses, such as liver disease. In lupus erythematosus, there is a circulating anticoagulant that elevates the PT/PTT but does not cause bleeding; Instead, it can cause excessive clotting. Heparin causes elevation of the PTT, while warfarin (Coumadin) causes elevation of the PT (and INR).
4. **Thrombin time.** Assays for functional fibrinogen level; can be used to assess the effect of heparin.
5. **Fibrinogen and fibrin split products (FSP).** In DIC, fibrinogen is decreased and FSP are increased.
6. **Bleeding time.** Evaluates platelet function. Uremia, liver disease, and recent aspirin therapy may adversely affect function. von Willebrand's disease also causes elevation of the bleeding time.
7. **Peripheral blood smears.** May reveal fragments and helmet cells in DIC and TTP.
8. **Type and crossmatch.** If needed.
9. Save one or two tubes of blood drawn before starting therapy in case it is necessary to work up the patient for a coagulopathy.

C. Radiographic and Other Studies

1. **Chest radiograph.** If there are indications of intrathoracic or mediastinal bleeding.
2. **Bone marrow biopsy.** May be performed at some point to assess platelet production.

V. Plan. Assess the rate of bleeding and differentiate between mechanical bleeding and true coagulopathy. Almost all external bleeding that is mechanical can be controlled by applying direct pressure or by elevation. Treatment of a medical coagulopathy requires the laboratory studies previously discussed to make the correct diagnosis and institute appropriate treatment. Treat patients acutely with intravenous fluids and blood, as indicated by their blood loss and volume.

A. Thrombocytopenia

1. Use random donor platelet transfusion (usually 5–10 units) at a time for a platelet count of 20,000/mm^3 or less. More can be given when there is ongoing bleeding. Patients receiving multiple platelet transfusions will develop antibodies and do better with HLA-matched single donor platelets. Immunocompromised patients should receive irradiated platelets to avoid a graft-vs-host reaction.
2. **Drug reaction.** Identify, then discontinue the responsible drug and transfuse platelets if necessary. Heparin and penicillins (infrequently) can cause thrombocytopenia.
3. **ITP.** The platelets function normally, and no treatment is usually needed until the platelet count is < 10,000/mm^3. Chronic ITP is treated with prednisone, cyclophosphamide (Cytoxan), azathioprine, or danazol. The best long-term results are with splenectomy. When platelets are transfused before splenectomy, they disappear rapidly.
4. Document functional defect with bleeding time.

B. von Willebrand's Disease

1. **Cryoprecipitate** (see Section VI, page 405).
2. **DDAVP.** A vasopressin analog that increases von Willebrand factor levels (see Section IX, page 477).

C. Hemophilia A. The half-life of factor VIII is about 12 h. One U/kg of factor VIII transfused raises the body activity about 2%. Load a patient with 50 U/kg IV, then give 25 U/kg every 12 h. Cryoprecipitate contains 20 times as much factor VIII as FFP. There is also a factor VIII concentrate.

D. Hemophilia B. FFP or plasma enriched in prothrombin complex is frequently used.

E. DIC. The key is to treat the underlying cause. Support the bleeding patient with FFP, platelet transfusions, and blood transfusions.

F. Vitamin K Deficiency/Liver Disease. If immediate treatment is needed, transfuse with 2–4 U of FFP and follow the PT/PTT. In all cases, begin treatment with vitamin K 10 mg SQ every day for 3 d.

16. COLOSTOMY PROBLEMS

I. Problem. A 68-year-old patient 6 d after abdominoperineal resection has problems with the function of his colostomy.

II. Immediate Questions

A. How old is the colostomy, and what type of colostomy is it? A new colostomy can retract into the wound, whereas obstruction tends to be a problem with an older colostomy. Loop or "double barrel" colostomies are usually temporary, whereas "end" colostomies are frequently permanent.

B. What kind of appliance is on the colostomy? A poorly fitting appliance can cause leakage and skin irritation.

C. What color is the mucosa? Check for mucosal ischemia in the immediate postoperative period.

D. What is the volume and nature of the output? A colostomy that has been working and suddenly stops should be approached differently than one that has never worked. The majority of colostomies are left-sided, end, descending colostomies. In the first few postoperative days, the output is scant and usually blood-tinged. When peristalsis resumes, the appliance will usually become filled with gas before the discharge of liquid feces, usually around the third or fourth postoperative day. High output from a stoma can be caused by outlet stenosis, intra-abdominal infection, recurrence of disease, or resection of an excessive length of bowel.

E. Is there a mass in the area of the colostomy? This may represent a parastomal hernia or an abscess.

III. Differential Diagnosis. There are a variety of potential problems with stomas that are discussed in two groups: new stomas and existing stomas. Problems with new stomas are likely to arise in the first few days after surgery.

A. New Stoma Problems

1. **Stomal retraction.** This condition is a surgical emergency. If the stoma should retract into the peritoneal cavity, it could lead to fecal spillage. Immediate operative intervention is usually required if the stoma retracts below the fascia.
2. **Stomal necrosis.** Superficial necrosis is of limited short-term significance, although it can lead to an eventual stricture. Full thickness necrosis can be a surgical emergency when it involves bowel below the level of

the fascia. Necrosis is caused by compromise of the stoma's blood supply.

3. **Stomal bleeding.** Intraluminal bleeding may be caused by mucosal trauma, proximal suture lines, or unrelated diseases (PUD, angiodysplasia). Peristomal bleeding may be arising from the skin, muscle, stomal mesentery, or from intra-abdominal hemorrhage.
4. **Parastomal hernia or prolapse.** Usually caused by a large fascial defect. Colostomies created emergently for obstructed dilated colon are often associated with hernias. These can be electively repaired with mesh. In some cases, the stroma must be moved (or closed).

B. Existing Stoma Problems

1. **Impaction/obstruction.** This should be obvious from the history and from examination of the stoma with a gloved finger.
2. **Bleeding.** See Problem 10, page 41.
3. **Mucosal slough.**
4. **Poor fitting appliance**/skin irritation.
5. **Parastomal hernia.**
6. **Stenosis.** Often associated with a high output of liquid and detected by examination with a gloved, well-lubricated finger. Can be at the level of the skin or the fascia.
7. **Abscess.** Leakage of stool into the surrounding subcutaneous tissue can cause an abscess. If an incision and drainage are not performed, necrotizing fasciitis can develop.

IV. Database

A. Physical Exam Key Points

1. Examine the stoma. Look for ischemia, retraction, stenosis, bleeding, parasternal abscesses, and parastomal hernias. Ischemia can be detected by pressing the transparent colostomy bag gently against the stoma and using a penlight to assess the color. A glass blood tube can be inserted into the stoma to allow inspection of the mucosa inside. In addition, a viable stoma will usually transilluminate, unlike a nonviable stoma. The stoma normally will appear edematous with a dull pink-brown color for the first few days. A pale tan color usually signifies ischemia. Black mucosa with a faint greenish tint signifies necrosis, and no visible mucosa signifies retraction. If the mucosa or surrounding site is bloody, quantify the rate of bleeding and look for a local source. A digital exam of the stoma should be done when stenosis is suspected.

2. Examine the abdomen for signs of peritonitis or obstruction.

B. **Laboratory Data.** Order a CBC and a PT/PTT when bleeding is a problem. (A CBC is also useful when an abscess is suspected).

C. **Radiographic and Other Studies**
1. **Abdominal films.** Look for evidence of a bowel obstruction (air-fluid levels, etc) at the level of the stoma or proximally.
2. A Gastrografin enema can be obtained through the colostomy to look for obstructing lesions. Gastrografin is also a cathartic. Barium is used infrequently.

V. **Plan.** The treatment of stomal problems depends on the nature of the problem and its etiology. Although some stomal problems are purely cosmetic, there are a few that require rapid evaluation and treatment.

A. **Stomal Ischemia.** Limited superficial ischemia may resolve with observation. More extensive ischemia (particularly when subfascial) should be treated with reoperation to revise the stoma, correcting any technical or mechanical problems that led to the ischemia (tight fascia, kinked mesentery).

B. **Stomal Retraction.** If the stoma retracts fully into the abdominal cavity, immediate operation is required.

C. **Fecal Impaction.** This is usually caused by dehydration, narcotics, or lack of bulk in the diet. It is managed by warm colostomy irrigation, gentle cathartics, and it is prevented in the long term by stool softeners, increased dietary fiber, adequate fluid intake, and laxatives.

D. **Bleeding.** If a site of bleeding is visible (skin or mucosa), it can often be corrected with a bedside cautery, silver nitrate, or a suture. Use caution with cautery, because colonic gas may be flammable. Gastrointestinal bleeding needs a full evaluation. (see Problem 10, page 41).

E. **Appliance Problems.** Consultation with an enterostomal care specialist can often be helpful to select the best appliance for the patient. Protective paste or Stomahesive may be needed to protect skin.

F. **Stenosis.** Usually responds to early digital dilatation, although reoperation may be needed when the stoma retracts and stenosis is at the level of the fascia.

G. **Continuous Colostomy Drainage.** Many patients are unhappy with the continuous discharge of fecal contents. Often the colon can be "trained" to evacuate only after

nerve roots can result in colonic dysmotility (Ogilvie's syndrome aka pseudo-obstruction of the colon).

D. Other Causes. Inactivity, poor fluid intake, and laxative abuse predispose to constipation. Electrolyte disturbances (hypokalemia) rarely may cause dysmotility.

IV. Database

A. Physical Exam Key Points

1. **Vital signs.** Fever and tachycardia suggests an infectious cause.
2. **Abdominal exam.** Determine the presence or absence as well as the quality of bowel sounds. Look for distention and palpate for masses. Determine if pain is present at rest or with palpation. Determine if there is rebound tenderness or any other peritoneal signs (tenderness to light percussion, bumping the bed).
3. **Rectal exam.** Is there hard stool in rectum? Is there blood or a mass?
4. **Neurologic exam.** Examine for evidence of a previous stroke or of other neurologic disease.

B. Laboratory Data

1. **Fecal occult blood.** Occurs with benign and malignant tumors, ischemia, and ulcers.
2. **Serum electrolytes.** Hypokalemia is an infrequent cause of bowel dysmotility.
3. **CBC.** Leukocytosis may indicate infection. Anemia may indicate GI bleeding, which could suggest a neoplasm.
4. **Arterial blood gas.** Indicated to look for acidosis when ischemia is suspected (refractory metabolic acidosis is the hallmark of advanced ischemia or infarction). A lactic acid level may similarly be helpful.

C. Radiographic and Other Studies

1. Mild constipation and impaction usually need no further studies.
2. Abdominal films should be ordered if obstruction is suspected (see Problem 1, page 1).
3. **Contrast studies and abdominal CT scan.** These are usually needed when there is evidence of chronic constipation or when there is evidence of blood in the stool (see Problem 10, page 41).

V. Plan. Medications that predispose patients to constipation (narcotics, anticholinergics) should be stopped whenever possible. Correct existing electrolyte abnormalities with specific attention paid to hypokalemia.

A. **Prevention.** Postoperative and bedridden patients benefit from stool softeners (sodium docusate), fiber-rich diet (fruits, vegetables, or bran, or supplemented with agents such as psyllium), and adequate fluid intake. The patient should also be out of bed and ambulating as soon as possible.

B. **Laxatives and Enemas.** Mild constipation can be treated in a variety of ways depending on physician preference: motility stimulant (bisacodyl), laxatives (milk of magnesia), or gentle enemas (Fleet enemas, tap water, soap suds). Lactulose syrup is an excellent laxative for chronic constipation. Gastrografin enemas can be used if all else fails. Doses can be found in Section VII, Commonly Used Medications. In general, laxatives are contraindicated in the presence of obstruction.

C. **Disimpaction.** Gentle digital disimpaction (well-lubricated, **double**-gloved finger) is required when the patient is unable to pass hard stool. This procedure can then be followed up with careful retention enemas (soap suds or mineral oil may be used) and then using stool softeners to prevent recurrence.

D. **Other.** Perforation, acute obstruction, and sepsis require emergency operation. For partial obstruction (no obstipation), gentle clearing with enemas followed by contrast studies or colonoscopy is indicated.

19. COUGH

I. **Problem.** A patient being treated with IV antibiotics for cellulitis complains of a cough.

II. **Immediate Questions**

A. **Is the patient bringing up sputum with the cough? What are the characteristics of the sputum?** A productive cough is more suggestive of significant infection than a nonproductive one, particularly if the sputum appears purulent. The presence of blood in the sputum raises a host of other issues (see Problem 36, page 146).

B. **Is the patient tachypneic or dyspneic?** A cough does not usually require urgent or emergent action. One exception is the patient with chronic pulmonary or cardiac disease who may suffer respiratory compromise with a new acute pulmonary event.

C. **Is the cough acute or chronic?** In patients with a chronic cough, the key is to determine whether the nature or characteristic of the cough has changed. In the absence of other respiratory complaints, a new cough in a smoker may represent cancer.

D. **Is the patient immunocompromised?** Ask specifically about medications (steroids, chemotherapeutics) or secondary conditions (diabetes, AIDS, cancer) that predispose to serious pulmonary infections.

E. **Is the cough associated with any specific activity?** A cough that occurs with recumbency may signify pulmonary edema. Coughing during sleep may be from aspiration. A cough that follows eating or drinking could also be from aspiration, if the patient has a swallowing disorder or fistula.

III. **Differential Diagnosis.** There are many reasons for a cough.

A. **Inflammatory**

1. **Acute.** Bacterial, viral, fungal, and acid-fast organisms are causative agents. These should be associated with infection, such as leukocytosis, fever, viral exanthem, and purulent sputum. Some sputum characteristics are noteworthy: rust-color with pneumococci, currant jelly with *Klebsiella* species, and foul-smelling with anaerobic organisms.
2. **Chronic.** Chronic bronchitis occurs almost exclusively in smokers and is defined as a chronic productive cough for at least 3 mo a year for 2 y. Occasionally, a patient on angiotensin-converting enzyme inhibitor therapy for hypertension may have a chronic cough, and this cough may be coincidental with the current disease.

B. **Mechanical.** Coughing may be caused by inhaled irritants or by intrinsic or extrinsic diseases.

1. **Inhalation**
   a. **Foreign body aspiration:** Presents as localized wheezing in a patient with a depressed level of consciousness.
   b. **Particulate aerosols.**
   c. **Aspiration of gastrointestinal secretions:** Nighttime or early morning coughing spells are characteristic.
   d. **Allergens in sensitive persons.**
2. **Intrinsic**
   a. **Pulmonary edema:** Can be cardiogenic or noncardiogenic. Typical symptoms include acute dyspnea and copious frothy sputum.
   b. **Interstitial lung disease:** Restrictive disease by PFTs and diffuse interstitial changes on chest radiograph.

c. **Bronchogenic carcinoma:** Risk factors are smoking and asbestos exposure. Symptoms include weight loss and hemoptysis.

d. **Bronchial adenoma:** There usually are no systemic symptoms. Hemoptysis is possible.

3. **Extrinsic**

a. **Thoracic aneurysm:** Can cause bronchial or tracheal compression.

b. **Lymphadenopathy:** Secondary to sarcoidosis, chronic infection, lymphoma, or cancer. There are often associated systemic symptoms (fever, fatigue, etc).

c. **Neuroenteric cysts or pulmonary sequestration:** This should be considered in the pediatric population. A CT scan may be helpful.

C. **Chemical.** These cause topical irritation.

1. Smoke inhalation.
2. Toxic fumes.

IV. Database

A. Physical Exam Key Points

1. **Vital signs.** Check the temperature and respiratory rate. The use of accessory respiratory muscles and nasal flaring suggest severe distress.
2. **Pulmonary**

a. **Stridor:** Represents upper airway obstruction or epiglottitis.

b. **Rhonchi:** Seen with bronchitis and inhalation injuries.

c. **Signs of consolidation:** Such as bronchial breath sounds, egobronchophony, and tactile fremitus occur in pneumonia.

d. **Rales:** These are the hallmarks of pulmonary edema.

e. **Localized wheezing/rhonchi:** May signify a foreign body or an obstructing neoplasm.

3. **Cardiac.** Signs of cardiac failure (cardiomegaly, S3 gallop).
4. **Skin/extremities.** Cyanosis and clubbing are typical in chronic obstructive respiratory disease (COPD). Rash can be seen in some viral illnesses.

B. Laboratory Data

1. **CBC.** A leukocytosis and left shift suggests infection.
2. **Calcium.** Hypercalcemia is a paraneoplastic syndrome in some bronchogenic carcinomas.
3. **Arterial blood gas.** If indicated by dyspnea or cyanosis.

4. **Arterial carboxyhemoglobin.** In cases of smoke and carbon monoxide inhalation.

C. **Radiographic and Other Studies**
   1. **Chest radiograph.** This should reveal pulmonary edema, neoplasm, pneumonia, interstitial lung disease, hilar lymphadenopathy, and in some cases, an aspirated foreign body (eg, teeth, coins). Acute aspiration may not be apparent on a chest radiograph for 6–12 h.
   2. **Sputum.** Look at the gross appearance noting color, viscosity, odor, and amount. Gram's stain, acid-fast stain, fungal stains, and appropriate cultures are essential. Obtain sputum cytology when a pulmonary neoplasm is considered.
   3. **PPD skin test.** When tuberculosis is possible.
   4. **Pulmonary function tests (PFT).** There is a restrictive pattern (decreased total lung capacity and vital capacity) in interstitial lung disease.
   5. **Bronchoscopy.** Helpful to evaluate and biopsy a neoplasm, to obtain samples for culture, to lavage and clear secretions, or to remove a foreign body.

V. **Plan.** Attempt to obtain a sputum sample even when told that a cough is nonproductive. Order a chest radiograph. When patient is dyspneic, obtain a room air ABG and begin oxygen therapy.

A. **Infectious Conditions.** (See Section IX for drug dosages).
   1. **Unknown community-acquired pneumonia.** Treat with penicillin G (for pneumococcal infections) or erythromycin (for mycoplasma or pneumococcal infections).
   2. **Community acquired/compromised host (COPD/Alcoholic).** Use a cephalosporin or tetracycline.
   3. **Hospital acquired.** Use two agents (an aminoglycoside and oxacillin or an aminoglycoside and a cephalosporin).
      a. **Anaerobic:** Penicillin G or clindamycin.
      b. **Mycoplasma:** Erythromycin or tetracycline.
      c. **Tuberculosis.** Isoniazid and rifampin.
      d. **Immunosuppressed patient:** (eg, after transplant).
         i. Requires coverage for *Legionella* (erythromycin) plus an aminoglycoside plus PCN/or a cephalosporin.
         ii. After a specific organism has been identified by Gram's stain and culture, antibiotic therapy should be adjusted appropriately.

iii. *Pneumocystis carinii* pneumonia is particularly prevalent in AIDS patients and is treated with trimethoprim/sulfamethoxazole or pentamidine.

e. **Coccidioidosis or blastomycosis or histoplasmosis:** Dependent on regional exposures.

B. **Pulmonary Edema**
1. Oxygen.
2. Upright posture.
3. **Diuretics.** The usual choice is furosemide 20–40 mg IV. When the patient is on chronic oral furosemide (Lasix), give 1–2 times the normal dose IV. Hypokalemia should be anticipated and treated.

C. **Nonproductive Cough.** Can be associated with viral upper respiratory infections or tracheal irritation.
1. **Cough suppressant**
   a. Most prescription suppressants are based on codeine.
   b. **Dextromethorphan:** A codeine derivative that acts centrally.
   c. Avoid cough suppressants in patients with a productive cough.
2. **Expectorants.** There is no clear evidence of value. Guaifenesin (Robitussin) is used most often. There are a multitude of preparations combining a cough suppressant, expectorant, and an antihistamine.

20. CVP (CENTRAL VENOUS PRESSURE/ LINE PROBLEMS)

(Central venous catheterization techniques are discussed in Section III, page 340).

I. **Problem.** The central venous pressure (CVP) catheter placed in a patient to undergo total hip replacement in the morning is not functioning.

II. **Immediate Questions**

A. **What is the appearance of the tracing?** A CVP tracing should have a slowly undulating waveform that varies with the patient's respirations. If there is no waveform, the catheter may be clotted. In the absence of a transducer, the column of fluid in the manometer should fluctuate with respirations.

B. **Can blood be aspirated from the line?** Inability to aspirate blood doesn't imply that a catheter can't be used for fluid infusions. It may mean the tip is against the vessel wall, but it also may indicate a kinked or clotted line.

C. **How long has the line been in place?** The longer a line has been in place, the higher the incidence of infection.

D. **Is the line in the correct position?** This must be evaluated on a chest radiograph. The tip should be at the junction of the superior vena cava and the right atrium. Catheters placed farther into the right atrium occasionally cause atrial or ventricular arrhythmias (if the catheter tip slips through the tricuspid valve into the right ventricle). If there is any question, get a new film and compare it to the postplacement radiograph.

E. **Is there bleeding from the site?** This may represent a local problem or a diffuse coagulopathy.

III. Differential Diagnosis

A. **Clotted Catheter.** This happens more frequently with slowly running lines or with capped lines periodically flushed with heparin.

B. **Incorrect Positioning.** Evaluated by chest radiograph. Subclavian lines occasionally go up into the neck (the tracing will not fluctuate with respiration). Rarely, a line will move after being correctly positioned.

C. **Kinked Catheter.** These include kinking of the line at the skin entry site or kinking under the clavicle because of the angle into the vein. This can usually be seen as an acute bend on radiograph.

D. **Other Mechanical Problems.** Cracking of the catheter at the hub or a loose connection.

E. **Flush Line or Transducer Malfunction.** Can be easily ruled out by checking the system. The nursing staff can be very helpful in evaluating this problem.

F. **Infected Catheter.** Any question of sepsis originating in a central venous line requires expeditious evaluation. The best approach is to draw cultures through the catheter, remove the line, and culture the tip.

IV. Database

A. Physical Exam Key Points

1. **Vital signs.** Fever signifies infection, whereas tachycardia and hypotension may represent excessive bleeding, tension pneumothorax, or hemothorax.
2. **HEENT.** Tracheal deviation may indicate an expanding hematoma or tension pneumothorax, especially when seen immediately after CVP line placement.
3. **Lung.** Diminished breath sounds may indicate a pneumothorax, hemothorax, or hydrothorax (which can

occur if fluid is infused through a central line that has gone through the vein into the pleural space).

4. **Check line site.** Inspect for evidence of cellulitis, bleeding, catheter kinking, or leakage from a cracked hub. Check the transducer and flush line.

B. Laboratory Data

1. Obtain cultures from both the catheter and from peripheral blood (see subsection V-E below).
2. Check a CBC or coagulation profile if bleeding is present.

V. Plan. In general, replacing the line will usually solve problems associated with the line itself. Unless the line is infected, it can be changed over a guidewire. Be sure to carefully suture it in place to avoid kinking at the hub. All line manipulations should be performed using sterile technique and with the patient in the Trendelenburg (head down) position to prevent air embolization. After removing a central line, patients should be kept flat or in Trendelenburg for several minutes. The site should be covered with an occlusive dressing, because air embolization is still possible.

A. Clotted Catheter. A new line thought to be clotted can often be declotted safely with a syringe. The decision to attempt to declot a catheter should be approached cautiously because the clot may become an embolus. The catheter can be gently aspirated or flushed with a 1-mL tuberculin syringe. The smaller the diameter of the syringe, the greater the hydraulic pressure generated. Use heparin flush solution (10–100 U/mL). One can also use small doses of streptokinase to declot a line (See Section IX, page 532 for dose), in appropriate clinical circumstances.

B. Kinked Catheter. Inspection of the site may reveal a kinked catheter that can be easily corrected by repositioning the skin sutures using sterile technique. A subclavian catheter that is kinked under the clavicle must be replaced. Placing an internal jugular (IJ) line is safer than placing a subclavian line; however, it is difficult to keep a sterile dressing on an IJ line, and IJ lines tend to move and kink more.

C. Misdirected Catheter. Usually requires removal and replacement, often to another site. Fluoroscopy can be used to reposition a line when this problem is detected during placement.

D. Bleeding. Site bleeding can usually be controlled with direct pressure.

E. Workup of the Infected Catheter. Draw one blood culture from the line, one from a peripheral site, and evaluate the colony counts at 24 h as described by Mosca. When the colony count from the culture is 5 or more times greater than the peripherally drawn culture, the line is implicated as the culprit and must be replaced at another site.

F. Hints for Catheter Insertion. (See Section III, page 340). There are many "tricks" to inserting a central venous catheter, most of which are personal preferences rather than proven helpful tools. Experience and consistency are the key.

1. The most common insertion sites are subclavian and internal jugular (IJ). IJ lines are difficult to fix to the skin and difficult to keep covered with a sterile dressing. Femoral lines are acceptable when there is no upper-body alternative or when rapid access is needed during CPR. Femoral lines have no risk of pneumothorax; the risk is low with IJ lines and is at least 1% with subclavian lines.
2. For subclavian line insertion, the patient is placed in Trendelenburg position, frequently with a roll between the scapulas. This presumably makes the vein more prominent and simplifies puncture. Recent evidence in the literature, however, contradicts this commonly held view. The needle is passed below the clavicle and aimed toward the sternal notch. After obtaining a good blood return (make sure it is venous), the syringe is removed, carefully holding the needle still. Watch for spontaneous blood return. A guidewire is then passed through the needle and the needle removed. The guidewire should pass easily. Remember that if the guidewire goes into the right ventricle, there may be arrhythmias. The skin is nicked with a scalpel, and the catheter passed over the guidewire. After removing the guidewire, it should be nearly straight. Affix the catheter at the hub to the skin.
3. The internal jugular vein is approached by having the patient turn their head away from the side approached. The needle is inserted two fingerbreadths above the clavicle, in the V-shaped area between the two heads of the sternocleidomastoid muscle. Aim for the ipsilateral nipple. Identifying the vein with a small needle (22 or 20 gauge), before inserting the large needle (16 gauge) to pass the guidewire, may reduce the risk of significant bleeding from inadvertent carotid artery puncture.
4. There are four signs that help you verify placement of a central line:
   a. Easy aspiration of blood through the syringe.

b. Easy passing of the guidewire.
c. After removal, the guidewire should be nearly straight.
d. Blood should aspirate easily through the catheter after placement.

5. Small portable ultrasound units can simplify placement of IJ lines. They are less useful for subclavian line insertion.

21. DEATH

I. **Problem.** On a cold night, a homeless man is brought to the emergency room unresponsive and pulseless after being found on a park bench.

II. **Immediate Questions**

A. **Is the patient responsive?** See Problem 11, page 47 and Problem 17, page 81.

B. **Is the patient cold from exposure?** If the core body temperature is less than 32.2 °C, the patient is hypothermic and must be warmed. Warm air ventilation, warming blankets, warming the bladder (irrigate the Foley), gastric lavage, and warm intravenous fluids are all effective. The most effective warming is done on cardiac bypass, which is generally not indicated with a core temperature over 30 °C.

C. **What medications or drugs has the patient taken?** Overdosage of narcotics and alcohol may cause coma and cardiac arrhythmias.

D. **Is the patient brain dead?** Death cannot be pronounced until the patient has been warmed to 32.2 °C, and a full 20 min of ACLS protocol CPR has been given (see page 48).

E. **Does the patient have a declaration of agreement regarding organ donation?** If vital signs are restored by CPR but the patient is ultimately declared brain dead, alert the organ transplant coordinator. When the patient has no declaration, the next of kin can allow procurement if the patient is an acceptable candidate. Respiration and cardiac function must be supported until procurement.

F. **Are the family or close friends available?** The family should be notified when a patient's hospital course changes markedly. In the acute setting, many health care workers suggest that families **not** be informed of the patient's unexpected death over the phone but be asked to come to the hospital immediately. For chronically ill patients, it may be appropriate to inform the family of the patient's death by telephone.

G. Is rigor mortis present? If so, resuscitation is not appropriate.

III. Differential Diagnosis. History obtained from family members, witnesses, and EMS personnel may help you make a diagnosis.

A. See Problem 11, page 47 and Problem 17, page 81 for a complete list of acute causes.

B. Intoxication and metabolic disorders. Among the causes of coma and cardiopulmonary arrest, these are common and can be reversible if corrected in time. CPR must continue (according to ACLS protocol) unsuccessfully for 20 min before pronouncing the patient dead.

C. Hypothermia. Core temperature below 32 °C can be protective against hypoxic neurologic damage. Attempt to rewarm and resuscitate the patient.

IV. Database

A. Physical Exam Key Points

1. **Evaluate Brainstem Function.** There is no brainstem function in brain death.
   a. **Pupillary light reflex**
   b. **Corneal reflex:** Use a cotton-tipped applicator.
   c. **Oculocephalic reflex (doll's eyes):** Tested by holding the upper eyelids open and flexing then quickly extending the neck. If the eyes move in a direction opposite to the movement of the head, the brainstem is intact. This should not be done unless a cervical spine fracture has been definitively ruled out.
   d. **Oculovestibular reflex (cold calorics):** Gives information similar to the oculocephalic reflex but without a risk of cervical spine injury. First, make sure there is no tympanic membrane perforation. Next, raise the head of the patient's bed 30 degrees and inject 60–100 mL of ice water into an ear. If the brainstem is intact, there will be conjugate deviation of the eyes toward the irrigated ear. This may take up to 5 min to occur. The contralateral ear may be tested after waiting 15 min.
   e. **Apnea test:** This test should only be done when the diagnosis of brain death is reasonably assured, because hypercarbia can lead to an increase in ICP and precipitate herniation. Before starting the test, administer 100% oxygen for 15 min. Also insert a

suction catheter (or other tubing) into the trachea and use this to administer 6 L/min of oxygen during the test to limit hypoxia. The ventilator should be set so that the patient's Pco_2 is > 40 mm Hg before the test is started. Obtain a baseline ABG, then disconnect the ventilator and wait (usually about 5 min) until the patient breathes, becomes hypotensive, develops arrhythmias, or the Sao_2 falls below 80 mm Hg. Immediately draw a second ABG and reconnect the ventilator. If the patient has not taken a breath, and the second blood gas reveals a $Pco_2 \geq 60$ mm Hg, apnea can be attributed to brain death. If the test must be stopped (hypotension, arrhythmias, hypoxia) before the Pco_2 reaches 60 mm Hg, another method must be used to determine brain death.

f. **Oropharyngeal reflex (Gag reflex)**

2. **Motor Response to Deep Central Pain.** Decerebrate and decorticate posturing are not consistent with brain death, while spinal reflexes may remain intact.
3. **Chest.** Listen for spontaneous respirations.
4. **Skin.** Any patient arriving at the emergency department with livor or rigor mortis or with injuries obviously incompatible with life, (eg, decapitation) is dead, and CPR should not be started.

B. **Laboratory Data.** If needed to determine cause of death.

1. **CBC.** Sepsis, anemia.
2. **Serum electrolytes.** Arrhythmogenic abnormalities, uremia, glucose.
3. **Drug screen.** Alcohol, barbiturates, opiates, or benzodiazepines. If present, you may need to wait before determining brain death.
4. **Arterial and venous blood gases.** Acid-base abnormalities.

C. **Radiographic and Other Studies.** To diagnose the inciting cause of death.

1. **Chest radiograph.** Pneumothorax, hemothorax, etc.
2. **Head CT.** For all comatose patients.
3. **ECG.** Arrhythmia, EMD.
4. **EEG,** blood flow study, brain scintigraphy, or cerebral angiography may or may not be necessary to augment the clinical exam.

V. Plan

A. **Resuscitation.** See Problem 17, page 81 and Problem 11, page 45.

Following full resuscitation and thorough investigation of possible causes and their treatment, when patients have no response to CPR (for 20 min of ACLS protocol), they can be pronounced dead. Make sure that temperature, intoxicant and brain death criteria are met, when applicable. Do not electrically cardiovert a hypothermic patient. Hypothermia causes refractory ventricular fibrillation that is reversible with warming. It may be reasonable to attempt to resuscitate a child after a prolonged arrest (particularly if hypothermic) as children are more resilient to hypoxic injury than adults.

B. **Pronouncing Death.** Confirm death and note the time.

C. Maintain support of ventilation and circulation when the patient is a potential organ donor.

D. **Notification**
   1. Attending physician, chief of service, primary care provider, and appropriate physicians.
   2. **Next of kin.** It is appropriate to have a family designate contact remaining family members once the designate has been notified.
   3. **Transplant coordinator.** If appropriate, they should be made aware of a potential donor before the declaration of death. The coordinator generally makes arrangements to approach the family regarding organ procurement to eliminate the burden on the caregiver and the possible appearance of a conflict of interest to the family. Studies have shown that families are more likely to consent to donation when they are initially approached by a transplant coordinator, instead of the patient's physician.
   4. **Morgue.** The transfer usually is arranged by the nursing staff. Allow time for the family of the deceased to view the body in the patient's room before transferring the patient to the morgue.
   5. **Coroner.** Laws regarding definition of "coroner's cases" differ among states. The medical examiner will usually investigate all traumatic, perioperative, and suspicious deaths.

E. **Preparation.** Most institutions have standard "mortuary packs" containing a plastic shroud and state death certificate. All IV lines, chest and endotracheal tubes, and other invasive devices are left in place. The ETT is disconnected but not removed. IV lines are tied off or capped. The nursing staff usually completes this task.

F. **Documentation**
   1. **Discharge summary.** The patient needs to be formally discharged.
   2. **Death certificate.** Do **not** list cardiopulmonary arrest as the cause of death—this is how everyone dies. Give

the main reason for hospitalization as the primary cause of death, eg, adenocarcinoma of the lung. Other events contributing to death can be listed secondarily, eg, pneumonia, acute renal failure.

G. **Reflection.** If you felt particularly close to the patient, do not forget that you also are allowed to grieve. Families will appreciate a kind word, and communicating with them provides a sense of closure. Be honest and forthright in providing explanations and in answering questions. Although families should be involved in prospective decision making whenever possible, **avoid being too critical or analytic of decisions made after the fact.** This does not bring the family peace and may lead to unnecessary litigation. There is an appropriate time and place to objectively analyze the patient's course, decisions that were made, and measures that could have been effective in preventing death. This should be done at Surgical Morbidity and Mortality Conference, and in Peer Review and Sentinel Event Reviews that are standard procedure at US hospitals.

22. DIARRHEA

I. **Problem.** A 56-year-old man develops diarrhea 2 d after an aortobifemoral vascular graft is placed.

II. **Immediate Questions**

A. **What are the patient's vital signs?** Tachycardia may indicate volume depletion. Hypotension and fever suggest sepsis. Tachypnea may be a direct effect of sepsis or a compensation for metabolic acidosis (as occurs with bowel ischemia or infarction).

B. **How much diarrhea is the patient having? Is it bloody?** Bloody diarrhea may be seen after ischemic injury to the bowel, and also with colonic neoplasms (carcinoma and villous adenoma), infections (*Shigella, Clostridium difficile, others*), and other inflammatory states.

C. **Is this an acute or chronic problem?** In a patient who has not had surgery, acute diarrhea is usually caused by infections, medications, or mesenteric ischemia. After abdominal surgery, one day of diarrhea is common as the patient's ileus resolves. Antibiotic-associated colitis (*C difficile* colitis) should be considered when diarrhea lasts longer. Ischemic colitis is specifically associated with aortic surgery, particularly when the inferior mesenteric artery is ligated.

Chronic diarrhea does not usually require urgent treatment and can be worked up electively.

D. **What medications is the patient taking?** Many medicines cause diarrhea. Antibiotics can cause diarrhea by altering the colonic flora leading to malabsorption or *C difficile* overgrowth (pseudomembranous colitis, a toxin-induced diarrhea).

E. **Is there a history of pelvic radiation therapy?** Radiation therapy is commonly used for certain malignancies (cervix, prostate, rectal) and can cause chronic diarrhea.

III. Differential Diagnosis

A. Acute Diarrhea

1. **Infectious.** Rare causes of acute diarrhea in the surgical patient include viral, bacterial and parasitic infections (*Salmonella, Shigella, Campylobacter, Yersinia*).
2. **Ischemic.** Mesenteric ischemia can be a catastrophic cause of diarrhea and should be viewed as a surgical emergency. Abdominal distention is accompanied by severe pain, loss of bowel sounds, and bloody diarrhea. This condition is usually seen in elderly, critically ill, hypotensive patients, or in patients with arrhythmias. It is also seen in vascular surgery patients after aortic cross-clamping and ligation of the inferior mesenteric artery.
3. **Gastrointestinal hemorrhage.** Blood acts as a cathartic (see Problem 10, page 41).
4. **Drug induced.**
   a. Quinidine, digoxin, colchicine, antacids (magnesium based), chemotherapeutic agents (methotrexate, adriamycin) and laxatives. Opioid withdrawal also causes diarrhea.
   b. Antibiotics cause diarrhea by altering the normal flora and causing malabsorption, or by inducing *C difficile* overgrowth and toxin production (pseudomembranous enterocolitis). Many antibiotics may cause pseudomembranous colitis; the most frequently implicated are cephalosporins and ampicillin (because of their common use), and clindamycin.

B. Chronic Diarrhea

1. **Inflammatory.** Regional enteritis (Crohn's) and ulcerative colitis cause diarrhea as can radiation.
2. **Neoplastic.** Colon cancer can cause diarrhea from partial colonic obstruction. Villous adenoma can occasionally cause a copious watery (secretory) diarrhea.
3. **Endocrine.** Diarrhea can be found with carcinoid syndrome, hyperthyroidism, and in the islet-cell tumors (gastrinoma, Zollinger-Ellison syndrome, and VIPoma [Vasoactive-Intestinal Polypeptide hormone-secreting tumors]).

4. **Postoperative.** Diarrhea can be seen after gastrectomy (dumping), significant small and large bowel resections, and pancreatic surgery.
5. **Pancreatic.** Exocrine pancreatic dysfunction leads to malabsorption and steatorrhea.
6. **Paradoxic.** Fecal impaction may result in diarrhea because only liquid stool can be expelled past the point of impaction.
7. **Other.** Psychogenic, irritable bowel syndrome, lactose intolerance, radiation induced.

IV. Database

A. **History.** Determining the frequency of diarrhea, the quality and quantity of loose stools, associated abdominal pain, and the use of medicines and laxatives may aid in making a diagnosis. If the diarrhea stops with fasting, malabsorption is likely; diarrhea that persists is usually categorized as secretory.

B. **Physical Exam Key Points**

1. **Vital signs.** An irregular pulse may indicate atrial fibrillation, a possible source of emboli and mesenteric ischemia.
2. **Abdominal exam.** Pain is rarely seen with diarrhea. When present, bacterial infections, such as *Shigella* and *Yersinia,* and mesenteric ischemia must be considered. Distention is seen with gastroenteritis, partial bowel obstruction, and with bowel ischemia. Bowel sounds vary, but absent sounds may indicate more advanced ischemia or infarction.
3. **Rectal exam.** Must always be performed to rule out neoplasm or impaction and to check for occult blood.
4. **Skin.** Jaundice, spider angiomata, palmar erythema should be looked for as signs of alcohol abuse, which is also associated with pancreatic insufficiency.

C. **Laboratory Data**

1. Check stool for occult blood using a Hemoccult or other test kit. Serial exams increase the sensitivity.
2. Order a stool culture for enteric pathogens and examine for ova and parasites, fecal leukocytes (see page 324), and *C difficile* toxin assay.
3. **CBC.** Monitor the hematocrit, especially when there is evidence of gastrointestinal bleeding. Look for leukocytosis as evidence of infection or perforation.
4. **Electrolytes.** Severe diarrhea may dangerously alter the serum electrolytes. Hypokalemia and bicarbonate loss may lead to metabolic acidosis with a normal anion gap (see page 284).

5. **Arterial blood gas.** Appropriate to assess metabolic acidosis, especially if mesenteric ischemia is suspected.
6. **Stool electrolytes.** Potassium, sodium, and bicarbonate determinations help guide fluid replacement in severe cases. See Section IV, page 381 to guide replacement.

D. **Radiographic and Other Studies**
1. **Sigmoidoscopy/Colonoscopy.** This should be performed in patients with diarrhea who are suspected of having pseudomembranous colitis despite negative stool cultures and toxin assays. Classic findings are yellow plaques or confluent pseudomembranes. Patients with a mass on rectal exam should undergo sigmoidoscopy and biopsy of the suspicious area. In addition, ischemic injury in the left colon can often be seen through a sigmoidoscope.
2. **Nasogastric aspiration.** An NG tube should be placed to rule out upper GI bleeding if diarrhea is grossly bloody or melanotic.
3. **Abdominal and chest radiographs.** Look for evidence of obstruction or ileus (dilated loops and air-fluid levels), or perforation (free air, best appreciated on an upright chest radiograph), air in the portal system (pylephlebitis from intra-abdominal sepsis or mesenteric ischemia) and pancreatic calcifications.
4. Diagnostic laparoscopy or exploratory laparotomy should be considered in a patient with a history and physical exam suspicious for ischemic bowel.
5. **Arteriography.** This can help to determine the etiology of ischemic bowel (eg, embolus, thrombosis, or low flow), although most patients are diagnosed by colonoscopy or surgery. Exploratory laparotomy should be the initial diagnostic study in any patient with peritoneal signs.
6. **ECG.** Rarely, mesenteric embolization can occur from atrial thrombus in atrial fibrillation or after myocardial infarction.

V. Plan

A. Fluid and Electrolytes

1. Significant dehydration can occur with acute diarrhea. Shock requires careful, yet aggressive, rehydration, and this may be aided by a central venous catheter or, rarely, with a pulmonary artery catheter. Alpha-adrenergic agents (norepinephrine, Neo-Synephrine, etc) may cause or exacerbate mesenteric ischemia; neverthe-

less, they may be needed to support the blood pressure of critically ill patients.

2. Frequent loose stools of toxic or endocrine origin (carcinoid) often require fluid replacement with additives, such as bicarbonate, to duplicate the electrolyte makeup of the diarrhea. See Section IV, page 381.

B. Stop Possible Causative Medications and Antibiotics

C. Antidiarrheal Agents. (Medication doses can be found in Section IX, page 441).

1. **Narcotics.** Tincture of opium, diphenoxylate with atropine (Lomotil), loperamide (Imodium), codeine, and paregoric can be used carefully to control diarrhea. These agents reportedly prolong infectious diarrhea. In addition, they should not be used in cases of impaction or partial obstruction (beware of low-lying neoplasms).
2. **Bismuth subsalicylate (Pepto-Bismol).** Shown to control some types of diarrhea, in part by inhibiting prostaglandin synthesis.
3. Kaolin and pectin do not work in most cases.
4. Dietary changes.
   a. Avoid lactose-containing foods.
   b. Try a clear liquid diet for 24–48 h.
   c. Advance the diet slowly.

D. Antibiotics

1. **Bacterial diarrhea.** Trimethoprim-sulfamethoxazole or ciprofloxacin cover most causes of infectious enterocolitis, although treatment should ideally be based on cultures. Most cases of bacterial diarrhea are self-limited; antibiotics are not necessary except to treat *Shigella, C difficile,* and any cause in an immunocompromised patient.
2. **Pseudomembranous colitis.** Treat with vancomycin 125 mg PO every 6 h or metronidazole 500 mg PO every 6 h, usually for 7 d. IV metronidazole or vancomycin may be used, although the oral route is preferred. When pseudomembranous colitis is strongly suspected, start empiric therapy while waiting for the result of the toxin assay or stool culture.

E. Operation. Exploratory laparotomy, laparoscopy, bowel resection, embolectomy, or mesenteric artery bypass may be indicated. Resection is required for colonic malignancies, villous adenoma, some complicated cases of inflammatory bowel disease, gangrene, and perforation. Resection may be possible (after localization) for some carcinoid and islet-cell tumors.

F. **Other**
   1. **Control GI bleeding.** See Problems 10 and 34, pages 41 and 137.
   2. **Disimpaction.** Done manually with a doubly gloved finger and adequate lubrication.
   3. **Pancreatic insufficiency.** Give replacement enzymes (pancrease, Viokase, etc).
   4. **Control thyrotoxicosis.** PTU or methimazole, iodide, β-blockers, dexamethasone.
   5. Inflammatory bowel disease is treated with steroids, sulfasalazine, and other immunosuppressive agents.
   6. Proton pump inhibitors (for hyperacidity and diarrhea) and surgery.

23. DRAIN OUTPUT-CHANGING AMOUNT

I. **Problem.** You are notified that a patient, 2 d after a hepatic lobectomy, has a 3-fold increase in the output from a Jackson-Pratt drain during the prior 8 h.

II. **Immediate Questions**

A. **Exactly where is the drain? What operative procedure was performed?** To begin to manage problems with drains, one must know the basic facts, including the location of the drain and the expected character and volume of output. For example, a drain placed in the gallbladder bed after a cholecystectomy should have a different output (low-volume serosanguineous drainage) compared with a T-tube placed during a common duct exploration (much higher volume bilious drainage)

B. **What is the nature of the drain fluid?** There are a limited number of body fluids that can account for an increase in drain output. The list includes serum, blood, pus, lymph (chyle), bile, pancreatic juice, intestinal contents, urine, or CSF. Some of these fluids can be identified by gross visual inspection and others by laboratory analysis.

C. **Are there any new symptoms associated with the change in drain output?** Ask specifically about pain, signs of infection, hypotension, and abdominal distention.

D. **What is the pattern of postoperative drainage?** Variations in drain output may reflect either a change in the ability of the drain to function or a change in the amount of fluid produced. For example, if an unexpectedly low output is followed by an increased output, it may reflect a sudden outflow of accumulated fluids. Also, a change in the output from one drain may affect the output from other drains in the same area.

E. **Has there been any change in the patient's activities coincident with changing drain output?** A patient started on oral intake would be expected to have increased drainage of pancreatic secretions, thoracic duct flow, or T tube output. Also, physical activity increases drainage after lymph node dissection. A change in position may lead to an increase in chest tube output from accumulated fluid.

III. **Differential Diagnosis.** The list below contains the more commonly used surgical drains, states the purpose of the drain, and points out specific problems to be expected. Drain management is neither mysterious nor complicated, but rather a simple plumbing matter with a finite number of possible explanations for a given situation.

A. **Extremity/lymph node dissection (axillary, inguinal) drains.**
   1. The purpose is to prevent the accumulation of lymph and serous fluid, which can lead to discomfort, drainage, and wound separation.
   2. Increased output is usually lymph and is often associated with increased motion of the associated extremity. Output will decrease when the extremity is immobilized, but this is rarely necessary.

B. **Mediastinal tubes.** Placed during open heart surgery.
   1. Their function is to identify excessive bleeding and prevent cardiac tamponade.
   2. Increased output is usually bloody and may be due to a specific bleeding point.
   3. A sudden decrease in output may be due to an obstructed tube and may precede tamponade.

C. **Chest Tubes (pleural).** (See also Problem 13, page 66).
   1. Their function is to drain blood, pus, air, or fluid from the pleural cavities.
   2. If the output increases when a patient begins to eat, consider injuries of the esophagus or thoracic duct.

D. **Hepatic/Biliary Tube**
   1. **Hepatectomy**
      a. Lymph, bile, and blood drain from the cut surface of the liver, and bile can leak from the ligated hepatic duct.
      b. **Examine for bile:** Often multiple drains are present so be aware of the total output.
   2. **Cholecystectomy** (often not drained).
      a. Drains help to identify and prevent collections from bile leaks and bleeding, although they are rarely used in uncomplicated procedures.
      b. Examine the drainage for bile.

3. **Common duct exploration.**
   a. T-tubes are used to stent a choledochotomy, prevent bile leaks, and provide a path for further diagnostic or therapeutic inquiries (cholangiogram or extraction of retained stones). A suction drain is frequently placed next to a T-tube. The T-tube is removed in 10–14 d (after a tract develops); the suction drain is removed in 2–3 d (if there is no bile leak). Be certain to remove the correct tube.
   b. Increased output may signify distal obstruction from a retained stone, edema, or the start of oral intake.

E. **Pancreatic Procedures**
1. Used when pancreatic parenchyma is divided (pancreatic resection, trauma) or when the ductal system is opened (eg, a Puestow pancreaticojejunostomy) to prevent the accumulation of pancreatic fluid.
2. Drain output increases with feeding or with distal duct obstruction.

F. **Esophageal Procedures**
1. Drains function to identify leaks and evacuate potentially irritating/infectious fluid.
2. **Output increases with an anastomotic leak.** Look for saliva or refluxed gastrointestinal contents.

G. **Urinary Tract Procedures**
1. Drains are used after radical cystectomy and urinary diversion, radical prostatectomy, or other procedures where the collecting system or bladder had been opened. They prevent urinoma formation and, in the case of a concomitant node dissection, lymphocele formation.
2. Increased output may be urine leaking from an anastomotic site or lymph.

IV. Database

A. **Physical Exam Key Points**
1. Examine drainage fluid for its color and characteristics, looking for blood, pus, or bile. Also look at the tube for clots or other obstructing material.
2. **Lungs.** Listen for changes in breath sounds (with chest tubes).
3. **Cardiac.** Increased jugular venous pressure, pulsus paradoxus, or quiet heart sounds suggest cardiac tamponade.
4. **Abdomen.** Tenderness, abdominal distention, or a fluid wave may be present with accumulating fluid.
5. **Extremities.** Examine for collections of undrained fluid at the surgical site. A groin lymphocele can cause peripheral swelling.

B. Laboratory Data

1. **CBC.** When considering infection or bleeding.
2. **Hematocrit of drainage fluid.** A small amount of blood mixed with a lot of serum may look grossly like blood. Compare the drainage hematocrit to the blood hematocrit.
3. **Gram's stain.** All drains eventually become colonized with bacteria. This may not represent a true infection, however obtaining a Gram's stain and culture of the drainage may help to guide antibiotic selection by identifying the emergence of resistant bacteria or yeast.
4. **Electrolytes.** May help to identify the source of drainage.
   a. **Amylase:** Markedly elevated in pancreatic secretions, also present in saliva.
   b. **Triglycerides:** Elevated in thoracic duct lymph.
   c. **Creatinine:** If the drained fluid is urine, creatinine will be markedly elevated.
   d. **pH:** Pleural fluid pH < 7.2 may be associated with an empyema.
   e. **LDH and protein:** See Section III for a discussion of ascitic fluid (paracentesis) and pleural fluid (thoracentesis).
   f. **Bilirubin:** May be from the biliary tree or proximal small intestine.

C. Radiographic and Other Studies

1. **Chest radiograph.** Particularly helpful when mediastinal or chest tubes stop draining to see whether fluid is collecting.
2. **Plain films.** Most drains are marked with a radiopaque stripe so that the drain position can be verified with plain films.
3. **Contrast studies.** A T-tube cholangiogram is routinely done after common duct exploration. Contrast can be injected through drains to identify fistulas, leaks, or cavities of accumulated fluid.

V. Plan. Identify the type of drain, location, and type of fluid draining; formulate ideas about the likely source of fluid.

A. Emergency Management. Drains do not usually require emergent or urgent management with the exception of mediastinal tubes placed after cardiac surgery.

1. **Increased output.** This is almost always blood. Document the rate of bleeding by accurately noting the output every 30–60 min and by following serial hematocrit determinations. Measure coagulation parameters and correct as necessary with FFP and platelets. Notify the

senior staff and operating team about the rate of bleeding as it may be necessary to bring the patient back to the operating room.

2. **Decreased output.** A sudden decrease in output may be the result of a clot in the tube. With mediastinal tubes, this may lead to cardiac tamponade. If the patient's blood pressure falls, give a fluid bolus and be prepared to open the lower portion of the wound and evacuate clot gently from the retrosternal space.

B. Routine Management

1. Accurately record the amount, characteristics, and lab analysis of increasing drain output.
2. If there is a lot of output, replace part or all of it with appropriate fluids.
   a. **Pancreatic, biliary & small bowel:** See Section IV.
   b. **Mediastinal drainage:** Transfuse the patient when clinically indicated. Mediastinal and pleural drainage are occasionally collected, spun down, and given back to the patient, using a "cell-saver" device.
3. Some drains are designed to be used with suction; however, suction will occasionally lead to persistent drainage. It may then be appropriate to put drains on "passive" (gravity) drainage to decrease the volume.
4. Remember that drain management is an area where individual idiosyncrasies abound. Never pull a drain unless you believe it is appropriate and the surgeon in charge wants it pulled.

24. DRAIN OUTPUT-CHANGING CHARACTER

I. Problem. A 45-year-old male, 2 d after cholecystectomy, now has bilious drainage from a right flank Penrose drain.

II. Immediate Questions

A. What are the characteristics of the drainage? Is it bloody, bilious, serous, serosanguineous, purulent, or urine-like?

B. What kind of drainage was there previously? A drain that had serous drainage and is now draining blood is an obvious cause for concern. Similarly, when serous drainage begins to look like urine, stool, or bile, the patient may have a new fistula or anastomotic leak.

C. How much is draining? You need to know this to determine when to pull a drain. When the output is high, fluid may need to be replaced, and this is addressed in Problem 23, page 103.

D. **What was the operation and where was the drain placed?** These questions help you to determine whether the drainage is appropriate or of concern and to identify potential sources for new or increased drainage.

III. Differential Diagnosis.

III. Differential Diagnosis. Clearly, the differential diagnosis depends on the characteristics of the drainage and the location of the drain. For a further discussion of drainage, see Problem 23, page 103.

A. **Bloody Drainage.** Of obvious concern after any surgical procedure. Read the operative note to see if there is any mention of a "generalized ooze" of blood at the end of the procedure.

B. **Serous Drainage.** Usually of no concern a few days after surgery. An increased volume of drainage may be a result of irritation from the drain.

C. **Purulent Drainage.** Indicates infection.

D. **Bilious Drainage.** May indicate an anastomotic leak after a duodenal, pancreatic, biliary, or gastric procedure. If noted after a cholecystectomy, the source may be an accessory liver duct (duct of Luschka), an injured common bile duct, loss of a tie or clip from the cystic duct stump, or, rarely, a duodenal injury.

E. **Intestinal Drainage.** Of obvious concern after any operation. A fistulogram (injecting contrast through the tract) can confirm the diagnosis.

F. **Urine Drainage.** Can be difficult to differentiate from serum. Injecting methylene blue or indigo carmine dye IV can help. Filling the bladder (with a Foley) differentiates bladder fistulas from ureteral fistulas.

G. **Chylous Drainage.** Indicates injury to the thoracic duct.

IV. Database

A. Physical Exam Key Points

1. **Vital signs.** Signs of infection (tachycardia, fever) and volume loss.
2. **Abdomen.** Check for signs of peritonitis.
3. **Wound.** Examine for cellulitis, pus, or seroma.

B. Laboratory Data

1. **CBC.** Check the white blood count and hematocrit. Remember that the white count may be mildly elevated for up to 24 h after surgery without an infection.
2. **Coagulation profile.** The PT/PTT, platelets, and fibrin split products help to explain excessive bleeding.

3. **Send drain fluid for chemistry analysis as appropriate.** See Problem 23, page 103.

C. **Radiographic and Other Studies**
   1. **Angiogram.** May help to localize a bleeding site if the bleeding is rapid (rate of bleeding at least 1 mL/min).
   2. **Fistulogram.** Useful to identify the origin of cutaneous fistulas.
   3. **CT scans and ultrasound.** May localize undrained fluid collections.

V. Plan

A. **Support patients who are bleeding.** Administer fluids and/or blood to maintain the patient's blood pressure. Identify and control the bleeding site with an operation or angiogram or by correction of a coagulopathy.

B. **Antibiotics.** Indicated for purulent drainage and for certain fistulas, such as colovesical fistulas.

C. **Reoperation.** May be needed, either urgently (with an incompletely drained or infected collection) or delayed (which improves the chances of successfully repairing many intestinal fistulas).

D. **Drain Abscesses.** Continuous drainage is essential until the abscess is completely cleared. If a collection persists despite apparently adequate drainage, an additional drain (or drains) is needed. This can often be placed percutaneously using ultrasound or CT guidance. When there are multiple abscesses or when an abscess is loculated, operative intervention may be required.

E. **Replace fluids as needed.** (see Section IV, page 381).

25. DTs (DELIRIUM TREMENS)

I. **Problem.** A 55-year-old intoxicated man is admitted with abdominal pain and an elevated amylase. Narcotic analgesia is initiated. On the third hospital day, he is found talking to the walls and shaking violently.

II. Immediate Questions

A. **What are the patient's vital signs?** Hypertension, tachycardia, and fever may represent signs of autonomic overactivity, common in delirium.

B. **What is the patient's mental status?** An altered level of consciousness and impaired cognitive function define delirium. Delirium can present as unresponsiveness, but hallucinations and confusion are the predominant symptoms. These coupled with autonomic hyperactivity are typical of delirium. As a general rule, visual hallucinations, "pink elephants," are characteristic of toxic psychosis (EtOH, etc), and auditory hallucinations are more commonly associated with psychiatric illness.

C. **What is the status of the patient's airway?** Any patient with an altered level of consciousness is at increased risk of aspiration.

D. **What medications is the patient taking?** Pay particular attention to addictive substances.

E. **Is there a history of drug or alcohol abuse?** This can be the key to the diagnosis.

III. **Differential Diagnosis.** Delirium is a manifestation of diffuse cerebral dysfunction. A focal neurologic deficit suggests a structural abnormality (stroke, brain tumor, etc). The differential diagnosis of delirium is more extensive than the following list indicates and includes any source of diffuse cerebral dysfunction (see also Problem 14, page 70). The patient appearing delirious may be suffering from a very wide range of problems. The patient described may be delirious on the basis of any of the following diagnoses.

A. **Withdrawal Syndromes**
   1. **Delirium tremens.** A potentially life-threatening form of alcohol withdrawal, DTs must be considered for any patient known to be a heavy drinker who develops delirium 3–4 d after hospitalization. For the patient not known to be a drinker, other causes must be investigated.
   2. **Barbiturate withdrawal.** Indistinguishable from DTs clinically.
   3. **Opioid withdrawal.** Occurs up to 48 h after cessation of the responsible agent (most rapid with heroin), and symptoms include restlessness, rhinorrhea, lacrimation, nausea, diarrhea, and hypertension.

B. **Metabolic Abnormalities**
   1. **Electrolyte abnormalities.** Chronic vomiting, pancreatitis, renal failure, and severe liver disease can all cause electrolyte and metabolic abnormalities, which can manifest as delirium.
   2. **Hypoxia.** Congestive heart failure can produce hypoxia and delirium in an indolent fashion.
   3. **Drug intoxication.** Check the urine for the presence of suspected drugs (opiates, benzodiazepines, cocaine).

C. **Endocrine Abnormalities.** Abnormal thyroid and adrenal cortical function can cause delirium as can hypoglycemia from an insulin overdose (accidental or intentional) or from an insulin-secreting tumor. Check for the C-peptide of insulin to distinguish an insulinoma from surreptitious use. Diabetic ketoacidosis and hyperosmolar coma should also be considered.

D. **CNS Infections.** Meningitis and encephalitis can cause delirium.

E. **ICU Psychosis.** "Post pump psychosis," or "Post pericardiotomy syndrome," was initially described in patients after coronary bypass procedures. This is commonly seen in elderly patients in the ICU after many different procedures.

F. **Sepsis.** Any cause of sepsis can lead to altered mentation. In elderly patients, an altered mental status may be the first or only sign of sepsis.

IV. Database

A. Physical Exam Key Points

1. **Vital signs.** Tachycardia is a common manifestation of withdrawal.
2. **Neck.** Look for jugular venous distention (CHF) and thyroid masses or a goiter (hyperthyroidism).
3. **Chest exam.** Listen for rales or rhonchi as signs of CHF or pulmonary edema (hypoxia causes delirium).
4. **Abdomen.** Check for bladder distention, a common cause of agitation in the elderly patient.
5. **Skin.** Profuse sweating is typical of DTs.
6. **Neurologic exam.** Mental status changes define delirium. Hallucinations, confusion, and disorientation are typical. Reflexes will be exaggerated but symmetrical. Pupils are reactive. Any focal findings on motor, sensory, deep tendon, or cranial nerve examination point to a structural abnormality, either spinal or intracranial.

B. Laboratory Data

1. **Electrolytes and glucose.** Look for hyponatremia and hypoglycemia, which are potentially life threatening. Hypercalcemia also changes a patient's affect and may cause frank psychosis.
2. **ABGs.** Obtain if hypoxemia is likely.

C. **Radiographic and Other Studies.** History, physical exam, and simple tests usually provide the underlying diagnosis for delirium. A chest radiograph might show cardiomegaly and pulmonary edema. Evaluation of the CNS by head CT scan or lumbar puncture is occasionally necessary, especially in the septic patient or the patient with focal neurologic findings. Rarely is an electroencephalogram (EEG) useful.

V. Plan

A. Prevention. The patient at risk for DTs should be treated while hospitalized with around-the-clock benzodiazepines, most commonly oxazepam (15–30 mg PO every 4–6 h), lorazepam 1 mg PO/IV every 8 h, or ethanol (small quantities PO or IV).

B. Delirium tremens. Alcoholics may have other potential causes of delirium, most notably electrolyte abnormalities (from vomiting) and hepatic encephalopathy.

1. Start with IV benzodiazepines (diazepam 5–10 mg IV every 4–6 h) followed by oral treatment with diazepam, chlordiazepoxide, or oxazepam in the nonvomiting patient.
2. Restrain the patient to prevent injury. The prone position decreases the risk of aspiration.
3. Use intravenous fluid to correct volume and electrolyte abnormalities. Supplement intravenous fluids with thiamine (100 mg), multivitamins, and folate (1 mg) ("banana bag") to replete wasted stores in these often malnourished patients.
4. Treat seizures with phenytoin or paraldehyde.

C. Hypoxia

1. **Oxygen.** Mask or nasal prong therapy may be necessary. Check pulse oximetry.
2. **Morphine sulfate and diuretics (furosemide).** These are used in the setting of pulmonary edema.
3. **Digoxin or dopamine and nitrates.** May be needed for pulmonary edema caused by congestive heart failure.

D. Other

1. **Narcotic withdrawal.** This can be treated with relatively high doses of minor tranquilizers or with methadone (10–20 mg PO, q2–6h). Clonidine may be used as alternate therapy to combat autonomic symptoms of withdrawal.
2. **Drug intoxication.** Usually, a safe and supportive environment suffices until the drug wears off. Minor or major tranquilizers can be used, especially in the violent patient.
3. **Endocrine abnormalities.** These are treated as indicated.
4. **CNS infections.** Use appropriate antibiotics, with or without surgical drainage, as indicated.
5. **ICU psychosis.** Make an attempt to keep the patient oriented. Attempt to reproduce a normal day-night environment and allow for adequate sleep. Agitation can be

controlled with oral or parenteral haloperidol (Haldol). TV or radio programs, a large wall calendar, family pictures, and optimally, a companion help to orient the patient. Avoid benzodiazepines (which can have a paradoxic effect).

6. Thiamine prophylaxis should be given to patients with a history of alcohol abuse.
7. **Sepsis.** Treat with appropriate antibiotics and fluid resuscitation.

26. DYSPNEA

I. **Problem.** A patient on the trauma service with a diagnosis of myocardial contusion complains of difficulty breathing.

II. **Immediate Questions**

A. **What was the patient doing when the dyspnea occurred?** Dyspnea on exertion is usually from myocardial ischemia (angina, acute MI, myocardial contusion), or COPD, although cardiac tamponade and pneumothorax are occasionally responsible. Dyspnea associated with a reclining position (ie, orthopnea) suggests CHF.

B. **Did the dyspnea begin abruptly, or did it have a gradual onset?** Acute dyspnea is often related to a specific event, such as a pulmonary embolus, pneumothorax, or myocardial infarction.

C. **What is the baseline respiratory status of the patient?** A complaint of "not getting enough air" in a well-trained athlete indicates a more serious problem than a similar complaint in a chronic smoker with emphysema. Inquire specifically about work and recreational activities and exercise tolerance (carrying groceries, climbing stairs).

D. **Are there other symptoms such as chest pain coincident with the dyspnea?** A patient may focus on their shortness of breath and not disclose chest pain or pressure unless asked. However, dyspnea may be the only evident symptom of an acute myocardial infarction.

E. **Is there wheezing or stridor?** Both acute asthma attacks and anaphylactic reactions are potentially lethal unless they are diagnosed and treated expeditiously.

F. **Is there a history of asthma or other pulmonary conditions?**

III. **Differential Diagnosis.** Dyspnea may be classified as acute or subacute/chronic. Within each category, there are pulmonary and cardiac mechanisms.

A. Acute

1. Pulmonary

a. Pneumothorax: Traumatic pneumothoraces are associated with rib fractures and bleeding (hemo-pneumothorax) and can progress (tension pneumothorax) in minutes to hours. Spontaneous pneumothoraces usually occur in males with a tall thin body habitus.

b. Pulmonary embolus: Maintain a high index of suspicion. Risk factors include immobilization, recent surgery, obesity, neoplastic disease, and estrogen use.

c. Asthma or allergic reactions: Wheezing suggests asthma. Anaphylactic reactions are identified by stridor, atopic history, hives, and facial edema (see Problem 5, page 23).

d. Aspirated foreign body. This is usually diagnosed by history, but in young or mentally impaired patients, you may need to rely on the physical exam and on radiographic studies.

e. Reflux with aspiration: See Problem 8, page 32.

2. Acute myocardial infarction. Usually associated with chest pain or pressure—but not always. Remember this when the patient is older than 50 or has cardiac risk factors.

3. Anxiety attack. An uncommon cause of shortness of breath, further complicated because it is frequently associated with chest pain. Often tachypnea cycles with period of normal breathing, and tachypnea may resolve when patients are not aware they are being observed. Don't rush to make this diagnosis without considering organic causes.

B. Subacute/Chronic

1. Pulmonary

a. COPD: These patients usually have a smoking history with baseline dyspnea on exertion. In progression of baseline dyspnea, look for evidence of an infectious process.

b. Pneumonia: Often associated with leukocytosis, fever, productive sputum, and chest radiograph changes (infiltrates).

c. Interstitial lung disease: Chest radiograph and pulmonary function tests are diagnostic.

2. Cardiac

a. Congestive heart failure: Physical exam shows an elevated jugular venous pressure, rales, peripheral edema, a cardiac gallop, and displacement of the left ventricular impulse. Dyspnea is associated with lying down (orthopnea).

IV. Database

A. Physical Exam Key Points

1. **Vital signs.** Fever may signify infection, but may also be seen with a pulmonary embolus. Tachypnea may accompany hypoxia, embolus, or a pneumothorax. Check oxygen saturation as soon as possible.
2. **Lung.** Observe the respiratory rate, the work of breathing, and the use of accessory muscles. Listen for wheezes, stridor, rales, evidence of consolidation, and decreased breath sounds. Tracheal shift may indicate a pneumothorax.
3. **Cardiac.** Is there elevated jugular venous pressure, displacement of the left ventricular impulse, or a new murmur of mitral regurgitation? Check for pulsus paradoxus.
4. **Extremities.** Leg swelling is evidence for deep venous thrombosis. Evaluate for cyanosis.
5. **Neurologic.** Confusion and drowsiness may signify severe hypoxia.

B. Laboratory Data

1. **CBC.** Leukocytosis suggests infection. Anemia impairs oxygen delivery.
2. **ABG.** Documents the level of respiratory compromise and guides therapeutic decisions. Look for an A-a gradient, which suggests a pulmonary embolus.
3. **Sputum Gram's stain/culture.** In patients with pneumonia or tracheobronchitis.
4. **Blood chemistries.** May reveal evidence of renal failure. Tachypnea may be a manifestation of respiratory compensation for metabolic acidosis.

C. Radiographic and Other Studies

1. **Chest radiograph.** Of obvious importance. If a patient is in distress, obtain an immediate portable chest radiograph (upright if possible). Look for pulmonary edema, pneumothorax, effusion, or pneumonia.
2. **ECG.** Always obtain an ECG when there is any question of myocardial ischemia.
3. **Pulmonary function tests.** Not applicable to the acute situation but helpful in patients with chronic lung disease.
4. **$\dot{V}/\dot{Q}$ scan.** A ventilation/perfusion scan may document a pulmonary embolism.
5. **Spiral CT with IV contrast.** Detects large centrally located pulmonary emboli. May be more easily obtained than an angiogram on an urgent basis.

6. **Pulmonary angiogram.** This is the "gold standard" in the diagnosis of pulmonary emboli. It is particularly helpful for equivocal cases (eg, an intermediate $\dot{V}/\dot{Q}$ scan and a strong clinical suspicion).
7. **Radionuclide angiogram.** This documents the left ventricular ejection fraction, which can be helpful in assessing patients with congestive heart failure.
8. **Exercise tolerance test.** Useful if episodes of dyspnea are related to ischemic heart disease.
9. **Echocardiography.** Identifies valvular disease, akinesis, failure, etc.

V. Plan

A. Emergent Therapy

1. **Oxygen supplementation.** If a patient is short of breath, institute oxygen therapy. Start with a 100% face mask, if the patient is very symptomatic, then gradually decrease the inspired oxygen keeping the arterial oxygen at least 60–80 mm Hg (on ABG) or the oxygen saturation > 90% (with pulse oximetry). Long-term oxygen therapy at more than 50% can cause pulmonary toxicity. Do not worry about suppression of hypoxic drive (chronic lung disease) in the acute situation. Patients with a history of COPD and CO_2 retention may be at increased risk to lose their "hypoxic drive" to breathe, but it is impossible to predict which patients may be affected. Remember that no facemask completely seals the airway (patients breathe around it), so that a 100% nonrebreather mask may only deliver as much oxygen as an endotracheal tube with 40% FiO_2. When a patient remains hypoxic with a 100% facemask, intubate the patient.
2. A stat portable chest radiograph, ECG, and ABG are usually indicated if the cause is not immediately obvious.

B. Specific Urgent/Immediate Treatments

1. **Asthma/COPD exacerbation.** Ask the respiratory therapist to administer a bronchodilator. Options include metaproterenol (Alupent) 0.3 mL in 2–3 mL NS, and ipratropium (Atrovent) 0.5 mL in 3 mL NS. Some patients have their own inhaler (eg, Proventyl).
2. **Anaphylaxis.** Refer to Problem 5, page 23.
3. **Myocardial ischemia.** If immediate evaluation is consistent with myocardial ischemia, give sublingual nitroglycerin and oxygen. Refer to Problem 12, page 54.
4. **Acute congestive heart failure.** Treat with oxygen, diuretics (IV Lasix 10–40 mg dependent on prior exposure), nitroglycerin, and sit the patient upright if blood pressure allows.

5. **Pneumonia.** Treat with antibiotics and pulmonary toilet.
6. **Pneumothorax.** Place a chest tube as outlined in Section III, page 346. Needle decompression may be necessary for a tension pneumothorax.

Remember, if the airway is compromised or the above steps fail to stabilize symptoms, proceed with endotracheal intubation.

27. DYSURIA

I. **Problem.** A patient complains of dysuria 4 d after an uncomplicated radical neck dissection.

II. **Immediate Questions**

A. **How long has the dysuria been present?** Knowing the time course of any illness can provide clues to the cause. If the illness is more chronic, check on any previous urinalysis available.

B. **What is the patient's urologic history; specifically, is there any history of infections or stone disease?** Some patients, especially females, are prone to recurrent urinary infections. Urethritis or prostatitis may be present in males.

C. **Are there any associated voiding symptoms?** Fever, chills, and back pain are often signs of upper urinary tract infection (pyelonephritis). Frequency, urgency, and pain on urination suggest lower urinary tract infection (cystitis, prostatitis, urethritis).

D. **Has the patient recently had a Foley catheter removed?** A catheter may cause cystitis or urethritis. Mild urethral irritation usually resolves within a day but can be treated with oral pyridium if the patient has substantial discomfort.

III. **Differential Diagnosis**

A. **Urinary Tract Infection**

1. **Upper.** Pyelonephritis typically presents with CVA tenderness, although patients occasionally have dysuria.
2. **Lower.** Cystitis is associated with urgency and frequency. Gonorrhea and *Chlamydia* are common causes of urethritis. Prostatitis may be acute (associated with fever, chills, and signs of sepsis) or chronic (associated with voiding symptoms or recurrent urinary tract infections).

B. **Vaginitis.** Can present with dysuria. It is caused by *Candida, Trichomonas,* and *Gardnerella*. Atrophic vaginitis is a problem in postmenopausal women.

C. **Genital Infections.** Include herpes and condylomata.

D. **Chemical Irritants.** Allergic reaction to a variety of agents (some foods, deodorant, douches).

E. **Postprocedure.** A frequent complaint after bladder catheterization or cystoscopy, which usually resolves spontaneously when no infection intervenes.

F. **Urethral Syndrome.** Dysuria and voiding complaints without evidence of a urinary tract infection. Seen commonly in women and often related to eating certain foods.

G. **Miscellaneous.** Urethral stricture, bladder tumor, urolithiasis, and interstitial cystitis.

IV. Database

A. Physical Exam Key Points

1. **Abdominal exam.** Look for suprapubic tenderness or costovertebral angle tenderness.
2. **Genitalia.** Evaluate the urethral meatus, urethra, testicles, and epididymis in men. Vaginal discharge suggests vaginitis. Females may require a formal pelvic exam if the cause is not readily apparent.
3. **Rectal exam.** Mandatory to evaluate the prostate and rule out prostatitis. Be aware that vigorous exam of an acutely inflamed prostate can induce bacteremia and may be contraindicated in the presence of a high fever and chills.

B. Laboratory Data

1. **Urinalysis and culture.** Pyuria (>5 WBC/HPF), the presence of leukocyte esterase or nitrites and a positive culture suggest a urinary tract infection.
2. **Hemogram.** Leukocytosis and a left shift will be seen with acute pyelonephritis and acute prostatitis and not normally seen in urethritis, chronic prostatitis, or cystitis.
3. **Culture and Gram's stain of urethral discharge.** Thayer-Martin media should be used if gonorrhea is suspected. *Neisseria gonorrhoeae* can be seen as a gram-negative intracellular diplococci on Gram's stain.
4. **Urine cytology.** Dysuria may be a subtle manifestation of transitional cell carcinoma.

C. **Radiographic and Other Studies.** Full urologic evaluation (excretory urography, cystoscopy, etc) may be required for definitive diagnosis, but is rarely performed acutely.

V. Plan

A. **Positive Urinalysis.** This is enough of a reason to start antibiotic therapy. If the patient is otherwise healthy and not systemically septic, then oral antibiotics (such as trimethoprim/sulfa, amoxicillin, or a quinolone) may be sufficient.

B. **Systemic Sepsis.** When a patient has fever, chills, nausea, malaise, or hypotension (often associated with acute pyelonephritis or prostatitis), obtain appropriate cultures (blood and urine), then start intravenous antibiotics. A third-generation cephalosporin (cefoperazone, ceftazidime, etc), or ampicillin with an aminoglycoside are good choices until the culture and sensitivities are available.

C. **Chronic Prostatitis.** May have a positive urine culture, although patients are usually not septic. Treatment is a 3-wk course of trimethoprim/sulfa or a quinolone.

D. **Vaginitis.** Should be treated appropriately; nystatin vaginal cream or suppositories for *Candida,* oral metronidazole for *Trichomonas,* dienestrol (AVC) cream for atrophic vaginitis.

E. **Other Infections.** Treated with appropriate antibiotics.
   1. **Gonococcal urethritis.** Many regimens are available (procaine penicillin G 4.8 million U IM plus probenecid 1 g PO, ceftriaxone 250 mg IM, ampicillin 3 g PO) followed by a 7-d course of tetracycline.
   2. **Nongonococcal urethritis (NGU)** ***(Chlamydia).*** Doxycycline 100 mg PO bid or tetracycline 500 mg PO qid for 7–10 d.

F. **Symptomatic Relief.** Symptomatic relief of dysuria can usually be achieved using phenazopyridine (Pyridium) 100–200 mg PO tid (turns the urine orange) while workup or treatment is in progress. A small subset of patients with dysuria are sensitive to excessively alkaline or acidic urine that may vary with diet.

28. EPISTAXIS

I. **Problem.** A 45-year-old hypertensive patient, 1 d after a laparoscopic cholecystectomy, complains of a nosebleed that has lasted for 2 h.

II. **Immediate Questions**

A. **What are the patient's vital signs?** Hypertension is usually a response to epistaxis rather than a cause. Tachycardia usually represents agitation but occasionally indicates significant blood loss in this setting. Each patient should therefore be checked for orthostatic hypotension.

B. **Is there a history of prior nosebleeds or any recent trauma?** The new onset of epistaxis may be a sign of intranasal disease. Recurrent epistaxis is usually traumatic, especially in younger patients.

III. **Differential Diagnosis.** Epistaxis has multiple causes. Obscure causes, such as hematologic malignancies and coagulation disorders, will not be discussed in detail. Ninety percent of epistaxis has its origin in the anterior portion of the nasopharynx.

A. **Trauma.** Blunt trauma to the nose often causes epistaxis that ceases spontaneously. Self-inflicted digital trauma (nose-picking) is a very common cause. The source is almost always an anterior site called the Kiesselbach's triangle, a submucosal mat of blood vessels located on the anterior-most aspect of the nasal septum.

B. **Hypertension.** Hypertension may make control of bleeding more difficult, but is rarely, if ever, a cause of bleeding in itself.

C. **Intranasal Causes.** An adult patient with a new epistaxis (in the absence of trauma) may have an intranasal lesion. These include polyps and benign and malignant tumors. Typically, no anterior source of bleeding is apparent. Local infections may also be responsible. Juvenile angiofibroma, a locally aggressive tumor that appears as a purple polypoid mass, should be considered in pubescent males.

D. **Systemic Illnesses and Medications.** Patients who take anticoagulants, such as warfarin, or have end stage liver disease can develop epistaxis when their prothrombin time is overly prolonged. Renal failure and aspirin interfere with platelet function. Obscure causes of epistaxis include leukemia, hemophilia, and chemotherapy-induced thrombocytopenia. Arteriosclerosis commonly predisposes to posterior epistaxis in elderly patients.

IV. **Database**

A. **Physical Exam Key Points**

1. **Vital signs.** Hypertension often improves as the patient relaxes. Orthostatic hypotension can be found after significant nasal hemorrhage. Patients with chronic hypertension should be treated after the acute episode.
2. **Skin.** Look for petechiae and ecchymoses, which may suggest a systemic problem.
3. **Nose.** Examination of the nasal cavity should be performed with a headlamp or mirror and a nasal speculum. Look for a bleeding site, examining as much of the mucosa as possible. Briefly examine the contralateral nasal cavity. Topical cocaine can be used to control bleeding when examination is difficult.

B. **Laboratory Data**

1. **Coagulation studies.** These are only occasionally useful, but may reveal over-anticoagulation.

2. **CBC.** The hematocrit may not accurately reflect acute blood loss. Look for unsuspected thrombocytopenia.

V. Plan

A. Initial Control of Bleeding. A quiet atmosphere, upright position, bilateral alar pressure, and 5% cocaine applied locally constitute the initial approach to control bleeding. Cocaine acts as both a vasoconstrictor and anesthetic.

B. Cauterization and Anterior Packing

1. **Silver nitrate sticks.** If examination reveals a likely bleeding source, silver nitrate sticks can be used to cauterize the site after initial control has been achieved.
2. **Anterior nasal packing.** An anterior pack can be placed if cauterization is not successful and is often placed anyway as reinforcement. Start by inserting a piece of Gelfoam over the bleeding site, and then layer bacitracin-impregnated Nu-Gauz into the nose. Tape a drip pad to the nose. Packing can usually be removed in 2–4 d. Patients who have packing should be started on antibiotics (ampicillin or erythromycin) to prevent sinusitis.

C. Posterior Packing. Persistent bleeding with no localized anterior site requires posterior packing and admission to the otolaryngology service. In addition to admission, these patients require antibiotics (as above), oxygen, and analgesia, usually with narcotics. Three methods are used commonly to place posterior packs.

1. A 14-Fr Foley catheter can be passed into the nasopharynx, inflated with saline, and gently drawn into the choanae.
2. Specialized nasal balloons are available (Nasal-Stat).
3. A pack made of 4 × 4 cotton gauze can be placed. This method is more complicated. Three 4 × 4 gauze sponges are rolled and tied with 3 large silk ties. A rubber catheter is passed into the nose and pulled out the mouth with a clamp. Two sutures from the pack are tied to the catheter and then pulled up into the nasal pharynx, guided with a finger. An anterior pack is then placed and the posterior pack sutures tied. The remaining pack sutures are pulled out the mouth and taped to the face. This allows removal of the pack in 4–5 d.

D. Recurrent bleeding. Recurrent bleeding after removal of a posterior pack is an indication for either angiography with embolization of the causative vessel or endoscopic cauterization. When this fails, surgery is needed to ligate the internal maxillary artery plus, possibly, the anterior and posterior ethmoid arteries.

29. EPIDURAL CATHETER PROBLEMS

I. **Problem.** A nurse reports the inadvertent dislodgement of an epidural catheter in a patient 1 d after a radical nephrectomy.

II. **Immediate Questions.** Lumbar epidural catheters, usually placed for intraoperative anesthesia, are also used for postoperative analgesia. A pump (or intermittent injection) is used to infuse narcotics or local anesthetics into the extradural space via a soft catheter.

A. **When was the last dose of epidural narcotic?** Long-acting narcotics (eg, morphine) can provide reliable analgesia for 12–18 h after each epidural dose.

B. **Is the patient in pain?** Arrange to start IV narcotics with a PCA (patient-controlled analgesia) pump or IM narcotics (prn injections) as normally done with patients who have not received epidural narcotics after surgery. There is a risk of respiratory depression with epidural narcotics, and this risk is increased when IV or IM narcotics are used at the same time. If the patient is in pain but received epidural narcotics before the catheter came out, you may wish to wait 10–15 min to see whether the epidural injection will be adequate. If you choose to give IV or IM narcotics soon after epidural narcotics, monitor the patient closely for an hour or two.

C. **Is the patient otherwise stable?** Delayed respiratory depression can occur from systemic absorption of narcotics. Local anesthetics injected into the epidural space can occasionally cause a sympathetic block and hypotension. Unintentional intravascular injection can exacerbate both of these complications. Although unusual, subarachnoid injection can lead to delayed cardiovascular collapse (usually 15–30 min after injection).

D. **Is the catheter tip intact?** A retained epidural catheter tip can lead to infectious complications, such as an epidural abscess. The tip of the catheter is marked by a black dot.

III. **Database**

A. **Physical Exam Key Points**

1. **Vital signs.** Compare the patient's vital signs with their vital signs before their last epidural injection. Both respiratory depression and hypotension can have an insidious onset, sometimes hours after the last epidural dose.
2. **Chest.** Check breath sounds for depth and rate.
3. **Neurologic.** Check mental status, determine the level of anesthesia, if still present, as well as motor and sensory function. The patient should be able to move their feet and feel your touch. Rarely, epidural hematomas

can occur, causing symptoms of an epidural mass that requires immediate neurosurgical decompression.

4. **Catheter exit site.** Examine for bleeding and signs of infection.
5. **Catheter tip.** Examine the tip to make sure the entire catheter has been removed. Document this in the chart.

B. Laboratory Data. Generally of little value unless coagulopathy or cardiopulmonary complications arise.

C. Radiographic and Other Studies. Usually not needed.

IV. Plan

A. Ensure that no complications of epidural anesthesia have occurred.

1. **Overmedication.** If the patient is oversedated, arrange to decrease the amount or frequency of dosing (you may need to speak with the anesthesia staff); make sure to provide adequate monitoring and support for the patient. Because of the risk of overmedication, patients receiving epidural anesthesia should remain in a monitored setting.
2. **Hematoma.** Diagnose and correct any coagulopathy and contact the neurosurgical service immediately.
3. **Inadvertent subarachnoid puncture.** Can cause a severe frontal or occipital headache that is exacerbated by sitting up. The initial treatment includes bed rest, caffeine, and analgesics. When the headache lasts more than 24 h, a "blood patch" procedure can be performed by the anesthesiologist. This generally provides relief within 30 min, and can be repeated if there is no improvement. When the pain persists, an alternate explanation for the headache must be sought (migraine, meningitis, cortical vein thrombosis, intracranial hemorrhage).
4. **Urinary retention.** This is infrequently seen with epidural anesthesia; use a Foley catheter to drain the bladder.
5. **Itching.** Commonly seen. Treat with Benadryl 25–50 mg IM or PO.

B. Analgesia. If the epidural catheter is not providing adequate pain relief, use additional IV, IM, or PO analgesics. Make sure you know the last dose given through the catheter to avoid overmedication.

C. Wound care. Cover the site with a sterile, dry dressing and inspect daily for signs of infection.

D. Positioning. Patients should remain recumbent for a few hours after catheter removal to prevent a "spinal headache."

30. FALL FROM BED

I. **Problem.** The day after an open reduction and internal fixation of a humeral fracture, a 60-year-old man fell out of bed while trying to go to the bathroom. He has a laceration on his forehead.

II. **Immediate Questions.** Most falls from bed are not associated with serious injury. However, they are extremely upsetting to the patient and the patient's family. Every fall from bed warrants a complete evaluation, documentation of the incident, and thorough search for injury. Pay attention to the "ABCs."

A. **Is the patient able to speak?** Quickly assess the airway and mental status by having the patient answer the question "What happened?"

B. **Is the patient back in bed?** To avoid further injury, log roll patient onto a back board, use in-line traction or cervical immobilization before placing patient back in bed. Assume that the patient has a cervical spine injury and place the patient in a soft cervical collar.

C. **Is the patient in pain?** Pain will guide you to the obvious injuries. Perform a thorough physical exam, as with a trauma patient.

III. **Differential Diagnosis.** History obtained from the patient, visitors, and staff may be helpful in determining the underlying reason for the fall. Specific injuries will not be covered here. Head injury, skeletal fractures and dislocations lead the list. Review the patient's medication list, focusing on any recent medications the patient may have received.

A. **Delirium.** See Problem 25, page 109 for a complete list.

B. **Dementia.** A preexisting risk factor for falling that should be recognized to prevent falls. A minimental status examination may be helpful.

C. **Acute Change in Neurologic Status.** See Problem 14, page 70 and Problem 17, page 81.

D. Delayed recovery from anesthesia.

E. Musculoskeletal weakness in postoperative period.

IV. **Database**

A. **Physical Exam Key Points**

1. **Vital signs.** Check for fever (which can cloud the sensorium), hypotension (a factor for' septic or cardiogenic

shock), arrhythmias, as well as the respiratory rate and pattern.

2. **HEENT.** Closely examine the scalp and face for signs of head injury, perform a cranial nerve exam, and examine the teeth.
3. **Neck.** JVD, C-spine tenderness, nuchal rigidity.
4. **Chest.** Listen for bilateral breath sounds, wheezing, consolidation, cardiac murmurs, and palpate the ribs.
5. **Abdomen.** Tenderness suggests an abdominal injury.
6. **Skin.** Bruising, lacerations.
7. **Extremities.** Is there tenderness or obvious fractures? Check IV lines.

B. Laboratory Data

1. **CBC.** Anemia, infection.
2. **Serum electrolytes.** Hypo- and hyperglycemia, kalemia, calcemia, natremia, and magnesemia; uremia, ammonia.
3. **Cardiac enzymes.** If MI suspected.
4. **Toxic drug screen.** If clinically indicated.
5. **Arterial and venous blood gases.** Acid-base disorders, hypoxia.
6. **Cultures.** Blood, urine, and sputum, if infection is suspected.

C. Radiographic and Other Studies

1. **ECG.** If an MI is suspected or an arrhythmia is noted.
2. **Chest radiograph.** When a respiratory or infectious source is likely and also to check for fractures. Rib detail films may be needed as rib fractures are hard to see on standard chest radiographs.
3. **Head CT.** For a change in mental status.
4. **Plain radiographs.** For tender extremities or joints to check for a fracture or dislocation.
5. **Lumbar puncture.** If indicated.(Check for nuchal rigidity)
6. **EEG.** If indicated.
7. **Pulse oximetry.** A noninvasive means of checking hypoxia.

V. Plan. Overall, look for and treat the underlying cause for the fall. See Problem 17, page 81 and Problem 14, page 70 for specific treatment plans.

A. Fractures and dislocations should be splinted and the orthopedic service contacted for definitive care and follow-up. Always check for distal pulses before and after splinting.

B. Lacerations should be cleaned and sutured. Provide local wound care for abrasions.

C. When a C-spine injury is suspected, immobilize the neck and keep the patient flat until the spine can be evaluated radiographically.

D. **Prevent Further Injury.** Mild sedation may be warranted (perform a brief mental status exam with Glasgow Coma Scale [GCS] before sedation). Make sure that the side rails of the bed are up and that the patient is able to reach and use the nurse call button. Use restraints when necessary. Weak or elderly patients may benefit from physical therapy (to improve their strength and balance) and a bedside commode (to minimize the distance they must to walk to use the toilet).

E. **Incident Report.** Document the incident in the chart and complete the appropriate forms for risk management.

31. FEVER

I. **Problem.** You are notified that a patient on another service who had a gastrectomy for cancer has a fever of 38.9 °C.

II. **Immediate Questions**

A. **How many days postop is the patient?** Most medical students know the mnemonic for postoperative fever: "The Five Ws: wind, water, walk, wound, wonder drugs." When the patient is female, you may also consider the uterus (womb). The time since operation helps to focus one's attention on the likely diagnosis. These five causes, in order from the mnemonic, are pneumonia, urinary tract infection, thrombophlebitis, wound infection, and drug reaction.

B. **What is the fever pattern?** Check the chart for the previous 2–3 d to see any emerging or changing fever patterns. Spiking fevers are often associated with infections in a closed space (ie, abscesses). Continual fevers are often found with vascular involvement, such as infected prosthetic grafts or septic phlebitis.

C. **Does the patient have chills/rigors with the fever?** Often rigors are associated with more serious fevers and indicate bacteremia. Fevers associated with drug reactions or atelectasis usually do not have associated rigors.

D. **Did the patient have fevers before the operation?** A patient may have a chronic disease associated with fever (lymphoma, etc). Even if the patient does not have one of these diagnoses, remember them when no other source can be found for the fever.

E. **Has the patient recently stopped taking an antipyretic agent?** Occasionally a new fever has been suppressed in patients taking aspirin, acetaminophen, or NSAIDs. Noting this may be of importance in diagnosing the fever.

F. **Has the patient recently been taking antibiotics?** Find out why, which drug, the start of treatment, and the time of the last dose.

G. **Are there any associated complaints, such as cough, dysuria, diarrhea, abdominal pain, or pain around any IV sites or incisions?** These may point to the cause of the fever.

H. **Is the patient immunocompromised?** This could be a neutropenic fever.

III. **Differential Diagnosis.** A febrile patient seen in an emergency room or in an outpatient setting usually has an acute infection that is readily diagnosed from associated complaints. This is not true of febrile patients on a surgical service. Most of these patients have a postoperative fever, although occasional patients (postoperative or otherwise) have a fever of unknown origin (defined as a temperature of at least 38.5 °C daily for at least 3 wk and no diagnosis after 1 wk of in-hospital investigation). The differential diagnosis of postoperative fever and fever of unknown origin is given below.

A. **Postoperative Fever**
   1. **Atelectasis.** The fever is usually < 39° C and occurs in first 12–48 h postop.
   2. **Urinary tract infection.** Typically occurs 3–5 d postop following urinary tract manipulation (with a Foley catheter).
   3. **IV catheter infection.** The longer a catheter is left in, the higher the risk of infection.
      a. **Peripheral:** The site will often appear infected.
      b. **Central:** Diagnosed by culturing the catheter tip. A positive blood culture for gram-positive cocci should lead to a high degree of clinical suspicion.
   4. **Deep venous thrombosis.** The fever is usually low grade (37.5–38.5 °C). Pulmonary embolus may also have an associated low grade fever.
   5. **Wound infection**
      a. **Early:** Infections occurring within 12–36 h of surgery are usually caused by *Clostridium* species or *Streptococcus* species. These infections are characterized by drainage that appears like "dirty dishwater," that is, thin, serous drainage. When there is concern about the possibility of these types of infections, rapid surgi-

cal wound exploration and debridement is mandatory along with appropriate antibiotic coverage. There is no place for watchful waiting or observation pending culture results in these rapidly spreading highly lethal infections.

b. **Late:** Most wound infections and abscesses occur 5–8 d postop, and common organisms include *Staphylococcus* species, *E coli*, *Pseudomonas* species, and others.

6. **Drug reaction.** Most commonly caused by antibiotics (penicillins, cephalosporins).
7. **CNS origin.** Central fever occurs in trauma patients with head injuries, and meningitis occurs as a complication of spinal anesthesia.
8. **Thyroid storm.** Following thyroidectomy for Graves' disease.
9. **Blood transfusion.** See Problem 68, page 247.
10. **Postpericardiotomy syndrome.** Usually seen 5–7 d after cardiac surgery.
11. **Anastomotic bowel leak.** Usually seen 7–10 d postop. Most patients have signs of peritoneal irritation.
12. **Otitis, sialadenitis, sinusitis.** Especially in patients with long-term nasogastric tubes.
13. **Parotitis.** Rarely seen in patients who have been NPO for a prolonged time.
14. **Addisonian crisis.**
15. **Acalculous cholecystitis.** May be seen after prolonged periods of being NPO (where the gallbladder does not empty); this condition is associated with trauma and other severe illnesses.
16. **Pancreatitis.**
17. ***Clostridium difficile* enterocolitis.** Typically diffuse green, watery, foul-smelling, or bloody diarrhea.
18. **Diabetic ketoacidosis.** Systemic infections put diabetes out of control.

B. **Fever of Unknown Origin**

1. **Infections**
   a. **Granulomatous:** Caused by *Mycobacterium* or fungal agents.
   b. **Endocarditis:** Especially with valvular heart disease.
   c. **Abscess:** Hepatic, subphrenic renal or pelvic.
   d. **Parasites:** May have frequent temperatures and eosinophilia.
2. **Neoplastic.** Fevers can be a part of a "paraneoplastic syndrome."
   a. Lymphoma.
   b. Renal cell carcinoma.
   c. Hepatic metastatic disease.

3. **Connective tissue disease**
   a. Systemic lupus erythematosus.
   b. Rheumatoid arthritis (usually juvenile).
   c. Polymyalgia rheumatica.
4. **Miscellaneous**
   a. Drug reaction.
   b. Recurrent pulmonary emboli/pelvic or deep vein thromboses.
   c. Inflammatory bowel disease.

IV. Database

A. Physical Exam Key Points

1. **Vital signs.** Document all fevers rectally. Check orthostatic vital signs.
2. **Skin.** Examine wounds and all past and current IV sites.
3. **HEENT.** Check for sialadenitis, otitis, and pharyngitis.
4. **Pulmonary.** Listen for rhonchi, rubs, and evidence of consolidation.
5. **Abdomen.** Palpate for right upper quadrant tenderness or peritoneal signs.
6. **Trunk.** Is there costovertebral angle tenderness?
7. **Extremities.** Rule out deep venous thrombosis (pain, swelling, etc).
8. **Wound.** Check the wound for erythema, a fluid collection, subcutaneous air, crepitation, and tenderness. If the wound is relatively recent, remember to use strict aseptic technique. Culture any drainage.
9. **Pelvic examination.** To look for evidence of a pelvic source.

B. Laboratory Data

1. **Hemogram.** Leukocytosis and left shift suggest infection. Anemia may be seen with endocarditis.
2. **Electrolytes.** Hyponatremia and hyperkalemia occur in an addisonian crisis.
3. **Thyroid hormone levels,** T_3 and T_4.
4. **Urinalysis,** Gram's stain and culture.
5. **Throat culture** if indicated.
6. **Wound culture** if indicated.
7. **Blood cultures** should be obtained, ideally from different sites at different times. If there is a central line, drawback blood cultures through the central line, or remove the line and culture the tip. Line exit site cultures are rarely helpful. Multiple cultures on different days may be best for endocarditis.
8. **Sputum Gram stain** and culture if indicated.
9. **Stool for fecal leukocytes** and *C difficile* toxin assay.

C. **Radiographic and Other Studies**
1. **Chest radiograph.** Linear densities occur with atelectasis; infiltrates with pneumonia; wedge-shaped infarction can occasionally be seen with pulmonary emboli.
2. **ECG.** ST elevations in postpericardiotomy syndrome.
3. **Venous Dopplers/Venogram.** If deep venous thrombosis suspected.
4. **Abdominal CT.** For evaluation of intra-abdominal abscess. Ultrasound is good for hepatic or subphrenic abscesses but a CT scan is the procedure of choice (if available and if the patient can be moved).
5. **Abdominal Ultrasound.** In acalculous cholecystitis, there may be thickening of the gallbladder wall and pericholecystic fluid.
6. **HIDA scan.** May be useful in acute acalculous cholecystitis, although unreliable if the patient has not eaten.
7. **Other nuclear scans.** Using gallium- or indium-labeled WBCs may help identify an otherwise elusive abscess. These are not normally used as a primary diagnostic modality with surgical patients. Recent surgery can lead to enough inflammation to cause a false-positive scan.

V. **Plan.** The primary goal is to diagnose and treat the underlying cause. A second goal is to treat the fever. Antipyretics can be given with caution after cultures are obtained. In some cases, proper management can prevent a fever.

A. **Treatment of Specific Causes**
1. **Atelectasis and pneumonia**
   a. Incentive spirometry, ambulation and coughing are general measures to both treat and help prevent atelectasis and pneumonia.
   b. For pneumonia, antibiotics are empirically started, based on the Gram's stain, and adjusted on the basis of culture results. Antibiotics should be tailored to the susceptibility pattern of organisms at your particular hospital, because most hospital-acquired pneumonias are caused by nosocomial organisms.
2. **Urinary tract infection.** See Problem 27, page 117.
3. **IV catheter sepsis**
   a. **Peripheral:** Remove all suspicious catheters and apply heat to the area. Cefazolin or dicloxacillin can be used to cover *Staphylococcus* if required. Observe for suppurative phlebitis, which usually requires vein excision.
   b. **Central:** Optimally remove the line, and treat with antibiotics (cephalosporin, oxacillin, or vancomycin)

for 1–2 d while awaiting culture results. (see Problem 20, page 90). If you obtain peripheral cultures and cultures drawn through the line (obtained in Isolator tubes), you can compare the number of colonies. If the number of colonies in the line culture is less than 5 times the number in the peripherally obtained culture, the line is not the source of sepsis.

4. **Thyroid storm.** Treat with propylthiouracil (PTU) 400 mg q6h, sodium iodide 250 mg PO/IV q6h, propranolol 1 mg/min IV for 2.8 min, and hydrocortisone 100 mg IV.
5. **Postpericardiotomy.** Use indomethacin 25–50 mg tid with food or antacids.
6. **Addisonian crisis.** Treat with 100 mg hydrocortisone IV q8h.
7. **Wound infection.** Open the wound carefully, culture any drainage, and pack the wound with saline-moistened gauze. Dress the wound with dry gauze. Change 3 times daily. Notify the attending surgeon when there is evidence of fascial dehiscence, as operative intervention may be necessary. When dealing with clostridial infections or any form of necrotizing fasciitis, rapid surgical debridement in the operating room is mandatory.
8. ***C difficile* colitis.** (See page 98).

B. **Treatment of Fever**

1. **Antipyretics.** Acetaminophen 650 mg PO/pr q4–6h is preferred, because aspirin inhibits platelet function. Fever does not necessarily require treatment unless the patient is uncomfortable or tachycardic.
2. **Maintain adequate hydration.** Fever increases baseline fluid requirements 500 mL per 24 h for each degree centigrade above 38.3 °C (101 °F).
3. **Cooling blanket.** Useful for lowering the body temperature.

C. **Preventive Measures**

1. **Atelectasis.** Have smokers quit for a few weeks before an elective operation. Teach patients incentive spirometry preoperatively.
2. **Intravenous catheters.** Change peripheral IVs routinely every 2–3 d or sooner if the patient gets recurring phlebitis.
3. Deep venous thrombosis
   a. Early ambulation should be encouraged.
   b. For high risk patients (obesity, prior DVT, neoplasia), consider subcutaneous heparin.
   c. Many surgeons routinely use sequential compression stockings in any patient undergoing a proce-

dure that requires general or regional anesthesia. These are used postoperatively until the patient is ambulatory. Bedridden preoperative patients may also benefit.

4. **Blood transfusion.** The administration of acetaminophen 650 mg and diphenhydramine (Benadryl) 25–50 mg IM or PO, given about 30 min before transfusion, may blunt the febrile response in patients with a history of transfusion reaction.
5. **Thyroid storm.** Use SSKI (saturated solution of potassium iodide) [KI] 2 drops tid and propranolol 20–40 mg PO qid for 7–10 d before surgery.

32. FOLEY CATHETER PROBLEMS

(Bladder catheterization is discussed in Section III, Bedside Procedures.)

I. **Problem.** The Foley catheter is not draining 2 d after a sigmoid colon resection.

II. **Immediate Questions**

A. **What has the urine output been?** If the urine output has slowly tapered off, then the problem may be oliguria rather than a nonfunctioning Foley catheter. A Foley catheter that has never put out urine may not be in the bladder.

B. **Is the urine grossly bloody; are there any clots in the tubing or collection bag?** Clots or tissue fragments, such as those present after a prostate or bladder resection, can obstruct the flow of urine in a Foley catheter. Similarly, bladder trauma during an abdominal operation can lead to hematuria.

C. **Is the patient complaining of any pain?** Bladder distention often causes severe lower abdominal pain; bladder spasms are painful and may cause urine to leak out around the catheter rather than through the catheter.

D. **Was any difficulty encountered in catheter insertion?** Problematic urethral catheterization should raise concern that the catheter may not be in the bladder.

E. **How is the catheter secured in place?** Sometimes a suture or wire may restrict the flow, or the catheter may have been damaged during placement. Has anyone tried to flush the catheter? This often helps to relieve the obstruction from a clot or debris.

III. Differential Diagnosis

A. Low Urine Output. This may be a result of dehydration, hemorrhage, acute renal failure, as well as a host of other causes (see Problem 56, page 213).

B. Obstructed Foley Catheter

1. Kinking of the catheter or tubing.
2. **Clots, tissue fragments.** Most common after transurethral resection of the prostate or bladder. Grossly bloody urine suggests a clot has formed. "Tea-colored" or "rusty" urine suggests an organized clot may be present even though the urine is no longer grossly bloody. Bleeding will often accompany "accidental" catheter removal where the catheter is removed with the balloon inflated. Bleeding may also suggest a coagulopathy.
3. **Sediment/stones.** Chronically indwelling catheters (usually 1 mo) can become encrusted and obstructed. Calculi can lodge in the catheter.

C. Improperly Positioned Foley Catheter. These problems are much more common in males. In traumatic urethral disruption associated with a pelvic fracture, the catheter can pass into the periurethral tissues. Strictures or prostatic hypertrophy may cause the end of the catheter to be positioned in the urethra and not the bladder.

D. Bladder Spasms. The patient may complain of severe suprapubic pain or pain radiating to the end of the penis. With a spasm, urine may leak around the sides of the catheter. Spasms are common after bladder or prostate surgery or surgery around the bladder. Spasms may be the only catheter complaint or may be so severe as to obstruct the flow of urine.

E. Bladder Disruption. Resulting from blunt abdominal trauma, operative complication, or caused by severe distention secondary to a blocked catheter.

F. Inability to Deflate the Foley Balloon. This is rare with modern catheters. All catheters should be tested before use.

IV. Database

A. Physical Exam Key Points

1. **Vital signs.** Check for tachycardia and hypotension, which are characteristic of hypovolemia.
2. **Abdominal exam.** Determine if the bladder is distended (suprapubic dullness to percussion with or without tenderness); a distended bladder suggests an

obstructed Foley catheter. Percuss the bladder to help identify distention. Small bedside ultrasound units are available for nurses to assess bladder filling.

3. **Genital exam.** Bleeding at the meatus suggests urethral trauma (either before Foley insertion or from partial removal of the catheter with the balloon inflated).
4. **Rectal exam.** A "floating prostate" suggests urethral disruption. This usually accompanies a pelvic fracture secondary to blunt trauma.
5. **General.** Look for signs of hypovolemia causing low urine output, such as skin turgor, mucous membrane appearance, etc.

B. Laboratory Data. Most problems are mechanical in nature so that laboratory data is rarely helpful.

1. **BUN, serum creatinine.** Elevations may be seen with cases of renal insufficiency.
2. **Coagulation studies.** Abnormal when there is severe bleeding.

C. Radiographic and Other Studies. Plain radiographs are rarely helpful. Abdominal ultrasound may demonstrate hydronephrosis in cases of obstructive uropathy; bladder ultrasound may confirm distention.

V. Plan

A. First, be sure the catheter is functioning. As a rule of thumb, a catheter that will not irrigate is in the urethra and not in the bladder. Start by gently irrigating the catheter with aseptic technique using a catheter-tipped 60-mL syringe and sterile normal saline. This may dislodge any clots obstructing the catheter. If sterile saline cannot be satisfactorily instilled and aspirated, the catheter should be replaced. Use extreme care when irrigating or changing the catheter in any patient who has undergone bladder or prostate surgery.

B. If the catheter irrigates freely, workup the patient for anuria. See Problem 56, page 213.

C. Bladder spasms can be treated with oxybutynin (Ditropan), propantheline (Pro-Banthine) or belladonna and opium (B&O) suppositories. (See dosage in Section IX, page 441). Be **sure** to discontinue these medications before removing the catheter to allow normal bladder function.

D. Techniques to deflate a balloon that will not empty include:

1. Injecting 5–10 mL mineral oil into the inflation port. This will cause balloon rupture (in latex catheters) in 5–10 min. Follow-up cystoscopy is recommended to make sure there are no retained fragments.

2. **2.** Threading a 16–Fr central venous catheter or a 0.035–in guidewire into the inflation channel (after the valve is removed). This may bypass the obstruction or allow the balloon to be perforated.
3. **3.** As a last resort, puncturing the balloon with an ultrasound-guided transvesical needle may be needed.

33. HEADACHE

I. Problem. A 42–year-old man complaining of a headache comes to the clinic 4 d after inguinal hernia repair performed under spinal anesthesia.

II. Immediate Questions

A. What does the headache feel like? Is it similar to previous headaches? A patient complaining about "the worst headache of his life," perhaps associated with vomiting and stiff neck, may have a subarachnoid bleed or meningitis. Unlike most other causes of headache, these require emergent attention.

B. What makes the headache better or worse? Spinal headaches typically become worse as the patient sits up and get better when the patient lies flat.

III. Differential Diagnosis

A. Spinal Headache. Relatively common after spinal anesthesia or lumbar puncture, these are caused by a slow leak of CSF. The use of smaller spinal needles has reduced the incidence of such headaches.

B. Sinusitis. Often associated facial pain that can be reproduced by applying pressure over the sinus.

C. Vascular

1. **Cluster headaches and migraine headaches.** These are usually recurrent and unilateral.
2. **Subarachnoid hemorrhage.** Often leads to severe headache and nuchal rigidity.
3. **Others.** Giant cell arteritis, subdural and epidural hematoma may cause headaches.

D. Tension. This is by far the most common cause of headaches. Patients usually describe a constant, band-like pressure, often occipital and frequently associated with muscular tension in the neck.

E. Neoplastic. Rarely causes headache in the absence of other focal neurologic abnormalities.

F. Meningitis. Nausea, vomiting, headache, fevers, and a stiff neck are hallmarks of this disease.

G. **Other.** Fever, dehydration, trauma, hypertension, and systemic viral illnesses can cause headache.

IV. Database

A. **History.** Determine if the patient had a recent operation under spinal anesthesia. Is there a history of similar headaches and associated symptoms, such as scotomata or nausea and vomiting?

B. **Physical Exam**

1. **Vital signs.** Check the temperature and blood pressure.
2. **Head and neck**
   a. Nuchal rigidity may indicate subarachnoid irritation or meningitis.
   b. Injected conjunctiva and excessive tearing are common with migraines.
   c. Percuss sinuses looking for tenderness.
   d. Tenderness over the temporal artery is associated with temporal arteritis.
   e. Papilledema suggests increased intracranial pressure (eg, a space-occupying lesion).
   f. Tight trapezius muscles are associated with tension headaches.

C. **Laboratory Data**

1. **CBC.** An elevated white count may indicate infection.
2. **Erythrocyte sedimentation rate (ESR).** A nonspecific test, but often elevated in temporal arteritis.

D. **Radiographic and Other Studies**

1. **Head CT scan.** A scan of the head can be performed if subarachnoid hemorrhage is suspected or in new-onset severe headaches to rule out an intracranial mass. Sinusitis can also be detected by CT scan. A CT is indicated when the neurologic exam reveals focal findings. If the headaches are recurrent and typical for migraines or cluster headaches, a CT scan is usually not necessary.

V. Plan.

A careful history and exam reveal the benign nature of most headaches. The most common treatment is acetaminophen or aspirin as needed. Occasionally, narcotic pain medication may be needed.

A. **Spinal headaches.** Headaches after lumbar puncture for spinal anesthesia can be very persistent. The initial treatment is rest in a supine position, analgesics, and IV hydration. Refractory spinal headaches can be treated by injecting an autologous blood "patch" into the epidural space to seal the dural leak.

B. Migraine

1. **Acute therapy for a mild-moderate migraine.** Standard analgesics are usually effective, including NSAIDs, Fiorinal, Midrin, and butorphanol nasal spray (once in each nostril, repeat in 3–5 h).
2. **Acute therapy for a severe migraine.** Use sumatriptan (Imitrex) 6 mg SQ or dihydroergotamine (DHE 45) 1 mg IM, repeat 2 times at 1–h intervals if needed.
3. Some migraine patients require chronic prophylaxis with β-blockers, tricyclic antidepressants (amitriptyline), or methysergide.

C. Intracranial Tumor or Subarachnoid Hemorrhage. Obtain urgent neurosurgical consultation.

D. Infections. Acute sinusitis can be treated with oral antibiotics, such as trimethoprim/sulfamethoxazole. Frontal sinusitis may need to be drained by an ENT physician. Meningitis requires urgent treatment with high dose antibiotics.

34. HEMATEMESIS

Immediate Actions

Treat these patients like a trauma patient!

1. Assess **A**irway, **B**reathing, and **C**irculation.
2. Obtain vital signs.
3. Intubate if necessary.
4. Ensure large-bore IV access and begin IV fluid or blood resuscitation.
5. Place an NG tube.

I. Problem. A patient admitted for an elective Le Veen shunt suddenly begins vomiting blood.

II. Immediate Questions

A. What are the blood pressure and orthostatic signs? The initial management focuses on maintaining intravascular volume and perfusion pressure.

B. Are there any bleeding tendencies? Review available history, physical exam, and lab data regarding any correctable coagulation problem (PT, PTT, platelet count).

C. Are there any stigmata of alcohol abuse? Look for signs of portal hypertension (ascites, caput medusae, etc.) and an elevated blood alcohol level.

D. **Did the patient retch or vomit before the hematemesis began?** A Mallory-Weiss tear is the fourth most common cause of hematemesis in most series.

E. **Does the patient have any history of aortic disease or a prior aortic vascular procedure?** Although an uncommon cause of hematemesis, aortoduodenal fistula should always be included in the initial differential diagnosis of upper GI bleeding when the patient has a history of prior aortic surgery. Primary aortoduodenal fistula (in the absence of prior aortic surgery) has been reported but is extremely rare and almost always fatal.

III. **Differential Diagnosis.** Hematemesis is virtually always associated with bleeding proximal to the ligament of Treitz. The converse, however, is certainly not true (see Problem 10, page [41]). Esophageal varices, ulcer disease, gastritis, and Mallory-Weiss tears account for 90–95% of episodes of hematemesis.

A. **Esophagus**
   1. **Esophageal varices.** This is the most common cause of upper GI bleeding. It is associated with cirrhosis and portal hypertension.
   2. **Mallory-Weiss tear.** Usually a mucosal tear at the gastroesophageal junction, associated with severe retching with or without vomiting.
   3. **Esophagitis.** Caused by gastroesophageal reflux (GERD). Patients usually have a history of heartburn, waking up with an acidic taste or food in the mouth, and worsening of symptoms with recumbency.
   4. **Esophageal tumors.** These may be benign, squamous carcinomas, or adenocarcinomas.

B. **Stomach**
   1. **Gastritis.** Significant hematemesis may occur with alcoholic gastritis or stress-induced (ICU) gastritis.
   2. **Gastric ulcer.** Symptoms can include severe pain, abdominal distension, nausea and vomiting.
   3. **Gastric tumors.** Rarely demonstrate bleeding. Associated with weight loss and inability to tolerate food.
   4. **Gastric varices.** Almost always associated with esophageal varices. Usually caused by portal hypertension; occasionally caused by splenic vein thrombosis without portal hypertension.

C. **Duodenum**
   1. **Duodenal ulcer**
   2. **Aortoduodenal fistula.** Almost exclusively seen after aortic reconstruction.
   3. **Postendoscopic sphincterotomy.**

D. Hemobilia. Usually caused by hepatic tumors, vascular malformations (AVMs), biliary trauma, and iatrogenic causes.

E. Systemic Causes

1. **Coagulopathy** (DIC, leukemia, etc).
2. **Osler-Weber-Rendu.** Associated with multiple telangiectases.
3. **Peutz-Jeghers.** Associated with multiple hamartomas.

F. Non-GI source. Nasopharyngeal bleeding (see Problem 28, page [119]).

IV. Database

A. Physical Exam Key Points

1. **Vital signs.** Obtain orthostatic vital signs in addition to supine pulse and blood pressure measurements. (Determine the pulse and blood pressure after the patient has been in the supine position for 5 min. Next, have the patient stand or dangle their legs off the side of the bed. At 1 min, determine the pulse and BP. A drop in BP of 10–20 mm Hg or an increase in pulse of 10 beats per minute suggests volume depletion.) Supine tachycardia or hypotension suggests a higher degree of hypovolemia.
2. **Skin.** Cool, moist, pale skin indicates volume loss. Look for evidence of alcohol abuse, such as spider angiomata or palmar erythema, and for signs of systemic disease, such as multiple bruises, telangiectases, or hamartomas of the lips and oral mucosa.
3. **HEENT.** Is there evidence of epistaxis suggesting a nasopharyngeal source?
4. **Abdomen.** Look for scars from prior ulcer, vascular, or other procedures, and for signs of portal hypertension (hepatosplenomegaly, caput medusa, or ascites). Does the patient have abdominal tenderness or peritoneal signs?
5. **Rectal.** Check for gross blood or melena. Perform a guaiac test.
6. **Genitourinary.** Testicular atrophy and gynecomastia suggest cirrhosis.

B. Laboratory Data

1. **CBC.** Obtain serial hematocrits (about every 4h) and document the time drawn and relation to transfusions.
2. **Platelet count.** Keep the platelet count above 40,000.
3. **PT/PTT.** Helps to identify coagulopathies. The PT can also be used to track liver synthetic function.
4. **Renal function.** Should be determined as a baseline.
5. **Liver function tests.** Identifies the presence and extent of liver disease.

6. **Blood bank specimen.** Remember to type and crossmatch the patient for up to 6–10 U of PRBCs, when you draw blood for the patient's initial lab work.

C. **Radiographic and Other Studies**
   1. **Chest radiograph.** Look for mediastinal air (in Boerhaave's syndrome), evidence of aspiration, free air under the diaphragm (with a perforated ulcer).
   2. **Upper endoscopy.** This is the diagnostic and therapeutic procedure of choice. The endoscopist should be contacted immediately for urgent esophagogastroduodenoscopy (EGD). If the patient's stomach is full (with food or blood), protect the patient's airway (with intubation or 6–8 h of NG suction) before administering sedation for EGD.
   3. **UGI series.** This test may be used when endoscopy is unavailable and when bleeding has stopped. It interferes with endoscopy and angiography, so it is not usually a first-line study.
   4. **Angiogram.** Rarely used unless endoscopy does not identify the source.

V. **Plan.** The normal algorithm is to treat patients for volume loss, establish a diagnosis, and then implement specific therapies. Eighty-five percent of cases of UGI bleeding resolve without operative intervention. Regardless of diagnosis, continued bleeding requires appropriate surgical intervention

A. **Initial Management.** Make sure there is at least one large-bore IV (18 gauge or larger). If the patient needs blood for hypotension or rapid bleeding, one 18–gauge IV will be inadequate (as in trauma). Central lines are helpful to monitor CVP or to infuse crystalloid. For blood transfusion, a short peripheral 16–gauge IV is better.
   1. **Type and crossmatch** the patient for packed red blood cells (6 U minimum).
   2. **Place an NG tube.** This documents ongoing bleeding and clears the stomach for endoscopy. Irrigate the stomach until free of clots. Use an Ewald tube if necessary.
   3. **Monitor volume replacement.**
      a. Always chart the serial hematocrits and the timing and amount of transfusions, because these indicators reflect the rate of bleeding, which is the major criterion in many instances for deciding whether surgery is needed.
      b. Foley catheter. Try to keep the urine output more than 30 cc/h.
      c. A central line or a Swan-Ganz catheter may be needed, especially in patients with cardiac/respiratory disease.

4. Correct any coagulopathy with platelets or FFP as indicated.
5. Consider intubation to protect the patient from aspirating.

B. **Specific Treatment.** After acute bleeding is stabilized.
   1. **Ulcer**
      a. **Administer antacids** via the NG tube q1–2 h.
      b. **IV H_2-receptor blockers (cimetidine, ranitidine).** May prevent rebleeding but probably does not stop ongoing bleeding.
      c. **Endoscopic coagulation or heater probe.** When this fails to control bleeding, the patient will need surgical intervention. Note that bleeding from a posterior duodenal ulcer usually arises from the gastroduodenal artery and is particularly concerning. Massive bleeding or active bleeding from a "visible vessel" will usually require surgical intervention.
   2. **Stress gastritis**
      a. Antacids and IV H_2-receptor blockers.
      b. **Endoscopic coagulation.** When this fails, the patient may need urgent surgical resection.
   3. **Esophageal varices**
      a. Injection sclerotherapy by endoscopy.
      b. IV Octreotide.
      c. Balloon tamponade (Sengstaken-Blakemore or Minnesota Tube) when sclerotherapy is unsucceful. Should be placed only if you are experienced with these devices, as there are many complications (aspiration, respiratory arrest, and esophageal rupture).
      d. Consider emergency portocaval shunt or TIPS procedure (radiographic transjugular intrahepatic portocaval shunting).
      e. In rare circumstances, other surgical procedures may be indicated (eg, splenectomy, division and reanastomosis of esophagus, etc.).
   4. **Mallory-Weiss tear**
      a. Bleeding usually stops spontaneously.
      b. Endoscopic coagulation, surgical oversewing, and angiographic embolization are all accepted treatments.

35. HEMATURIA

I. **Problem.** A 51–year-old patient has blood in his urine 3 d after undergoing a vagotomy and pyloroplasty.

II. **Immediate Questions**

A. **Is it gross or microscopic hematuria?** Microscopic hematuria may have been present for a long time and suggests a chronic process, whereas most patients notice and are concerned by gross hematuria.

B. **Does the patient have a Foley catheter or ureteral stents in place?** Foley catheters commonly cause hematuria by irritating the bladder mucosa; however, other causes should be investigated when urine remains bloody after the catheter has been removed. Stents are often placed perioperatively (by cystoscopy) for difficult pelvic cases and can cause minor bleeding.

C. **Has the patient recently undergone abdominal surgery?** Unexpected hematuria the night after surgery may implicate a ureteral, renal or bladder injury.

D. **Does the patient have abdominal pain or fever?** Abdominal pain may suggest an inflammatory or infectious process, particularly when accompanied by fever. Renal colic typically radiates from the flank into the groin.

E. **Is the urine output adequate?** Urine output is the best indicator of renal function and overall perfusion. A sudden decrease in the urine output may indicate an abrupt change in renal function or perfusion, or an outflow obstruction caused by clots or a catheter malfunction.

F. **Does the patient have symptoms of urinary tract infection?** Dysuria, frequency, and urgency are common symptoms associated with urinary tract infections.

G. **What is the history?** A recent cystoscopic procedure (TURP or transurethral resection of a bladder tumor) may explain the bleeding (microscopic hematuria may persist 2–3 mo after TURP). If there is a prior history of a bladder tumor, consider a recurrent tumor. Chemotherapy with agents such as cyclophosphamide (Cytoxan) may cause acute hemorrhagic cystitis and is associated with bladder cancer many years later.

H. **If the patient is female, when was her last period?** Menses will often contaminate the urinalysis.

III. Differential Diagnosis

A. **Foley Catheter Irritation/Trauma.** This should be a diagnosis of exclusion, reached after thorough consideration of alternative possibilities (see Problem 32, page 132.)

B. **Stone.** Hematuria can be caused by a calculus anywhere in the urinary tract (from the kidney to the urethra). It is usually associated with severe abdominal pain, especially when the stone is in the ureter.

C. **Infection.** A urinary tract infection can occasionally cause hematuria. It is important to obtain a clean catch specimen for urinalysis and culture.

D. **Tumor.** Painless hematuria is the sine qua non of bladder tumors and can also occur with renal cell carcinoma or prostatic carcinoma.

E. **Trauma.** Posttraumatic hematuria can be caused by injuries to the kidneys, ureters, bladder, or urethra (secondary to pelvic fractures). A Foley catheter should **not** be inserted in any patient suspected to have a urethral injury (ie, blood at the urethral meatus) until a retrograde urethrogram has been performed to rule out a urethral tear. Iatrogenic trauma should be considered in any patient that has undergone surgery anywhere near the urinary tract.

F. **Excessive Anticoagulation.** This is a common cause of hematuria in anticoagulated patients and requires medication adjustment.

G. **Structural Abnormalities.** Polycystic kidneys and medullary sponge kidneys can bleed; however, it is important to rule out other potential causes of hematuria in patients with known structural abnormalities.

H. **Prostatic Hypertrophy or Cancer.** These are commonly considered in older men, but other causes must be ruled out as well.

I. **Glomerulonephritis.** Red cell casts are often seen on urinalysis.

J. **Enterovesical Fistula.** As with other fistulas to the urinary tract, hematuria is uncommon. Pneumaturia and recurrent urinary tract infections usually lead to this diagnosis.

K. **Vascular.** A variety of vascular problems cause hematuria, including renal infarction, renal vein thrombosis, and A-V malformations.

L. **Renal Papillary Necrosis.** Predominantly a disease of diabetics.

M. **Drugs.** Especially cyclophosphamide, which can cause hemorrhagic cystitis.

N. **Radiation Cystitis.** Commonly seen in patients with rectal or genitourinary malignancies who have been treated with radiation.

O. **Hemorrhagic Cystitis.** Usually a complication of chemotherapy with cyclophosphamide and may predispose to transitional cell carcinoma.

P. **Systemic Diseases.** Systemic lupus erythematosus, hemolytic-uremic syndrome, and Goodpasture's syndrome (see Problem 36, page 146) are all associated with hematuria.

Q. Tuberculosis. Although most patients with TB in the United States have pulmonary tuberculosis, renal involvement does occur. Hematuria is less common than sterile pyuria in these patients.

R. Sickle-cell Anemia. African-American patients with no other cause for hematuria should be evaluated for sickle-cell disease.

S. Contamination. Often caused by menses or dysfunctional uterine bleeding. Check a catheterized specimen to exclude this possibility.

T. Benign Essential Hematuria. This is a diagnosis of exclusion after extensive workup reveals no pathology to explain clinical bleeding.

IV. Database

A. Physical Exam Key Points

1. **Abdominal.** Examine for masses and tenderness that may accompany tumors, infection, sickle cell disease, and inflammatory processes. Flank (costovertebral angle) tenderness suggests ureteral obstruction (from a stone) or pyelonephritis.
2. **Urethral meatus.** Look for gross blood at the meatus, especially in men with pelvic fractures.
3. **Rectal exam.** This may reveal a "free floating prostate" in trauma patients with urethral disruption. Prostatic carcinoma or prostatitis may also be detected.
4. **Pelvic exam.** To exclude cervical bleeding or vaginal pathology.

B. Laboratory Data

1. **Urinalysis.** Red cell casts are associated with upper tract (kidney) bleeding. Myoglobinuria (from crush or electrical injury) may be confused with hematuria (this is diagnosed with blood on the UA, but a zero RBC count).
2. **Clotting studies.** To determine if anticoagulation is a cause of hematuria.
3. **Hemoglobin electrophoresis.** To screen for sickle cell disease as a cause of hematuria.
4. **CBC.** To determine the hematocrit and platelet count.
5. **Urine cytology.** May diagnose transitional cell carcinoma, but not renal cell or prostate carcinoma. Many clinical labs offer "localization" studies whereby the site of bleeding can be identified as renal or postrenal on the basis of RBC morphology.

6. **Urine Culture.** To rule out bacterial infection. Check acid-fast stains on several urine specimens to identify tuberculosis of the urinary tract.
7. **BUN and creatinine.** Baseline renal function should be determined.

C. **Radiographic and Other Studies**
1. **Abdominal plain radiograph.** Most urinary calculi are calcified and visible on plain radiographs.
2. **Excretory urography (IVP).** Usually the first diagnostic test performed after laboratory studies for patients with a suspected urinary calculus.
3. **Retrograde urethrogram/cystogram.** This test should be performed before Foley insertion when there is a suspicion of urethral disruption or bladder rupture (in trauma patients).
4. Other appropriate studies include a CT of the abdomen (especially in trauma patients or patients suspected of having a ureteral stone), an ultrasound (to look for hydronephrosis) with or without color-flow Doppler, a renal perfusion scan, angiography, and cystoscopy.

V. **Plan.** The treatment for hematuria depends on the cause, which can take several days to ascertain. The "standard workup" in the adult is the physical exam, UA, urine culture, urine cytology, intravenous pyelogram, and cystoscopy. Hematuria rarely causes significant blood loss, and as long as renal function and urine output are not impaired, the workup is generally not an emergency.

A. **Gross Hematuria with Clots.** This usually arises from the bladder and is treated with a large irrigating "3–way" Foley catheter, (such as 24–26 Fr, 30 mL balloon). Irrigate out the clots with a 60-mL syringe, because clots can perpetuate the bleeding (this can also be a problem with blood in the stomach or peritoneal cavity.). Continuous irrigation with normal saline will often be necessary to keep the urine clear until the source of bleeding is corrected.

B. **Specific Treatments**
1. **Urinary tract infection.** Treated with appropriate antibiotics. A follow-up urinalysis is needed to document the resolution of hematuria. Recurrent UTIs need further workup.
2. **Urolithiasis.** When the stone is expected to pass spontaneously, (usually less than 1 cm), expectant therapy with analgesics and hydration is customary. Strain the urine to look for the stone. If the stone does not pass, urology consultation (for ureteroscopy) should be obtained.

3. **Tumors.** Requires complete evaluation, usually with abdominal CT and other studies, as indicated by urologic consultation.
4. **Tuberculosis.** Treated with antibiotics. Long-term follow-up with IVPs is needed because strictures (often 5–10 y after treatment) can lead to loss of renal funtion.
5. **Collecting system abnormality.** Requires further workup, usually retrograde ureteropyelogram and cystoscopy, then management as indicated.
6. **Coagulopathy.** Adjust the dose of anticoagulant or treat with fresh frozen plasma as indicated.
7. **Glomerulonephritis.** Usually managed medically, although a kidney biopsy may be needed.
8. **Hemorrhagic cystitis.** Managed with saline irrigation and occasionally alum irrigation. Refractory, life-threatening cases may require formalin instillation in the operating room, or cystectomy.

36. HEMOPTYSIS

I. **Problem.** A 50-year-old male smoker admitted for elective aortofemoral bypass shows you a specimen of bloody sputum he just coughed up.

II. **Immediate Questions**

A. **What are the vital signs?** Fever may signify pulmonary infection. Orthostasis, hypotension, and tachycardia signify significant blood loss. Tachycardia associated with tachypnea and decreased oxygen saturation may indicate a pulmonary embolus.

B. **Has this happened before?** Ask about the onset, amount of blood, a history of epistaxis or chronic hemoptysis, and pain on coughing.

C. **Is the patient a smoker?** Smoking makes cancer and chronic bronchitis more likely.

D. **What volume of blood was coughed up?** Massive hemoptysis is defined as more than 500 mL blood loss in a 24–h period.

E. **Does the patient have a history of TB or pneumonia?** Although TB is uncommon, it frequently causes hemoptysis.

III. **Differential Diagnosis**

A. **Pulmonary Sources**

1. **Neoplastic**

a. **Bronchial carcinoma:** Early cancers cause streaked sputum; advanced cancers may erode into pulmonary vessels causing severe hemorrhage or exsanguination.

b. **Bronchial adenoma:** These are uncommon, often highly vascular lesions.

2. **Infectious**
   a. Tuberculosis.
   b. Fungal infections (ie, coccidiomycosis).
   c. Bacterial pneumonia rarely produces more than blood-streaked sputum. *Klebsiella* pneumonia is known for bloody sputum. *Serratia marcescens* produces a reddish sputum that can be confused with blood.
   d. Chronic bronchitis. Usually caused by smoking.
   e. Bronchiectasis.
3. **Vascular**
   a. **Pulmonary infarction from emboli:** Hemoptysis may be accompanied by dyspnea and pleuritic chest pain. A venous duplex scan can be quickly obtained to identify lower-extremity deep venous thrombosis. A negative duplex scan does not exclude the possibility of pelvic vein thrombosis however.
   b. **Vascular aneurysms:** Thoracic aortic aneurysms rarely erode into the bronchial tree resulting in rapid exsanguination.
4. **Trauma.** Pulmonary contusion (after blunt trauma) or laceration (after penetrating trauma) can cause hemoptysis.
5. **Foreign body aspiration.**
6. **Mitral stenosis.** Pulmonary vessels can rupture with severe pulmonary hypertension.

B. **Nonpulmonary Sources.** Some patients cannot differentiate coughed-up blood from other sources, such as gastrointestinal, oral, or nasal.

C. **Systemic Causes.** Hemoptysis is rarely the sole site of hemorrhage in a patient with a bleeding diathesis. Other systemic causes of hemoptysis include vasculitis, the leukemias, idiopathic thrombocytopenic purpura (ITP), Henoch-Schönlein purpura (HSP), Goodpasture's syndrome, and lupus erythematosus.

IV. Database

A. Physical Exam Key Points

1. **Vital signs.** Regular and orthostatic.
2. **HEENT.** Look carefully for an oral or nasal source of bleeding.
3. **Chest.** Listen for decreased breath sounds, or for a pleural rub that may signify an effusion or pulmonary in-

farction. If the patient has sustained trauma, you may find a contusion, rib fracture, subcutaneous emphysema, or audible changes (from pneumothorax or hemothorax).

4. **Cardiac.** Irregular beats may signify atrial fibrillation and an atrial source of emboli. Mitral stenosis is heard as a low, rumbling diastolic murmur.
5. **Abdomen.** If the patient is tender, the bleeding may be hematemesis (from peptic ulcer disease), which is easily confused with hemoptysis.
6. **Extremities.** Evidence of DVT or cyanosis may be present.

B. Laboratory Data

1. CBC with attention to the hematocrit and platelet counts.
2. Coagulation studies.
3. Sputum examination.
   a. **Sputum culture and Gram's stain:** A properly collected specimen will have few epithelial cells. Large numbers of epithelial cells suggests that the specimen contains more saliva than sputum.
   b. **AFB culture and stain**
   c. **Sputum cytology**
4. **Renal function.** Check the patient's BUN and creatinine, as renal dysfunction usually accompanies hemoptysis in Goodpasture's syndrome.

C. Radiographic and Other Studies

1. **A chest radiograph is mandatory.** It may reveal an infiltrate, infarct, obstructing lesion, contusion, pneumothorax, hemothorax, rib fracture, or aortic aneurysm.
2. **Chest CT scan.** Will further define suspicious lesions seen on routine chest radiograph.
3. **Bronchoscopy.** Although not as readily available as a chest radiograph, bronchoscopy will often identify the source of hemoptysis. This should be performed after the acute bleeding subsides, although rigid bronchoscopy can be used to evaluate a patient with persistent bleeding.
4. **Angiogram.** When a patient has a thoracic aneurysm (seen on radiograph or CT), angiography can be used to identify an aortobronchial fistula when the bleeding source was not seen on bronchoscopy. Pulmonary angiography is the gold standard for making or excluding the diagnosis of pulmonary emboli and is particularly helpful when $\dot{V}/\dot{Q}$ scans and spiral CT scans are equivocal.
5. **Electrocardiogram.** To confirm the diagnosis of atrial fibrillation in a patient with an irregular pulse.

6. PPD skin test to identify TB.
7. **Nuclear ventilation/perfusion ($\dot{V}/\dot{Q}$) scan.** Indicated in the initial evaluation if pulmonary embolus is suspected.

V. Plan

A. Immediate Management.
With significant hemorrhage, the patient should be monitored in the ICU.

1. Establish venous access with large bore (16 gauge or larger) IVs, begin volume replacement as for any patient with blood loss. Send specimens to the blood bank for type and crossmatch.
2. Because these patients are at significant risk for asphyxia, the airway should be protected and endotracheal intubation considered.
3. Perform gastric lavage with a nasogastric tube when evaluation cannot differentiate between GI and pulmonary hemorrhage.
4. Be sure the nurse collects and quantifies all bloody sputum.
5. Obtain pulmonary consultation for urgent bronchoscopy.

B. Specific Plans

1. **Neoplasm.** Pulmonary resection should be performed when feasible. This may be necessary on an emergent basis when there is massive bleeding.
2. **Infection.** Antibiotics should initially be started empirically. Subsequent antibiotics should be given according to culture results. Tuberculosis or fungal cavities that are bleeding may require urgent surgical excision.
3. **Vascular**
   a. Pulmonary infarction from embolization should be treated with heparin to prevent further embolization, although this may exacerbate bleeding. A Greenfield filter may be necessary when anticoagulation fails or is contraindicated. Streptokinase or urokinase can be considered in the nonoperative patient, as can thoracotomy and embolectomy in the salvageable but unstable patient.
   b. **Aneurysm:** Sentinel bleeding from an eroding aneurysm may precede exsanguinating hemorrhage. Resection should be attempted, with prosthetic replacement, when possible.
   c. **Innominate artery fistula:** This occurs when a tracheostomy tube erodes into the innominate artery. This is a life-threatening problem usually heralded by minor sentinel bleeding episodes. Carefully eval-

uate all tracheostomy patients who have had even minor bleeding. During acute hemorrhage, temporary control can be obtained by overinflating the tracheostomy cuff or by pressing the innominate artery up against the sternum (pass your finger in front of the trachea behind the suprasternal notch).

4. **Trauma**
   a. Blunt trauma can cause rib fractures and flail chest with underlying pulmonary contusion and laceration. In this setting, hemoptysis often results in severe respiratory decompensation. Mechanical ventilation with positive pressure and aggressive pulmonary toilet is the treatment. In general, blood in the airway is less problematic than the damage caused by the pulmonary contusion.
   b. Penetrating trauma resulting in hemoptysis should be initially treated with tube thoracostomy; persistent bloody chest tube drainage or hemoptysis mandates exploratory thoracotomy. Bronchial tree disruption can cause hemoptysis and requires urgent thoracotomy.
5. **Foreign body.** Rigid bronchoscopy is usually successful in retrieving foreign bodies from the tracheobronchial tree.
6. **Massive hemoptysis**
   a. Thoracotomy and resection are sometimes needed in cases of massive hemoptysis.
   b. Placement of a double lumen endotracheal tube allows you to protect one lung while localizing and/or treating the site of bleeding in the other lung. The affected lung can also be intentionally collapsed to shunt blood to the ventilated nonbleeding lung.
   c. Bronchoscopy with balloon tamponade can also be used when available.

37. HICCUPS (SINGULTUS)

I. **Problem.** A patient admitted for right upper quadrant pain with possible cholecystitis develops hiccups for 4 h.

II. **Immediate Questions**

A. **Is there any new or increased abdominal pain?** Hiccups may be associated with a variety of significant intra-abdominal diseases so a careful evaluation of associated abdominal symptoms is needed.

B. **Is there any shoulder pain or pain with respiration?** A second major category of hiccup-related disorders is diaphragmatic irritation. Both referred pain to the shoulder or pleuritic pain may point to a diaphragmatic process, such as a subphrenic abscess, cholecystitis, or pneumonia.

C. **Does the patient have any cardiac history or symptoms?** Although unusual, hiccups may be the only symptom of a transmural myocardial infarction. Always remember this, especially if a patient with hiccups looks gravely ill.

D. **Does the patient have any emotional problems?** Hiccups are a common manifestation of anxiety and other psychogenic causes, usually in women. Inquire about previous problems with hiccups.

III. **Differential Diagnosis.** Hiccups are usually a short-term innocuous complaint, and they are often a result of aerophagia caused by rapid eating, drinking, or laughter. Even when chronic, it may not be possible to find a cause. Some of the organic causes are listed below.

A. **Diaphragmatic/Phrenic Nerve Irritation**
1. Subphrenic abscess
2. Pneumonia/pleuritis
3. Myocardial infarction
4. Pericarditis
5. Peritonitis
6. Metastatic implants on the diaphragm
7. Lung tumors
8. Postoperative

B. **Gastrointestinal Diseases**
1. Gastric dilatation
2. Hiatal hernia
3. Pancreatitis

C. **Metabolic Diseases**
1. Uremia
2. Diabetes
3. Alcohol abuse

D. **CNS Dysfunction.** "Central hiccups" are caused by posterior fossa tumors or infarction or encephalitis. In neonates, hiccups may indicate a seizure.

E. **Psychogenic.** The hallmark is that hiccups stop when the patient is asleep.

IV. **Database**

A. **Physical Exam Key Points**
1. **Vital signs.** Spiking temperatures may indicate an abscess.
2. **Pulmonary.** There may be decreased diaphragmatic excursion that may accompany diaphragmatic irritation

(from a subphrenic abscess, pulmonary infiltrate or effusion) or evidence for an infiltrate or effusion.

3. **Cardiac.** Listen for a pericardial friction rub.
4. **Abdomen.** Distention (either ascites or gaseous), pain, peritoneal signs, hepatosplenomegaly, and tympany (especially over the gastric area), may suggest a diagnosis. "Punch tenderness" over the lower ribs occurs with diaphragmatic irritation.

B. Laboratory Data

1. **CBC.** When considering infection.
2. **Renal function tests.** An increased BUN and creatinine suggest uremia.
3. **Glucose.** A glucose tolerance test may be needed at some point to diagnose diabetes.
4. **Amylase.** Elevated in pancreatic disease.

C. Radiographic and Other Studies

1. **Chest radiograph.** Identifies elevation of the diaphragm, effusions, infiltrates, or tumors.
2. **Abdominal radiographs.** Gastric dilatation may be seen on this study or on chest radiograph.
3. **ECG.** To rule out ischemic changes if clinically indicated.
4. **Ultrasound/CT abdomen.** May reveal subphrenic fluid collections or other diseases.
5. **CT chest.** Chest tumors may irritate the phrenic nerve.

V. Plan. Problems identified (myocardial infarction, gastric dilatation, subphrenic abscess) should be treated appropriately. There are a variety of individual or "home remedies" to manage hiccups. Those listed below are found to have withstood at least some objective scrutiny.

A. Mechanisms to Interfere with Respiration. Low P_{CO_2} accentuates hiccups whereas high P_{CO_2} inhibits them. Maneuvers to increase P_{CO_2} are:

1. Breathholding.
2. Drinking water rapidly.
3. Rebreathing from a paper bag.

B. Mechanisms to Alter Afferent Pathways

1. Stimulate the nasopharynx with cotton swab.
2. Swallow a teaspoon of dry granulated sugar.

C. Pharmacologic Management

1. **Chlorpromazine.** 25–50 mg PO/IM q6h.
2. **Perphenazine.** 4–8 mg PO or 5 mg IM q8h.
3. **Metoclopramide.** 10 mg PO q6h for several days.

38. HYPERCALCEMIA

I. Problem. The clinical laboratory calls to tell you that one of your patients, a 45–year-old male scheduled for surgery in the morning, has a serum calcium of 12.5 mg/dL (normal 8.5–10.5 mg/dL).

II. Immediate Questions

A. Is the patient symptomatic? "Stones, bones, abdominal groans, and psychic overtones" is a phrase used often to describe the symptoms of hypercalcemia. Delirium, confusion, lethargy, nausea and vomiting, abdominal pain, symptoms of kidney stones, such as CVA tenderness, and bone pain occur with significant hypercalcemia (ionized calcium greater than 3.0 mmol/L).

B. Does the patient have a history of hyperparathyroidism? The patient may have a history of asymptomatic hypercalcemia or chronic renal failure and may have been worked up in the past.

C. Has the patient had recent surgery? Adrenal surgery (hypoadrenalism), in particular, and long-term immobilization can cause excessive bone resorption and hypercalcemia. A recent parathyroidectomy (for hyperparathyroidism) may have been unsuccessful.

D. What IV fluids and medications are currently being given? Oral calcium supplementation rarely causes hypercalcemia in the absence of another disease. Ask about IV calcium, lithium, thiazide diuretics, and Vitamin D (particularly dihydroxy D3).

E. Is there any history of cancer? Bone metastases cause hypercalcemia. Hypercalcemia can also be caused by a paraneoplastic syndrome (where the cancer secretes a substance that mimics PTH).

F. Is there a history of peptic ulcer disease? A condition known as milk alkali syndrome occurs when a patient tries to relieve ulcer symptoms by drinking excessive amounts of milk.

G. Is there a history of granulomatous disease? TB, coccidiomycosis, histoplasmosis and sarcoidosis can cause hypercalcemia.

III. Differential Diagnosis. (See also Section II, page 293)

A. Hyperparathyroidism (HPT). About 20% of patients with hypercalcemia will have associated hyperparathyroidism. Primary hyperparathyroidism is diagnosed by showing that the calcium and parathormone levels are simultaneously elevated.

B. **Malignant Neoplasm.** Bone metastases from metastatic cancer are the most frequent cause of hypercalcemia, although paraneoplastic syndrome also occurs (typically with multiple myeloma, lung, breast, and renal cancers).

C. **Thiazide Diuretics.** Hydrochlorothiazide causes increased renal resorption of calcium.

D. **Granulomatous diseases.** These produce a vitamin D metabolite.

E. **Vitamin D Intoxication.** There should be a history of chronic ingestion.

F. **Milk-alkali syndrome.** Caused by the excessive intake of alkali and calcium in the treatment of peptic ulcer disease. This has become rare now that we have a number of over-the-counter H_2 blockers and magnesium-based antacids that are more effective than milk.

G. **Hyperthyroidism.**

H. **Adrenal Insufficiency.**

I. **Paget's disease.** Usually with secondary hyperparathyroidism.

J. **Acute tubular necrosis (diuretic phase).**

K. **Acromegaly.**

L. **Excessive calcium administration.**

M. **Long-term immobilization.**

IV. Database

A. Physical Exam Key Points

1. **Vital signs.** Hypertension may accompany hypercalcemia.
2. **Cardiac.** Arrhythmias may include bradycardia or tachycardia. Sudden death is possible with very high calcium levels (over 15 mg/dL).
3. **Chest.** Breast carcinoma may be suggested by a mass or a scar from a prior mastectomy.
4. **Abdomen.** Check for masses.
5. **Bones.** Tenderness to palpation may indicate metastatic disease.
6. **Nodes.** Lymphadenopathy is present with cancer or granulomatous disease.
7. Neurologic weakness, hyperactive reflexes, impaired mentation (stupor, delirium).
8. **Skin.** Evidence of pruritus.

9. **Rectal exam.** May show evidence of a prostate cancer (a common cause of bone metastases).

B. **Laboratory Data**

1. **Serum calcium and albumin.** Confirm elevation on a repeat determination. **Caution:** The units of calcium measurement may differ in different institutions (mg/dL vs mEq/dL). When the albumin is not normal, a corrected calcium level must be determined (see page 293). Symptoms usually appear at levels of 12 mg/dL (or ionized level > 3.0 mmol/L).
2. **Phosphorous.** Usually low in hyperparathyroidism except if renal failure is present.
3. **Potassium, magnesium.** Decreases may be associated with a high serum calcium level.
4. **Arterial blood gases.** Look for acidosis with hyperchlorhydria.
5. **Alkaline phosphatase.** Elevated in hyperparathyroidism with bone disease.
6. **Renal function.** Secondary and tertiary hyperparathyroidism are related to renal failure. In addition, renal insufficiency exacerbates hypercalcemia in all patients.
7. **Parathyroid hormone (PTH) level.** Increased in primary and secondary hyperparathyroidism; often decreased in hypercalcemia not caused by hyperparathyroidism.

C. **Radiographic and Other Studies**

1. **Chest radiograph.** May show hilar adenopathy with sarcoidosis or lymphoma.
2. **Abdomen radiographs.** May show renal stones with hyperparathyroidism.
3. **Skull.** Look for the typical punched-out lesions of multiple myeloma.
4. **Bones.** May show osteolytic lesions of metastatic cancer, evidence of osteitis fibrosa cystica (brown cysts in bone), or subperiosteal resorption on the radial aspect of second and third phalanges and distal clavicles.
5. **IVP.** Used to confirm the presence of renal stones with hyperparathyroidism and, rarely, renal cell carcinoma, which may have associated hypercalcemia.
6. **Barium swallow.** The esophagus can be displaced by a parathyroid adenoma, although there are better tests available for identifying an adenoma (technetium sestamibi, ultrasound).
7. **ECG.** Hypercalcemia is associated with a shortened QT interval and prolonged PR interval.
8. **Cortisone suppression test.** No response in hyperparathyroidism, but metastatic cancer, myeloma, sar-

coid, vitamin D intoxication, milk-alkali syndrome, and adrenal insufficiency usually respond with a decrease in calcium.

V. Plan

A. Initial Management. First, lower the serum calcium (when necessary), then control the underlying cause.

1. **Levels < 12 mg/dL.** Management is usually directed only at the underlying cause.
2. **Moderate elevation (12–15 mg/dL).** Treat with hydration and loop diuretics initially (see below).
3. **Severe hypercalcemia (> 15 mg/dL) or any symptomatic patient regardless of level.** A life-threatening emergency requiring more rigorous therapy (as described below).

B. Specific Plans

1. Restrict calcium intake, encourage mobilization, and treat the underlying disorder. Avoid calcium carbonate antacids (e.g., Tums®), vitamins A and D, and thiazide diuretics (hydrochlorothiazide).
2. **Saline diuresis.** This should be done only after the patient is adequately hydrated. Use IV normal saline and furosemide to produce at least 100–200 mL/h of urine. Sodium increases calcium excretion by competing for resorption in the distal tubule. In the presence of renal or cardiac failure, this must be done with caution. Monitor serum calcium, phosphate, potassium, magnesium, and BUN.
3. **Furosemide** can be given 20–40 mg IV q2–4h to bring the Ca level below 12 mg/dL after hydration. Carefully monitor serum potassium during diuresis and replace as necessary.
4. **Corticosteroids.** These are ineffective in patients with primary HPT and may take 1–2 wk to work in patients with malignancies. Prednisone 5–15 mg PO daily is a fairly typical dosing.
5. **Bisphosphonates.** Pamidronate (preferred bisphosphonate) 90 mg during 24 h or etidronate 7.5 mg/g IV daily for 3 d followed by 5–20 mg/kg/d PO. These are potent inhibitors of bone resorption due to cancer. Do not use them in renal failure. Their onset of action is delayed by 4–5 d.
6. **Calcitonin** (salmon) inhibits bone resorption and works quickly but only minimally reduces the amount of hypercalcemia (max reduction is 0.5 mmol/L). Give 4 U/kg q12 h.

7. **Dialysis.** May be the first treatment in patients with renal failure; usually the last treatment in other patients, unless there is life-threatening hypercalcemia and other treatments have failed.
8. **Other agents.** Mithramycin, used only as a last resort, because its use may be complicated by aplastic anemia. Give 25 μg/kg during 4 h.

39. HYPERGLYCEMIA

I. **Problem.** An elderly woman who has just undergone hemicolectomy has a high urine output and is complaining of thirst. A stat serum glucose is 285 mg/dL (normal 70–105 mg/dL).

II. **Immediate Questions**

A. **Is there a history of diabetes?** Diabetic patients who usually take insulin will need a portion of their usual daily dose even while taking nothing by mouth (usually 50% of their morning dose before surgery). Surgical stress may temporarily create insulin requirements in the non-insulin-dependent diabetic (epinephrine and cortisol levels increase after surgery, and both antagonize insulin). If a patient has no history of diabetes, look for other causes (sepsis, TPN, glucocorticoids, and other medications).

B. **What are the vital signs?** Fever and hyperglycemia are early signs of sepsis and may be the only signs of sepsis. As a general rule in any diabetic patient, new-onset hyperglycemia or a sudden increase in serum glucose should be viewed as a warning of possible infection.

III. **Differential Diagnosis.** (See also Section II, page 305).

A. **Diabetes**

1. **Insulin-dependent (IDDM) (type I) (formerly called juvenile diabetes).** Insulin-dependent diabetics require insulin even when taking nothing by mouth.
2. **Non-insulin-dependent (NIDDM) (type II) (formerly called Adult Onset Diabetes or AODM).** Surgical stress often aggravates diabetes. Thus, patients controlled with diet or oral hypoglycemic agents may develop a worsening of their diabetes, requiring temporary treatment with insulin.

B. **Hyperosmolar Coma.** Nonketotic hyperglycemic syndrome characterized by impaired consciousness, extreme dehydration, occasional seizures, and extreme hyperglycemia that is not accompanied by ketoacidosis. It is a complication of NIDDM and has more than a 50% mortality rate.

C. **Sepsis.** Glucose intolerance is often an early sign of sepsis in the critically ill patient.

D. **Hyperalimentation.** Typical central parenteral nutrition solutions contain 20–35% glucose. When TPN is first started or advanced too quickly or administered in excessive amounts (greater than nutritional requirements), hyperglycemia can develop.

E. **Gestational Diabetes.** Some women develop hyperglycemia during pregnancy.

F. **Other Causes**
   1. **Medication.** Steroid use causes insulin resistance in many patients; other agents include oral contraceptives.
   2. Cushing's syndrome.
   3. Pancreatic disease or resection.

IV. Database

A. **Physical Exam Key Points**
   1. **Vital signs.** Fever and tachycardia suggest infection, and hypotension suggests sepsis. Kussmaul respiration (deep, rapid respiratory pattern) may be seen with severe ketoacidosis.
   2. **HEENT.** A fruity odor on the breath may signify ketoacidosis.
   3. **Lungs.** Listen for evidence of pneumonia.
   4. **Abdomen.** Exclude intra-abdominal causes of sepsis.
   5. **Neurologic.** Obtundation may indicate ketoacidosis in a diabetic patient.

B. **Laboratory Data.** Significantly elevated chemsticks should be confirmed with a serum glucose determination, and electrolytes should be assessed to rule out ketoacidosis.
   1. **Serum electrolytes.** Potassium and phosphorus must be monitored closely in diabetic ketoacidosis (DKA).
   2. **Arterial blood gas.** When considering sepsis or DKA, determine the serum pH and Po_2.
   3. Serial serum ketones and anion gap are useful in following up the management of DKA.
   4. **CBC.** An elevated leukocyte count may indicate infection.
   5. Cultures of blood, urine, central lines, etc, should be done when infection is suspected.
   6. **Urine glucose.** Thresholds for spilling glucose in the urine vary widely; confirm hyperglycemia with a serum glucose when any doubt exists.

C. **Radiographic and Other Studies.** These studies should be selected on the basis of clinical impression. For example, infection in the postoperative hyperglycemic patient may be evaluated with a chest radiograph when a pulmonary source is suspected, or an abdominal CT scan if an intra-abdominal abscess is considered likely.

V. Plan

A. **Initial Management.** Control the serum glucose quickly and safely and treat any predisposing infection appropriately.

B. **Specific Plans**

1. **Sliding scale insulin.** Small doses of subcutaneous regular insulin can be given every 4–6 h on the basis of rapid evaluation of blood sugars using a glucometer or chemsticks. This is the best way to achieve good control of sugars in the NPO patient. Typically, a serum glucose of < 200 mg/dL is considered adequate control. A typical sliding scale is as follows: for glucose < 80 mg/dL, call MD; 81–150 mg/dL, no insulin units; 151–200 mg/dL, 2 U of regular human insulin SC; 201–250 mg/dL, 4 U; 251–300 mg/dL, 6 U; 301–350 mg/dL, 8 U; greater than 350 mg/dL, call MD. Any chemstick > 400 mg/dL should be confirmed with a stat serum measurement from the lab. It is safer to start with a low dosing scale as described above. More resistant diabetics may need higher doses.
2. **Diet.** Caloric and carbohydrate restriction are important, particularly for obese patients. The usual diet is an 1800 cal/d ADA (American Diabetes Association) diet for females and a 2000 cal/d ADA diet for males.
3. **Oral hypoglycemic agents.** Many type II diabetics, normally controlled on these medications, require insulin after an operation. Nevertheless, most are discharged on their usual medication.
4. **Severe glucose intolerance in sepsis and DKA.** Aggressive therapy is warranted, usually in an ICU setting. Patients with DKA have tachypnea, dehydration, ketones on their breath, and abdominal pain, with hyperglycemia, hyperketonemia, and metabolic acidosis.
   a. **Precipitating factors:** In the surgical patient, infection precipitates severe glucose intolerance. It should be appropriately treated.
   b. **Dehydration:** Typically, patients become volume depleted, often because of severe glycosuria. Rehydrate the patient starting with dextrose free saline. Increased urine output may be a result of an osmotic

diuresis and not a reflection of the patient's true volume status. Volume status must be assessed by other means, such as a central venous pressure.

c. **Potassium:** Potassium levels will go down as DKA improves. Insulin causes glucose and potassium to move intracellularly, thus decreasing serum levels. Because most patients are total body potassium depleted, it is usually necessary to start replacing potassium with the second bag of IV solution infused.

d. **Bicarbonate:** Correct severe acidosis with intravenous bicarbonate. Insulin must be continued until the serum bicarbonate normalizes. You may need to administer both insulin and glucose simultaneously.

e. **Insulin:** Start with a 10–20 U IV bolus and follow this with a continuous drip. The infusion rate will vary, but should be started at 2–5 U/h and adjusted as needed. Finger stick glucose should be checked frequently (q2h) while using an insulin drip.

f. **Dextrose:** Normal saline should be changed to 5% dextrose when serum glucose levels decrease to 300 mg/dL.

g. **Maintenance insulin:** Once IV therapy has controlled severe hyperglycemia, maintenance insulin will be needed. Subcutaneous administration should be performed twice a day, to achieve better control, often with a combination of NPH and regular insulin. The starting dose can be calculated by adding daily insulin requirements (total up the sliding scale insulin administered the previous day) and giving 2/3 in the morning, and 1/3 at bedtime with 2/3 NPH and 1/3 regular insulin. Patients on hyperalimentation can receive maintenance insulin by adding it directly to the solution. You may need to adjust the dose as some insulin sticks to the IV tubing.

40. HYPERKALEMIA

Immediate Actions

1. ECG monitoring is essential with severe hyperkalemia (> 6.5 mEq/L).
2. Administer 10% calcium gluconate 10–20 mL IV to protect the heart from dysrhythmias.
3. Begin maneuvers to decrease the potassium level as noted below.

I. Problem. A patient on the trauma service with a crush injury has a potassium of 7.1 mmol/L on the second hospital day (normal 3.5–5.1 mEq/L).

II. Immediate Questions

A. What are the vital signs? Check these first because hyperkalemia can lead to life-threatening arrhythmias.

B. What is the patient's urine output? Renal failure (with inability to excrete potassium) is the most common cause of acute hyperkalemia on a surgical service. Evaluate the patient's urine output and recent renal function chemistries. Ensure that there is no obstruction to urinary flow.

C. Is the patient receiving potassium in an intravenous solution? A bag of IV solution may contain 20–40 mEq/L of potassium, and hyperalimentation solutions may contain more. When beginning the initial evaluation of an abnormal potassium value, stop all exogenous potassium until the problem is solved.

D. Is the lab result accurate? In the previous example, hyperkalemia is an almost expected outcome. However, abnormally elevated potassium levels are often entirely unexpected or inconsistent. If the lab doesn't notify you, inquire about hemolysis of the specimen, which can falsely elevate the potassium.

E. Is the patient on any medication that could elevate the potassium? If the patient is receiving spironolactone, triamterene, or indomethacin, stop these medications immediately.

III. Differential Diagnosis. Laboratory tests measure the extracellular potassium concentration, which is the level that correlates with the harmful consequences of hyperkalemia. Extracellular hyperkalemia can be caused by the redistribution of potassium from intracellular stores (where 98% of the total body potassium is located) or by a real increase in total body potassium.

A. Redistribution

1. **Acidosis.**
2. **Insulin deficiency.**
3. **Digoxin overdose.**
4. **Succinylcholine.** This can cause chronically debilitated patients, patients with muscle diseases, and burn patients to mobilize potassium from muscle.
5. **Cellular breakdown.**
   a. **Crush injury (rhabdomyolysis).**
   b. **Hemolysis.**

B. Increased Total Body Potassium

1. **Renal causes.**
   a. **Acute renal failure.**
   b. **Chronic renal failure:** Potassium will not usually be elevated until endstage disease, (creatinine clearance typically < 20 mL/s).
   c. **Renal tubular dysfunction:** Associated with renal transplantation, lupus erythematosus, sickle cell disease, or myeloma.
2. **Mineralocorticoid deficiency.**
   a. **Addison's disease.**
   b. **Hypoaldosteronism (hyporeninemic).**
3. **Drug-induced.** Common causes:
   a. **Spironolactone.**
   b. **Triamterene.**
   c. **Indomethacin:** Thought to interfere with renal prostaglandin levels.
   d. **Cyclosporine.**
   e. **Potassium supplement excess.**
   f. **Heparin:** Reported to decrease aldosterone synthesis.

C. Pseudohyperkalemia

1. Hemolysis of the specimen.
2. Prolonged tourniquet occlusion before drawing blood.
3. **Thrombocytosis/leukocytosis:** White blood cells and platelets release potassium as the clot forms.

IV. Database

A. Physical Exam Key Points

1. **Cardiac.** Bradycardia, ventricular fibrillation, and asystole occur with markedly elevated potassium levels.
2. **Neuromuscular.** Hyperkalemia causes tingling, weakness, flaccid paralysis, and hyperactive deep tendon reflexes. Unfortunately, cardiac arrest often precedes these symptoms.

B. Laboratory Data

1. **Electrolytes, BUN, and creatinine.** Diagnostic of hyperkalemia and renal failure.
2. **Arterial blood gas.** A nonanion gap acidosis is associated with hyperkalemia.
3. **Platelet count, white blood count.** Elevations may yield factitious hyperkalemia. With significant platelet and WBC elevations, order a plasma potassium level.
4. **Cortisol levels or ACTH stimulation test.**
5. **Digoxin level.** If indicated.
6. **Myoglobin level in serum/urine.** Check in crush injuries.

C. **Radiographic and Other Studies**

1. **ECG.** This is the second most important test after the potassium level, and a means to separate pseudohyperkalemia from actual elevations of potassium. As the potassium increases, the ECG will show peaked T waves, flat P waves, prolonged PR interval, and a widened QRS complex progressing to a sine wave and arrest.
2. **Ultrasound.** Helps to identify several causes of renal insufficiency. It may show hydronephrosis (with an obstructed ureter), a dilated bladder (urethral or bladder outlet obstruction),or renal atrophy (chronic renal disease).

V. **Plan.** Treatment is dictated by the severity of hyperkalemia as judged by the serum potassium level and the ECG. In general, aggressive treatment is indicated for a serum potassium > 6.5–7 mmol/L or when ECG changes are present. The first priority is to counteract the membrane effects of hyperkalemia, then move potassium into cells, and finally remove potassium from the body.

A. **Counteract membrane effects.** Protect the heart by administering calcium gluconate 10% 10–20 mL IV during 3–5 min while monitoring the ECG. Be careful with patients on digitalis, because arrhythmias may occur.

B. **Transfer Potassium to the Intracellular Compartment**

1. **Sodium bicarbonate 1 ampule (44 mEq) IV.** May repeat 1–2 times every 20–30 min. This is most effective in acidotic patients, but also works in normal patients.
2. **Insulin/glucose.** One ampule of D50W and 10 units of regular insulin given IV over 5 min.
3. The two methods listed above can be combined by mixing one liter D10W with 3 ampules of sodium bicarbonate. Give over 2–4 h with regular insulin 10 units SQ every 4–6 h.
4. **Beta-agonists.** Albuterol (given by nebulizer every 4 h) will drive potassium intracellularly.

C. **Remove potassium from the body**

1. **Kayexalate (exchange resin)**
   a. **Oral:** 30 grams in 30–70 mL of 70% sorbitol every 4–6 h.
   b. **Rectal:** 50–100 g in 200 mL water given as a retention enema for 30 min every 2–4 h.
2. **Dialysis:** Peritoneal or hemodialysis.
3. **Furosemide:** Monitor the urine output and volume status carefully after administering furosemide IV.

D. Remove all potassium from intravenous fluids.

E Any ECG changes should incite prompt transfer to a monitored bed or ICU.

F. Consider inserting a Foley catheter to assess urine output and eliminate the possibility of lower urinary tract obstruction.

G. **Chronic Therapy.** For patients with chronic renal failure, use a potassium-restricted diet (40–60 mEq/d). Addison's disease usually requires glucocorticoid and mineralocorticoid therapy.

41. HYPERNATREMIA

(See also Section II, page 323)

I. **Problem.** The clinical lab calls to tell you that an 85–year-old female patient has a serum sodium of 155 mmol/L (normal 136–145 mmol/L).

II. **Immediate Questions**

A. **Is the patient alert and oriented, or is the patient seizing?** Symptoms of hypernatremia usually do not appear until the level is > 160 mmol/L (irritability, ataxia, anorexia, cramping). Levels > 180 mmol/L may result in confusion, stupor, or seizure. The more rapid the change in sodium level, the more likely it will be symptomatic.

B. **What medications is the patient taking?** Diuretics can cause water loss leading to hypernatremia. Many IV antibiotics contain large amounts of sodium.

C. **What are the intake/output values for the past few days?** A loss of total body water by fluid deprivation (inadequate administration of fluids) can cause hypernatremia.

D. **Are there underlying conditions?** Certain diseases, most notably diabetes insipidus (after pituitary surgery, head injury or nephrogenic disease), are associated with hypernatremia. Cardiac bypass patients can develop hypernatremia from water loss secondary to ADH inhibition.

E. **Is the lab value accurate?** As with any unexpected lab result, the lab may be in error. Consider repeating the test.

F. **What IV fluids are being administered?** Check the sodium content. Is the patient receiving adequate free water (usually 35 mL/kg per 24h in adult)?

III. **Differential Diagnosis.** Hypernatremia is usually caused by a loss of total body water, and is rarely associated with an increased total body sodium.

A. **Inadequate Fluid Intake.** Water deprivation (comatose or postoperative patients).

B. **Increased Water Loss.** Most body fluids are hypotonic (with respect to sodium); thus excessive loss leads to hypernatremia.

   1. **Nonrenal losses**
      a. **Gastrointestinal losses:** NG suction, diarrhea, fistulas.
      b. **Pulmonary losses:** There may be significant insensible losses, especially in intubated patients who are not receiving adequate humidification.
      c. **Cutaneous Losses:** Insensible losses increase in the febrile patient 500 mL every 24 h for each degree centigrade increase above 38 °C. Air-filled or heated beds also increase cutaneous losses.
   2. **Renal losses**
      a. **Diuretics.**
      b. **Hypercalcemic nephropathy.**
      c. **Hypokalemic nephropathy.**
      d. **Diabetes insipidus (true vs nephrogenic).**
      e. **Acute tubular necrosis:** Polyuric phase.
      f. **Postobstructive diuresis:** Usually caused by the relief of long-standing bilateral renal obstruction.
      g. **Diabetes mellitus:** Caused by osmotic diuresis (water loss) from glycosuria.
      h. **ADH inhibition (water loss) via baroreceptor activation.**
      i. **Drugs:** Including lithium, ethanol, phenytoin, colchicine, and mannitol.

C. **Administration of Hypertonic Saline.** Hypertonic saline is almost never needed in general surgical patients. It is occasionally used in neurosurgical patients.

D. **Increased Mineralocorticoids or Glucocorticoids**

   1. **Primary aldosteronism.**
   2. **Cushing's syndrome.**
   3. **Ectopic ACTH production.**
   4. **Over-administration of exogenous steroids.**

IV. Database

A. Physical Exam Key Points

1. **Vital signs.** Orthostatic blood pressure changes, tachycardia, and decreased weight suggest volume loss.
2. **Skin.** Check turgor. Mucous membranes may be dry with volume contraction. Note any "cushingoid" features.

3. **Neurologic exam.** Look to see if the patient is irritable, weak, twitches, or experiences seizures.
4. **History.** The history and physical exam can give insight into the degree of fluid deficit. With volume loss of 5% or less, the patient may complain only of thirst. With volume loss between 5% and 10%, the patient will be lethargic, with sunken eyes, decreased skin turgor, absent tears, and orthostatic hypotension. Above 10% loss, the patient will be hypotensive and hyperventilatory.

B. Laboratory Data

1. **Serum electrolytes.** Electrolyte disorders often involve more than one extracellular ion. An elevated BUN may indicate dehydration.
2. **Serum osmolality.** Increased with volume loss.
3. **Urine osmolality.** Hypertonic urine suggests extrarenal fluid loss, while isotonic or hypotonic urine suggests renal losses.
4. **Spot urine sodium.** When < 20 mEq/L, this suggests extrarenal volume losses.
5. **Hematocrit.** May be elevated with dehydration because of hemoconcentration.

V. Plan. The overall plan is to replace free water slowly to bring the serum sodium concentration down to normal levels. Volume repletion is especially important in patients with orthostatic hypotension. Correction should be done slowly to prevent the development of cerebral edema, which can precipitate seizures.

A. Determine the volume of free water needed to correct the serum sodium from the actual total body water (TBW).

$$\text{Water Deficit} = (0.6 \times \text{weight in kg}) - \text{TBW}$$

$$\text{TBW} = \frac{140}{\text{Serum Na}} \times (0.6 \times \text{weight in kg})$$

Administer the fluids over a 24–h period as 5% dextrose in water. Alternatively, if a patient is receiving 5% dextrose in 0.45 N saline, the extra free water can be given by increasing the rate of administration or by changing it to 5% dextrose in 0.2 N saline.

B. Identify and Treat the Underlying Cause of Hypernatremia.

1. Replace unusually large nonrenal losses of free water, such as small bowel or pancreatic fistula drainage (see Section IV, page 381).

2. Treat diabetes mellitus with insulin (see Problem 35, page 141)
3. Treat diabetes insipidus with adequate free water or with vasopressin.

42. HYPERTENSION

I. **Problem.** After vagotomy and antrectomy, a 45–year-old man has a blood pressure of 190/110 in the recovery room.

II. **Immediate Questions**

A. **What is the heart and respiratory rate?** Postoperative pain is often manifested by tachycardia and hypertension; the addition of tachypnea should alert you to the possibility of hypoxia, especially in the presence of agitation. Bradycardia and hypertension suggests increased intracranial pressure (Cushing's sign).

B. **Is there a history of hypertension?** Mild blood pressure elevations are often seen in hypertensive patients after large intraoperative fluid infusions; this is rarely worrisome in the absence of other findings.

C. **Is the patient having chest pain?** Significant hypertension can stress patients with coronary artery disease; it can cause angina or infarction and requires rapid control. Aortic dissection is also an emergency; although rare, it typically presents in hypertensive patients with back and chest pain.

D. **What medications is the patient taking?** Patients with well-controlled hypertension occasionally stop their medications at the time of surgery, leading to postoperative hypertension. To prevent this, most cardiac medications and antihypertensives, with the exception of diuretics, should be given in their usual doses with a small sip of water the morning of the operation. Carefully check the rates of all IV solutions. Sympathomimetic agents, steroids, and oral contraceptives can cause hypertension.

III. **Differential Diagnosis.** There are six surgically correctable causes of hypertension: coarctation of the aorta, pheochromocytoma, Cushing's syndrome, primary hyperaldosteronism, unilateral renal parenchymal disease, and renovascular hypertension.

A. **Postoperative**

1. **Pain-induced.**
2. **Fluid overload.**
3. **Hypoxia.**

4. **Vasospasm.** Patients become cold during surgery for a number of reasons (room temperature, cold IV fluids, refrigerated blood, sympathetic block). After surgery, patients "clamp down" (vasoconstrict) to warm up. Vasospasm may also occur after aortic cross-clamping.
5. **Carotid sinus reflex disturbance.** May augment postoperative hypertension following a CVA (cerebrovascular accident) and can lead to intracerebral hemorrhage.

B. **Essential Hypertension.** There is no cause found in 90–95% of patients with chronic hypertension.

C. **Secondary Hypertension**
1. **Renal.** Vascular or parenchymal.
2. **Endocrine.** Pheochromocytoma, Cushing's syndrome.
3. **Drug-induced.** Oral contraceptives, amphetamines, ketamine, and other sympathomimetic agents.
4. **Pregnancy.** Preeclampsia or eclampsia.
5. **Coarctation of the aorta.**
6. **Increased intracranial pressure.** Typically caused by trauma, tumors, and subarachnoid hemorrhage; usually associated with hypertension and bradycardia (Cushing's reflex).
7. **Polycythemia vera.**
8. **Baroreceptor stimulation.**

D. **Factitious.** Using too small a blood pressure cuff on an obese arm may falsely elevate readings.

IV. Database

A. **History.** Start with a careful history to identify preexisting hypertension, the type of treatment, medications, and other predisposing factors.

B. **Physical Exam Key Points**
1. **Vital signs.** Measure the blood pressure in both arms. In postoperative patients, check the core body temperature (especially in the recovery room).
2. **HEENT.** Papilledema, retinal hemorrhages, or exudates may be present. Papilledema represents increased intracranial pressure or malignant hypertension.
3. **Lungs.** Listen for rales indicating pulmonary edema and congestive heart failure.
4. **Abdomen.** Is there a pulsatile mass (with aneurysm) or a bruit (with renovascular hypertension)?
5. **Neurologic exam.** Focal changes may represent cerebral ischemia.

C. **Laboratory Data**
1. **Arterial blood gas.** Should be performed if there is any question about hypoxemia.

2. **Urinalysis, BUN, serum creatinine.** Because hypertension can accompany renal insufficiency, evaluate the patient's renal function.
3. **Serum catecholamines, urinary VMA, and metanephrines.** Only if one suspects pheochromocytoma.
4. A dexamethasone suppression test can be obtained later to test for Cushing's syndrome (see page 301.

D. Radiographic and Other Studies

1. **Electrocardiogram.** Should be performed routinely in most elderly patients after major cardiac, thoracic, or vascular surgery, and in patients with a history of heart disease after any major operation. In the presence of hypertension, the ECG may show ischemic changes in the absence of symptoms.
2. **Pulmonary artery catheter.** This is not routinely indicated. It can help to determine the cardiac output and pulmonary capillary wedge pressure in critically ill hypertensive postoperative patients.
3. New-onset hypertension in patients younger than 30 y and older than 60 y or with hypertension refractory to medical treatment should have a thorough evaluation for secondary causes of hypertension. This often includes renal arteriography, selective renal vein renin measurements, renal ultrasonography (renovascular hypertension), determination of urinary VMA and metanephrine (pheochromocytoma), serum potassium (aldosteronoma), and serum cortisol (Cushing's syndrome).

V. Plan

A. Emergent Management. Severe hypertension (ie, hypertensive encephalopathy, malignant hypertension, and dissecting aortic aneurysm) is usually treated emergently with sodium nitroprusside (Nipride). Esmolol is an easily titratable, rapidly acting β-blocker that can be used instead of nitroprusside, or to treat tachycardia in patients on nitroprusside. Other agents used to control acute hypertension (diazoxide, labetalol or hydralazine) are harder to titrate. With evidence of myocardia ischemia, use IV nitroglycerin.

1. **Sodium nitroprusside 0.5–10 μg/kg/min IV infusion.** Titrate to effect. Monitor for thiocyanate toxicity and methemoglobinemia.
2. **Nitroglycerin 5–100 μg/min.** Titrate to effect.
3. **Esmolol** 5 mg/min IV push (in a patient monitored with an arterial line) until the BP is brought down to a reasonable range, then 20 μg/min by IV drip, titrated to effect.

4. **Nifedipine 10–20 mg PO/SL.** Often a useful oral adjunct to lower blood pressure immediately. Unfortunately, this use has been associated with an increased risk of myocardial infarction.

B. **Preoperative.** The goal is to obtain good control of blood pressure before performing elective procedures.
   1. **Obtain an ECG.** Look for signs of ischemia, failure, or a recent MI (which can be asymptomatic).
   2. All blood pressure and cardiac medications, except diuretics should be given on the morning of the operation.
   3. Weight loss and a low-salt diet are a good first step.
   4. Typical staged therapy includes starting with a β-blocker or thiazide diuretic. Thiazides work better in African-American patients. When a second agent is needed, add the first-line agent that was not used. When there are contraindications to the use of β-blockers (eg, asthma, heart failure), central antiadrenergic agents (eg, methyldopa, clonidine) or antialpha adrenergic agents can be used. Third-line drugs include hydralazine, prazosin, and angiotensin-converting enzyme inhibitors (captopril). Hydralazine can cause reflex tachycardia in the non-beta-blocked patient. Calcium-channel blockers are also frequently used. Drug doses are listed in Section IX, page [441].

C. **Postoperative**
   1. Ensure adequate oxygenation and pain relief and warm the patient with blankets or heating blanket if necessary.
   2. Mild postoperative hypertension can be treated with a variety of agents. Sublingual nifedipine (10–20 mg) was the most commonly used agent until recent studies concluded that calcium-channel blockers increased the risk of myocardial infarction. Nitroglycerin is safe but less effective. β-Blockers are effective and safe, except in patients with heart failure. Hydralazine 5–10 mg IV can be used for elderly patients. Sedatives and pain control are often all that are needed to control mild hypertension. Mild persistent hypertension can be further managed by adding a diuretic, such as furosemide, to the treatment regimen temporarily to help excrete mobilized fluids. A pregnant hypertensive patient should be treated with methyldopa, which seems to be safe for the fetus. Always exclude eclampsia before treating hypertensive pregnant patients.
   3. Severe hypertension (for example, after major vascular surgery), often requires parenteral administration of vasodilators; rarely, parenteral β-blockers are used if

there is a significant history of coronary artery disease and/or myocardial infarction without heart failure. The vasodilator of choice is sodium nitroprusside.

4. Newly diagnosed hypertensive patients need appropriate follow-up after discharge.

43. HYPOCALCEMIA

(See also Section II, page 293)

I. **Problem.** A patient admitted to the trauma service with multiple injuries after a motor vehicle accident has a serum calcium level of 7.7 mg/dL (normal, 8.5–0.5 mg/dL).

II. **Immediate Questions**

A. **Are there any symptoms relevant to hypocalcemia?** Asymptomatic hypocalcemia usually does not require treatment. Signs and symptoms of hypocalcemia may include perioral and peripheral (fingers and toes) paresthesias, Chvostek's sign (twitching of the lip with tapping on the cheek), Trousseau's sign (carpopedal spasm after application of a blood pressure cuff), confusion, muscle twitching, tetany, or seizures.

B. **Is there a history of surgery?** Look for scars from a previous neck operation because surgical removal or infarction of the parathyroids is the most common cause of true hypocalcemia. Any patient that receives large volumes (several liters) of fluid during or after surgery will drop their calcium and albumin to very low levels. Although the ionized calcium is much more reliable, awake, asymptomatic patients rarely need treatment. A patient with normal parathyroid function can mobilize a nearly endless supply of calcium from their bones. If you can't assess the patient clinically (intubated, sedated), or the patient has a reason to be hypocalcemic (multiple blood transfusions in a short period of time), treat until the ionized calcium reaches the normal range. Don't be surprised if the serum calcium doesn't change much even with treatment in this setting.

C. **Does the low calcium level represent the true calcium level?** Most laboratories report the total serum calcium. However, a decrease in the serum albumin of 1 g/dL will decrease the protein bound calcium by 0.8 mg/dL. Obtain serum albumin values and correct for the total calcium level appropriately or measure the ionized calcium.

Corrected Ca = [(normal albumin − patient's albumin) × 0.8] + patient's measured serum Ca

III. Differential Diagnosis

A. **Parathyroid Hormone (PTH) Deficits** due to surgical excision (can occur 12 h to 5 d postop), injury, or irradiation of the parathyroids.

B. **Pseudohypoparathyroidism:** Resistance to PTH at the tissue level. PTH level is elevated and can be suppressed by calcium infusion.

C. **Vitamin D Deficiency**
   1. **Malnutrition.**
   2. **Malabsorption**
      a. Pancreatitis.
      b. Postgastrectomy.
      c. Short-gut syndrome.
      d. Laxative abuse.
      e. Sprue.
      f. Hepatobiliary disease with bile salt deficiency.
   3. **Defective metabolism**
      a. **Liver disease:** Failure to synthesize 25(OH) vitamin D.
      b. **Renal disease:** Failure to synthesize 1–25 dihydroxy vitamin D.
      c. **Anticonvulsive Treatment:** Phenobarbital and phenytoin produce inactive metabolites of vitamin D.

D. **Magnesium Deficiency.** Results in decreased PTH release and activity; correcting the magnesium deficit will often correct the calcium level.

E. **Calcium Loss/Displacement**
   1. **Hyperphosphatemia.** Increases bone deposition of calcium.
      a. Acute phosphate ingestion.
      b. Acute phosphate release by rhabdomyolysis, tumor lysis.
   2. **Acute Pancreatitis.**
   3. **Osteoblastic metastases.** Especially breast and prostate.
   4. **Medullary carcinoma of the thyroid.** Resulting from increased thyrocalcitonin.
   5. **Decreased bone resorption.** Agents such as actinomycin, calcitonin, mithramycin.
   6. **Alkalosis** causes increased binding of calcium to plasma proteins.

IV. Database

A. **Physical Exam Key Points**
   1. **Skin.** Dermatitis, eczema with chronic hypocalcemia.

2. **HEENT.** Cataracts may be present; laryngospasm is rare but life-threatening. Look for surgical scars on the neck.
3. **Neuromuscular.** Confusion, spasm, twitching, facial grimacing, hyperactive deep tendon reflexes, and depression.
4. **Clinical tests for hypocalcemia**
   a. **Chvostek's sign:** Present in 5–10% of patients with normal calcium levels. Tap on facial nerve near the zygoma of patient's jaw (the cheek) and observe for twitching.
   b. **Trousseau's sign:** Inflate a blood pressure cuff higher than the systolic pressure for 3 min and observe for carpal spasm.

B. **Laboratory Data**
1. **Serum electrolytes.** Particularly calcium, phosphate, potassium and magnesium. Calcium must be interpreted in terms of the serum albumin. Hypomagnesemia and hyperkalemia may potentiate the symptoms of hypocalcemia.
2. **Serum albumin.** Use to adjust the calcium level as previously noted. A low albumin should not affect the ionized calcium level.
3. **Renal function tests (BUN and creatinine).** May reveal evidence of chronic renal insufficiency.
4. The combination of hypocalcemia with a high serum phosphate usually indicates hypoparathyroidism.
5. **Parathyroid hormone levels.**
6. **Vitamin D levels.** 25 hydroxy and 1,25 dihydroxy vitamin D levels.
7. **Urinary cyclic AMP levels.** This gives an index of parathyroid function and is increased with elevated PTH levels.
8. **Fecal fat.** To look for steatorrhea.

C. **Radiographic and Other Tests**
1. **ECG.** Hypocalcemia prolongs the QT interval.
2. **Bone films.** There are bone changes in renal failure or with osteoblastic metastases.

V. **Plan.** Assess the patient for tetany, which can potentially progress to laryngeal spasm or seizures and requires urgent treatment. Otherwise, establish the diagnosis by blood tests of calcium, albumin, magnesium, phosphate and PTH and begin appropriate therapy.

A. **Acute Treatment.** Give 200–300 mg of elemental calcium rapidly.
1. **10% calcium gluconate.** One 10-mL ampule contains 90 mg of calcium. Give 20–30 mL total IV. This may

take a little time, but it is safer than using calcium chloride, when the patient is stable enough to wait.

2. **10% calcium chloride.** One 10–mL ampule contains 360 mg of calcium. Give 10 mL IV, ideally through a central line. If calcium chloride infiltrates during administration through a peripheral line, it can cause tissue necrosis.

B. **Chronic Treatment.** With primary parathormone deficiency, the goal is to give 2–4 g of oral calcium daily, then add vitamin D if necessary. In a vitamin D disorder, supplement with vitamin D. You may need to use 1–25 dihydroxy vitamin D (Rocaltrol) in patients with renal disease. The use of aluminum phosphate gels (eg, ALTernaGEL) will limit phosphate absorption.

1. **Calcium carbonate.** 240 mg of calcium per 600 mg tablet.
2. **OsCal-500.** A 1.25 g calcium carbonate tablet provides 500 mg of elemental calcium.
3. **Dihydrotachysterol vitamin D2.** 0.25–1.0 μg/d.

C. **Magnesium Deficiency**

1. 1–2 g of 10% magnesium sulfate IV over a 20 min period or 40–80 mEq $Mgso_4$/L IV fluid.
2. For chronic replacement, use magnesium oxide 600 mg 1–2 tablets qd.

44. HYPOGLYCEMIA

(See also Section II, page 305)

I. **Problem.** A nurse notifies you that a 40-year-old man has a serum glucose of 40 mg/dL (normal fasting, 70–105 mg/dL).

II. **Immediate Questions**

A. **Is the patient diabetic and on insulin?** Hypoglycemia is commonly caused by the inadvertent administration of too much insulin to a diabetic, or the administration of insulin to a diabetic patient who is not eating.

B. **What medications is the patient taking? Do they include any oral hypoglycemic agents?**

C. **What IV fluids are running? Was TPN recently stopped (abruptly stopping TPN rarely causes reactive hypoglycemia)?** If the patient is receiving hyperalimentation, how much insulin has been added? Is the patient receiving IV fluid without dextrose (eg, NS)?

D. **What is the patient's diagnosis?** There are certain rare diseases associated with hypoglycemia, such as retroperitoneal sarcoma, insulinoma, and paraneoplastic syndromes (especially squamous cell carcinoma of the lung). Pancreatic transplant recipients can have hypoglycemia secondary to dysfunctional autoregulation postoperatively. Liver transplant patients are commonly hypoglycemic after surgery because the liver is the site of stored glycogen.

E. **Is the patient awake, alert, comatose, or diaphoretic?** Stupor or coma suggest a degree of hypoglycemia that can potentially cause permanent neurologic damage. Diaphoresis and tremulousness are usually a manifestation of catecholamine discharge.

III. Differential Diagnosis

A. Medications

1. **Insulin.** There may be an administration error; for example, inadvertent administration of an excessive dose, an additional dose, a wrong preparation, IV administration of a dose ordered subcutaneously, or administration to the wrong patient.
2. **Oral hypoglycemic agents.** Tolbutamide, chlorpropamide, acetohexamide, and others.
3. **Others.** Pentamidine, ethanol, and MAO inhibitors are infrequent causes.

B. Severe Liver Failure/Resection Extensive Hepatic Destruction.

C. Insulinoma.
Check serum insulin and glucose levels simultaneously. These are suggested by Whipple's triad: symptoms of hypoglycemia, a documented serum glucose < 50 mg/dL, and relief of symptoms with the administration of glucose.

D. Sudden Discontinuation of TPN.
This is more of a theoretical than an actual problem. In fact, most patients can easily tolerate the sudden discontinuation of TPN.

E. Retroperitoneal Sarcomas.
These tumors can rarely cause hypoglycemia.

F. Paraneoplastic Syndrome.
Hypoglycemia can be caused by the secretion of insulin or insulin-like substances by tumors, especially small-cell carcinoma of the lung.

G. Surreptitious Insulin/Oral Hypoglycemic Administration.

H. Reactive Functional Hypoglycemia.

I. Alimentary Hypoglycemia.
Found in 5–10% of patients who have undergone partial to complete gastrectomies. It results from rapid gastric emptying.

J. Factitious Hypoglycemia. A rare but possibly confounding diagnosis, it is found in patients with WBC > 40,000, where leukocytes continue to metabolize glucose after blood drawing (in a red- topped tube). These patients will have asymptomatic hypoglycemia. Thus, any patient with a very high WBC count should have their serum glucose determined from blood collected in a tube that contains sodium fluoride (gray top), which inhibits white cell metabolism.

K. Hormone Deficiencies. Glucocorticoids, growth hormone, thyroid hormone, glucagon, panhypopituitarism.

L. Miscellaneous. Sepsis, alcoholism or severe malnutrition.

IV. Database

A. Physical Exam Key Points

1. **Vital signs.** Tachycardia may be caused by the adrenergic response to hypoglycemia.
2. **Skin.** Diaphoresis is also an adrenergic response.
3. **Neurologic exam.** Assess orientation and level of consciousness.

B. Laboratory Data

1. **Serum glucose.** The most important diagnostic test is the serum glucose level. Values < 50 mg/dL are diagnostic in the presence of symptoms. Rapid glucose measurements using reagent strips, glucometers, and fingerstick blood samples may be helpful but should be confirmed with a serum level.
2. **Urine glucose levels.** Usually of little help in this setting.
3. **Serum insulin levels.** Elevated with both insulinoma and surreptitious insulin administration.
4. **C-peptide levels.** Reflects endogenous insulin production. An elevated C-peptide, with an elevated serum insulin level suggests an insulinoma. If the serum insulin is increased and the C peptide level is decreased, insulin overdosage or surreptitious insulin administration is likely.

C. Radiographic and Other Studies. Used to work up clinically suspected tumors. Arteriography is often more useful than CT in localizing a pancreatic insulinoma. Intraoperative ultrasound is helpful when preoperative studies are negative.

V. Plan.

In acute cases, increase the serum glucose and eliminate the patient's symptoms, then identify the cause.

A. Administer Glucose. Do not wait for the results of the serum glucose (drawn before treatment) if you strongly suspect the diagnosis. The mainstay of initial therapy is glucose, given orally if the patient is awake, alert and able to take fluids, or intravenously otherwise.

1. **Oral.** Give orange juice with or without additional sugar.
2. **Parenteral.** Give one ampule of D50 (dextrose 50%) IV push. If there is no change, give another ampule of D50. If the patient doesn't respond at this point, you should question the presumptive diagnosis of hypoglycemia and consider other possibilities.
3. When you can't obtain IV access, give glucagon 0.5–1 mg IM or SQ. Vomiting may occur.
4. Start a maintenance IV of D5W at 50–100 mL/h to help prevent a recurrence of hypoglycemia. Follow up with serial glucose measurements after the initial episode.

B. Adjust Medications. Reevaluate the current dosing schedule of insulin or oral hypoglycemic agents.

C. Workup of Hypoglycemia. After treating the acute episode, look for the underlying cause. Serum insulin levels, C-peptide levels, liver function tests, glucose tolerance tests, and appropriate radiographic tests should be considered.

D. Liver Resection. Patients should be maintained on IV fluids containing 10% dextrose and should have frequent serum glucose determinations after liver resection.

45. HYPOKALEMIA

(See also Section II, page 318)

I. Problem. A 72–year-old man on long-term diuretics for heart failure develops abdominal distention and an ileus. His serum potassium is 2.5 mEq/L (normal 3.5–5.1 mEq/L).

II. Immediate Questions

A. What medications is the patient taking? Loop diuretics (furosemide, as an example) are kaliuretic and cause significant renal potassium wasting. Thiazide diuretics can cause hypokalemia, but the level is rarely dangerous, except when digoxin is used concomitantly (hypokalemia potentiates digitalis toxicity). Amphotericin B causes potassium wasting by direct renal toxicity.

B. Is there a history of vomiting, NG suction, or diarrhea? Gastrointestinal losses are common causes of hypokalemia in the surgical patient.

C. What are the vital signs? Look for an irregular pulse, which could represent new premature atrial or ventricular contractions (PACs and PVCs). Hypokalemia increases myocardial irritability and an ECG is important. Check the urine output and urine electrolytes.

D. Is the patient symptomatic? Symptoms of hypokalemia include weakness, nausea, vomiting, and abdominal tenderness.

III. Differential Diagnosis

A. Potassium Losses

1. Gastrointestinal

- **a.** Prolonged NG suction without replacement can cause hypokalemia through direct losses, induced renal losses, and through potassium shifts into cells due to the development of metabolic alkalosis. This is the most common electrolyte abnormality in surgical patients.
- **b.** Intractable vomiting (same mechanism as NG suction).
- **c.** Bowel obstruction can result in hypokalemia through the pooling of secretions and inefficient potassium absorption.
- **d.** Diarrhea, fistula, villous adenoma.

2. Renal

- **a. Diuretics:** Especially loop diuretics, such as furosemide.
- **b.** Renal tubular acidosis results in hypokalemia when K^+ is secreted and H^+ is absorbed.
- **c. Antibiotics:** Carbenicillin and others. Amphotericin B may also cause magnesium wasting.
- **d.** Postobstructive diuresis or the diuretic phase of acute tubular necrosis (ATN).

B. Potassium Redistribution

1. **Alkalosis.** Cation balance requires that as H^+ moves out of cells to correct alkalosis, K^+ moves in.
2. **Insulin.** Insulin causes the coupled transport of glucose and potassium into cells.

C. Inadequate Intake. This is usually iatrogenic (from the administration of potassium free IV fluids over a prolonged time period). In the absence of other losses, normal daily potassium requirements (with normal renal function) are 40–60 mEq per 24h.

IV. Database. Because potassium is the principal intracellular cation, hypokalemia usually represents a significant loss of body potassium. Thus, a serum level of 3.0 mEq/L (mmol/L) often represents a total deficit of 100–200 mEq in the adult.

A. **Physical Exam Key Points**

1. **Cardiac.** An Irregular pulse may represent a new arrhythmia (PAC, PVC) or digoxin toxicity.
2. **Abdomen.** Look for evidence of distention and listen for bowel sounds. Obstruction can cause hypokalemia; rarely, ileus results from hypokalemia and thus exacerbates the condition. Vomiting may cause hypokalemia, and vomiting can occasionally be caused by digitalis toxicity.
3. **Neurologic exam.** Severe hypokalemia can cause blunting of reflexes, paresthesias, and paralysis.

B. **Laboratory Data**

1. **Serum electrolytes.** Hypocalcemia and hypomagnesemia may coexist.
2. **Arterial blood gas.** Severe electrolyte abnormalities often have accompanying acid-base defects. Renal tubular acidosis and metabolic alkalosis often result in hypokalemia.
3. **Urine electrolytes.** Renal potassium wasting can be evaluated with a simple "spot" determination of urine K^+, Na^+, and osmolality (see page 331).This is only useful when the patient is not taking diuretics.
4. Digoxin level, if appropriate.

C. **Radiographic and Other Studies.** An ECG and a rhythm strip should be done on any patient with evidence of digitalis toxicity, new PACs, or new PVCs, as manifested by a new irregular pulse. T wave flattening, U waves, and S-T segment changes all occur with hypokalemia.

V. **Plan.** More severe cases of hypokalemia, (levels < 3.0 mmol/L) or those cases associated with ECG abnormalities should be treated aggressively because of the potential for life-threatening arrhythmias. Potassium should be aggressively replaced after verifying that the patient has good renal function.

A. **Parenteral Replacement**

1. **Indications.** Should be considered in patients with digoxin toxicity, significant arrhythmias, severe hypokalemia (< 3.0 mmol/L), and in those who cannot take oral replacement (NPO, ileus, nausea, and vomiting). Parenteral administration is ideally given via a central venous catheter. Most hypokalemia can be safely corrected in a slow, controlled fashion with oral supplementation.
2. **Replacement.** Add 10–40 mEq/L of potassium chloride to peripheral IV fluids. Administering more than 40 mEq/L causes pain and phlebitis, although 60 mEq/L is occasionally used in emergent circumstances. Alterna-

tively, dilute between 10 and 20 mEq KCl in 50–100 mL D5W or NS and infuse over 1 h through a central line, with doses repeated as needed for severe depletion or life-threatening hypokalemia. Special care must be taken to ensure slow infusion of these high doses.

3. **Monitoring.** Check serum levels frequently (every 2–4 h) to avoid hyperkalemia. ECG and ICU monitoring is required for arrhythmias or for rapid infusions of KCl.

B. **Oral Replacement.** (see also Section IX, page 521). Generally indicated for asymptomatic patients with mild levels of potassium repletion (3.0 < K < 4.0 mEq/L). Oral replacements come in liquids, powders, and pills. Slow release pills typically contain > 10 mEq per tablet and are thus more useful for maintenance than for repletion therapy. Replacement normally requires 40–120 mEq/d in divided doses depending on the patient's weight and level of hypokalemia. Maintenance therapy, if needed, should be given in doses of 20–40 mEq daily, using the preparation best tolerated by the patient. For patients with normal renal function, it is difficult to induce hyperkalemia by the oral administration of potassium. Remember to avoid the use of potassium supplements in patients on potassium-sparing diuretics (eg, triamterene, spironolactone, amiloride).

C. **Replace Ongoing Losses.** Large amounts of nasogastric drainage should be replaced mL for mL with D5 1/2 NS plus 20 mEq/L KCl every 4–6 h.

D. **Refractory Cases.** Rarely, hypokalemia may not be correctable because of concomitant hypomagnesemia or hypocalcemia. Replace calcium as described in Problem 43, page 171.

46. HYPONATREMIA

(See also Section II, page 323)

I. **Problem.** An elderly woman admitted for a mastectomy has a sodium of 119 mEq/L on routine admission labs (normal, 136–145 mEq/L).

II. **Immediate Questions**

A. **Does the patient have any CNS symptoms?** Brain cells become edematous in a hypoosmotic state. Inquire about lethargy, agitation, disorientation, or obtundation. Neurologic manifestations are usually evident when the Na level is ≤ 120 mEq/L.

B. **Are there any recent sodium levels?** The rate of development of hyponatremia correlates directly with the severity of symptoms it produces. Acute changes in sodium are more likely to produce severe symptoms.

C. **Does the patient take diuretics?** Hyponatremia is common in elderly patients undergoing loop diuretic therapy (eg, furosemide).

D. **Is the hyponatremia real, or is it a laboratory artifact?** High concentrations of osmotic agents and space-occupying compounds alter the reported laboratory value of sodium. This is also known as pseudohyponatremia. Note the concentration of glucose and triglycerides and adjust the measured sodium up to true levels (as described below).

E. **Has the patient had recent surgery?** Surgery and anesthesia often result in an inappropriate ADH secretion for 2–3 d. This leads to mild hyponatremia in most patients and to significant hyponatremia when the patient has been given an excessive amount of free water.

F. **What is the patient receiving for IV fluids?** The long-term administration of hypotonic fluids can lead to the gradual development of hyponatremia.

III. **Differential Diagnosis.** First determine whether the patient has true hyponatremia or a laboratory artifact. Hyponatremia may then be classified according to the volume status of the patient: hypovolemic, euvolemic, or hypervolemic. Hypovolemic hyponatremia may be further classified by serum and urine chemistries.

A. **Laboratory Artifact (Pseudohyponatremia)**
   1. **Osmotic agents.** Hyperglycemia is most common. Adjust the serum sodium up 1.6 mEq/L for every excess 100 mg/dL of glucose greater than the reference value of 100 mg/dL.
   2. **Space-occupying compounds.** Lipids (hyperlipidemia) are the most common. The lab can ultracentrifuge the specimen to find the corrected plasma level.

B. **Hypovolemic Hyponatremia**
   1. **Spot urinary Na < 10 mEq/L**
      a. **GI fluid losses:** Vomiting or diarrhea. In surreptitious vomiting or bulimia the urinary chloride is usually < 10 mEq/L.
      b. **Third space fluid loss:** As seen in pancreatitis or peritonitis.
      c. **Burns.**
   2. **Urinary Na > 10 mEq/L**
      a. **Diuretic usage:** Caused by thiazides (eg, hydrochlorothiazide) and loop diuretics (eg, furosemide) and often associated with hypokalemia and

alkalosis; with surreptitious diuretic use, the urinary chloride is > 20 mEq/L.

b. **Renal disorders:** Medullary cystic disease, polycystic disease, and chronic interstitial nephritis can result in hyponatremia.

c. **Addison's disease:** Hyperkalemia and low urinary potassium are also found.

d. **Osmotic diuresis:** Most commonly owing to glucose, mannitol, or ketones (as in diabetic ketoacidosis [DKA]).

C. Euvolemic Hyponatremia

1. **SIADH.** The diagnosis of SIADH (Syndrome of Inappropriate Antidiuretic Hormone) is based on the finding of low serum osmolality, elevated urine sodium, and slightly concentrated urine (osmolality near sodium).
   a. **Postoperative:** Anesthesia and surgical procedures commonly cause an increased secretion of ADH for several days. The TURP (transurethral resection of the prostate) syndrome is caused by excessive fluid absorption from water used for irrigation during transurethral surgery.
   b. **Tumors:** Small-cell lung cancer is most often responsible.
   c. **Pulmonary infections:** Such as TB and other bacterial pneumonias.
   d. **CNS disorders:** Trauma, tumors, and infections.
   e. **Stress:** Including perioperative stress.
   f. **Drugs:** Oral hypoglycemics, chemotherapeutics (cyclophosphamide, vincristine), psychiatric drugs (haloperidol, tricyclic antidepressants), and clofibrate.
2. **Hypothyroidism.**
3. **Hypopituitarism.**

D. Hypervolemic Hyponatremia

1. Congestive heart failure.
2. Cirrhosis.
3. Renal disease.
   a. Chronic renal failure.
   b. Nephrotic syndrome.
4. Psychogenic polydipsia.

IV. Database

A. Physical Exam Key Points. As apparent from the differential diagnosis, close attention should be paid to the patient's volume status.

1. **Vital signs.** Evaluate for orthostatic hypotension. (A drop in blood pressure > 10 mm Hg or a pulse increase

of > 10 BPM is highly suggestive of volume depletion). Tachypnea may suggest volume overload and pulmonary edema.

2. **Skin.** Check for decreased skin turgor and dry mucous membranes as expected with dehydration. Edema suggests volume overload. Jaundice and caput medusae are evidence of cirrhosis.
3. **HEENT.** Evaluate the patient's jugular venous pressure by elevating the bed 45 degrees (veins are flat with volume depletion and markedly engorged with volume overload).
4. **Lungs.** Rales may be heard with volume overload.
5. **Heart.** An S_3 gallop murmur suggests volume overload.
6. **Abdomen.** Hepatosplenomegaly, ascites, and other signs of cirrhosis may be present. A hepatojugular reflex may be present in CHF.
7. **Neurologic exam.** Hyperactive deep tendon reflexes, altered mental status, confusion, coma, or seizures usually indicate a sodium level of < 120 mmol/L.

B. Laboratory Data

1. **Electrolytes.** There may be abnormalities involving many of the electrolytes on the SMA-7.
2. **Spot urine electrolytes and creatinine.** Obtain before any diuretic treatment.
3. **Urine and serum osmolality.** Serum osmolality will be normal in cases of laboratory artifact but decreased in true hyponatremia.
4. **Liver function tests.** To detect liver disease.
5. **Arterial blood gases.** Acidosis/alkalosis may be present.
6. Thyroid function.
7. Cortisol levels, ACTH stimulation test.
8. Cultures (blood and sputum).

C. Radiographic and Other Studies

1. **Chest radiograph.** Look for evidence of CHF or a lung tumor.
2. **Head CT scan, if indicated.**
3. **Water load test.** Bring the serum sodium to a safe level by fluid restriction. Then challenge the patient with 20 mL/kg of water PO. Collect urine hourly for 5 h. When < 75% of intake volume is excreted or when urine osmolarity fails to decrease to less than 200, then SIADH is present.

V. Plan. The underlying cause of the hyponatremia and the presence and severity of symptoms guide therapy. Aggressive therapy for severe symptoms (eg, coma) will be discussed as well as specific therapies for certain diagnoses.

A. **Acute Therapy**
   1. **Normal saline and furosemide 1 mg/kg IV.** Use the combination of normal saline and diuretics to achieve a net negative volume balance. Document carefully the volume in and the volume out. Supplement fluids with potassium as needed.
   2. **Hypertonic saline (3%) is rarely, if ever, needed.** Many institutions have banned its use entirely because of serious complications.

B. **Specific Therapies**
   1. **Hypovolemic hyponatremia**
      a. For almost all causes, treat by repleting volume and sodium. (Normal saline IV infusion).
      b. In cases of diuretic abuse, also replace lost body potassium.
   2. **Euvolemic hyponatremia.** The patient is not edematous.
      a. **SIADH:** Restrict water to between 800 and 1000 mL daily. Administer demeclocycline for increased urine Na or urine osmolarity.
      b. **Hypothyroidism:** Treat with thyroid replacement.
      c. **Hypopituitary:** Treat with hormone replacement.
   3. **Hypervolemic hyponatremia.** The patient is edematous. Restrict IV and oral fluids. Check urine sodium (usually (< 10 mEq/L).
      a. **CHF:** Treat with digoxin, diuretics, and water restriction.
      b. **Nephrotic syndrome:** Steroids, water restriction, and increased protein intake are commonly used.
      c. **Cirrhosis:** Treat with water restriction, diuretics, and a portosystemic shunt when indicated. The urine sodium is usually > 20 mEq/L.
      d. **Renal failure:** Treat with water restriction and dialysis if indicated.

47. HYPOTENSION (SHOCK)

Immediate Actions

1. Assess the airway and breathing. Intubate if necessary.
2. Ensure large-bore IV access and begin a 500-mL LR bolus.
3. Control external hemorrhage (when present) with direct pressure.
4. Use the Trendelenburg position.
5. See Figure I–11, page 60.

I. **Problem.** A 40-year-old female who underwent total abdominal hysterectomy earlier that day has a blood pressure of 80/50 mm Hg.

II. Immediate Questions

A. **What is the patient's pulse?** Tachycardia suggests hypovolemia. Hypotension with a low or normal pulse suggests adrenergic blockade from anesthesia or other pharmacologic agents. Patients with pacemakers and/or heart disease may not be able to raise their pulse in response to hypovolemia.

B. **What were the blood pressure readings preoperatively?** A normal resting systolic blood pressure of 80–90 mm Hg is occasionally seen in very thin women. Again, the pulse rate should help you identify hypovolemia. Always double-check any arterial line blood pressure readings with a careful cuff determination.

C. **When was the patient's surgery?** Hypovolemia and bleeding should be at the top of the differential diagnosis after surgery, particularly on the first postoperative night.

D. **What is the cardiac rhythm?** Abnormal atrial and ventricular rhythms can cause hypotension. Atrial fibrillation is particularly common 2–3 d after surgery. Hypotension with bradycardia suggests heart block.

E. **What is the patient's mental status?** See if the hypotension is affecting critical organ perfusion.

F. **What medications is the patient taking?** A patient on β-blockers may have a lower pulse and may be unable to develop reflex tachycardia in response to hypovolemia. Narcotics and some sedatives can induce hypotension. Anaphylactic reactions may be caused by medications or intravenous contrast agents (see Problem 5, page 23). Epidural anesthesia may occasionally cause hypotension.

G. **What is the fluid balance?** Urine output generally reflects the volume status of the patient. A decreasing urine output with hypotension suggests poor renal perfusion. Be sure that the patient has been adequately hydrated and that excessive losses (such as NG drainage) are being replaced.

H. **Is there any obvious bleeding source?** Inquire about blood on the dressings, bloody NG drainage, increased chest tube or mediastinal tube output.

I. **Addisonian Crisis (Adrenal Insufficiency).** Check for this condition especially after adrenal surgery or radical nephrectomy. Any patient who has taken steroids during the last year may have a blunted adrenal response to the stress of surgery.

J. **Is there underlying sepsis?** There may be bouts of hypotension throughout the septic episode, usually with secondary tachycardia.

III. **Differential Diagnosis.** As a rule of thumb, a systolic blood pressure of 90 mm Hg or less in an adult is considered hypotension. Hypotension may cause shock, a state characterized by inadequate tissue perfusion. Shock can be classified as hypovolemic, neurogenic, vasogenic, and cardiogenic. Each type is presented below:

A. **Hypovolemic.** A condition often seen in surgical patients.

1. **Hemorrhagic**

   a. **Traumatic:** Patients in shock often have significant blood loss that may be obvious or may be inapparent (into the chest, abdomen, or retroperitoneum; into fracture sites such as the pelvis and long bones; or into soft tissues).

   b. **Postoperative:** Drains may reveal bleeding, but, as with trauma, there are many places for blood to hide.

   c. **Others:** Disseminated intravascular coagulation, GI tract bleeding, a ruptured aneurysm, a ruptured ovarian cyst, or an ectopic pregnancy (in female patients) should be considered.

2. **Fluid losses.** From repeated vomiting, diarrhea, profuse sweating, extensive burns, and "third space losses" (eg, pancreatitis, bowel obstruction). It can also be a result of inadequate hydration during surgery with continued vasodilatation and evaporative losses from an open abdomen.

B. **Neurogenic.** Seen in patients with spinal cord trauma. It is characterized by hypotension and a normal pulse. These patients will usually have a normal urine output after fluid administration, however they may require large amounts of fluid due to loss of sympathetic tone.

C. **Vasogenic.** Septic shock, anaphylactic reactions, or adrenocortical insufficiency may cause decreased vascular tone (low systemic vascular resistance). In surgical patients, septic shock is usually a hyperdynamic state with high cardiac output and low peripheral vascular resistance.

D. **Cardiogenic.** "Pump failure" (usually from myocardial infarction, occasionally from cardiopathy, valvular disease, or septal rupture), arrhythmias (atrial fibrillation, complete heart block), tension pneumothorax, cardiac tamponade and pulmonary embolus can lead to cardiogenic shock.

IV. **Database**

A. **Physical Exam Key Points**

1. **Vital signs.** Confirm arterial line pressure readings with a cuff pressure. Tachycardia is the usual response to hypotension, with bradycardia suggesting heart block.

Irregularity of the pulse suggests an arrhythmia. Tachypnea may indicate hypoxia or acidosis resulting from poor perfusion or early sepsis. Fever suggests sepsis; however, elderly or immunosuppressed patients may be afebrile, and other patients may rarely be hypothermic despite being septic.

2. **Skin.** Good skin turgor and moist mucous membranes suggest adequate hydration; cool, clammy skin may indicate shock.
3. **Neck.** Check for jugular venous distention. Bulging neck veins are seen with congestive failure, pericardial tamponade, or tension pneumothorax.
4. **Chest.** Rales occur with congestive heart failure; wheezing and stridor with anaphylaxis; decreased breath sounds with hemothorax or pneumothorax. Rib tenderness (from fractures) is associated with hemo- or pneumothorax and sternal tenderness with pericardial tamponade (such as in steering wheel trauma).
5. **Cardiac.** Check for new murmurs, arrhythmias, or rubs. Heart sounds may be muffled with cardiac tamponade.
6. **Abdomen.** Distention, a pulsatile mass, flank ecchymoses, or active bleeding at drain sites or wound dressings may suggest the cause.
7. **Rectal exam.** Check for gross (hematochezia) or occult blood.
8. **Pelvic exam.** Pelvic fractures can result in a large amount of blood loss. The pelvic exam (in females) may reveal a gynecologic cause.
9. **Extremities.** Absent or "thready" pulses are consistent with shock; long bone fractures (especially the femur) may result in significant bleeding (1–2 U) into soft tissues. Examine IV sites for evidence of infection. Edema is often seen with CHF.
10. **Neurologic exam.** Mental status changes suggest poor central perfusion. A loss of motor and sensory function occurs with spinal cord trauma.

B. Laboratory Data

1. **CBC.** Serial hematocrit determinations are essential, because the hematocrit may not drop for some time after an acute bleed.
2. **Serum electrolytes.** An Addisonian crisis causes hyperkalemia with hyponatremia.
3. **Coagulation panel (PT, PTT, platelet count).** If excessive bleeding from DIC is suspected, check the fibrinogen and fibrin split products.
4. **Arterial blood gases.** Early sepsis may cause tachypnea, which leads to respiratory alkalosis; acidosis may

indicate inadequate tissue perfusion; hypoxia may require ventilatory support.

5. **Cardiac injury panel.** Troponin levels may reveal evidence of myocardial injury (see Section II, page 327).
6. **Pregnancy test.** Especially if a ruptured ectopic pregnancy is suspected.
7. **Blood.** Should be typed and crossmatched immediately.

C. Radiographic and Other Studies

1. **Chest radiograph.** Look for evidence of CHF, cardiac enlargement, pneumothorax, or hemothorax.
2. **ECG.** Myocardial ischemia may show flipped T waves or S-T segment depression; arrhythmias may be noted.
3. **Pulmonary artery catheter.** A PA catheter is helpful in managing a patient in whom fluid overload would be particularly dangerous. By using a PA catheter, filling pressures are measured directly, avoiding iatrogenic pulmonary edema. PA pressures help to differentiate cardiogenic from hypovolemic or vasogenic shock. For diagnostic and insertion details, see Section III, page 368.
4. **Angiogram.** This may help to identify bleeding sites (especially for GI tract bleeding). A pulmonary angiogram may be needed to diagnose a pulmonary embolus with an equivocal $\dot{V}/\dot{Q}$ scan.
5. **Nuclear ventilation/perfusion ($\dot{V}/\dot{Q}$) scan.** This is commonly used to diagnose a pulmonary embolus.
6. **Echocardiogram.** This may be helpful to examine valves (mitral stenosis, aortic insufficiency, etc), pericardial fluid, and intracardiac thrombi.
7. **Blood, sputum, urine cultures.** These should be ordered in cases of suspected sepsis.
8. Perform a peritoneal tap, thoracentesis, or culdocentesis when indicated (see Section III, page 368).

V. Plan. Reestablish adequate tissue perfusion as soon as possible if the patient is in shock. In general, a blood pressure of > 90 mm Hg and urine output of at least 0.5 mL/kg/min is acceptable.

A. Emergency Management. See Figure I–11, page 60 for useful algorithm.

1. Control external hemorrhage with direct pressure.
2. Establish good venous access, and closely monitor the patient in shock.
3. Trendelenburg position (supine with feet higher than head) may improve cerebral perfusion and blood pressure immediately.

4. Except for cardiogenic shock, replace volume immediately with IV crystalloid (normal saline, lactated Ringer's, etc).
5. Use a Foley catheter to monitor urinary output.
6. Use supplemental oxygen or ventilatory support when needed. Correct severe acidosis with IV sodium bicarbonate.
7. Insert a CVP line or PA catheter to manage volume replacement and to accurately diagnose the cause of the shock.

B. Hypovolemic Shock. Restore intravascular volume.

1. Place two large-bore (18–gauge or larger) IVs.
2. **Administer fluids.** Use blood if the hematocrit is low or crystalloid (normal saline or lactated Ringer's) when blood is not available or when the hematocrit is adequate (ie, > 30%).
3. Titrate fluids by following the blood pressure and urine output.
4. A CVP line or PA catheter may help to guide fluid administration. Avoid using central lines as resuscitation lines. A short large-bore peripheral line will allow a much faster rate of fluid administration.
5. Do not use pressor agents (eg, dopamine) unless there is persistent hypotension despite adequate cardiac filling pressures ("a full tank," wedge pressure > 12 mm Hg). Hypotension with low filling pressures (wedge pressure < 6 mm Hg) should be treated primarily with volume (intravenous fluids). Use a CVP line or PA catheter to ensure adequate volume when using pressor agents.
6. If a patient remains hypotensive after you restore their volume, reconsider the diagnosis of hypovolemic shock, or consider the possibility of a secondary event (an MI occurring as a result of shock). Treat persistent shock (after restoring volume) by increasing the cardiac output (with epinephrine or dopamine) or by increasing the peripheral vascular resistance (with norepinephrine, Neo-Synephrine, or, to a lesser extent, epinephrine).

C. Neurogenic Shock

1. Start by administering fluid. This does not correct the loss of vascular tone but increases the BP by increasing the cardiac preload and output. Avoid volume overload.
2. Low-dose dopamine may help support blood pressure, although some patients need a stronger alpha agonist (eg, Neo-Synephrine).

3. A major neurologic injury may not be obvious at the time of presentation in an unconscious trauma patient.

D. **Vasogenic Shock**
   1. **Septic shock.** Treatment is directed at the underlying infection.
      a. Measure the cardiac output and systemic vascular resistance (typically high cardiac output with low systemic resistance) with a PA catheter (see Section III, page 368).
      b. Administer IV fluids to support blood pressure and urine output.
      c. Culture aggressively to identify the pathogen.
      d. Treat the underlying cause of sepsis. Initiate appropriate antibiotics, consider laparotomy or percutaneous drainage of an abscess if indicated.
      e. Use pressors as needed. The first-line consideration is usually dopamine. Dopamine is discussed in Section IX, page 481. Use the lowest effective dose of dopamine to maintain blood pressure and urine output. Physiologic effects of dopamine are as follows:

3–5 μg/kg/min—Renal and splanchnic vasodilatation via dopamine receptors
5–10 μg/kg/min—Positive inotrope via β-1–receptors
> 10 μg/kg/min—Peripheral vasoconstriction via α-receptors.

   2. Anaphylactic shock, see Problem 5, page 23.

E. **Cardiogenic Shock**
   1. Cardiac output is maximized by the judicious use of inotropic (dopamine or dobutamine) agents. Dobutamine is the drug of choice for pump failure. Pulmonary edema is treated with diuretics (eg, furosemide) and vasodilators (eg, nitrates).
   2. Myocardial ischemia is acutely treated with oxygen, pain relief (morphine), and nitrates.
   3. Identified and appropriately treated arrhythmias ensure a return to normal sinus rhythm.
   4. Pulmonary embolus

48. HYPOXIA

I. **Problem.** An intubated patient has become hypoxic after the morning chest radiograph and is not responding to 100% FIO_2.

II. **Immediate Questions**

A. **Are the monitoring devices accurately connected?** Determine whether the patient is cyanotic and/or in respiratory distress. Monitor cardiac output and SaO_2 (pulse oximetry) continuously.

B. **Is the airway secure?** After you reposition the patient for a chest radiograph, the endotracheal tube may have advanced into the right mainstem bronchus, or the cuff may have ruptured or moved above the vocal cords, necessitating repositioning of the endotracheal tube or reintubating the patient.

C. **Are the breath sounds equal?** Absence of breath sounds indicates a lung collapse, a pneumothorax, or a mucous plug.

D. **Is the chest moving symmetrically?** Pain from a rib fracture, lung injury, or an incision can cause splinting and decreased air movement.

E. **Does the patient have a history of pulmonary disease or congestive heart failure?** Knowledge of the patient's medical history or medications may be helpful.

F. **Is the patient alert?** Severe hypoxia will alter the patient's mental status. Opioid overdose may cause hypoventilation.

III. **Differential Diagnosis.** Alveolar-arterial ([A-a] or [A-a]DO_2) gradient is useful to determine the cause and the severity of the oxygenation defect (see the following section, "Database"). It is best used in the ventilated patient.

A. **Low Inspired Oxygen Tension.** This is seen in high altitude situations, such as mountain climbing or improper ventilator settings. The A-a gradient is normal.

B. **Hypoventilation.** This may be caused by CNS depression from a drug overdose, a CVA, a spinal cord injury, chest wall failure from circumferential burns, splinting, neuromuscular disease (Guillain-Barré, myasthenia gravis, tetanus), or may have begun as a compensatory mechanism for metabolic alkalosis or airway obstruction. The A-a gradient is normal.

C. **Diffusion Impairment.** This may be caused by carbon monoxide poisoning or pulmonary fibrosis. The A-a gradient is increased.

D. **Ventilation.** There may be a perfusion imbalance(nonventilated alveoli pulmonary embolism, fat emboli, pneumonia, COPD, ARDS, pulmonary contusion, asthma, atelectasis, TB, pneumothorax). The A-a gradient is increased.

E. **Right to Left Shunt.** This may be caused by pulmonary edema, nitroglycerin, or cardiac anomalies (patent ductus arteriosus, patent foramen ovale, arterial septal defect, or ventricular septal defect.) The A-a gradient is increased.

IV. Database

A. Physical Exam Key Points

1. **Vital signs.** Is the hypoxia associated with tachycardia or bradycardia? What is the respiratory rate? Is the patient hypo- or hypertensive? Tachypnea, tachycardia, and hypertension are common early indicators of respiratory distress.
2. **Chest.** Listen for equal breath sounds to identify pneumothorax, intubation of right mainstem bronchus, consolidation, or mucus plugging. Asthma will cause poor air movement and wheezing. Palpate for rib fractures.
3. **Heart.** Listen for a murmur, suggesting valvular disease or CHF.
4. **Skin and nailbeds.** Look for cyanosis and signs of emboli.
5. **CNS.** Confusion and agitation are signs of inadequate CNS perfusion.
6. **Respiratory equipment.** Inspect for loose connections and incorrect settings.

B. Laboratory Data

1. Obtain an arterial blood gas and mixed venous blood gas.
2. **CBC.** Check for anemia.
3. **Cardiac enzymes.** Test when an MI is suspected.
4. Alveolar-arterial gradient (A-a or [A-a]DO_2) is a useful calculated value that determines the difference in the alveolar oxygen and the arterial oxygen content in the pulmonary capillary bed. The normal difference is 20–65 mm Hg on 100% O_2.
   - **a.** Place the patient on 100% O_2 (FIO_2 = 1.0) for 20 min.
   - **b.** Obtain a peripheral ABG.
   - **c.** A-a gradient (in mm Hg) = Atmospheric pressure (760 mm Hg) minus partial pressure of H_2O (47 at 37 °C) minus arterial PCO_2 minus arterial PO_2.
   - **d.** The larger the gradient, the more severe the defect. Gradients greater than 400 mm Hg are severe.

C. Radiographic and Other Studies

1. **Chest radiograph.** May be useful to evaluate pneumothorax, pleural effusion, pulmonary edema, and to check the position of the endotracheal tube.
2. **ECG.** An acute myocardial infarction will decrease cardiac output; right heart strain may indicate a pulmonary embolism.

3. Perform a nuclear ventilation-perfusion scan, a spiral CT scan, or a pulmonary angiogram if a pulmonary embolism is suspected.
4. **Chest CT.** Newer-generation spiral CT scans can help to identify pulmonary emboli and other types of chest pathology. Try to stabilize the patient before going to CT.

V. **Plan.** Overall, the underlying cause should be ascertained while improving the patient's oxygenation. The patient should be transferred to a monitored setting.

A. **Increase FIO_2.** Many respiratory aids are available to provide supplemental oxygen (for example, nasal cannula, ventimask, or a face tent). When there is any question about the patient's ability to protect their airway or maintain sufficient ventilation, they should be intubated and started on mechanical ventilation. When an acceptable level of oxygenation has been achieved, gradually decrease the FIO_2 level as tolerated. Remember that oxygen at high concentrations can lead to atelectasis (by eliminating nitrogen from alveoli) and oxygen toxicity.

B. Pneumothorax or other mechanical problems should be diagnosed and treated as rapidly as possible. Insertion or manipulation of a chest tube and endotracheal tube should be followed by a chest radiograph to ensure their proper position.

C. **Airway Care.** Clear the airway with suctioning and postural drainage.

D. **Atelectasis.** This should be treated by incentive spirometry and chest physiotherapy or with increased tidal volume and PEEP (in intubated patients).

E. **Bronchodilators.** These can be used to relieve bronchospasm and increase the clearance of secretions. Inhalational metaproterenol, IV theophylline and oral or subcutaneous terbutaline are the most commonly used agents. Asthma that is refractory to these may require steroids.

F. **Other Medications.** Antibiotics, inotropic agents and anticoagulation should be used as indicated.

49. INABILITY TO VOID (URINARY RETENTION)

I. **Problem.** A 66–year-old man with severe suprapubic pain comes to the emergency department after not being able to void for almost 24 h.

II. Immediate Questions

A. **What are the patient's vital signs?** Fever and tachycardia may be signs of acute bacterial prostatitis.

B. **What medications is the patient taking?** Pharmacologic causes of acute urinary retention are common and are discussed further below.

C. **Is there any history of voiding problems, such as hesitancy, urgency, frequency, or nocturia?** These symptoms suggest a bladder outlet obstruction in males (prostatic hypertrophy, stricture). When patients have gross hematuria, obstruction may result from clots.

D. **Has the patient had recent surgery?** Patients who have had recent prostate or bladder surgery may bleed in the postoperative period and develop clot retention; patients who have had abdominoperineal resection can develop a neurogenic bladder. Male patients commonly develop urinary retention due to pain and increased sympathetic outflow (closes the bladder neck) in the immediate postoperative period (particularly after herniorrhaphy and anorectal surgery).

E. **Is there a history of neurologic problems?** A herniated disk, spinal cord injury, or a stroke can affect bladder function.

III. Differential Diagnosis

A. **Pharmacologic.** Medications that cause retention include major tranquilizers (phenothiazines), antihypertensives (ganglionic blockers, methyldopa), anticholinergic agents (cold preparations), and narcotics.

B. **Neurologic.** Pelvic or lumbar spine trauma can result in urinary retention (detrusor contraction is dysfunctional while bladder sensation is intact). Other causes include pelvic surgery (APR) and neuromuscular diseases. Temporary acute urinary retention is commonly seen are after spinal anesthesia and after operative procedures performed in the inguinal, genital, or anal region.

C. **Anatomic.** Prostatic enlargement, from benign prostatic hypertrophy, is the most common cause of urinary retention in older men. Other anatomic causes include prostate cancer, acute prostatitis (history of perineal pain and fever), and urethral stricture (history of episodes of sexually transmitted diseases or instrumentation). Psychiatric patients occasionally insert foreign bodies into their urethra. In a patient with a history consistent with urolithiasis (flank pain radiating to the groin, nausea and vomiting), consider an obstructing calculus at the bladder neck. Gross hematuria can result in clot retention. Trauma patients may have urethral disruption, usually from a pelvic fracture (eg, blood at the meatus, "floating prostate"), which may cause urinary retention.

IV. Database. Ask about medications, infections, previous operative and urologic procedures, a psychiatric history, and recent trauma or injury.

A. Physical Exam Key Points

1. **Rectal exam.** Specifically determine the presence of focal or generalized prostatic enlargement. Tenderness may indicate prostatitis. Note the quality of anal sphincter tone as an indicator of pelvic nerve function. A high-riding "floating" prostate may indicate urethral disruption.
2. **Genital exam.** Look for purulent (infectious) or bloody (traumatic) meatal discharge.
3. **Abdomen.** Palpate gently and percuss the lower abdomen to identify bladder distention.
4. **Neurologic.** Check the deep tendon reflexes, the cremasteric reflex, normal local sensation, and the presence of the "anal wink" (squeezing the glans penis will result in involuntary contraction of the anal sphincter, indicating an intact pelvic reflex arc).

B. Laboratory Data

1. **CBC.** WBC elevation may indicate infection (prostatitis).
2. **Serum electrolytes, BUN, creatinine.** Long-standing urinary retention can lead to renal dysfunction.
3. **Urinalysis and urine culture.** Note the presence of blood or crystals. The urine culture should be positive with acute bacterial prostatitis.
4. Culture urethral discharge.

C. Radiographic and Other Studies

1. **Excretory urography/VCUG.** This may be helpful when blood is found on urinalysis or if urolithiasis is suspected. When the creatinine is elevated, start with ultrasound (to look for upper tract obstruction).
2. **Retrograde urethrogram.** This is the best test to identify a urethral stricture or urethral disruption.
3. **Cystoscopy.** Indicated in most patients with anatomic and neurologic causes for urinary retention. It is usually performed after Foley catheter decompression.

V. Plan

A. **Catheterization (see page 338).** First, attempt decompression by passing a 16–18 Fr Foley catheter gently into the urethra. When this fails, try a coude tip (elbow tip) catheter, which will sometimes pass more readily in males. Injection of 30 mL of water-soluble jelly into the urethra may also help to pass the catheter. Rarely will filiform and followers or a suprapubic cystostomy be required. Decompression should be performed gradually to minimize postobstructive diuresis. Do not perform catheterization in a trauma patient with blood at the meatus or a floating prostate unless urethral disruption has been ruled out with a retrograde urethrogram.

B. **Antibiotics.** Cystitis, pyelonephritis, and acute prostatitis should be treated with appropriate antibiotics. Obtain cultures before starting antibiotics. Fluoroquinolones are a good empiric choice for urinary tract infections.

C. **Fluid and Electrolyte Management.** Care should be taken to monitor serum electrolytes, especially if postobstructive diuresis follows decompression of the obstruction. This should not be a significant concern with acute retention caused by spinal anesthesia, operation, or prostatitis, but it is seen in patients with chronic obstruction from prostatic hypertrophy. Patients with an elevated BUN and creatinine are more prone to this problem. The diuresis occurs because obstructed kidneys have an impaired concentrating ability; there is also an osmotic diuresis caused by the chronic retention of waste products. Untreated postobstructive diuresis can result in vascular collapse due to hypovolemia. To prevent this, monitor the urine output and vital signs closely after decompressing the bladder. Initially, use maintenance IV fluids without potassium. Physiologic diuresis is common, but a high urine output in a hypotensive patient suggests postobstructive diuresis. Check electrolytes and replace mL/mL with IV fluid similar to the urine electrolyte profile; then gradually change to $^1/_2$ mL/mL and taper the IV from there.

D. **Postoperative.** Once they are ambulatory, many patients will be able to void without difficulty. This is especially true in patients who have undergone painful groin or anorectal procedures. Limiting narcotics may help. Alpha-blockers (terazosin, doxazosin) may help to relax the bladder neck and restore normal voiding.

E. **Cystoscopy.** Cystoscopy and urodynamic studies are usually performed in patients with chronic urinary retention, but are rarely needed in acute cases.

50. INSOMNIA

I. **Problem.** A patient hospitalized for 14 d of intravenous antibiotics for fasciitis complains of lying awake for hours at night.

II. Immediate Questions

A. **Is the patient bothered by pain?** Most surgical patients experience some degree of pain, either from surgery or from their underlying disease. Painful stimuli coupled with the disruptive situation of being in the hospital (noise, interruptions, roommates, strange bed) can understandably produce insomnia. Make sure a patient is receiving adequate pain medication in addition to sleeping medication.

B. **What are the patient's sleep habits during the day?** When a patient sleeps for extended periods during the day, they may find it difficult to fall asleep at night. Discuss this matter with the patient and with the social services and recreational therapy departments (if available).

C. **Does the patient routinely take sleeping medications?** Patients become tolerant to most sleeping pills with 1–2 wk of use. Subsequent to this, sleep may be fitful with medication but impossible without it. Take a detailed drug history to assess the contribution of withdrawal or tolerance to the insomnia.

D. **Does the patient have difficulty lying down?** Ask the patient specifically about shortness of breath (orthopnea) and calf pain (ischemic rest pain) as possible causes for disrupted sleep.

E. **What is the patient's sleep pattern?** Depression is associated with early morning awakening; anxiety usually causes difficulty in getting to sleep.

F. **Does the patient use recreational drugs or abuse alcohol?** Withdrawal may lead to insomnia and hallucinations.

III. Differential Diagnosis

A. Medical Causes

1. **Pain.** Inadequate control is often correctable.
2. **Congestive heart failure.** Orthopnea is the key symptom.
3. **Peripheral vascular disease.** Ischemic rest pain indicates advanced disease.
4. **Hyperthyroidism.**
5. **Sleep apnea syndrome.** This is most often seen with morbid obesity. Patients often awaken with a sense of panic and complain of chronic lethargy.

B. Drug or Toxin

1. Tolerance to sleeping medications or tranquilizers.
2. **Alcohol abuse.** With secondary chronic disruption of appropriate sleep patterns.

C. Psychiatric

1. **Depressive illness.** Either bipolar or unipolar.
2. **Anxiety.**

D. Situational

1. **Noise.** Is the patient's bed close to the nursing station? Does the patient have a noisy roommate?
2. **Anger.** Does the patient indicate unexpressed anger toward the staff or family?
3. **Anxiety.** Does the patient indicate either appropriate or inappropriate anxiety about their medical condition, possible operation or discharge?

IV. Database. The key to diagnosing insomnia is the history, including an evaluation of the mental status of the patient. Other studies add little except in rare cases.

A. Physical Exam Key Points

1. **Neurologic exam.** Make note of the patient's mental status. Evaluate for anxiety or depression.
2. **Cardiopulmonary.** Listen for rales, a displaced PMI, or a gallop rhythm to suggest CHF.
3. **Extremities.** Check for decreased or absent pulses, pallor on elevation, and dependent rubor.

B. Laboratory Data. The cause of insomnia can usually be determined without ordering laboratory tests.

1. **Screening chemistries.** Hepatic and renal function tests may be useful.
2. **Thyroid hormone levels.** When clinically indicated.

C. Radiographic and Other Studies

1. Chest radiograph This may be helpful when indicated for cough or CHF.
2. Obtain an ankle-brachial blood pressure index and other vascular studies when indicated.
3. Refer the patient to the Sleep lab for chronic sleeping difficulty and to rule out sleep apnea.

V. Plan

A. Etiology. Determine the cause of the insomnia, whether medical, psychologic, or situational. Most cases of insomnia will be from situational causes or a result of the patient being in the hospital. For this reason, you should include a prn sleeping medication order with all admission and postop orders unless specifically contraindicated. Any specific medical problem should be treated, and pain should be adequately controlled.

B. Specific Treatments

1. **Oral sleeping medication.** Frequently used agents are
   a. Diphenhydramine (Benadryl) 25–50 mg PO or IM. This often helps patients with mild insomnia.
   b. Temazepam (Restoril) 15–30 mg PO.
   c. Flurazepam (Dalmane) 15–30 mg PO. This used to be the standard order until it was found to have prolonged and cumulative effects.
   d. Chloral hydrate 500–1000 mg PO.
   e. Triazolam (Halcion) 0.125 or 0.25 mg PO. Use 0.125 for elderly patients. This is a popular choice, although memory loss has been associated with long-term use.
   f. Zolpidem (Ambien) 5 or 10 mg PO. A new nonbenzodiazepine agent that does not distort the natural sleep cycle.
2. **Nonoral sleeping medications**
   a. Chloral hydrate 500–1000 mg per rectum.
   b. Nembutal 100 mg per rectum.
   c. Diphenhydramine (Benadryl) 25–50 mg IM.
   d. Ativan can be given sublingually or IM.
3. **Nonmedical treatments.** These are often as effective as drugs. Discuss apprehensions with the patient or having the patient's room changed.
4. Sleep apnea is usually managed by nighttime nasal CPAP support.

51. IRREGULAR PULSE

Immediate Actions

1. Assess the ABCs. Intubate if necessary. Check the vital signs. Administer O_2.
2. Assess the impact on hemodynamic stability. Hypotension associated with arrhythmia requires rapid action.
3. Ensure IV access.
4. Assess the mental status before proceeding further for a baseline.

I. Problem. On routine check of vital signs, a nurse discovers that a 75-year-old man, status postamputation, has an irregular pulse.

II. Immediate Questions

A. **What is the pulse rate?** The pulse rate can suggest the nature of an arrhythmia. For instance, the ventricular rate in atrial fibrillation is rarely greater than 150 bpm, whereas in supraventricular tachycardias, it is usually greater than 150 bpm.

B. **What are the other vital signs?** You must know if the irregular pulse is associated with hemodynamic instability (hypotension).

C. **What medications is the patient taking?** Diuretics induce hypokalemia, which increases myocardial irritability. Check for cardiac medications, particularly antiarrhythmics.

D. **Is there a history of cardiac disease?** The patient may have a history of ischemia or arrhythmias. Postoperative arrhythmias are rare in individuals younger than 40–45 years. Mitral stenosis is often seen with atrial fibrillation.

E. **Is the rhythm regular, irregular, or irregularly irregular?** Although an ECG is necessary to formally evaluate the rhythm, a quick check of the pulse is helpful. Obtain an old chart and compare the ECG/rhythm strips.

F. **What are the laboratory results (chemistry, CBC, TSH)?** Electrolyte abnormalities, anemia, hypo- and hyperthyroidism may lead to arrhythmias.

III. Differential Diagnosis.

Remember that an irregular pulse is a result of a disease process, not a diagnosis.

A. **Impulse Formation Disorders**
   1. **Premature atrial and ventricular contractions.**
   2. **Sinus arrhythmia.** A benign variation of a normal pulse.
   3. **Escape beats.** These are seen particularly in bradycardias.
   4. **Extrasystoles.** These show as a constant interval between a sinus beat and the extrasystole. They are abolished by exercise.
   5. **Atrial fibrillation.** Commonly associated with many types of underlying heart disease (ischemic, valvular). P waves are absent on the ECG, there is an irregularly irregular ventricular rate, and flutter waves may also be seen.
   6. **Pacemaker malfunction.**
   7. **Sick sinus syndrome.**
   8. **Paroxysmal atrial tachycardia with variable block.** The atrial rate is 140–250 bpm with a variable ventricular response.

B. Conduction Disorders

1. **Sinoatrial block.** This can be associated with ischemia or caused by digoxin toxicity.
2. **Partial AV block.** Mobitz type I (Wenckebach) or type II second-degree block.
3. **Pulsus alternans.** This is indicated on the ECG as a regular rhythm with alternation in amplitude of equally spaced beats.

C. Myocardial Ischemia. The first evidence of asymptomatic myocardial ischemia (or infarction) is often an arrhythmia.

D. Pulmonary Disease. Supraventricular arrhythmias occur in up to 40% of patients after cardiac surgery and in nearly as many patients after other thoracic (pulmonary) procedures. A pulmonary embolus can occasionally present with atrial fibrillation or other arrhythmias.

E. Pericardial Disease. Constrictive pericarditis and tamponade can cause an irregular pulse.

IV. Database

A. Physical Exam Key Points

1. **Vital signs.** What is the pulse rate and regularity? Tachypnea may suggest a pulmonary embolism.
2. **Heart.** A rub is associated with pericarditis or a transmural infarction; murmurs suggest valvular disease.
3. **Neck.** Look for jugular atrial waves, venous distention.
4. **Blood pressure.** Check for pulsus paradoxus, associated with constrictive pericarditis, pericardial tamponade, or severe asthma. The pulse rate is grossly irregular at first, but is easily related to respiratory variations. A positive test shows a greater than 10 mm Hg fall in blood pressure with inspiration, as measured by cuff.

B. Laboratory Data

1. **Electrolytes.** Electrolyte abnormalities, especially potassium, can cause a variety of arrhythmias.
2. **Arterial blood gases.** Hypoxia can cause arrhythmias and may be associated with pulmonary embolism.
3. **Cardiac Panel (Troponin I, CPK, LDH, isoenzymes, AST).** Look for evidence of myocardial ischemia.
4. **Digoxin level.** This is particularly important for the patient already on digoxin.
5. Other drug levels (quinidine, procainamide) as indicated.
6. **Thyroid hormone levels.** Hyperthyroidism can lead to arrhythmias (T_4, TSH).

C. Radiographic and Other Studies

1. **12–lead electrocardiogram/rhythm strip.** This is essential to evaluate any arrhythmia. Atrial fibrillation will be

an obvious diagnosis on ECG. Look for signs of acute ischemia. Compare the new ECG with the old ECGs.

2. **Chest radiograph.** Look for signs of CHF, cardiomegaly, primary pulmonary disease, and pneumothorax. A central line that is in too far may cause arrhythmias.
3. **Ultrasound.** This can help to identify intracardiac mural thrombus in a patient with chronic atrial fibrillation, valvular disease, or a pericardial effusion.
4. **Nuclear ventilation/perfusion ($\dot{V}/\dot{Q}$) scan/CT angiography.** When pulmonary embolus is suspected, see an experienced radiologist for interpretation of these studies.

V. Plan

A. Overall Plan. Eliminate the arrhythmia by treating the underlying cause. It is imperative to rapidly treat any patient who is hemodynamically compromised (hypotensive) or symptomatic (shortness of breath or chest pain) from the arrhythmia. An otherwise stable patient can be treated more conservatively.

1. Start O_2 on any patient with an arrhythmia.
2. Establish IV access if not already present.

B. Specific Plans. Drug dosages are discussed in detail in Section IX, page 441.

1. **Sinus arrhythmia.** No treatment is needed.
2. **Atrial fibrillation**
   - **a.** Treat hypokalemia or hypoxia.
   - **b.** Administer digoxin.
     - **i.** Give 1.0 mg over 24 h in divided doses as 0.5 mg, then 0.25 mg, then 0.25 mg.
     - **ii.** Follow with a daily maintenance dose.
     - **iii.** If rate control is imperative, the 1.0 mg may be given more rapidly.
     - **iv.** Adjust the dose for patient size and for renal failure.
   - **c.** Administer verapamil 0.25 mg IV push; repeat in 10 minutes when rate control is still not achieved.
   - **d.** Pronestyl can be used for chemical cardioversion after treatment with digoxin. Quinidine can be useful. These medications may also be helpful in maintaining a sinus rhythm.
   - **e.** A patient with hemodynamic compromise should be electrically cardioverted.
3. **Pulmonary embolus**
   - **a.** A ventilation/perfusion scan or a spiral CT is usually done first.

b. When the question of pulmonary embolus remains after a negative or "low probability" scan, obtain a pulmonary angiogram—the "gold standard" of diagnosis.

c. Treat with heparin (bolus followed by constant drip to maintain PTT > 1.5–2 times control). Streptokinase, urokinase, and t-PA can be used to lyse the embolus if the patient has not had recent surgery. Hemodynamically unstable patients and symptomatic patients (angina, hypoxia, right heart strain on ECG) need rapid aggressive anticoagulation.

d. If the patient can't be anticoagulated or if the patient has a pulmonary embolus while anticoagulated, insert a Greenfield filter.

4. **Myocardial infarction.** The usual supportive therapy is indicated: monitoring, oxygen, pain relief (morphine), nitrates, and prophylactic lidocaine.

52. IV (INTRAVENOUS) ACCESS PROBLEMS

I. **Problem.** A 40-year-old intravenous drug abuser enters the hospital with abdominal pain and protracted vomiting. There are no available veins for IV access for rehydration.

II. **Immediate Questions**

A. **What is the nature of the patient's illness?** Patients requiring immediate IV access (eg, hypotension with shock) should undergo percutaneous central line placement or cutdown in the absence of large peripheral veins. Do not waste time looking for small peripheral veins. Always have a well-formulated plan to be used for vascular access. Are you going to attempt an internal jugular, a femoral or a subclavian approach? Consider the possibility of a bleeding diathesis or coagulopathy before inserting a central venous line.

B. **Is there a history of IV drug abuse or a history of prolonged hospitalization? What routes of access were used on other occasions?** Chronically hospitalized patients often lose usable peripheral veins after multiple IVs and venipunctures.

III. **Differential Diagnosis.** Peripheral intravenous access may be poor in the following situations:

A. **Intravenous Drug Abuse.**

B. **Obesity.**

C. **Prior Chemotherapy.**

D. **Prolonged Hospitalization.**

E. **Lymphedema.** After mastectomy or axillary lymphadenectomy for other reasons.

F. **Anasarca.**

G. **Hypotension and Hypovolemia.**

IV. Database

A. **Physical Exam Key Points**

1. **Upper extremities.** Look for needle marks indicating previous IV access. Look for an antecubital vein.
2. **Vital signs.** Hypotension or other signs of shock often cause peripheral veins to collapse.

B. **Laboratory Data.** These are usually not helpful in solving the problem. Consider a hematocrit and platelet count with children, as even a small amount of blood loss can be significant in a child.

V. Plan.

IV access should be approached in the following order in both emergent and elective situations. (see also Section III, pages 354, 340, 377).

A. **Peripheral (Arm).** Start distally and work proximally. These are standard IV lines, and are the lines of choice in trauma situations because 14–16 gauge catheters allow for rapid fluid repletion, more so than central lines. Antecubital lines can be used, although immobilization of the elbow can cause discomfort. For elective IV line placement, use the following method: Inflate a blood pressure cuff to just above the patient's systolic pressure for 5–10 min, then release the cuff. This often causes a reflex that dilates the extremity veins. Alternatively, place warm towels or a heating pad on the arm for a few minutes to dilate the veins. Lower-extremity lines should be avoided, because they do not work well or last for more than a few hours with patients who are ambulatory. There is also a higher incidence of thrombophlebitis.

B. **External Jugular.** Simple 1–2″ angiocatheters can be placed in the external jugular vein without difficulty and with little or no patient risk. Placing the patient in the Trendelenburg (head down) position and gently occluding the vein just above the clavicle will usually dilate it.

C. **Central Lines.** Percutaneous puncture should be attempted in the following order:

1. Internal jugular (IJ).
2. Subclavian.
3. Femoral (technically not central).

Experience with a particular route of access, however, is also an important determinant.

IJ and subclavian lines are useful for measuring central venous pressure. Femoral lines are easier to insert but have an increased risk of infection. They are less reliable for delivery of medications after cardiac arrest because of the poor lower-extremity circulation during CPR. Femoral lines are adequate for short-term use for fluid resuscitation, particularly after trauma.

D. Cutdowns. Three veins are readily accessible by cutdown techniques, as described on page 377.

E. Other. For small children with no IV access, a large needle can be inserted directly into the tibial marrow for fluid resuscitation and medications. This clearly represents a technique of last resort, to be used only for pediatric patients near death. The incidence of osteomyelitis in survivors is relatively high.

F. Clotted Catheter. Occasionally, clotted catheters can be cleared by gentle irrigation with agents such as urokinase (see page 538).

53. NAUSEA/VOMITING

I. Problem. A patient complains of nausea and then vomits repeatedly 1 wk after a colectomy for diverticulitis.

II. Immediate Questions

A. Are there any associated symptoms, particularly gastrointestinal? Nausea and vomiting may accompany a wide spectrum of illnesses covering most body systems. Inquire about related concurrent symptoms to focus the differential diagnosis. Specifically ask about abdominal pain, abdominal distention, diarrhea, constipation, and obstipation.

B. What is the appearance and odor of vomitus? Sometimes the vomited material can suggest the nature of the underlying dysfunction. First, look and test for blood (see Problem 34, page 137). Feculent vomitus suggests stasis or distal obstruction. Bilious vomit merely implies a patent pyloric channel. Retching or repeated vomiting can lead to a Mallory-Weiss tear, in which case the vomitus changes from bilious to bloody.

C. Is the vomiting related to eating or any specific medications? The patient may have a postoperative ileus or obstruction. Has their diet changed recently? Vomiting 1–2 h after eating (especially if the vomit is partially digested food) points to gastric stasis or a gastric outlet obstruction.

Vomiting concurrent or immediately after eating is often psychogenic. Certain medications can cause vomiting, such as narcotics or nonsteroidal anti-inflammatory drugs (NSAIDs). Does the patient have antiemetics prescribed to accompany the narcotic medications?

D. **Is the vomiting projectile?** Projectile vomiting is often associated with CNS dysfunction. However, it may also occur with certain types of food poisoning.

E. **Does the patient have a nasogastric drainage tube in place?** Confirm its proper functioning and positioning. Check the blue sump for a sucking sound. If not heard, inject air or water to flush the tube. If there is still no sucking sound, reposition the tube.

III. Differential Diagnosis.

A. Gastrointestinal

1. **General**
   - a. Peritonitis.
   - b. Postoperative ileus.
   - c. Mechanical obstruction at any level.
   - d. Gastroenteritis.
2. **Stomach**
   - a. Gastric outlet obstruction.
   - b. Peptic ulcer disease.
   - c. Gastric atony.
3. **Hepatobiliary/pancreas**
   - a. Biliary colic or acute cholecystitis.
   - b. Pancreatitis.
   - c. Hepatitis.
4. **Colon**
   - a. Diverticulitis.
   - b. Malignant obstruction from colorectal cancer.
   - c. Appendicitis.

B. Metabolic

1. Uremia.
2. Hepatic failure.
3. Metabolic acidosis.
4. **Electrolyte abnormalities**
   - a. Hypercalcemia.
   - b. Hyperkalemia.

C. Endocrine

1. **Diabetes.** Gastroparesis.
2. Adrenal insufficiency.
3. Hypothyroidism.

D. Drug/Toxin

1. Alcohol abuse.

2. Botulism.
3. Food poisoning (eg, staphylococcal).
4. Food or drug allergy.
5. Narcotics, especially codeine.
6. Nonsteroidal anti-inflammatory drugs (eg, ibuprofen).
7. Chemotherapeutic agents.

E. **Cardiopulmonary**
1. **Acute myocardial infarction.** Particularly inferior MI.
2. Congestive heart failure.

F. **Genitourinary**
1. Renal colic.
2. Pelvic inflammatory disease.
3. Pregnancy.

G. **Nervous System**
1. Space-occupying CNS lesion; increased intracranial pressure.
2. Migraine headache.
3. Labyrinthitis.

H. **Acute Febrile Illnesses.** Particularly in the pediatric age group.

IV. Database

A. Physical Exam Key Points

1. **Vital signs.** Check for orthostatic signs, fever, and tachycardia.
2. **HEENT.** Check for pharyngitis, otitis, or other evidence of acute infections, papilledema.
3. **Skin.** Decreased turgor and dry mucous membranes suggest dehydration. Look for evidence of jaundice.
4. **Abdomen.** Listen for bowel sounds, palpate for abdominal distention and tenderness. If the patient has pain out of proportion to physical findings, consider ischemic bowel.
5. **Rectal exam.** Check for stool impaction, positive fecal occult blood, masses, or fluctuance (suggestive of an abscess).
6. **Neurologic exam.** Mental status changes may signify a CNS lesion or a severe electrolyte disorder.
7. **Pelvic exam.** The patient may have PID.

B. Laboratory Data

1. **CBC.** May be helpful for signs of infection or blood loss.
2. **Urinalysis and urine culture.** May reveal infection or blood (with stones).
3. **Chemistries.** General screening includes electrolytes, BUN, creatinine, calcium, and liver function tests.
4. **Amylase.**

5. Arterial blood gases if indicated.
6. Urinary HCG to diagnose pregnancy.

C. **Radiographic and Other Studies**

1. **KUB and upright abdominal films.** Obtain abdominal films in most patients with vomiting and in all patients with abdominal distention.
2. **Chest radiograph.** This can be helpful to aid in the diagnosis of pneumonia, CHF, and to find evidence of aspiration. A pleural effusion can be seen with pancreatitis. Look for free air on an upright film.
3. **ECG.** Obtain when considering myocardial ischemia.
4. **Abdominal ultrasound/HIDA scan.** Is there a possibility of biliary colic?
5. **UGI series/upper endoscopy.** Both can identify a gastric outlet obstruction. Use water soluble contrast (Gastrografin) instead of barium.
6. **Barium enema/colonoscopy.** Perform if there is colonic disease or obstruction.
7. **CT of the head.** Obtain when an intracranial lesion is suspected.
8. **CT of abdomen and pelvis.** Best for identifying masses and abscesses (which can cause obstruction); occasionally it is able to identify the site of an adhesive small-bowel obstruction.

V. **Plan**

A. **Overall Plan.** Assess the patient for hypovolemia and begin appropriate fluid resuscitation. Make the patient NPO. Screen for drug allergies or reactions. Narcotics are common offenders in the postoperative surgical patient. Treat electrolyte abnormalities.

B. **Abdominal Causes.** Always make the patient NPO and treat them with IV fluids. Place a nasogastric tube when there is persistent vomiting, mechanical obstruction, or abdominal distention. Proceed with your diagnostic workup.

C. **Nonabdominal causes,** such as metabolic disorders, labyrinthitis, minor infections (eg, acute viral gastroenteritis). Assess volume status, administer intravenous fluids as needed, and treat the underlying disorder. If the patient is not obstructed, treat the vomiting with antiemetics. Frequently used antiemetics include

1. Prochlorperazine (Compazine) 10 mg IM or PO every 6 h.
2. Trimethobenzamide (Tigan) 250 mg PO every 6–8 h, 200 mg IM or PR every 6–8 h.
3. Promethazine (Phenergan) 12.5–25 mg PO every 8 h, or 25 mg IM every 8 h.

4. Meclizine (Antivert) 25–50 mg PO every 8–2 h. This is useful for nausea in patients with labyrinthitis or vertigo.
5. Metoclopramide (Reglan) 10 mg IV or PO every 6 h. This is particularly useful in diabetic patients or other patients with poor gastric emptying that is not due to obstruction.
6. Granisetron hydrochloride (Kytril) 10 μg/kg IV over 5 minutes before chemotherapy. Related agents may help chemotherapy-induced nausea and vomiting.
7. Zophren. Start with 4 mg IV. This is very effective after chemotherapy; it is also useful after anesthesia.

54. NASOGASTRIC TUBE MANAGEMENT-BLOODY DRAINAGE

I. **Problem.** A 43–year-old male has bloody output from his nasogastric tube 2 d after small bowel resection for a Meckel's diverticulum.

II. **Immediate Questions**

A. **How long has the NG tube been in place?** A tube that has been placed recently may have bloody drainage from the trauma of insertion or gastric surgery. An old tube may show blood from local mucosal irritation. If the tube was placed after gastric surgery, there may be anastomotic bleeding.

B. **How much bloody drainage has there been?** A tube that passes large amounts of bright red blood obviously requires more concern than one that passes a few red streaks.

C. **Has the patient had recent or remote upper gastrointestinal surgery?** If the surgery is recent, there may be bleeding at a new anastomotic site, or there may be a marginal ulcer at an old anastomotic site.

D. **Is the patient receiving antacids? What is the pH of the drainage?** The presence of acidic gastric secretions increases the likelihood of developing gastritis. Specifically, the pH should be kept > 4.0 for mucosal protection.

E. **How are the patient's blood pressure and pulse?** Hypotension and tachycardia are indicative of a volume loss that needs to be corrected promptly.

III. **Differential Diagnosis**

A. **Insertion Trauma.** This is usually nasopharyngeal.

B. **Mucosal Irritation.** This often results from a tube that has been in place for some time. There is usually an associated acidic pH.

C. **Suture Line Disruption or Hemorrhage.** Look for this in a patient who had recent surgery.

D. **Swallowed Pharyngeal Blood.** This may occur in trauma patients with facial fractures.

E. **Ulceration (Curling, Cushing, preexisting).** Look for associated conditions: burns, head injury, and so forth.

F. **Gastric erosion/gastritis/esophagitis/variceal bleed.**

G. **Coagulopathy.** This can have a physiologic or pharmacologic cause.

IV. Database

A. Physical Exam Key Points

1. **Vital signs.** Look for tachycardia and hypotension as evidence of sepsis or excessive blood loss.
2. **Abdomen.** Look for peritoneal signs, epigastric tenderness or gastric distention.
3. **HEENT.** Look for evidence of pharyngeal bleeding.

B. Laboratory Data

1. **CBC.** Check for excessive blood loss.
2. **PT/PTT and platelet count.** May be useful to rule out a coagulopathy.

C. Radiographic and Other Studies

1. **Upright chest radiograph.** Look for free intra-abdominal air. Mediastinal air suggests esophageal perforation, which can occur from endoscopy or after forceful vomiting (Boerhaave's syndrome).
2. **pH.** Check the pH of the gastric fluid. Is it < 4.0?

V. Plan

A. **Overall Plan.** First, determine whether the bleeding is serious enough to require aggressive therapy.

B. Specific Plans

1. For life-threatening upper GI bleeding, establish venous access and begin fluids. A CVP line may be helpful, especially in elderly patients. Hypotensive patients will require vigorous fluid and blood replacement. Transfer the patient to the ICU.
2. **Begin antacid therapy.** Use Maalox 30 mL every 2 h via NG tube. Intravenous H_2-receptor blockers (cimetidine, etc) may also be used. Sucralfate can also help, particularly with gastritis.
3. **Irrigate the NG tube with saline.** The temperature is not important. Irrigation allows you to assess the rate of bleeding. It also removes clots from the stomach,

which, if left inside, can lead to distention and persistent bleeding.

4. The presence of peritoneal signs or new free intra-abdominal air requires emergency laparotomy.
5. Perform an upper GI endoscopy when bleeding persists (see Problem 34, page 137).

55. NASOGASTRIC TUBE MANAGEMENT—CHANGE IN THE AMOUNT OF OUTPUT

I. **Problem.** A 56–year-old woman with pancreatitis has a sudden increase in the amount of nasogastric tube aspirate on the fifth hospital day. Another patient had minimal NG aspirate after a small bowel resection 3 d ago.

II. **Immediate Questions**

A. **Is there associated abdominal distention?** If a patient develops an ileus or obstruction, the amount of aspirate will increase.

B. **Is the output bilious?** Bilious NG output indicates bile reflux into the stomach or that the nasogastric tube has been placed distal to the pylorus.

C. **Is the tube functioning?** Tubes often become obstructed with mucus or antacids. Listen for a whistle, which indicates patency.

D. **Is the patient passing flatus or stool?** Often, decreased NG output correlates with return of bowel function.

E. **Is an NPO patient surreptitiously taking PO fluid?** This occurs with recalcitrant patients and patients with psychiatric histories. Often excessive amounts of "ice chips" are given to patients with NG tubes and can cause high NG tube outputs.

III. **Differential Diagnosis**

A. **Increased Output**

1. **Tip of tube distal to pylorus.** The tube aspirates all biliary and pancreatic secretions as well as gastric output.
2. Check for gastric bowel obstruction or small-bowel obstruction.
3. Gastric secretions increase after stopping H_2-receptor blockers, such as cimetidine.
4. **Surreptitious ingestion.**

B. **Decreased Output**

1. There may be return of normal bowel motility and function.

2. Check for an obstructed or kinked tube.
3. Was the patient started on an H_2-receptor blocker, which decreases gastric secretion or agents that improve motility and gastric emptying, such as metoclopramide?
4. The tube may be in the esophagus (above the GE junction) or coiled in the oropharynx.

IV. Database

A. Physical Exam Key Points

1. **Abdomen.** Listen for bowel sounds and their quality. No sounds may indicate an ileus or a far-advanced obstruction. High-pitched, hollow sounds indicate obstruction. Distention occurs with an obstruction or ileus.
2. **Mouth.** Check that the tube is not coiled or kinked in the mouth or throat.
3. **Rectal exam.** Is stool present?
4. **Tube.** Check its patency and function by flushing with air or saline.

B. Laboratory Data

1. **Serum electrolytes.** Carefully monitor the patient's hydration and potassium and bicarbonate levels during nasogastric suction.
2. **Nasogastric aspirate.** A pH > 6 indicates the use of antacids or that the tip of the tube is distal to the pylorus.

C. Radiographic and Other Studies

1. **Upright chest radiograph.** Look for a large stomach bubble, indicating poor gastric emptying. Check the position of the tube.'
2. **Upright and flat abdominal radiographs.** These may show distended bowel, indicating an ileus or obstruction.
3. **Contrast swallow.** To identify a gastric outlet obstruction or partial small-bowel obstruction, order a Gastrografin or dilute barium swallow. Serial radiographs will show normal or delayed emptying and the passage of contrast. Contrast should **not** be used in the presence of ileus or complete obstruction.

V. Plan.

The first priority is to determine that the nasogastric tube is functioning properly and is in a proper position. **Note:** Do not reposition a nasogastric tube without a full understanding of why the tube was placed and what was done at surgery.

A. Position. The tube should be in the stomach without a kink on radiograph.

B. Function. Sump tubes should whistle continuously on low suction. Most tubes need to be flushed with saline (30 mL) every 3–4 h to maintain patency. Flush the tube with 40 mL of air while auscultating over the gastric area to determine its function and positioning.

C. **Increased Output**
   1. **Poor gastric emptying (no obstruction).** Try metoclopramide 10 mg IV every 6 h. Erythromycin can also be used.
   2. **Distal obstruction.** Continue NG suction; consider further workup and surgery to relieve obstruction.
   3. **Ileus.** Patience and a period of observation are necessary, especially if this occurs immediately postop. Correct electrolyte abnormalities, especially hypokalemia, with a parenteral solution. Continue NG suction. Look for an intra-abdominal abscess if the ileus persists.

D. **Decreased Output**
   1. This usually indicates the return of bowel function. Correlate this return with a physical examination and the passage of flatus or stool. Remove the tube if appropriate.
   2. Irrigate the tube to clear it, or advance it into the stomach if it is not positioned correctly.

56. OLIGURIA/ANURIA

I. **Problem.** A patient has sequential hourly urine outputs of 22, 15, 9, and 4 mL via an indwelling Foley catheter 1 d after an aortic aneurysm repair.

II. **Immediate Questions**

A. **What is the patient's volume status?** The most common cause of oliguria in the postoperative setting is hypovolemia. This must be distinguished from acute tubular necrosis (usually secondary to ischemia), which is also related to hypovolemia. Determine the intravascular volume status by assessing the (1) left-sided pressures from a pulmonary artery catheter; (2) central venous pressures; (3) change in body weight; and (4) findings from a physical exam; or (5) cumulative I/O records. Do not let an increase in body weight dissuade you if other assessments point to a decreased intravascular volume. Be sure that hypovolemia is not a result of hemorrhage.

B. **Did the patient suffer any periods of documented hypotension?** As previously mentioned, acute tubular necrosis needs to be considered in surgical patients. Review the operative record of the anesthesiologist, noting any intraoperative hypotension.

C. **What is the baseline renal function?** Look at the admission BUN and creatinine levels and any subsequent chemistries. Any insult to the kidneys will be amplified by chronic renal dysfunction.

D. **Is the patient taking any nephrotoxic drugs?** Aminoglycosides are the major offenders. Send off blood samples for testing drug levels and hold the next dose until the levels return. Has the patient received IV contrast dye from radiographic procedures?

E. **Is the patient taking any medications that are excreted by the kidneys?** Digoxin and antibiotics are the most important medications in this category. Either modify or hold the dose until renal function improves or drug levels become available.

F. **Is the Foley catheter patent?** Most nurses will think of this before you do, but flush the catheter at least once to make sure the oliguria is real (see Problem 32, page 132).

III. **Differential Diagnosis.** The differential diagnosis for acute oliguria is identical to that of acute renal failure and its causes may be viewed as prerenal, renal, or postrenal.

A. **Prerenal (Renal Hypoperfusion)**
   1. **Shock/hypovolemia**
      a. **Hemorrhage:** Traumatic or as a postoperative complication.
      b. Inadequate fluid administration.
      c. Sepsis.
   2. Apparent intravascular hypovolemia, a relative decrease in the effective circulating volume.
      a. **"Third space" losses:** These are very common in the initial postoperative period after major operations or with major burns. Prolonged exposure of bowels during a lengthy operative procedure may account for insensible losses from 4–6 cc/kg per hour of operative time. These fluid losses need to be replaced along with other intraoperative losses.
      b. Congestive heart failure.
      c. Cirrhosis may lead to hepatorenal syndrome.
      d. Nephrotic syndrome.
   3. **Vascular**
      a. Renal artery occlusion (acute or chronic).
      b. Aortic dissection.
      c. Emboli (eg, cholesterol).

B. **Renal**
   1. **Acute tubular necrosis**
      a. **Ischemic:** Secondary to shock, sepsis.

   b. **Toxins:** Medications (aminoglycosides), contrast media, heavy metals.
2. **Acute interstitial nephritis**
   a. **Drugs:** β-lactamase resistant penicillins, NSAIDs.
   b. **Hypercalcemia:** This can cause nephrocalcinosis.
3. **Acute glomerular disease**
   a. Malignant hypertension.
   b. Immune complexes.
   c. Systemic diseases (Wegener's, TTP, SLE, Goodpasture's syndrome).

C. **Postrenal**
1. Urethral obstruction (prostatic hypertrophy, catheter obstruction).
2. Bilateral ureteral obstruction (carcinoma or retroperitoneal fibrosis).

IV. Database

A. **Physical Exam Key Points**
1. **Vital signs.** Look for a change in body weight and other orthostatic signs suggesting fluid loss.
2. **Skin.** Inspect for decreased turgor, dry mucous membranes, or edema, suggesting dehydration.
3. **Cardiopulmonary.** Listen for rales, elevated venous pressure, cardiac gallop, or JVD.
4. **Abdomen.** Is there ascites, or is the bladder distended?
5. **Extremities.** Assess perfusion by color and temperature.

B. **Laboratory Data**
1. **Electrolytes, BUN, and creatinine.** If The ratio of BUN/creatinine is > 20:1, then the oliguria is likely prerenal; if the ratio is < 15:1 then the oliguria is likely renal. Hyperkalemia can be life-threatening and may accompany acute renal insufficiency.
2. **Urinalysis.** Protein and red blood cell casts suggest glomerular disease. Eosinophils are associated with hypersensitivity reactions. WBC casts may indicate glomerulonephritis.
3. **Spot or random urine electrolytes and creatinine.** Obtain lab results before giving diuretics. A urinary sodium < 20 mEq/L indicates a prerenal cause; a urinary sodium > 20 mEq/L suggests a renal cause. Calculate the renal function index (RFI) as urinary sodium × plasma creatinine divided by the urine creatinine. If the RFI is > 1, it is likely a renal cause; if the RFI is < 1, it is likely prerenal (see also Section II, page 331).
4. **CBC.** Look for evidence of infection or anemia.

5. **Drug levels.** Evaluate for any nephrotoxic drugs (eg, aminoglycosides), or any medications cleared through the kidneys (eg, digoxin).

C. **Radiographic and Other Studies**
   1. **Chest radiograph.** This may reveal congestive failure.
   2. **Central venous pressure line or PA catheter.** This will give useful information about the volume status.
   3. **KUB.** This may reveal obstructing renal calculi.
   4. **IVP.** A combination of an ultrasound, a renal scan, and retrograde studies will give more information than an IVP without nephrotoxic contrast media.
   5. **Ultrasound.** This is useful to examine the bladder and upper urinary tract for signs of obstruction, also to estimate renal size.
   6. **Renal scan.** Perform a technetium-labeled DTPA or MAG-3 nuclear medicine study to assess blood flow to the kidneys, especially if emboli are a concern.
   7. **Angiogram.** This may be useful to visualize the vascular anatomy, but is rarely needed acutely.
   8. **Renal biopsy.** This is occasionally needed to determine the specific diagnosis of a renal cause of oliguria. It is not needed immediately to treat oliguria.

V. Plan

A. **Overall Plan.** As a general rule, the minimal acceptable urine output in an adult is 0.5 mL/kg/h. As previously stated, oliguria in most surgical patients results from hypovolemia. In almost every case it is appropriate to give the patient a potassium-free volume challenge (eg, 500 mL of normal saline). For patients with fragile cardiorespiratory status, smaller boluses and central venous catheters should be used to monitor volume status. Also review the patient's medications, stop or alter all nephrotoxic or renally excreted drugs, and remove potassium from the IV fluids.

B. **Prerenal**
   1. Treat with volume boluses and increase the baseline IV rate.
   2. Monitor volume replacement with a central line, if needed.
   3. **Follow hourly urine output.** Give specific criteria for which you wish to be notified (eg, call house officer for a urine output lower than 25 mL/h).

C. **Renal**
   1. Monitor the volume status with a central line.
   2. Remove potassium from IV solutions unless it is documented to be low.

3. Attempt to increase the urine output once volume status is corrected.
    a. **Furosemide:** Use escalating doses to increase the urine output. One method is to start with 80 mg IV, then 160 mg IV, and then 320 mg IV. Review patient's previous creatinine levels. If elevated, fluid challenge may be warranted before the administration of Lasix. Higher doses are needed for patients who chronically use Lasix.
    b. **Mannitol:** 12.5–25 g (50–100 mL of a 25% solution) to induce an osmotic diuresis.
    c. **Dopamine:** 3–5 µg/kg/min to increase renal blood flow.
4. **Review medications.** Adjust doses or stop nephrotoxic drugs.
5. **Monitor electrolytes.**

D. **Postrenal.** This usually requires a urologic consultation. Ureteral stents or percutaneous nephrostomy may be needed. A blocked Foley catheter can be treated as outlined in Problem 32, page 132.

57. PARESTHESIAS

I. **Problem.** A 62–year-old male patient is complaining of paresthesias (tingling or "pins and needles") 1 d after right radical neck dissection.

II. **Immediate Questions**

A. **Where are the paresthesias?** A patient with paresthesias in an extremity and with known or likely peripheral vascular occlusive disease presents a different clinical dilemma than one with circumoral paresthesias.

B. **Does the patient have peripheral vascular disease?** Paresthesias are one of the "five Ps" of peripheral ischemia—the others being pain, pallor, pulselessness, and paralysis. Determine whether the patient has any of these other signs of vascular occlusive disease.

C. **Has the patient had these symptoms before?** It is important to determine if the condition was present preoperatively or is a consequence of a recent surgical procedure.

D. **Did the paresthesias appear suddenly or gradually?** Find out if they can be linked to a particular event, such as an operation. Was there any unusual positioning during the surgical procedure (see paragraph C below)?

E. **What does the operative wound look like?** Is there a hematoma or a mass causing compression in the neck?

III. Differential Diagnosis. Paresthesias may be reported as tingling, "pins and needles," or numbness.

A. Vascular Insufficiency. Paresthesias may be one of the early symptoms of vascular compromise, and immediate action may be necessary to save the affected extremity.

B. Hypocalcemia. Paresthesias primarily involve the lips, tongue, fingers, and feet. Hypocalcemia is a result of hypoparathyroidism after thyroid or parathyroid surgery (see Problem 43, page 171 for further suggestions regarding patient evaluation and therapy).

C. Operating Room Causes. People (eg, tired residents and students) leaning on the patient for prolonged periods in the operating room may lead to postoperative paresthesias in a peripheral nerve distribution. Improper positioning and padding of a patient's extremities is also a preventable cause. Check placement of pneumatic compression boots.

D. Neuroma. This would occur weeks postoperatively as a result of nerve injury during surgery.

E. Hyperventilation. This causes bilateral hand and finger tip numbness. Patients frequently have a history of previous hyperventilation.

F. Transient Ischemic Attack (TIA). Bilateral extremity numbness is common and may accompany speech and sight difficulties. A carotid bruit may be present. Residual neurologic deficits are rare.

G. Peripheral Neuropathy. This is the classic "glove and stocking" distribution often seen in patients with diabetes, alcoholism, or chronic renal insufficiency.

H. Nerve Compression. This may be from carpal tunnel syndrome or a dressing that is applied too tightly.

I. CNS tumors, neurosyphilis.

IV. Database

A. Physical Exam Key Points

1. **Vital signs.** Look for tachypnea associated with hyperventilation.
2. **Check peripheral pulses.** Use palpation and Doppler. Try to determine the patient's baseline.
3. **Look for causes of pressure in the area.** Dressings, casts, etc.
4. **Check for physical signs of hypocalcemia.** Chvostek's and Trousseau's sign (see Problem 43, page 171).

5. A **carotid bruit** may be present to suggest TIAs.
6. **Neurologic exam.** Signs of peripheral neuropathy include symmetric loss of pinprick sensation. Reflexes are decreased with nerve compression.

B. **Laboratory Data**
1. **Serum electrolytes and calcium.** These are useful to rule out hypocalcemia, renal failure, and diabetes.
2. **Arterial blood gases.** Hyperventilation can occasionally cause paresthesias, as seen in a respiratory alkalosis.

C. **Radiographic and Other Studies**
1. **ECG.** Look for atrial fibrillation, which predisposes to thrombi and embolization.
2. **Nerve conduction velocities.** Assessment may help to determine the diagnosis of nerve compression.
3. **Doppler ultrasound** may reveal blood flow in an extremity without a palpable pulse.

V. Plan

A. **Vascular Insufficiency.** Paresthesias are a serious symptom and require rapid therapy to save an extremity. Obtain an angiogram (see Problem 62, page 229), or reexplore the patient (after a recent vascular bypass).

B. **Hypocalcemia.** For the patient with paresthesias after thyroidectomy, administer oral or IV calcium. (see Problem 43, page 171).

C. **Transient ischemic attacks.** TIAs may be caused by platelet emboli from an ulcerated carotid plaque, and this can be treated surgically.

D. **Peripheral Neuropathies.** With alcoholism and diabetes, the neuropathy is usually chronic and irreversible.

E. **Dressings and Casts** should be revised as appropriate.

58. PHLEBITIS

I. **Problem.** A 32–year-old woman had an exploratory laparotomy for ovarian cancer. An IV in her arm has not been changed for 5 d, and the site is now red and painful.

II. Immediate Questions

A. **What are the patient's vital signs?** Fever can develop from both superficial thrombophlebitis and deep venous thrombosis.

B. **Can pus be expressed from the site?** Pus indicates a local infection, and sepsis with pus may indicate suppurative thrombophlebitis. Look for red streaks proximal to the IV site.

C. **What medications are being administered through the line?** Agents such as potassium and calcium can cause phlebitis. Peripheral parenteral nutrition may cause phlebitis when the concentration of glucose or lipids is too high. This is difficult to avoid unless you are only trying to administer 1000 cal/d.

III. **Differential Diagnosis.** Acute venous inflammation (thrombophlebitis) or occlusion (phlebothrombosis) can occur in superficial or deep veins. Deep venous thrombosis usually does not have a significant inflammatory component and is rarely infected. This discussion will be limited to inflammation and infection of superficial veins.

A. **Superficial Thrombophlebitis.** Acute inflammation without infection is the most common presentation. This occurs
1. At the site of an intravenous catheter, especially in the upper extremity.
2. From the extravasation of irritant medications, such as chemotherapeutic agents.
3. From an unknown cause, especially in the lower extremities.

B. **Suppurative Thrombophlebitis.** Persistent fever, sepsis, and positive blood cultures indicate a significant infection of the affected vein. Pus is expressed, and there may be daily increases in the length of vein involved despite local treatment. Superficial thrombophlebitis occurs rarely at upper-extremity IV sites, and slightly more commonly at emergent cutdown sites, especially in the lower extremities.

C. **Other**
1. Deep venous thrombosis (see Problem 65, page 238).
2. Septic thrombophlebitis of the subclavian vein.

IV. **Database**

A. **Physical Exam Key Points**
1. **Vital signs.** Look for signs of sepsis.
2. **Extremities.** Check all old intravenous sites. Palpate the calves for tenderness. Gently squeeze erythematous IV sites in an attempt to express pus.

B. **Laboratory Data**
1. **CBC.** Leukocytosis is present in suppurative superficial thrombophlebitis.
2. Obtain a culture and do a Gram's stain of any pus (eg, at an old IV site.

C. **Radiographic and Other Studies.** Venography is rarely indicated if a central vein infection (*Staphylococcus aureus, Staphylococcus epidermidis,* and *Candida* species are common), or deep venous thrombosis is suspected in a septic patient with no known source.

V. **Plan.** Prevention of thrombophlebitis by frequent rotation of IV sites should keep this problem at a minimum.

A. **Superficial Thrombophlebitis**
   1. Apply local heat, dry or moist.
   2. Elevate the limb.
   3. Administer NSAIDs.
   4. Consider administering heparin, if patient is an acceptable anticoagulation candidate.

B. **Suppurative Thrombophlebitis**
   1. Apply local treatment.
   2. Administer analgesics and anti-inflammatory agents.
   3. Intravenous antibiotics. These are usually broad-spectrum with good anti-staphylococcal coverage (nafcillin, etc).
   4. Persistent or progressing infection mandates exploratory venotomy and venectomy of the entire involved venous segment. This usually needs to be done in the operating room. Segments of vein should be sent to the pathology and microbiology departments, and the wound should be left open and packed.
   5. Consider administering heparin if the patient is an acceptable candidate for anticoagulation.

C. **Other.** Suppurative thrombophlebitis of a subclavian vein requires resection in the operating room and intravenous antibiotics.

59. POSTOPERATIVE PAIN MANAGEMENT

I. **Problem.** On the night of an open lung biopsy, the patient threatens to pull out his chest tube and leave the hospital because of severe incisional pain.

II. **Immediate Questions**

A. **Is there any evidence of a wound infection, hematoma, or other problem?** Early wound infections (*Clostridium, Streptococcus*) may be a factor when patients have more postoperative pain than expected. Also, a wound hematoma may amplify normal postop pain.

B. **What is the current pain medication regimen? What drug is being used? How much and how often has it been given?** When a patient complains of excruciating postop pain, then the current pain medication is inadequate. Titrate up the dose (amount and frequency), and ensure that the nurses are administering the medication appropriately. Consider using a PCA in awake patients. Expect pain after thoracotomy, midline abdominal, flank, and orthopedic incisions, especially in young, muscular patients. If the patient has had an epidural, discuss the case with an anesthesiologist before adding pain medications.

C. **Is there any history of narcotic use or abuse?** Tolerance to narcotics is a real phenomenon, and patients with a history of prior use occasionally need their doses elevated to alarmingly high levels to achieve pain control in the immediate postop period.

III. **Differential Diagnosis.** Discussions of postoperative pain almost always mean incisional pain.

A. **Inadequate Analgesic Regimen**

1. **Too small a dose.** When writing postop orders, take into account the size and age of the patient and the type of operation. If your orders specify a wide range for the dose, expect the nurse to begin at the lower end of the scale, so as not to overmedicate. The nurse will gradually increase the dose, and the patient's pain will gradually improve, although you should not make the patient wait too long for an adequate safe dose.
2. **Too long between doses.** Dosing schedules should be set by the half-life of the drug, which is usually 3–4 h in narcotics given IM or SC. Also make certain a patient knows to request a medication that is administered as needed. On the other hand, if the patient is still alert, breathing normally, and in pain after a drug has reached its peak effect (usually 15–30 min after IM administration), you can safely administer a supplemental dose without waiting for the half-life interval.
3. **Patient-controlled analgesia.** Dosing may be too low or lockout too long.

B. **Wound Complications**

1. Infections. Be alert for aggressive life-threatening infections (*Clostridium, Streptococcus,* necrotizing fasciitis) that may initially present only with pain.
2. Hematoma.
3. Dehiscence.

4. Nerve entrapment or excessive pressure from a dressing postop.
5. Compartment syndrome developing in an extremity.

C. **Drug-seeking Behavior.** Patients should usually be given the benefit of the doubt in the immediate postoperative period. However, if reported pain persists or increases with time, a contributing factor, including drug-seeking behavior, should be considered. Look for signs of drowsiness and disorientation due to overmedication.

IV. Database

A. Physical Exam Key Points

1. **Vital signs.** Fever and tachycardia suggest an infection. Hypertension and tachycardia suggest pain.
2. **Wound.** Look for signs of an infection (erythema, purulence, crepitation, margination, drainage) or a developing hematoma. Make sure the dressing is not the cause of the pain.
3. **Neurologic exam.** Observe for posturing, grimacing, splinting, and other body movements consistent with pain. Disorientation or obtundation is consistent with narcotic overdose or sepsis.

B. Laboratory Data

1. CBC, if infection is suspected.
2. Wound culture, if it is the suspected source.

C. **Radiographic and Other Studies.** Chest radiograph if indicated.

V. Plan

A. **Overall Plan.** Realize that pain management is part of the complete care of the surgical patient. Let the patient know you are concerned and are taking actions to improve pain control. Follow-up on any changes made.

B. **Pain Medications.** Medications are discussed in detail in Section IX, page 441.

1. **Morphine sulfate.** This is the gold standard for postop pain. The dose is 8–2 mg IM or SC every 3–4 h in most cases. In thoracic and orthopedic patients 12–15 mg are commonly needed. In the ICU, patients may be given
   1–4 mg IV every 1–3 h.
2. **Demerol.** Give 75–125 mg IM every 3 h. Although commonly used, Demerol has a higher incidence of respiratory complications than either morphine or Dilaudid.
3. **Dilaudid.** Give 2–4 mg IM or SC every 3–4 h.

4. **Percocet and Percodan (oxycodone), Vicodin (hydrocodone), and Tylenol No.3 or No.4 (codeine).** These are fairly standard oral analgesics used postop. Give one or two tablets PO every 4–6 h as needed.
5. **Hydroxyzine (Atarax, Vistaril).** Traditionally given as an adjunct to Demerol, 25–50 mg every 8 h. It potentiates the pain relief and minimizes the nausea associated with narcotics, although it is also sedating.

C. **Alternative Methods of Pain Control**
1. **Epidural narcotics.** An epidural catheter is left in place by the anesthesia team and is usually managed by the anesthesiologists. Always confirm who is to help with the catheter (particularly at night). Find out what medications can be given in addition to the epidural.
2. **Self-controlled IV pumps.** These can be used to infuse either boluses, continuous IV narcotics, or both and are controlled to some extent by the patient. This method is called PCA or "Patient-Controlled Analgesia." Orders are given for a number of milligrams per dose, lockout time (ie, minimum time interval between doses), and maximum dose per 4 h. A typical order is 3 mg, 15 min lockout, maximum 30 mg per 4 h. A continuous drip can be added to intermittent dosing.
3. **Nerve blocks.** Certain incisions (thorax, flank) can be extremely painful, especially in the first few hours postop. Infiltration with a long-acting anesthetic in the operating room at the end of the case can be helpful. For example, bupivacaine (Marcaine) can be used to infiltrate the intercostal nerves at the end of a thoracotomy.

60. PRURITUS

I. **Problem.** Three days after a low anterior resection a 49–year-old male is complaining of severe pruritus (itching) of both legs.

II. **Immediate Questions**

A. **What is the duration of the symptom?** An acute condition can more often be related to an exact cause, such as a change in medication, a new laundry soap, and so forth.

B. **Has the patient recently started taking any new medications, eating different foods, wearing different clothing, or using new deodorants, perfumes, or soaps?** These factors, and especially postoperative analgesics, are common causes of itching.

C. **Is there an associated rash or lesions?** These may also suggest the cause.

D. **Does the patient have any allergies?** Find out if there are any drug or food sensitivities listed on the patient's record.

III. Differential Diagnosis

A. **Skin Disorders.** Pruritus may be associated with visible skin lesions.
   1. Papulosquamous skin diseases.
   2. Vesicobullous diseases.
   3. Allergic reactions, eg, contact dermatitis (usually caused by soaps, detergents, etc).
   4. Infestations, eg, scabies.
   5. Infection, eg, viral exanthemas.

B. **Systemic.** Itching can be associated with a variety of systemic conditions without an associated rash.
   1. Dry skin. This may be related to cold weather, particularly in elderly patients.
   2. Liver disease. This often presents with jaundice and pruritus.
   3. Uremia. This may be unrelated to the BUN level.
   4. Hypothyroidism.
   5. Hyperparathyroidism.
   6. Diabetes mellitus.
   7. Gout.
   8. Hodgkin's disease, leukemias.
   9. Intestinal parasites, such as pinworms or hookworms.
   10. Drug reactions.
   11. Pregnancy.
   12. Polycythemia vera.
   13. Blood borne neoplasms

C. **Psychosomatic Pruritus.**

D. **Neurologic and Circulatory Disturbances.**

IV. Database

A. **Physical Exam Key Points.** Check the patient's skin (not just the affected area); examine the distribution of the rash and any skin lesions; carefully record the distribution and appearance. What looks like a rash may be a skin breakdown secondary to severe scratching of the pruritic area. Examine the skin carefully near IV sites.

B. **Laboratory Data**
   1. **Liver function tests.** These are useful to rule out liver disease.
   2. **BUN and creatinine.** These may reveal renal insufficiency and uremia.

C. Radiographic and Other Studies. A chest radiograph may show a new lung malignancy, a finding that can be associated with pruritus.

V. Plan

A. Overall Plan. Pruritus does not require immediate treatment unless caused by a significant systemic disease or early anaphylaxis. It is important to rule out major illness as a cause. The primary goal is to enhance the patient's comfort until the definitive diagnosis is available to dictate therapy.

B. Specific Measures

1. **Dry skin.** Ensure adequate skin hydration by bathing the patient daily in warm water, followed immediately by applying a skin moisturizer cream (Aquaphor, Eucerin). This will give some relief, especially if xerosis is the cause. Adding salt to the water may be of added benefit. Creams should not be applied in cases of chronic pruritus in the absence of a rash.
2. **Uremic pruritus.** For a patient with uremic pruritus, UV light and lidocaine IV may help.
3. **Cholestasis.** Cholestyramine may also help in pruritus secondary to hepatic disease.
4. **Medical treatment.** There are three oral medications useful in the treatment of symptomatic pruritus.
   a. Diphenhydramine (Benadryl) 25–50 mg PO or IV every 8 h.
   b. Cyproheptadine (Periactin) 4 mg PO tid.
   c. Hydroxyzine (Atarax) 25 mg PO tid or qid.

   Topical steroids range from mild (hydrocortisone), to midpotency (triamcinolone [Kenalog]), high potency (halcinonide [Halog]), and the highest potency (betamethasone dipropionate [Diprolene]).
5. **Discontinue** any medication causing pruritus, if possible.

61. PULMONARY ARTERY CATHETER PROBLEMS

(The technique of pulmonary artery catheterization is discussed in Section III, Bedside Procedures, page 368)

I. Problem. A pulmonary artery (PA) catheter inserted into a septic patient will not "wedge."

II. Immediate Questions

A. Has the catheter ever been in a good "wedge" position? Be sure that the catheter has worked properly in the past. Check the tip position on a chest radiograph. It may reveal that the catheter is no longer in the proper position (see below).

B. **Is the balloon working properly, or is there any problem with the monitor or transducer system?** Balloons can occasionally rupture. A pulmonary artery pressure tracing shows that the transducer system is otherwise intact.

C. **Flush all ports thoroughly and check the transducer before use.** Be certain that all of the air has been evacuated from the lines.

III. Differential Diagnosis

A. **Placement Problem.** The most frequent sites of catheterization are the internal jugular and subclavian veins. Fluoroscopy will help in certain cases, such as in patients who have undergone pneumonectomy and in patients with pacemakers where careful placement is mandatory. Placement problems include

1. Passage from the subclavian into the internal jugular or out the contralateral subclavian vein.
2. Looping in the right ventricle.
3. Knotting of the catheter.

B. **Functional Problems.** Functional problems develop relatively frequently after successful placement of a PA catheter.

1. **No waveform.** A thrombus may occlude the catheter.
2. **Cannot "wedge" catheter.** This is perhaps the most common problem. A small amount of repositioning is usually adequate to restore function and is particularly easy if the flexible plastic sheath was used at the time of the original placement.
3. **Balloon rupture.** Never use more than 1.5 mL of air to inflate the balloon. Make sure the wave form changes from a pulmonary artery tracing to a wedge as the balloon is inflated.

C. **Complications**

1. **Pneumothorax/hemothorax,** usually related to initial line placement.
2. **Infection.**
3. **Pulmonary artery perforation,** either immediate or delayed (very rare).
4. **Arrhythmias.** Ventricular ectopy is common as the catheter passes through the ventricle. Patients with left bundle branch block may develop complete heart block if the PA catheter causes right bundle branch block.

5. Check for pulmonary infarction, most often caused by a catheter tip that remains in a small pulmonary artery with the balloon inflated.

IV. Database

A. Physical Exam Key Points

1. **Look at the catheter and check all connections.** Make sure the patient's heart is level with the transducer.
2. **Check how much of the catheter is in the patient.** Even in large patients, a wedge waveform should be present by the time 60 cm is used (from a subclavian approach). If you haven't wedged the Swan-Ganz by 60 cm, start over or use fluoroscopy.

B. Laboratory Data

B. Laboratory Data Usually not needed.

C. Radiographic and Other Studies

1. **Check catheter position on a chest radiograph.** The tip is usually in the right main pulmonary artery. There should be a gentle curve as the catheter passes from the right atrium, through the tricuspid valve, into and out of the ventricle, and into the pulmonary artery. The catheter should not be farther than 5 cm from the midline. There is a greater incidence of pulmonary artery perforation when the catheter tip is in the left main pulmonary artery.

V. Plan.

V. Plan. Placement of a pulmonary artery catheter should be done with careful monitoring. Before placement, flush the catheter, then test the balloon (by inflating it with 1 mL of air and then deflating it). Connect the catheter to the transducer and test the electronics. Once connected, the tip of the catheter should be briskly tapped, revealing a high frequency, high amplitude waveform on the monitor.

A. Placement

1. Inflate the balloon in the superior vena cava to allow blood flow to carry the catheter out the right ventricular outflow tract. This is usually at about 20 cm via a subclavian approach. Plan to use the right internal jugular or left subclavian veins to facilitate the natural curve of the swan.
2. Be sure that the balloon is **deflated** whenever the catheter is being withdrawn and **inflated** when advancing the catheter.
3. As the catheter passes into the right ventricle, ventricular arrhythmias may develop and should be treated if persistent or associated with hemodynamic compromise. Some clinicians believe the safest course is to withdraw the catheter into the right atrium and give the patient a

bolus of lidocaine before replacing the catheter. These arrhythmias are usually short-lived and rarely persist after the catheter has been advanced into the PA.

B. Functional Problems. A nonfunctioning catheter should be replaced after certain maneuvers have been performed, even if the catheter has just been placed. Most functional problems develop because of thrombosis at the catheter tip or at other ports.

1. Flush nonfunctional ports frequently.
2. Test balloon. If the balloon is intact you should be able to remove the same volume of air that you carefully placed into the balloon. During use, however, passive deflation is safest.
3. Advance the catheter with the balloon inflated if the catheter won't "wedge." Use fluoroscopy (C-arm), if necessary.

C. Complications

1. Pneumothorax requires tube thoracostomy.
2. An infected catheter should be immediately removed. Antibiotics may be required with positive blood cultures.
3. Arrhythmias are treated with lidocaine; use a 1–mg/kg bolus. Withdraw the catheter into the right atrium until the drug is given.

62. PULSELESS EXTREMITY

I. Problem. Two days after a coronary artery bypass, a nurse examines an elderly patient and reports that he has no pulses in his right leg.

II. Immediate Questions

A. Is this an acute change for the patient? Look at the admission history and physical for prior documentation of pulses. Unfortunately, a complete vascular exam (at a minimum, checking femoral and pedal pulses) is often neglected. Ask the patient if they noted any acute changes in the extremity.

B. Are there any associated symptoms of pain or numbness in the involved extremity? Pain, pallor, pulselessness, paresthesias, and paralysis are the "Five Ps" for diagnosis of acute ischemia. Most patients with ischemia have pain and pallor. Paresthesias are an early sign, and paralysis is a late sign. Ask whether these symptoms are new, and if so, how rapidly they developed (see also Problem 57, page 217).

C. **Is there any history of claudication or any previous vascular surgery?** Significant peripheral vascular atherosclerosis may be the underlying cause of an acute arterial occlusion. Also, the degree of chronic obstruction determines the amount of collateral circulation to the extremity. This may have an effect on how well an acute occlusion is tolerated.

D. **What are the pulses in the other leg?** Chronic peripheral vascular occlusive disease is usually bilateral, and comparison of the pulses between the extremities may indicate the baseline status of the extremity in question. Some acute events may also be bilateral (eg, saddle embolus).

E. **Is there any history of palpitations or atrial fibrillation?** Atrial fibrillation is one of the leading causes of embolic arterial occlusion. Even if a patient is found to be in a sinus rhythm, ask about history of arrhythmias or digoxin use. A recent conversion to sinus rhythm may be the cause of an acute embolic event.

III. **Differential Diagnosis.** The majority of acute arterial occlusions occur in the lower extremity, as a result of embolic phenomenon. However, thrombosis, vasculitis, and even venous disease may cause an acute occlusion. Review the operative note for any intraoperative complications.

A. **Embolic Causes**

1. **Cardiac sources**

a. **Coronary artery disease.** Check patient's history for a prior myocardial infarction. Mural thrombi can embolize, leading to a pulseless extremity.

b. **Atrial fibrillation.**

c. **Rheumatic heart disease.** With this history, suspect mitral stenosis with atrial fibrillation.

d. **Prosthetic cardiac valves.**

e. **Endocarditis.**

f. **Atrial myxoma.**

2. **Peripheral sources**

a. **Aortic.** Mural thrombi can embolize from an aneurysm, leading to a pulseless extremity.

b. **Atheroemboli.** These are often associated with invasive procedures (cardiac catheterization) or from peripheral sources (aortic, iliac, popliteal); this phenomenon is known as blue toe syndrome or "trash foot."

c. **Paradoxical emboli.** These are venous clots that pass through a patent foramen ovale or other type of right to left shunt to become arterial emboli.

B. Thrombotic Causes. There is usually some degree of atherosclerotic occlusive disease with the addition of hypovolemia or a low flow or hypercoagulable state.

1. **Arterial occlusive disease.**
2. **Hypovolemia or low flow**
   - **a.** Trauma and resultant shock.
   - **b.** Dehydration.
   - **c.** Fever.
   - **d.** Sepsis.
3. **Hypercoagulable**
   - **a.** Malignancy.
   - **b.** Polycythemia.
   - **c.** Estrogen use.
   - **d.** Heparin-induced thrombosis.

C. Arterial Dissection.

D. Trauma. Either blunt or penetrating.

E. Vasculitis

1. **Takayasu's disease.** This often causes upper-extremity occlusions.
2. **Thromboangiitis obliterans.** This is usually found in young smokers (Buerger's disease).

F. Acute Femoral or Iliac Vein Occlusion. This may lead to phlegmasia cerulea dolens (a painful blue extremity).

IV. Database

A. Physical Exam Key Points

1. **Vital signs.** Look for orthostatic hypotension (for hypovolemia) or an irregular pulse (atrial fibrillation).
2. **Cardiac.** There may be a murmur with valvular diseases, endocarditis, or rhythm disturbances.
3. **Abdomen.** Listen for an abdominal bruit. Palpate for an aneurysm.
4. **Extremity exam.** Check the pulses and temperature of the affected extremity at all levels and compare results with those on the contralateral side. Examine for skin pallor or mottling, and look for a cutoff for the level of ischemia. Look for changes of chronic ischemia, such as hair loss or skin atrophy. Look also for areas of well-demarcated ecchymoses in the feet and toes suggesting "trash foot." Do not forget to feel for popliteal and femoral artery aneurysms. Use a Doppler probe if pulses are not readily palpable.
5. **Neurologic exam.** Focal signs, paresthesias indicate significant ischemia. Paralysis warrants immediate intervention to prevent limb loss.

B. **Laboratory Data**
   1. **Chemistries.** Hyperkalemia may be associated with tissue damage from ischemia.
   2. **CBC.**
   3. **PT/PTT.** This is helpful, especially for a patient on anticoagulant therapy (see pages 317 and 320).
   4. **Arterial blood gas.** Acidosis may be seen with poor perfusion.
   5. **Urinalysis.** The presence of hemoglobin with an absence of RBCs suggests myoglobinuria.
   6. **Urinary myoglobin level** appears with rhabdomyolysis and tissue loss.

C. **Radiographic and Other Studies**
   1. **Chest radiograph.** This is useful to identify cardiac or thoracic aortic disease.
   2. **ECG and rhythm strip.** This is important to identify arrhythmias.
   3. **Noninvasive vascular study.** Always check nonpalpable pulses with the Doppler. If a more sophisticated noninvasive lab is available, it can also be used.
   4. **Echocardiogram.** This helps to look for valvular disease, a ventricular aneurysm, a mural thrombus, or akinesis.
   5. **Cardiac thallium scan.** This scan evaluates for prior infarct, but is not usually needed in acute cases.
   6. **Angiogram.** This documents the site of obstruction and reconstitution from collaterals, and it occasionally shows aneurysms and other unrecognized visceral emboli. It may show a source of peripheral emboli.
   7. **Abdominal ultrasound.** This is an excellent noninvasive screening test for an abdominal aortic aneurysm or peripheral aneurysm.

V. Plan

A. **Overall Plan.** An acute arterial occlusion is a surgical emergency, requiring prompt diagnosis and early treatment to save the extremity. Be alert for the five "Ps" as described previously. Treat the patient with anticoagulation, volume as needed, and prepare the patient for the operating room. An angiogram is usually obtained before surgery, but in some cases, the diagnosis and the level of obstruction is obvious, and the patient can go directly to the operating room.

B. **Correct Volume Deficit.** If hypovolemia is a contributing factor, bolus the patient with IV fluid. Monitor the urine output and central filling pressures to guide therapy.

C. **Anticoagulation.** If there is any delay before surgery or an angiogram, load the patient with 10,000 units of heparin IV, then give a continuous infusion of 10 U/kg/h to prevent thrombus progression. Monitor the PT/PTT level (see Section II, pages 317 and 320). Some centers may use thrombolytic therapy (streptokinase, urokinase, tissue plasminogen activator) as a first-line treatment. In some cases, debilitated patients with significant operative risk are managed conservatively with anticoagulation only.

D. **Antibiotics.** These should be administered, especially when the patient has prosthetic graft in place.

E. **Protection of the Ischemic Extremity.** Position the limb in a mildly dependent position. Protect it from trauma.

F. **Operation.** Alert the appropriate senior staff, the anesthesiologist, and the patient's family as most acute occlusions will be managed by either embolectomy or bypass.

G. Postoperatively, observe for acidosis, hyperkalemia, myoglobinuria, and compartment syndrome, all of which may develop after extremity reperfusion. Also, monitor the pulses and perform a neurologic exam every 2 h.

63. SEIZURES

Immediate Actions

1. Assess the ABCs. Do not force anything into the mouth of a patient having seizures.
2. Prevent self-inflicted injuries.
3. Obtain IV access.
4. Single seizures usually end before therapy can be started. A patient in status epilepticus, however needs urgent therapy. Start with diazepam (Valium) 10 mg slow IV push (see following section, "Plan").

I. **Problem.** A 25–year-old male is found in bed having seizures 1 d after an appendectomy.

II. **Immediate Questions**

A. **Has the patient ever had seizures before?** A patient with a history of seizures is often on an antiseizure medication (or is supposed to be). In these patients, a common cause of seizures is the failure to take the prescribed medication.

B. **Is the patient taking any anticonvulsant medications? Has the patient been put back on all medications he**

was taking before admission? If the patient is NPO, be sure that an appropriate parenteral form is given. Check for other medications, as some of these can affect the blood levels of antiseizure medication, particularly diphenylhydantoin (Dilantin).

C. **Does the patient have a history of alcohol abuse or diabetes?** Alcoholic withdrawal and severe hypoglycemia mimic seizures.

D. **Was the seizure generalized or focal?** Focal seizures suggest a central nervous system cause.

E. **What are the results of the most recent lab tests?** These may reveal an obvious electrolyte abnormality. Are the serum levels of antiseizure medications therapeutic?

F. **Were there any witnesses?** Observers may indicate a prodrome, or whether the patient suffered any specific injury or fall.

III. **Differential Diagnosis.** The hallmark of the seizure is rigid stiffening of the muscles, loss of bladder control, and cyanosis with a postictal phase consisting of confusion, myalgia, lethargy, and headache.

A. **Idiopathic Epilepsy.** This is the most common cause of seizures, but it must be a diagnosis of exclusion in the acute situation.

B. **Tumors.** Either primary brain tumors or metastatic lesions can be responsible for seizures. Cancers of the breast, lung, or kidney, melanoma, and lymphoma are common causes.

C. **Infection.** In adults, intracranial infection can cause seizures, whereas in children any infectious process with systemic reaction (fever) can cause seizures.

D. **Trauma.** A careful history must be obtained. Was the patient found on the floor? Was the skull fractured?

E. **Alcohol/Drug Withdrawal.** This is common when patients are hospitalized, leading to sudden withdrawal (see Problem 25, page 109).

F. **Chronic Renal Failure.** This is associated with uremia.

G. **Anoxia.** Evaluate the arterial blood gases.

H. **Electrolyte Abnormalities.** These include hypoglycemia, hypomagnesemia, hypocalcemia, and hyponatremia with rapid correction.

I. **Collagen Vascular Disease.**

J. **Hallucinations.**

K. **Hypothyroidism.**

L. Degenerative Disease (eg, Tay-Sachs disease).

M. Vascular Lesions. Infarcts, emboli, hypertensive encephalopathy, carotid sinus disease, and subarachnoid hemorrhage can all result in seizures.

N. Syncope. Often what is thought to be a seizure is just a syncopal attack. Get a careful description from nurses and other witnesses about the event.

O. Hysteria. Psychiatric patients can have pseudoseizures.

P. Inadequate level of prescribed anticonvulsants. This is a common problem with phenytoin (Dilantin), where the level can be altered by the addition of almost any drug (aspirin, others).

IV. Database

A. Physical Exam Key Points

1. **Vital signs.** Fever suggests an infection; febrile seizures may be seen in children. Check the blood pressure and palpate the pulse to be sure the patient is stable.
2. **Do not interfere if the patient is spontaneously breathing.** Specifically, do not try to force something into the patient's mouth, such as a tongue depressor. This can injure you or the patient and is unnecessary.
3. **Check for aspiration.**
4. **Neurologic exam.** Look for focal signs that may help to diagnose the cause. Perform a complete exam including all cranial nerves, sensation, strength, DTRs, and mental status. There may be transient deficits after the seizure (the postictal state).
5. **Is there evidence of fecal or urinary incontinence?**

B. Laboratory Data

1. **Check the serum electrolytes,** calcium, magnesium, creatinine, and glucose levels to rapidly screen for metabolic causes.
2. **Arterial blood gases.** These should be assessed to rule out hypoxia as a cause.
3. **Check the drug levels** of any anticonvulsants being taken. Do this immediately as a patient who seizes with adequate drug levels will need to have new therapy instituted.
4. **Perform a CSF fluid analysis, if** indicated (see Section III, page 360.)

C. Radiographic and Other Studies

1. **Head CT scan.** If this is the patient's first seizure and there is no obvious cause, then a CT scan of the head is indicated. However, the scan does not need to be done

emergently, unless other evidence suggests a space-occupying lesion that may require emergent treatment.

2. **Lumbar puncture** may help if there is evidence of meningeal irritation. Be sure to check for increased intracranial pressure before the spinal tap.

V. Plan

A. General Plan. Support vital functions (the ABCs), and prevent self-inflicted injury during the seizure. This should be followed by a careful workup to determine the cause and institute appropriate therapy.

B. Specific Measures. (see Section IX, page 441, for a discussion of drugs listed below).

1. Monitor and support the patient's airway. The patient may turn blue during the seizure. As hypoxia worsens, neurologic function will eventually cease, ending the seizure. When this happens, rapidly open and clear the patient's airway. Begin ventilation, if necessary.
2. Establish IV access as soon as possible.
3. A single seizure will usually finish before the onset of any IV medication, and therefore does not need to be specifically treated. However, to treat a second seizure, or status epilepticus (repeated seizures with no regaining of consciousness between seizures), diazepam (Valium) IV may be given, usually as a 5–mg IV push (slowly), repeating at 10–15 min intervals as needed to control seizure activity.
4. Phenytoin (Dilantin) may be used if diazepam fails, or to prevent recurrent seizures after diazepam has led to temporary control. Phenytoin must be given slow IV push, no faster than 50 mg/min. Check levels daily first starting 24 h after the initial dose. The usual loading dose is 15–18 mg/kg IV.
5. Phenobarbital may also be used. It is given slowly IV, usually with a 120–240 mg (10–20 mg/kg in children) loading dose. Maintenance doses are given IV, IM, or PO to maintain therapeutic levels.
6. Be alert for the complications of aspiration and hyperthermia.
7. Anticonvulsants are not indicated for alcohol withdrawal seizures, but chlordiazepoxide (Librium) may be useful to control other symptoms of delirium tremens.
8. Refractory seizures that do not respond to the above management may require general anesthesia.

C. Treat Underlying Condition. After the acute seizure episode is controlled, treat the underlying condition. Treat electrolyte abnormalities as outlined in the specific "on call" problem. Treat any CNS lesion as appropriate.

64. SUPRAPUBIC CATHETER PROBLEMS

I. Problem. A patient has a suprapubic catheter that has stopped draining.

II. Immediate Questions

A. Does the patient have a full bladder? This should be determined by palpating for suprapubic fullness with associated tenderness.

B. Is the total urine output adequate? A gradual decrease in urine may suggest oliguria as opposed to an obstructed tube.

C. Is urine draining around the suprapubic tube, and is there blood or clots? This suggests that the tube is blocked or has pulled out of the bladder.

D. Why does this patient have a suprapubic catheter? Suprapubic cystostomy drains are placed surgically or percutaneously for bladder decompression. Temporary tubes placed emergently (ie, Cystocath, Stamey type, which have a small diameter [ie, 12–14 Fr]) can dislodge if not carefully secured. Tubes placed in the operating room intended for long-term use are usually of the Malecot variety and are of larger caliber (22–24 Fr). They are placed for a wide range of indications, such as a bladder injury, a urethral injury or obstruction, and a transplant neoureterocystostomy obstruction or stricture.

E. How long has the catheter been in place? A long-standing suprapubic tube usually will have a mature tract into the bladder, whereas a recently placed tube may not.

III. Differential Diagnosis

A. Systemic Causes. For a detailed discussion of low urine output (oliguria), see Problem 56, page 213.

B. Catheter Obstruction. This can be caused by blood clots or occasionally by debris (stone encrustation). Long-standing tubes can become coated with calcium deposits. Examine the catheter for kinks.

C. Catheter Tip Dislodgement. This is more of a problem with a recent suprapubic tube because the tract may be immature.

IV. Database

A. Directed History and Physical Exam. Check the patient's fluid status, vital signs, temperature, catheter exit site, catheter suture, and do an abdominal exam.

B. Laboratory Data. Lab studies are usually not necessary in acute cases.

V. Plan. The approach to a poorly functioning tube depends primarily on the age of the tube.

A. Recently Placed Tube. Attempt to flush the tube. A tube change probably should be done in the operating room because the tract is immature.

B. Chronically Indwelling Tube. A new tube of similar size can be placed because the tract is mature. When a tube is no longer needed, and the patient can void via the urethra, the tract will typically close within 48 h. Chronic tubes are generally replaced every 4–8 wk to prevent encrustation. An annual KUB radiograph is needed in these patients to look for stone formation in the bladder. Unless symptomatic, the colonization that accompanies a chronic suprapubic tube is generally not treated. The notable exception is that any colonization with stone-forming organisms (eg, *Proteus* species) must be treated.

65. SWOLLEN EXTREMITY

I. Problem. Three days after a knee replacement, a 49–year-old obese woman develops a swollen left calf and right ankle.

II. Immediate Questions

A. What are the vital signs? Tachycardia and fever may represent infection. Tachycardia and tachypnea may be manifestations of a pulmonary embolus.

B. Is the patient short of breath? Complaints of "not getting enough air" in a patient with a swollen extremity should raise concern for a pulmonary embolus or congestive heart failure.

C. Is the extremity or just the joint swollen? The latter would limit the diagnostic possibilities. Is there tenderness of the extremity or joint to palpation?

III. Differential Diagnosis

A. Venous Obstruction. Deep venous thrombosis (DVT), most of which remain clinically silent, occurs in a high percentage of immobile postoperative patients. Thrombus can form anywhere from the level of the calf to the pelvis. The major risk of DVT is pulmonary embolus (PE), which can lead to respiratory or cardiac arrest. Superficial thrombophlebitis can also occur in the upper or lower extremity (see Problem 58, page 219).

B. **Lymphatics Obstruction.** This is typically a result of a tumor involving the inguinal nodes; obstructed lymphatics produce diffuse, nontender nonpitting edema of the entire leg.
   2. **Destruction.** Operative removal of draining lymph nodes can produce extremity swelling acutely or years later, as typified by arm swelling after axillary node dissection. Radiation can also ablate lymphatic channels.

C. **Infection.** Cellulitis of the lower extremity, especially the "diabetic foot," can produce swelling to any level, depending on the extent of the infection. A foreign body with associated infection can also produce leg swelling.

D. **Congenital.** This is usually lymphedema, either lymphedema tarda or praecox.

E. **Other.** Causes of edema, such as renal failure, liver disease, and congestive heart failure, typically produce bilateral swelling, though early disease may be unilateral. Joint swelling suggests infectious or inflammatory arthritis.

IV. Database

Physical Exam Key Points

1. **Vital signs.** Tachypnea is a sign of a pulmonary embolus. Hypotension is a particularly worrisome sign.
2. **Extremities.** Check both extremities for swelling. Look for evidence of infection (eg, cellulitis, lymphangitis, or tender superficial veins). Palpate for calf tenderness and cords, which suggest DVT. Measure calf and thigh circumferences from a well-marked constant point on both legs as a baseline.
3. **Chest.** Listen for rales (congestive heart failure).
4. **Abdomen.** Look for ascites (liver disease).
5. **Axillary and inguinal nodes.** Has a lymphadenectomy been performed? Are nodes palpable (tumor)? Has there been recent breast surgery, or is there a breast mass?

B. Laboratory Data

1. **CBC.** This can be helpful, especially if infection is suspected.
2. **Serum electrolytes and glucose.** Inflammatory processes can affect the therapy of diabetics and patients with chronic renal failure.
3. **Coagulation panel (PT, PTT, platelet count).** Obtain a baseline before starting anticoagulant therapy; occult thrombocytosis may be evident, as well as DIC.

C. Radiographic and Other Studies

1. **Venogram.** This is the invasive standard for evaluating DVT. Doppler studies are noninvasive and much faster.

A spiral CT scan can detect pelvic vein thrombosis as well as pulmonary emboli. You will need an experienced radiologist to perform and interpret a venogram.

2. **Noninvasive venous studies** such as impedance plethysmography (IPG) are sometimes useful. Venous Doppler studies are also helpful, but expert interpretation is mandatory.
3. **Bone radiographs.**These may be useful if "diabetic foot" and cellulitis are suspected. They detect soft tissue air and osteomyelitis, as well as foreign bodies.
4. A CT scan of the abdomen and pelvis may identify a mass obstructing the iliac veins or vena cava.

V. Plan

A. Venous Obstruction

1. Prescribe bedrest with elevation of the involved extremity.
2. A baseline platelet count and activated partial thromboplastin time (PTT) should be done. In rare patients, heparin causes thrombosis and thrombocytopenia. Patients on heparin should have serial platelet counts to identify thrombocytopenia.
3. **Heparin.** A 5000–10,000 U IV bolus followed by 1000–1500 U/h continuous infusion should be administered to maintain PTT at 2–2.5 times the control value.
4. **Coumadin.** Coumadin should be started slowly so that all coagulation factors affected (II, VII, IX, and X—which have different half-lives) decrease at the same rate. Heparin should be continued for 3–5 d after starting Coumadin. The prothrombin time should be maintained at 1.5–2.5 times control values (INR, 2.0–4.5). Coumadin is normally given for 6 mo, or longer for recurrent episodes.
5. **Prevention.** Minidose heparin is useful for preventing DVTs when started preoperatively in high-risk patients, for example, those undergoing pelvic or orthopedic procedures, obese patients, patients with cancer, or patients with a history of DVT. The dosage is 5000 U given subcutaneously every 8–12 h. There are several forms of low-molecular weight heparin that may be as effective with a lower risk of bleeding, depending on the circumstances. One example is Lovenox, given 30 mg bid or 40 mg qd. Pneumatic stockings are available, and these intermittently inflate around the calves, presumably reproducing muscle contractions to improve venous flow (they also increase endogenous t-PA). Early ambulation also helps to prevent DVT.

6. **Superficial thrombophlebitis.** This is typically treated with local heat and nonsteroidal anti-inflammatory agents (see problem 58, page 219).

B. **Lymphatic Disease.** Local measures, such as heat and elevation, are of little benefit. Custom-made elastic stockings (eg, Jobst) are of some help. Intermittent pneumatic compression (at bedtime), may also give some relief.

C. **Infection.** Antibiotics should be started. Cover for *Staphylococcus* and *Streptococcus* species in upper-extremity infections, as well as gram-negative and anaerobic species in the lower extremity. Blood cultures should be obtained in the toxic patient. It may be difficult to differentiate cellulitis from DVT.

D. **Pulmonary Embolus.** Heparin and Coumadin are therapeutic options. Patients with DVT and contraindications to anticoagulation should probably be treated with a Greenfield filter, although this leaves the patient at risk for chronic lower-extremity swelling (postphlebitic syndrome) if the clot propagates.

66. SYNCOPE

I. **Problem.** A patient undergoing a preoperative evaluation for a mitral valve replacement has a syncopal episode in the radiology department.

II. Immediate Questions

A. **What was the patient doing when the episode occurred?** Vasovagal syncope or fainting from orthostatic hypotension can occur only in a sitting or standing position. Syncope while lying flat is almost always cardiac in origin. Vasovagal attacks are associated with heat, anxiety, pain, or a closed space. Syncope with exertion is often cardiac. Also ask the patient about syncope occurrence with coughing, turning or twisting the head, or getting up quickly.

B. **Was the syncope observed? Could it have been a seizure?** In determining the cause of a loss of consciousness, a seizure should always be in the initial differential diagnosis. Ask observers if they noticed evidence of seizures, examine the patient for tongue injuries (bites), and consider the patient's rate of return to baseline consciousness. Syncopal patients recover quickly, whereas seizure patients have a postictal period. Incontinence is indicative of a seizure.

C. **How did the patient feel immediately before the loss of consciousness?** Patients with vasovagal syncope normally have a presyncopal complex consisting of sweating, lightheadedness, and abdominal queasiness. Cardiac syncope and orthostatic hypotension are usually sudden in onset. Seizure episodes may have a preceding aura.

D. **Did anyone take the patient's pulse during the episode?** Vasovagal attacks are associated with bradycardia; orthostatic hypotension with tachycardia; and cardiac syncope with variable heart rates ranging from severe bradycardia in heart block to tachycardia (SVT, AF) as the cause for the syncope.

E. **Is the patient a diabetic? Is the patient insulin dependent?** Hypoglycemic events are an infrequent but readily treatable cause of syncope.

F. **What medications is the patient taking?** MAO inhibitors and antihypertensives can cause orthostatic hypotension if the dose is large enough. Pay close attention to administration of sedatives, especially during and after procedures.

III. Differential Diagnosis

A. Cardiovascular

1. **Reflex syncope**
   - a. Vasovagal (a simple faint).
   - b. Orthostatic hypotension is often associated with volume depletion or medications (ie, α-blockers, such as terazosin).
   - c. Carotid sinus syncope.
2. **Cardiac**
   - a. Mechanical
     - i. Aortic stenosis.
     - ii. Myocardial infarction.
     - iii. Mitral stenosis.
     - iv. Cardiomyopathy.
     - v. Pulmonary embolism.
   - b. **Electrical (dysrhythmias)**
     - i. AV block
     - ii. SVT/Ventricular arrhythmias
     - iii. Sick sinus syndrome
     - iv. Pacemaker-related

B. Noncardiovascular

1. **Neurologic.** Subclavian steal, seizure (see Problem 63, page 233).
2. **Metabolic.** Hypoxia, hypoglycemia, hyperventilation.
3. **Psychiatric.** Hysteria, panic.
4. **Pharmacologic.** Review the medication list

IV. Database

A. Physical Exam Key Points

1. **General exam.** Is the patient confused, lethargic, or anxious? Is there any obvious injury? Evidence of incontinence suggests a seizure.
2. **Vital signs.** Look for orthostatic changes. What is the heart rate and rhythm? A discrepancy in the blood pressure between both arms (ie, > 20 mm Hg) is suggestive of a subclavian steal syndrome.
3. **Neck.** Listen for carotid bruits and the carotid upstroke.
4. **Chest.** Listen for the murmurs of aortic stenosis, IHSS, and the rhythm. Crackles and wheezes may indicate aspiration associated with the episode or CHF.
5. **Rectal exam.** Check for heme positive stool or other evidence of an acute bleed.
6. **Neurologic exam.** Check for dysarthria, focal signs, and the patient's mental status.

B. Laboratory Data

1. **CBC.** This can be helpful, especially the hematocrit.
2. **Chemistry panel.** This should be done to determine the electrolytes and glucose level.
3. **Blood gas.** Hypoxia or hyperventilation (decreased CO_2, decreased pH) may be present.

C. Radiographic and Other Studies

1. **Chest radiograph.** Check the cardiac silhouette for evidence of heart failure or an effusion.
2. **ECG with a rhythm strip.** Look for a short PR interval, delta waves, or any other obvious sign of a rhythm disturbance.
3. **Echocardiogram.** This may reveal myxoma, valvular lesions, or mural thrombi.
4. **Reproduce syncope** with maneuvers such as coughing, turning the head, hyperventilation, or carotid massage.
5. **Holter monitor.** This can be useful to identify intermittent arrhythmias (over a 24–h period).

V. Plan

A. Overall Plan. Causes for syncope range from an inconsequential vasovagal attack to an emergent episode of heart block. Therefore, treatment is determined by the diagnosis. Always assess the patient for injury from a fall during syncope.

B. Specific Treatments

1. **Vasovagal.** Instruct the patient to put his head down at the onset of presyncopal symptoms.
2. **Orthostatic hypotension**

a. Assess for fluid volume loss (paying close attention for possible GI bleeding) and treat accordingly. The patient may need ICU care.
b. Instruct the patient to change positions slowly.

3. **Cardiac**
   a. **Treat the arrhythmia:** If tachyarrhythmia is causing hypotension, treat as outlined in Problem 67, page 244. Cardiac arrest rhythms are treated as in Problem 11, page 47.
   b. **Monitor the patient:** Often, a 24–h Holter monitor needs to be obtained for diagnosis. Assess the patient for hemodynamic stability; if unstable, place the patient in the ICU and consider central line placement or Swan-Ganz catheter for fluid status.

67. TACHYCARDIA

I. **Problem.** On a routine check of vital signs, a 68–year-old woman is found to have a pulse of 155 2 d after sigmoid colectomy.

II. **Immediate Questions**

A. **What is the patient's normal pulse?** It is important to have a frame of reference for evaluating tachycardia.

B. **What are the other vital signs?** Tachycardia plus hypotension in a postoperative patient suggests hypovolemia. Similarly, a fever can cause tachycardia. For a patient with tachycardia above 150 BPM with significant symptoms (eg, decreased consciousness, significant hypotension, chest pain or shortness of breath), cardioversion may be indicated. Otherwise, use medications to slow the rate, as per ACLS protocol. An ECG with a rhythm strip should be obtained before starting pharmacologic intervention or cardioversion when the patient is stable.

C. **Does the patient have underlying heart disease?** Is the rhythm regular or irregular (atrial fibrillation).

D. **What medications is the patient taking?** If the patient is on an antiarrhythmic, has the patient been receiving the appropriate dose? Diuretics and potassium supplements may cause electrolyte abnormalities and arrhythmias.

III. **Differential Diagnosis**

A. **Sinus Tachycardia**
   1. **Thyrotoxicosis.** Weight loss, irritability, and tremor are associated symptoms.

2. **Pheochromocytoma.** This is associated with headache, abdominal pain, hypertension, and sweating.
3. **Anxiety/Pain.** This is a normal physiologic response to catecholamine release.
4. **Drug-related.** Sympathomimetics, such as epinephrine, can cause tachycardia.
5. **Hypotension.** This can occur with hypovolemia.
6. **High-output states.** These can be the result of a rise in right atrial pressure from any cause, such as thyrotoxicosis, A/V fistula, anemia, pregnancy, or severe Paget's disease.
7. **Cardiac failure.** A drop in pulse pressure along with increased right atrial pressure leads to tachycardia.
8. **Fever related.**
9. **Sepsis.**
10. **Pneumothorax/pericardial effusion.**

B. Ectopic Tachycardia

1. **Paroxysmal atrial tachycardia.** This is often accompanied by palpitations and lightheadedness, with a rate of 140–250 BPM.
2. **Atrial flutter.** Rates are faster than in atrial or junctional tachycardia (rate 250–350 BPM).
3. **Ventricular tachycardia.** This is usually associated with ischemic heart disease, including acute MI; it also can be a forerunner of ventricular fibrillation.

IV. Database

A. Physical Exam Key Points

1. **Vital signs.** Check the pulse rate and regularity and the temperature. Hypotension is a major threat to life.
2. **Cardiac.** Look for evidence of cardiac failure (neck vein distention, S_3 gallop, etc.).
3. **Lungs.** Listen for evidence of cardiac failure, rales, or pneumothorax.
4. **Extremities.** Check for edema or cyanosis.

B. Laboratory Data

1. **Serum electrolytes.** The potassium level is critical.
2. **Arterial blood gases.** Rule out hypoxia.
3. **CBC.** Is there evidence of sepsis or anemia?
4. **Thyroid function tests.** If indicated.
5. **Cardiac enzymes.** Check a CK-MB or troponin I.

C. Radiographic and Other Studies

1. **ECG.** The most important piece of information will be the electrocardiogram because this allows for the correct diagnosis of the particular tachycardia.

2. **Chest radiograph.** This can reveal signs of cardiac failure or primary pulmonary problems.

V. Plan

A. General Plan. Establish the correct diagnosis. Remember that even late at night, a medical colleague usually will be glad to help you read a confusing ECG. It may be wise to transfer the patient to the telemetry or the intensive care unit.

B. Specific Plans

1. **Ventricular tachycardia.** This is perhaps the most important arrhythmia because it can rapidly lead to cardiac arrest and death (see Problem 11, page 47 and Figure I–9). It can be difficult to tell if a very rapid narrow complex rhythm is a supraventricular or ventricular tachycardia. When faced with this dilemma, try adenosine 6 mg IV (may repeat). This won't affect ventricular tachycardia but will lead to several seconds of asystole with SVT.
2. **Atrial flutter and fibrillation.**
   - **a.** If the patient is hemodynamically compromised, treat immediately with synchronized electrical cardioversion is indicated (20–50 J) along with IV diazepam for sedation.
   - **b.** Initially, attempt carotid massage to slow the heart rate and visualize flutter waves.
   - **c.** If the patient is stable, start pharmacologic therapy.
     - **i.** The first goal is to slow the ventricular response. This is accomplished with IV digoxin or verapamil.
     - **ii.** The second goal is to restore normal sinus rhythm. Quinidine may be used to do this once the ventricular response is lower. Procainamide is an alternative to quinidine (see Problem 51, page 199).
     - **iii.** Digoxin and verapamil should not be used in patients with the Wolff-Parkinson-White syndrome.
     - **iv.** Patients with chronic atrial fibrillation may not be convertible to sinus rhythm. Although verapamil acts faster than digoxin, its rapid clearance from the blood may require more frequent dosing.
3. **Paroxysmal atrial tachycardia.** This condition can be treated in a variety of ways.
   - **a.** Vagal maneuvers such as an ice bag on the face, induced vomiting, or carotid massage should be tried first. Be careful performing carotid massage in patients with carotid disease.

b. Verapamil given IV is also effective, usually starting with 2.5 mg IV push and giving added doses of 2.5 mg every 5 min to a total dose of 10 mg.

c. Combining verapamil with carotid massage is often effective. IV propranolol is also effective (but don't use propranolol and verapamil at the same time).

d. Synchronized DC cardioversion is an uncomfortable but effective therapy.

4. Sinus tachycardia. In the surgical patient, fever and hypovolemia are common causes of this condition. The key to the therapy of sinus tachycardia is treatment of the underlying condition. Hypovolemia should be associated with oliguria.

68. TRANSFUSION REACTION

I. Problem. During a transfusion of packed red blood cells, a patient's temperature rises to 38.5 °C.

II. Immediate Questions

A. Vital signs. Check for hypotension or tachypnea, which are signs of a significant reaction. Fever is the most common manifestation of a transfusion reaction.

B. Does the patient have back or chest pain? Other symptoms include chills, diaphoresis, hypersensitivity reactions (hives, wheezing, pruritus), exacerbation of congestive heart failure, hemoglobinuria, bleeding/DIC, discomfort at the infusion site, or facial flushing. An acute coagulopathy can also develop from a major transfusion reaction.

C. Has the transfusion been stopped? If not, do so, and maintain an open IV line with normal saline.

III. Differential Diagnosis. Differentiating a fever due to a transfusion reaction from other causes of postoperative fever is difficult. Assuming there is no other source, the following transfusion reactions are possible, in order of decreasing likelihood and increasing severity:

A. White Cell Antigens. Unlike washed red cells, packed cells contain relatively large numbers of leukocytes. Febrile responses to these cells are usually accompanied by urticaria.

B. Minor Protein Reactions. Allergic reactions to transfused serum proteins can cause fever, although anaphylaxis and acute pulmonary edema are possible.

C. ABO Incompatibility. This represents a potentially life-threatening problem, but it occurs rarely. Signs of this are seen after transfusion of relatively small quantities of blood.

D. Contaminated Blood. Bacterial contamination is rare but should be suspected when a high fever and hypotension develop early during a transfusion. This is often fatal.

IV. Database

A. Physical Exam Key Points

1. **Lungs.** Listen for rales and wheezing.
2. **Cardiac.** Examine for tachycardia and a new flow murmur.
3. **Abdomen.** Evaluate for pain, especially in the flanks.
4. **Skin.** Look for a rash or hives.

B. Laboratory Data

1. **Blood bank specimen.** Two freshly drawn clot tubes (red-top tubes) should be returned to the blood bank with the remaining untransfused blood. A repeat cross-match will be performed. In addition, most blood banks require a heparinized specimen to perform an indirect Coombs' test, looking for previous sensitization.
2. **Urinalysis.** Hematuria after a transfusion reaction represents hemoglobinuria after hemolysis from a major ABO incompatibility.
3. **CBC.** Schistocytes may be present in a transfusion reaction; a worsening anemia may develop in the face of massive red cell destruction.
4. **Serum for free hemoglobin and haptoglobin.** Free hemoglobin will be present with a reaction, and haptoglobin will be decreased.
5. **Other lab tests.** Coagulation studies and thrombocytopenia may indicate DIC. Monitor renal function by obtaining a BUN and creatinine along with serum electrolytes. Arterial blood gases rarely are indicated (except in cardiovascular collapse).

C. Radiographic and Other Studies. These are not routinely needed, but should be ordered if clinically indicated.

V. Plan

A. Immediately Stop Transfusion. Consultation with the blood bank pathologist usually is indicated to evaluate the reaction and to discuss any further transfusions.

B. Maintain IV Access. Monitor the urine output and vital signs closely.

C. **Send the Blood Bank Appropriate Specimens.** See the preceding section, "Laboratory Data." Make sure the bag is returned to the blood bank immediately.

D. **Mild Reactions.** There may be a fever without any evidence of more severe symptoms or hemolysis.
   1. Antihistamines (diphenhydramine 25–50 mg IM or IV) and acetaminophen may reverse mild allergic and febrile reactions.
   2. Transfusion can usually be restarted.

E. **Severe Reactions.** These usually signify that acute hemolysis has taken place. One of the major goals should be to prevent renal failure.
   1. **Circulatory support.** Maintain adequate blood pressure with volume or pressors. In the setting of marked hemolysis, diurese with furosemide or mannitol plus D5W to minimize renal injury. Also consider alkalinization of the urine with bicarbonate to further protect the kidneys.
   2. **Antibiotics.** These will be needed if examination of the remaining untransfused unit reveals evidence of bacterial contamination. Gram-negative bacilli are usually responsible.

F. **Known Reactions.** In patients with known febrile reactions to blood products, pretreat with antihistamines (diphenhydramine) or antipyretics or steroids to minimize the reaction. Blood bank products are discussed in Section VI, Blood Component Therapy.

69. TRAUMA ASSESSMENT & RESUSCITATION

Immediate Actions

Start with the ABCs of trauma:

1. **A**irway. Check for a clear airway. Evaluate the C-spine and assume injury until it is cleared. (In high-risk patients, you need a radiograph to rule out vertebral fractures, and flexion-extension views, or a normal clinical exam to rule out ligamentous injury). Intubate if necessary. (Try to avoid hyperextending the neck). Perform a cricothyrotomy if needed.
2. **B**reathing. Administer oxygen, ventilate, and vent any suspected pneumothorax (with a 14–gauge needle or chest tube).
3. **C**irculation. Obtain two large-bore (14–16 gauge) IVs, on opposite sides of the body, preferably in the upper extremi-

ties, and begin crystalloid infusion (LR) as fast as possible. Draw baseline lab work.

4. Evaluate the response to initial resuscitation. Begin the secondary survey once stabilized.
5. **D**isability. Perform a rapid neurologic assessment.
6. **E**xamine. Remove all clothing and quickly evaluate the patient.
7. Begin ECG monitoring.

I. **Problem.** An 18–year-old female involved in a motor vehicle accident has a blood pressure of 90/50 mm Hg and is combative.

II. **Immediate Questions**

A. **Is the patient able to talk?** Airway obstruction and major chest injuries are rapidly fatal and therefore are addressed first. If the patient is unable to talk, but is making ventilatory efforts, sweep the oropharynx with gloved fingers to remove debris. Suction the oropharynx. Grasp the symphysis (chin) and displace it anteriorly. Ventilate with a well-fitting mask and 100% oxygen for 2–3 min. If unsuccessful (oxygen saturation < 90%, no clinical improvement), then intubate with a No. 7 or 7.5 cuffed endotracheal tube. Rarely, patients who present with severe maxillofacial injury cannot be intubated orally and require an immediate surgical airway. A cricothyroidotomy made between the first laryngeal cartilage and cricoid is preferred over a formal tracheostomy because it is faster and safer. Use an assistant to maintain in-line stabilization of the neck during all airway maneuvers to minimize cord injury.

B. **Has the patient's ventilatory status improved?** Reevaluation is an essential part of trauma management to identify missed injuries. A patient in severe respiratory distress that has not improved with intubation should have chest tubes placed immediately, before a chest radiograph is performed. Flail chest, tension pneumothorax, tracheal or bronchial disruption are lethal injuries that are treatable.

C. **How long ago was the injury?** Assessing the degree of shock and planning fluid resuscitation are the next priorities. If the injury occurred 2 h ago and the degree of shock is mild, then massive or ongoing hemorrhage is unlikely.

D. **What is the blood pressure?** Blood pressure does not fall until more than 20% of the intravascular blood volume is lost. Compensatory mechanisms (vasoconstriction, increased heart rate, and contractility) allow blood pressure to be maintained in early shock.'

E. **What is the heart rate?** Tachycardia above 120 BPM should be considered a sign of hypovolemic shock in the trauma setting.

F. **Is the skin cool and moist?** Vasoconstriction of muscle and skin is an early compensatory mechanism. Epinephrine release causes sweating. Cool, moist skin is a reliable clinical sign of impending shock.

G. **What is the urine output?** Any patient with serious trauma should have their urine output monitored. Visceral vasoconstriction reduces renal blood flow and is reflected in diminished urine output.

H. **Are the external jugular veins distended?** A trauma patient who appears to be in hypovolemic shock by other parameters, but who has distended neck veins has cardiac tamponade or tension pneumothorax (SVC disruption is a rare cause). Check the heart sounds. Is the trachea deviated?

III. Database

A. **Physical Exam Key Points.** A history should be taken and a physical examination should be performed with the patient fully immobilized and completely exposed. It is particularly important to perform a thorough head-to-toe initial examination to avoid any missed injuries, such as unsuspected entrance and exit sites in penetrating injuries. Obtain an initial GCS before proceeding with the rest of the physical examination.

1. **Lungs.** Evaluate breath sounds, considering the possibility of pneumothorax.
2. **Heart.** Listen for tachycardia and muffled heart sounds.
3. **Abdomen.** Evaluate for distention (possible site of significant bleeding) and tenderness.

B. **Laboratory Data.** Send a complete blood count, coagulation studies, chemistries, a toxicology screen, a urinalysis, and a type and crossmatch sample from blood obtained while placing the first intravenous line. Send arterial blood gas. Send a repeat hemoglobin and hematocrit (serial Hcts) every 5–15 min in severely injured patients.

C. **Radiographic Studies.** Order a lateral C-spine with the collar on, an A-P pelvic film, an A-P supine chest radiograph, and other radiographs as indicated. Obtain an upright chest radiograph, if indicated, once it is safe to sit up the patient (after stabilizing or clearing the cervical spine and evaluating the thoracic and lumbar spine).

IV. Plan

A. **Fluid Resuscitation.** With moderate to severe hypovolemic shock, treatment is initiated as the evaluation is beginning. Large-bore, peripheral intravenous lines are started (two is the minimum required) at different sites. The upper extremities are preferred.

1. Cutdowns are placed easily in the saphenous vein at the ankles or the brachial and cephalic veins at the antecubital crease. An 8.5 Fr Swan-Ganz introducer can be placed percutaneously into the femoral vein at the groin. The use of large-bore lines (8.5 Fr introducers or cut IV tubing) allows the administration of 2 L crystalloid in < 15 min. Short catheters are best (thus subclavian CVP lines are not used at all).
2. Avoid placing percutaneous subclavian or internal jugular lines. These are very hard to place in hypovolemic patients with collapsed central veins. The added risk of iatrogenic pneumothorax is not warranted.
3. Trauma patients who need more than 2000 cc of crystalloid should be transfused with red blood cells. Type-specific blood is preferred, but if unavailable, universal type O should be given. Packed red blood cells are more viscous than whole blood. To infuse packed cells rapidly, dilute them first with normal saline.

B. **Secondary Assessment.** If the patient is hemodynamically stable and neurologically intact after initial resuscitation and assessment, then start your secondary assessment and reevaluation. If shock persists despite resuscitation, then ongoing hemorrhage is present, and immediate operative intervention may be indicated.

C. **Observation.** After completing your assessment, place an NG tube and Foley catheter (these steps are done simultaneously with a team approach). Don't insert a Foley catheter in a patient with a possible urethral injury (eg, pelvic fracture) until you check for blood at the urethral meatus and check for a free floating prostate on rectal exam. In these cases, urinary catheter placement is only performed after radiographic evaluation of the urethra (urethrogram and cystogram). Peritoneal lavage may be indicated at this time. Temperature monitoring should be started.

D. If a patient remains in shock despite aggressive resuscitation, you must rapidly determine the cause. Hypovolemic shock usually results from blood loss within the chest or abdomen, or from a massive pelvic injury. Cardiogenic shock may be due to tension pneumothorax or cardiac tamponade, both of which are easily treated (once suspected). The detailed secondary survey is begun once the patient is stabilized during the initial resuscitation phase. This includes a comprehensive examination and reevaluation of the patient.

70. VAGINAL BLEEDING

I. Problem. A young woman admitted for observation for possible appendicitis develops vaginal bleeding.

II. Immediate Questions

A. Is there any evidence of shock? Vaginal bleeding can be profuse. In some cases, the visible blood loss may represent only a fraction of the actual blood loss. Assess the patient for hypovolemia or shock.

B. Is there any pain associated with the bleeding? The most serious condition in the differential diagnosis of acute vaginal bleeding is ectopic pregnancy, and pain is always a predominant part of the patient's complaints. In fact, most causes of vaginal bleeding are also associated with pain or other gastrointestinal symptoms.

C. When was the patient's last period, and has she been sexually active since that time? Inquire about specific details of the menstrual history, regarding the most recent period, and any abnormal bleeding in the past. Obtain a complete sexual history, including contraceptive use and any associated symptoms of early pregnancy (morning sickness, fluid retention, etc).

D. Attempt to quantify the blood loss. The rate of bleeding has both diagnostic and therapeutic implications. If the patient can't estimate the volume of blood loss, ask about the number of pads or tampons used and the degree of saturation.

III. Differential Diagnosis

A. Normal Menstrual Period. This is clearly the most commonly encountered cause.

B. Dysfunctional Bleeding (Related to Menstrual Cycle)

1. Perimenopausal.
2. Inadequate luteal phase.
3. Oral contraceptives.
4. Endometriosis.

C. Pregnancy Related

1. Ectopic pregnancy.
2. Threatened or spontaneous abortion.
3. Retained products of gestation.

D. Neoplasia

1. Uterine fibroids.
2. Cervical polyps.
3. Carcinoma
   a. Endometrium.
   b. Cervix.
   c. Ovarian.

E. Infection

1. Pelvic inflammatory disease.
2. Vaginitis.

F. Trauma

G. Bleeding Diathesis. Bleeding is usually present at other sites as well.

IV. Database

A. Physical Exam Key Points

1. **Vital signs.** Check orthostatic signs for excessive blood loss; fever is a sign of infection.
2. **Skin.** Pallor suggests significant blood loss. Bruising and petechiae suggest a bleeding diathesis.
3. **Abdomen.** Observe for peritoneal signs, tenderness, and distention.
4. **Pelvic exam.** Examine for a mass in the vagina, cervix, uterus, or adnexa. Palpate for areas of tenderness, including cervical motion tenderness. Look for the source and rate of bleeding, and determine whether the cervical os is open or closed. Are tissue fragments present?

B. Laboratory Data

1. **CBC.** This should be ordered to look for leukocytosis, anemia, or thrombocytopenia. Serial Hcts should be obtained to assess the rate of bleeding.
2. **PT/PTT.** These should be ordered when coagulopathy is suspected. Check the fibrinogen and fibrin split products if DIC is suspected.
3. **Blood.** Type and crossmatch blood if indicated.
4. **Serum/urine HCG.** A pregnancy test will be positive with an ectopic pregnancy.
5. **Perform a Pap smear of cervix.**
6. **Order a cervical culture.**

C. Radiographic and Other Studies

1. **Culdocentesis.** Look for blood with an ectopic pregnancy or pus with PID.
2. **Pelvic ultrasound.** This identifies intrauterine and intratubal lesions (an ectopic pregnancy) or any pelvic mass.

3. **CT scan of pelvis.** This is a good method to detect or characterize a mass. An ultrasound is usually easier to obtain however. Ultrasound is clearly preferred in a pregnant patient (to avoid radiating the uterus).

V. **Plan.** Most vaginal bleeding does not require specific treatment because it represents normal menstrual bleeding.

A. **Overall Plan**

1. Resuscitate the patient from the acute blood loss as needed.
2. Establish large-bore IVs, administer crystalloid, type and crossmatch for blood, monitor the urine output, and follow serial hematocrits. Also make the patient NPO as an urgent operative procedure may be indicated.

B. **Specific Treatment.** Virtually all of the causes of significant vaginal bleeding require evaluation by the gynecology service. Ongoing bleeds require emergency consultation, whereas spotting or a bleeding episode that has resolved can be evaluated as above and seen on an elective basis, (depending on the diagnosis).

C. **Ectopic Pregnancy.** When lower abdominal pain is a part of the symptom complex and the patient is of child-bearing age, ectopic pregnancy must be ruled out even if the pregnancy tests are normal. The diagnostic procedure of choice is a pelvic ultrasound; if ultrasound is not available, then use culdocentesis.

71. VENTILATOR MANAGEMENT: AGITATION

(Ventilators are discussed in detail in Section VII, page 414)

I. **Problem.** A patient on a ventilator in the ICU—status post-craniotomy for a cerebellar lesion—has become agitated and is "bucking" the ventilator.

II. **Immediate Questions**

A. **What are the patient's most recent blood gases?** Hypoxia may be the cause of agitation, or there may be hypocarbia from tachypnea.

B. **When was the most recent chest radiograph?** Be sure there is a recent chest radiograph. Positive pressure ventilation can cause a pneumothorax, which can cause hypoxia, resulting in agitation. Placement of the ETT into the right mainstem bronchus can also cause hypoxia and agitation.

C. **What is the patient's respiratory rate?** Tachypnea is a common cause of "bucking" the ventilator.

D. What are the ventilator settings (mode, rate, PEEP, F_{IO_2}, TV)? IMV delivers a fixed number of breaths per minute. Assist control will cause the ventilator to deliver a full tidal volume with each patient-initiated breath.

III. Differential Diagnosis

A. Respiratory Decompensation. This must be ruled out first.

1. **Pneumothorax** or tension pneumothorax.
2. **Improper positioning of the endotracheal tube.** Either proximally or distally (usually down the right mainstem bronchus).
3. **Mucous plugging.** Tenacious secretions can obstruct the tube.
4. **Ventilator malfunction.** Have the respiratory therapist verify that the ventilator is working properly and delivering the preset parameters.
5. **Aspiration.** This can occur if the ETT cuff is only partially inflated.
6. **Sepsis.** Systemic sepsis can cause agitation.
7. **Other causes.** Consider CHF, pulmonary embolus, hiccups.

B. Inadequate Tidal Volume. Is the preset tidal volume sufficient for the patient (10–5 mL/kg)?

C. Insufficient Pain Medication or Sedation.

D. Status Epilepticus. This may be confused with agitation.

E. Tetanus.

IV. Database

A. Physical Exam Key Points

1. **Vital signs.** Check the blood pressure and respiratory rate.
2. **Neck.** Distended neck veins and tracheal deviation suggest tension pneumothorax.
3. **Lungs.** Listen for bilateral breath sounds, wheezing, or evidence of congestive heart failure.
4. **Chest.** Look for subcutaneous emphysema and symmetric excursion.
5. **Verify that the cuff** is inflated properly and listen for any air leaks.

B. Laboratory Data

1. **Arterial blood gases.** Look for hypoxia and hypercarbia.

2. **Serum electrolytes.** Check to complete the acid-base workup.

C. **Radiographic and Other Studies.** A chest radiograph is necessary to check endotracheal tube placement, rule out a pneumothorax, an effusion, etc. Therapy should not be delayed because of a pending radiograph.

V. Plan

A. **Obtain a new set of arterial blood gases and a STAT portable chest radiograph.** This should be the first step for any patient on positive pressure ventilation.

B. **Manually ventilate the patient with a bag and 100% O_2.**
   1. If the patient is easily ventilated, check for a mechanical ventilator problem.
   2. When there is increased resistance to ventilation, consider a pneumothorax. Be sure to check for bilateral breath sounds, etc. If there is evidence of a pneumothorax, and the patient is unstable, do not wait for the radiograph; place a chest tube immediately.
   3. When there is no evidence of pneumothorax, check the ET tube for obstruction. Consider replacing the tube if the obstruction cannot be relieved. If there is no obstruction, then consider sepsis, CHF, pulmonary embolus, or aspiration as a cause of decompensation.

C. **Treat Pain Appropriately.** Sedation may also be helpful. Use diazepam (Valium) IV, 2–5 mg IV every 2 h as a start. Other agents include lorazepam (Ativan), midazolam (Versed), and others. Depending on your institutional policies, propofol (Diprivan) may be a suitable sedating agent for acute situations.

D. **Patients "fighting" the ventilator can sometimes be calmed by increasing the tidal volume.**

E. **Remember that IMV mode delivers a fixed tidal volume at preset intervals, regardless of the patient's own respiratory rate.** This allows the patient to breathe more often than the preset rate without triggering the machine. Assist control will give a full breath at a preset tidal volume whenever the patient triggers the ventilator with an inspiration. Thus, a patient making frequent small inspiratory efforts will trigger the ventilator for a full breath each time, which can lead the patient to "fight" the ventilator. Controlled ventilation should not routinely be used on conscious patients, because it will not allow the patient to initiate any breaths on his own; the use of this modality in the conscious patient may lead to agitation.

F. **If the patient is alert, reassure the patient by carefully explaining the mechanical ventilator.** Often this helps to relieve the fears of an otherwise frightened patient and assists in ventilator management.

G. **Paralysis must be used with extreme caution, if at all.** Patients are occasionally paralyzed in critical situations where they remain hypoxic despite maximal ventilatory support. It is also used in tetanus. Paralytic agents such as succinylcholine or pancuronium bromide must be used with adequate sedation.

72. VENTILATOR MANAGEMENT: HIGH F_{IO_2}

(Ventilators are discussed in Section VII, page 414)

I. **Problem.** A mechanically ventilated trauma patient is maintaining a P_{O_2} of only 75 mm Hg on 90% inspired oxygen.

II. **Immediate Questions**

A. **What are the rest of the arterial blood gas values?** An elevated P_{CO_2} indicates hypoventilation. When ventilation, as reflected by minute ventilation, is not adequate to maintain P_{CO_2} in a normal range, and there is concomitant lung disease, hypoxemia may result.

B. **What does the chest radiograph show?** Significant atelectasis, pneumonia, pneumothorax, pleural effusion, pulmonary edema, pulmonary contusion, and ARDS can cause hypoxemia and result in high oxygen concentration requirements.

C. **What is the status of the endotracheal tube?** Mucous plugging could be occluding the tube. A cuff leak may not be allowing adequate inflation. If the tube is in too far, it may be down the right mainstem bronchus.

D. **What are the ventilator settings?** Poor oxygenation may sometimes be corrected by increasing PEEP. PEEP should be increased cautiously as it may impede cardiac output or cause barotrauma.

III. **Differential Diagnosis.** Causes of hypoxia can be classified into two main categories: problems causing a mismatch between ventilation and perfusion ($\dot{V}/\dot{Q}$ mismatch, shunt, and diffusion abnormalities) and pure hypoventilation.

A. **Ventilation and Perfusion Mismatches.** This is the most common cause of hypoxemia and high oxygen requirements. A 100% mismatch is termed a **physiologic shunt**.

1. Reactive airways (COPD, asthma).
2. Pneumonia.
3. Atelectasis.
4. Pulmonary embolus.
5. Pneumothorax.
6. Physiologic shunting seen in ARDS and pulmonary edema.
7. Anatomic shunting seen in congenital heart disease.
8. Sepsis. This is one of the most common causes of pulmonary shunting. Patients with acute sepsis are frequently sent for a $\dot{V}/\dot{Q}$ scan, long before they are cultured and started on antibiotics.
9. Mainstem intubation tube. An endotracheal tube may migrate down the right mainstem bronchus.
10. Pulmonary contusion.

B. **Hypoventilation.** A rare cause of hypoxemia.
1. Very low minute ventilation (low tidal volume, low rate, or both).
2. Increased dead space (unavoidable part of mechanical ventilation).
3. Muscle weakness in nonventilated patient.
4. Cuff leak.

IV. Database

A. Physical Exam Key Points
1. **Vital signs.** Fever, tachycardia, and hypotension may indicate sepsis.
2. **Cardiac.** Presence of an S_3 and tachycardia may indicate heart failure as a cause of pulmonary edema.
3. **Lungs.** A careful exam may reveal pulmonary edema (rales), decreased sounds (atelectasis, effusion, pneumothorax), egophony (pneumonia), or wheezing (asthma). Follow-up with a chest radiograph.
4. **Neck.** Look for jugular venous distention.

B. Laboratory Data
1. **Arterial blood gas.** Follow serially.
2. **CBC.** Verify that the hemoglobin and hematocrit are adequate.
3. **Cultures.** Order cultures of sputum, blood, urine, drains, and wounds as clinically indicated.
4. **Sputum exam.** Tenacious secretions are common in reactive airways disease. Purulent sputum indicates pneumonia, and frothy sputum suggests pulmonary edema. A Gram's stain is a quick and useful means to evaluate sputum.
5. **Mixed venous oxygen content.** Drawn from the pulmonary artery through a Swan-Ganz catheter, the mixed

venous oxygen tension should normally measure 40 mm Hg (approximately 70% saturated). Lower levels indicate that the oxygen delivery to tissues is inadequate, as would be found in major trauma and severe sepsis.

6. **Alveolar-arterial gradient.**

C. **Radiographic and Other Studies**

1. **Chest radiograph.** This is critical to understanding the nature of the problem. Look for evidence of
   a. ARDS.
   b. Pneumonia.
   c. Pulmonary edema.
   d. Atelectasis.
   e. Pneumothorax.
   f. Effusion.
   g. Endotracheal tube misplacement.
   h. Pulmonary contusion
2. **ECG.** Look for dysrhythmias, such as atrial fibrillation or flutter, which can be corrected. Ischemic changes may indicate infarction. When possible, compare with previous ECGs.
3. **$\dot{V}/\dot{Q}$ scan, spiral CT scan, or pulmonary angiogram.** Perform when a pulmonary embolus is suspected.
4. **CT scan of abdomen.** Order when sepsis is suspected.
5. **Bronchoscopy.** This should be used aggressively to clear tenacious mucous plugs causing atelectasis, and with lavage, biopsy, and brushings as diagnostic aids.
6. **Open lung biopsy.** This is rarely indicated; it may be used when hypoxemia and lung disease persist, despite aggressive medical therapy, and there is no clear cause of the lung disease.

V. **Plan.** The main objective is to provide adequate tissue oxygenation without subjecting the patient to the risks of oxygen toxicity. The goal is to keep F_{IO_2} below 60%, especially with long-term oxygen use.

A. **Correct Anemia.** Keep the Hct > 30% with transfusions.

B. **Correct Pulmonary Disease**

1. Treat pneumothorax with a chest tube.
2. **Pneumonia.** Use antibiotics and pulmonary toilet, including nebulizer treatments and chest physiotherapy (postural drainage).
3. **Atelectasis.** Ensure adequate tidal volume and frequent suctioning. Sighs set at 2 times the tidal volume 6–10 times an hour will help reduce the incidence of atelectasis.

4. **Asthma.** The use of bronchodilators, aminophylline, and steroids may help treat reactive airways.
5. **Effusion.** Perform a thoracentesis or tube thoracostomy.
6. **Pulmonary edema.** Administer diuretics with careful attention to fluid management.

C. **Pulmonary Toilet**
   1. Perform frequent suctioning.
   2. Perform saline lavage into the endotracheal tube.
   3. Provide an occasional large tidal volume ("sigh") by bagging before suctioning.
   4. Use bronchodilators (eg, metaproterenol), if needed.
   5. Chest physical therapy.

D. **Treat Sepsis.** Administer appropriate antibiotics and perform surgical drainage as required.

E. **Optimize Ventilator Settings**
   1. Place a radial arterial catheter for frequent arterial blood gas measurements.
   2. Adjust the rate and tidal volume to maintain a normal Pco_2.
   3. Start with high Fio_2 (0.9–1.0 mm Hg) and wean down to avoid oxygen toxicity.
   4. Positive end expiratory pressure (PEEP) should be added slowly. Complications are rare below 10–15 mm Hg of PEEP, but may include barotrauma and decreased cardiac output (caused by decreased cardiac blood return). It may be necessary to increase PEEP to high levels to allow Fio_2 to be decreased to safe levels. This trade-off results in higher mean and peak airway pressures. Consider a Swan-Ganz catheter for higher PEEP settings (> 10 mm Hg).
   5. **Sedation or paralysis.** Consider these in a patient fighting the ventilator who still requires mechanically assisted ventilation. Agitation interferes with adequate function of the ventilator. Remember that agents such as pancuronium (Pavulon) should not routinely be used alone. Pavulon induces paralysis but does not cause sedation or relieve pain. Use it along with morphine and/or diazepam.

F. **Maximize Hemodynamic State.** A pulmonary artery catheter may help in the management of a patient with respiratory failure.
   1. Maintain adequate filling pressures (15 mm Hg) with crystalloid or blood products. Give furosemide if the wedge pressure is above 20 mm Hg.

2. Increase the cardiac output(and cardiac index) if needed with dopamine or dobutamine.

G. **Heparin.** Administer when a pulmonary embolus is suspected. Inject heparin 5000–10,000–U bolus followed by continuous drip at approximately 1000 U/h to maintain an activated partial thromboplastin time (PTT) between 2–2.5 times control. Some centers are using thrombolytic therapy (streptokinase, urokinase, t-PA).

73. VENTILATOR MANAGEMENT: HIGH PEAK PRESSURE

(Ventilators are discussed in Section VII, page 414)

I. **Problem.** An intubated patient on the trauma service with multiple injuries from blunt trauma is continually setting off the peak pressure alarm.

II. **Immediate Questions**

A. **What is the arterial blood gas?** A change in peak pressure may represent a ventilator system malfunction, a decrease in sedation, or a new pulmonary event or condition. First, determine whether the patient is being ventilated adequately. Send off an arterial blood sample for blood gas determination immediately.

B. **Has the position of the endotracheal tube changed?** If the endotracheal tube has migrated into the right mainstem bronchus, the peak pressure will increase as the entire tidal volume is administered to one lung. Check the mark on the endotracheal tube at the lips and compare to previous positions. Obtain a chest radiograph.

C. **Are there increased secretions in the endotracheal tube?** Find out if the nurse has been suctioning increased or thicker secretions from the endotracheal tube. The tube may become partially obstructed with secretions, particularly in chronically intubated patients.

D. **Is there any subcutaneous emphysema?** An important cause for increased peak pressure in a patient on a ventilator is a tension pneumothorax, which can be associated with subcutaneous emphysema. The chest wall and neck can be palpated quickly for crepitus before a chest radiograph can be obtained. Also look for jugular venous distention or tracheal deviation.

E. **Has there been any change in the ventilator or the control settings?** Perhaps the peak pressure alarm was reset. Were other settings changed? Troubleshoot the ventilator with the assistance of the respiratory therapist and look for circuit disconnections, etc.

III. Differential Diagnosis. If the peak pressure alarm is sounded in a ventilated patient, there is either a ventilator problem or an increased resistance to the delivered tidal volume in the patient. Increased resistance can be a result of intrinsic pulmonary disease or a resistance to lung expansion from extrinsic compressive forces. Clinical situations can vary greatly, but in general, peak inspiratory pressures should be less than 20–30 cm water.

A. Ventilator Problems

1. Lowered peak pressure setting.
2. Incorrect ventilator circuit set-up.
3. Shift in the position of the endotracheal tube.

B. Intrinsic Pulmonary Problems

1. Obstruction of the endotracheal tube by secretions.
2. Pulmonary edema. ARDS, CHF can cause decreased compliance, and high pressures will be required to ventilate the patient.
3. Interstitial disease.
   a. **Malignancy:** Lymphangitic spread.
   b. **Fibrosis:** Such as bleomycin-induced.
4. Reactive airway disease. Asthma.

C. Extrinsic Pulmonary Compression

1. Pneumothorax or tension pneumothorax.
2. Pleural effusion or hemothorax.
3. Abdominal distention.
4. Chest wall or respiratory muscle contraction
   a. The patient may be bucking the ventilator because of anxiety, pain, or decreased sedation. However, agitation may be secondary to hypoventilation and hypoxia, so check the Pao_2.
   b. Coughing spasm.

IV. Database

A. Physical Exam Key Points

1. **Skin.** Look for cyanosis and crepitus (subcutaneous emphysema).
2. **Lungs.** Examine the secretions from the endotracheal tube noting the amount and viscosity. Listen for decreased or absent breath sounds, rales, and wheezes.
3. **Cardiac.** Listen for decreased heart sounds. Look for distended neck veins.
4. **Abdomen.** Is there marked distention or ascites?

B. Laboratory Data

1. Draw an arterial blood gas immediately.

2. **CBC.** Is there evidence of anemia or leukocytosis?

C. **Radiographic and Other Studies**

1. **Chest radiograph.** If the ventilator is not responsible for the problem, order a portable chest radiograph immediately. Look for a pleural effusion, pulmonary edema, a pneumothorax, or a new infiltrate. Check the endotracheal tube position (the tip should be 2 cm above the carina). If the patient already has a chest tube in place and it is on water seal, placing it on suction may help. Look for a pneumothorax, even if the patient has a chest tube in place.

V. Plan

A. **Overall Plan.** Initial therapy is to disconnect the patient from the ventilator and bag ventilate by hand. This maneuver allows for immediate hyperventilation, removes the ventilator as the source of the problem, allows manual assessment of pulmonary compliance, and allows the endotracheal tube to be irrigated and the patient to be suctioned of secretions. At the same time, draw an arterial blood gas, call for a portable chest radiograph, and check the ventilator. Decide whether the problem is the patient or the ventilator.

B. **Specific Problems**

1. **Hemo- or pneumothorax, effusion.** Treat with a tube thoracostomy. In urgent situations, a tension pneumothorax can be treated with a 14–gauge IV catheter inserted into the anterior chest at the level of the second or third intercostal space (see page 255).
2. **Endotracheal tube malposition.** Adjust the tube, retape, and repeat the chest radiograph to document its new position.
3. **Bucking the ventilator.**
   a. Give pain medication or sedation once hypoxia and mechanical problems have been ruled out.
   b. Change the ventilation to assist/control. Follow the blood gases as the patient may hyperventilate on this setting. Patients making small respiratory efforts will not do as well on assist/control (as on IMV) because the machine will be triggered by each small breath.
4. **For cases of fibrosis,** infiltrative disease, and ARDS being maximally treated, you may have to tolerate higher peak airway pressures to ventilate the patient. Adjust the alarm setting and follow up the patient closely for a pneumothorax (resulting from barotrauma).

74. VENTILATOR MANAGEMENT: LOW Po_2/HIGH Pco_2

(Ventilator Management is discussed in Section VII, page 414.)

I. **Problem.** An 83–year-old male has a Po_2 of 55 mm Hg 1 d after grafting of a ruptured abdominal aortic aneurysm.

II. **Immediate Questions**

A. **What are the current ventilator settings, and were there any recent changes in these settings?** Were settings for Fio_2, rate (IMV or Assist Control), PEEP or tidal volume changed? Find out when the last ventilator changes were made, and what the blood gas results were before those changes.

B. **What are the most recent blood gas results? What were the prior results? On what ventilator settings were they obtained?**

C. **What is the patient's respiratory rate?** Tachypnea is an important finding and suggests that the ventilator settings may not be providing enough ventilatory support.

D. **What operation has the patient had? What type of incision is there?** Thoracotomy incisions, flank and large abdominal incisions are the most painful and limit the patient's ability to breathe on their own much more, than for example, a median sternotomy.

E. **What are the patient's baseline blood gases (preop) on room air? What were the results of preop PFTs?** These should be done in a patient with emphysema or COPD, who may have baseline CO_2 levels that are often in the 50–mm Hg range.

F. **What is the peak pressure?** This allows the clinician to calculate compliance (tidal volume/peak pressure), thus following lung stiffness. A progressively stiffer lung may indicate ARDS as a cause for the low oxygen levels. Normal compliance is $>$ 100 mL/cm water.

G. **When was the most recent chest radiograph?** If not within a few hours, obtain a repeat chest film immediately.

III. **Differential Diagnosis**

A. **Mucous Plugging.**

B. **Pulmonary Edema.** Check the fluid balance over the last several days. Is the patient ahead on fluids? This may result in a lower Po_2.

C. **Ventilator Leak.** This is usually the result of a broken cuff. Be sure the patient is receiving all of the tidal volume delivered.

D. **Pulmonary Parenchymal Disease.** It is important to know about any preoperative diseases (COPD, emphysema, bronchitis, asthma).

E. **Inadequate Ventilatory Support.** Check the ventilator settings and Pco_2. Is the rate or tidal volume too low?

F. **Pneumothorax.** A simple pneumothorax can rapidly progress to a tension pneumothorax in a mechanically ventilated patient.

G. **Endotracheal Tube Malposition.** Evaluate on chest radiograph. Is the tube positioned past the carina?

H. **Aspiration.**

I. **Bronchospasm.** Check for wheezing on physical exam.

J. **ARDS.**

K. **Atelectasis/Pneumonia.**

L. **Pulmonary Embolus.** If you increase the $F\text{IO}_2$ and there is a minimal increase in saturation or Pao_2, there may be an acute $\dot{V}/\dot{Q}$ mismatch (shunt).

M. **Circulatory Problems.** Assess for CHF.

N. **Low hemoglobin.**

O. **Pulmonary contusion.**

IV. Database

A. Physical Exam Key Points

1. **HEENT.** Listen for an obvious air leak.
2. **Neck.** Look for distended neck veins with CHF, volume overload, or pneumothorax.
3. **Lungs.** Evaluate for bronchospasm or pulmonary edema. Check for subcutaneous emphysema, which can result from pneumothorax.
4. Look for equal expansion, tracheal deviation, and adequate breath sounds bilaterally.

B. Laboratory Data

1. **Arterial blood gas.** Follow serial studies.

C. Radiographic and Other Studies

1. **Chest radiograph.** Look for congestive heart failure, pneumothorax, endotracheal tube position, lobar infiltrate, collapse secondary to mucous plugging, or signs of ARDS.

2. **Nuclear ventilation/Perfusion scan ($\dot{V}/\dot{Q}$ scan).** If there is any question of a pulmonary embolus, then a $\dot{V}/\dot{Q}$ scan is indicated. An equivocal scan usually necessitates pulmonary angiography.

V. Plan. The goal of ventilatory support is to provide, in conjunction with alveolar exchange, adequate tissue oxygenation. Many times, sudden changes in PO_2 and PCO_2 in the absence of ventilatory changes are due to such phenomena as altered FIO_2, pneumothorax, mucous plugging, and so on. Consider bronchoscopy for severe mucous plugging if endotracheal tube suctioning is inadequate.

A. Hypoxemia. Aim for an FIO_2 between 40% and 50%, because at this level, there is minimal oxygen toxicity. In general, a PaO_2 of 60 mm Hg is acceptable, because at this level, hemoglobin is about 90% saturated. Cardiac output is also important, and you may need to place a Swan-Ganz for direct measurement. Urine output may be the best indicator of cardiac output, even if the patient has a PA catheter. Hypoxia may be treated by increasing oxygen delivery or by decreasing oxygen consumption.

1. **Increasing delivery**
   a. **Ventilatory**
      i. Increasing the FIO_2.
      ii. Decreasing the Shunt: This can be done by increasing PEEP. Remember that increasing PEEP can significantly affect cardiac output, so that a pulmonary artery catheter may be needed, especially with PEEP levels above 10–15 cm water.
   b. **Circulatory**
      i. Improve cardiac output.
      ii. There may be a physical obstruction to circulation, such as a pulmonary embolus. Treatment should be anticoagulation or thrombolytic therapy, after diagnosis by imaging studies as previously discussed.
   c. **Hemoglobin**
      i. Transfuse to an acceptable range (usually to an Hct $> 30\%$).
      ii. Decreased consumption: Sedation, paralysis, and hypothermia can be combined in critical situations.

B. Hypercarbia. The adequacy of ventilation is based solely on the PCO_2 and can be affected by changes in the ventilatory rate and tidal volume.

1. Rule out mechanical problems such as leaks, plugging of the endotracheal tube, kinking, or malpositioning of the tube.
2. Tidal volume should be 10–15 mL/kg of body weight. Is the patient receiving the delivered volume? Hypoventilation (low minute volume) can raise P_{CO_2}.
3. Is the P_{CO_2} increased because of increased CO_2 production or excessive deadspace ventilation?
   a. Increased CO_2 production
      i. Sepsis: Treat appropriately (antibiotics, etc).
      ii. Hyperalimentation with a high percentage of carbohydrates or excessive calories.
   b. Increased deadspace: Deadspace refers to the ventilation of areas such as the ventilator tubing, endotracheal tube, nonperfused alveoli, and so on, where gas exchange cannot occur. Correct the following conditions when possible:
      i. Inadequate cardiac output.
      ii. PEEP causing overdistention.
      iii. Pulmonary emboli.
      iv. Vasoconstriction of pulmonary vessels by vasoactive medications.

75. WHEEZING

I. **Problem.** A 20–year-old has been admitted for laparoscopic appendectomy and begins wheezing in the anesthesia holding area.

II. **Immediate Questions**

A. **What are the vital signs?** A respiratory rate of 40/min may indicate the need for immediate treatment. Associated hypotension may suggest an anaphylactic reaction or an acute MI. Fever may point to an underlying infection or new pulmonary embolism.

B. **Were any diagnostic tests recently performed or medications recently administered?** A β-blocker given to a stable asthmatic may precipitate an acute attack of bronchospasm. Wheezing following the administration of a drug, such as penicillin or radiocontrast dye, suggests an anaphylactic reaction.

C. **For what condition was the patient admitted?** A patient admitted to rule out an MI may have developed acute pulmonary edema; whereas, a patient with a gastric ulcer may have gastric outlet obstruction and aspiration.

D. **Is there any history of asthma?** Childhood asthma may reactivate at any age given the right stimuli.

E. **Does the patient have any allergies to medications or other substances, such as shellfish?** It is prudent to inquire about any known allergies.

III. Differential Diagnosis

A. Diffuse Wheezing

1. **Acute bronchospasm.** This may be due to asthma, an exacerbation of chronic obstructive pulmonary disease (COPD), or an anaphylactic reaction.
2. **Aspiration.** This may trigger bronchospasm from mucosal irritation or from impacted foreign bodies.
3. **Cardiogenic pulmonary edema.** The primary finding in "cardiac asthma" may be wheezing. Other findings of pulmonary edema should be present and the chest radiograph will be diagnostic.
4. **Pulmonary embolism (PE).** Platelet factors may be released that not only cause shunting and hypoxemia, but may also cause transient bronchospasm.

B. Stridor (Upper Airway) Wheezing

1. **Laryngospasm.** This may be part of an anaphylactic reaction or secondary to aspiration.
2. **Laryngeal or tracheal tumor.** A history of dysphagia, hoarseness, cough, or weight loss and anorexia may be present.
3. **Epiglottis.** The patient will often be unable to speak and will be unable to swallow secretions.
4. **Foreign body aspiration.**
5. **Vocal cord dysfunction.** Bilaterally paralyzed vocal cords may result in severe stridor and dyspnea. A subgroup of patients recently has been recognized to have "factitious asthma" in which they voluntarily adduct their vocal cords for psychogenic reasons.

C. Localized Wheezing

1. **Tumors.** These may obstruct one bronchus leading to localized wheezing.
2. **Mucous plugging.**
3. **An aspirated foreign body.**

IV. Database

A. **Physical Exam Key Points.** Localization of wheezing allows categorization as outlined in the differential diagnosis.

1. **Vital signs.** A fever may indicate an infectious cause. A pulsus paradoxicus > 20 mm Hg indicates severe respiratory distress. Hypotension requires immediate assessment and action.

2. **HEENT.** Check the mouth carefully. Examine the neck for angioneurotic edema. Palpate the sternocleidomastoid muscles for accessory muscle use. Auscultate over the mouth and larynx in an effort to localize the wheeze.
3. **Chest.** Carefully auscultate for localized wheezing. Listen for bibasilar rales, which may be present in pulmonary edema. Rales, increased fremitus, and egophony suggest pneumonia.
4. **Cardiac.** Check carefully for evidence of an S_3 or S_4 gallop or jugular venous distention, which points to pulmonary edema.
5. **Extremities.** Clubbed fingers most likely indicate an underlying lung cancer or severe COPD. Cyanosis indicates underlying hypoxemia. Edema may signify chronic CHF.
6. **Skin.** Urticaria probably indicates an acute allergic reaction. A malar rash may indicate acute systemic lupus erythematosus (SLE), which can present with acute pneumonitis.

B. Laboratory Data

1. **Arterial blood gases.** An elevated Pco_2 indicates significant ventilatory failure. Also check for hypoxemia.
2. **Complete blood count (CBC).** An increased white blood cell (WBC) count may indicate an underlying infection; however, an increase in the WBCs without a left shift can be seen with an acute MI and PE. Eosinophilia suggests an allergic or asthmatic cause to the wheezing.

C. Radiographic and Other Studies

1. **Electrocardiogram (ECG).** An ECG may show an acute MI or ischemia. Other ECG changes can be present with a PE, including an S wave in I, Q wave in III and T wave inversion in III ($S_1Q_3T_3$), new right bundle branch block (RBBB), and right axis shift. There may also be a change in rhythm.
2. **Chest radiograph.** A PE severe enough to cause wheezing will always be evident on the chest film. Look for a pleural-based, wedge-shaped lesion. Also, Kerley B lines, bilateral pleural effusions, vascular redistribution, and cardiomegaly may suggest CHF or pulmonary edema. Look for localized infiltrates or masses suggesting other causes.

V. Plan. Treatment depends on the diagnosis. The differential diagnoses previously listed should enable the clinician to form a tentative categorization, on which to base initial therapy.

A. Bronchospasm (Asthma, COPD, Allergic Reaction)

1. Administer methylprednisolone (Solu-medrol) 200 mg IV stat dose.
2. Give nebulized albuterol (Ventolin) 0.5 mL (2.5 mg) or metaproterenol (Alupent) 0.3 mL of 5% solution in 3.0 mL normal saline stat and then every 2–4 h.
3. Administer a loading dose of aminophylline, 6 mg/kg (assuming the patient is not already on aminophylline) and then a maintenance IV dose of 0.2–0.6 mg/kg/h (15–30 mg/h) IV. Aminophylline is now considered to be of only modest acute benefit and may cause considerable worsening of arrhythmias. Therefore, initial dosing should be on the "low side" and blood levels need to be monitored closely.

B. Stridor

1. Administer methylprednisolone 200 mg IV stat dose.
2. Give Nebulized racemic epinephrine (Micronephrine) 0.5 mL in 3 mL normal saline.
3. Consider intubation or tracheostomy.

C. Pulmonary Edema

1. Administer furosemide (Lasix) 20–80 mg IV.
2. Give nitroglycerin 0.4 mg sl; or paste ½" on skin; or a nitroglycerin drip 10–20 μg/min and increase by 5–10 μg every 10 min.
3. Ensure afterload reduction with agents such as intravenous nitroprusside (Nipride) or oral agents such as captopril (Capoten) or enalapril (Vasotec).
4. Administer IV morphine for venodilation and to relieve anxiety. Be prepared to intubate the patient.
5. Oxygen. Start with 2 L by nasal cannula.

D. Miscellaneous. Treatment varies with the disease. Obviously, PE should be treated with anticoagulants. Suspected tumors require additional tests, such as bronchoscopy, before reasonable treatment can be initiated. Acute allergic reactions are best prevented by pretreatment with Benadryl IV.

76. WOUND DEHISCENCE

I. Problem. A nurse notifies you that there is a piece of fat poking out of a laparotomy wound in a patient who has had a bilateral adrenalectomy.

II. Immediate Questions

A. Is there a wound dehiscence, and if so, to what extent? Always evaluate the wound yourself as soon as possible. See how much of the wound has opened, how deep, and if there is an evisceration. Check the integrity of the fascia with a cotton-tipped applicator (an "open wound" is not a dehiscence unless the fascia opens).

B. Did any fluid leak from the wound? Look at the dressing and ask the nurse and the patient about the nature and amount of fluid. Serous or serosanguineous fluid is more ominous and suggests a true fascial dehiscence. Grossly bloody or purulent fluid is indicative of a superficial wound infection, a liquefying hematoma, or active bleeding in the superficial tissues.

C. Are there any predisposing factors to dehiscence? Sepsis, poor nutrition, diabetes, and steroids predispose to poor wound healing and increase the likelihood of dehiscence.

III. Differential Diagnosis. A wound dehiscence usually results from a combination of factors including technical problems, local wound problems, poor wound healing, and increased stress on the wound. The following list is not so much a differential diagnosis as a list of contributing factors.

A. Technical Problems

1. **Poorly placed sutures.** This can be caused by failure to take a full-thickness bite or reapproximating muscle instead of fascia.
2. **Inappropriate suture material.** A wound dehiscence can be caused by a simple mistake, such as not using a heavy enough gauge suture for an abdominal closure.
3. **Sutures tied too tightly.** This usually induces tissue ischemia, and the sutures will eventually rip through.
4. **Other technical errors.** Monofilament sutures (prolene, PDS) require many knots and fray if tension is applied incorrectly while tying.

B. Local Wound Problems

1. **Infection.** There may be a superficial wound infection or an intraperitoneal abscess.
2. **Hematomas.** These may predispose a wound to become infected.

C. Poor Wound Healing

1. Poor nutrition.
2. Diabetes.
3. Steroids. Endogenous or exogenous.
4. Uremia.
5. Chemotherapy.
6. Advanced malignancy.

D. Decreased Tension On Wound

1. Abdominal distention

a. Ascites.
b. Dilated bowel.
2. Vomiting or coughing.
3. COPD.

IV. Database

A. Physical Exam Key Points

1. **Incision.** Use sterile gloves, take off all the dressings, and examine the entire wound. Look for the leakage of fluid when the wound is palpated, and look for signs of infection. Examine for opening of the fascia with a cotton-tipped applicator.

B. Laboratory Data. Order a wound culture and Gram's stain if indicated.

V. Plan

A. Overall Plan. Determine by wound examination if there is an evisceration, fascial disruption without evisceration, or a superficial wound separation. In all cases, it is safe to make the patient NPO and start antibiotics (cephalosporins are used frequently) to cover at least skin organisms until a final plan is formulated.

B. Evisceration/Fascial Dehiscence. Cover the wound with saline-soaked sterile gauze and cover with a large sterile dressing. Prevent insensible losses at all times. Notify the senior staff and the operating room because evisceration requires operative repair.

C. Fascial Dehiscence Without Evisceration. If the overlying skin and subcutaneous tissues are intact but there is clearly a fascial defect, it may be treated by operative repair or observation with a resultant ventral hernia. Use an abdominal binder if the senior staff selects observation.

D. Superficial Wound Separation

1. **Healing** by secondary intention is mandatory when there is an associated superficial wound infection and is the safest management in any case. Open the wound to drain the pus or fluid, then treat with 2–4 wet-to-dry dressing changes per day (depending on the size of the defect, saline-soaked 4 x 4s are often used).
2. **Closure.** Some surgeons may attempt to reclose a superficial wound separation either immediately or following a period of wet-to-dry dressing changes. If this approach is used, realize that there is an increased risk of developing a superficial infection or spread of the infection to the fascial layer.

77. WOUND DRAINAGE

I. **Problem.** A patient has new drainage from a midline laparotomy incision 5 d after a small-bowel resection for ischemic bowel.

II. **Immediate Questions**

A. **How old is the wound, and what was the operative procedure?** The drainage may have been expected. If not, the timing of its appearance and the details of surgery can help elucidate the cause.

B. **Was there any prior drainage, and are drains present?** An increase in the drainage from a wound may occur because suction drains have stopped working.

C. **How was the wound closed? Were sutures, staples, or retention sutures used, or was the wound packed open?**

D. **What is the character of the drainage? Is it bloody, serosanguinous, or frankly purulent? Does it resemble intestinal contents?**

E. **How much drainage is there?** Quantification is essential especially to replace gastrointestinal tract losses in the presence of a fistula. Consider saving and weighing the dressings if it is critical to determine the volume.

III. **Differential Diagnosis**

A. **Wound Infection.** This is typically seen a few days postoperatively.

1. **Subcutaneous abscess.** This is most often due to *Staphylococcus* or *Streptococcus* species, although gram-negative rods may be present after colon surgery. A staphylococcal abscess takes at least 3 d to appear. *Streptococcus* species grows faster.
2. **Gas forming infections (*Clostridium* species, necrotizing fasciitis).** Severe pain may be the only sign, although crepitation may be present. This can be hard to diagnose, but it is a surgical emergency and must be promptly drained and débrided. *Clostridium* species may be the cause or, more commonly, there is a mixed gram-negative and microaerophilic gram-positive infection (particularly with diabetic patients).

B. **Impending Dehiscence.** Serosanguinous drainage after the first 24 postoperative hours is almost pathognomonic for wound dehiscence.

C. **Enterocutaneous Fistula.** This presents as draining intestinal contents. The fistula can have a high or low output. It is often caused by the inadvertent suturing of a segment of intestine during fascial closure. This usually follows several days of abdominal pain and fevers.

D. **Hemorrhage.** Excessive bleeding may exit through a fresh postoperative wound. DIC presents as bleeding from the wound as well as other sites (IV sites, etc).

E. **Pancreatic Fistula.** This can be postoperative or posttraumatic.

F. **Urinary Fistula.** This can be postoperative or posttraumatic, after radiation therapy, or from a neoplasm; it is rarely congenital.

G. **Ascitic Leak.** This can be minimized by closing one layer with a continuous running suture.

H. **Drain Malfunction.** When a surgically placed drain is not performing properly, the intended fluid may exit through the wound.

IV. Database

A. Physical Exam Key Points

1. **Vital signs.** Look for fever, tachycardia, and signs of sepsis.
2. **Abdomen.** Look for signs of peritonitis.
3. **Wound.** Examine the wound and surrounding area with sterile gloves. If there is any sign of purulent drainage, crepitus, cellulitis with fluctuance, immediately open the wound and inspect the drainage and fascial planes for integrity. Pay close attention to the adipose layer as well.

B. Laboratory Data

1. **CBC.** May reveal infection or indicate severe anemia from bleeding. Platelets may be decreased in DIC or in other causes of thrombocytopenia.
2. **Coagulation profile.** Check the PT, PTT, and fibrin split products, if DIC is suspected.
3. **Send drainage** for culture, Gram's stain, and amylase. Amylase may be elevated in an intestinal fistula but is markedly elevated in a pancreatic fistula.
4. **Drainage creatinine.** If the drainage is thought to be urine, the creatinine will be much higher than the serum level.

C. **Radiographic and Other Studies.** A fistulogram may be helpful to identify the origin of the drainage.

V. Plan

A. General Plan. Immediately treat any life-threatening complication such as evisceration (see page 273) while performing a diagnostic workup in less acute situations. Effluent from a wound should be sent for a Gram's stain, and culture. Send a sample of clear fluid for creatinine or amylase.

B. Specific Plans

1. **Wound infection.** The wound must be opened, which usually can be done at the bedside, and packed with saline-moistened gauze after evacuating pus in the wound. Remove enough skin closure staples or sutures to fully drain the area. In the presence of advancing local cellulitis or systemic signs of infection, antibiotics are indicated.
   a. ***Clostridium* species.** Treat with early debridement along with high dose IV penicillin.
   b. Gas forming nonclostridial infections are treated with broad spectrum antibiotics.
2. **Dehiscence.** Fascial dehiscence (indicated by serosanguinous wound drainage) can be watched if the skin closure remains intact. This results in a ventral hernia, which may require therapy at a later date. However, fascial dehiscence with eviscerated abdominal contents (intestine in the bed) requires prompt operative intervention (see Problem 76, page 271).
3. **Enterocutaneous fistula.** Ask your enterostomal therapist to fashion a bag to capture the effluent and protect the skin. A sump drain can be placed in the bag or in the wound to collect and remove the drainage. Quantify the drainage to determine whether the fistula is high output or low output. Charcoal or dye can be administered to confirm the diagnosis. Make the patient NPO, and use nasogastric suction for proximal intestinal fistulas. Remember to start early parenteral nutritional support. Fistulas generally appear after several days of abdominal pain and fever. Low-output fistulas often close spontaneously; high-output fistulas are more likely to require surgical intervention. Somatostatin may be of some benefit to reduce secretions.
4. **Pancreatic fistula.** Skin protection is essential. There can be serious nutritional deficits caused by pancreatic fistulas, as the fluid contains much protein. Since the alkalinization of duodenal contents is prevented by the fistulous drainage of pancreatic juice, these patients are at high risk for a peptic ulcer. A tube in the fistula opening may help to prevent premature closure of the skin.

5. **Hemorrhage.** Evaluate the patient's volume status. Replete volume with crystalloid, blood, or both. Remember that, despite bleeding, the hematocrit may not drop until you replace the lost volume with crystalloid. The decision to reoperate for bleeding depends on the clinical situation and the patient's overall status. There may be a bleeding vessel in the skin or subcutaneous fat and, if it can be seen, it can be cauterized at the bedside with a battery-powered cautery.

II. Laboratory Tests & Their Interpretation

This section is a selection of the most commonly used lab tests on a surgical service. If an increased or decreased value is not clinically useful, it is not listed. Because each laboratory has its own set of "normal" reference values, the normals given should be used only as a rough guide. The range for common normal values is given in parentheses and, unless specified, reflects normal adult levels.

ACTH (Adrenocorticotropic Hormone)

(8 AM: 20–140 pg/mL [SI: 20–140 ng/L]; midnight: approximately 50% of 8 AM value)

Increased: Addison's disease (primary adrenal hypofunction), ectopic ACTH production (oat cell and large cell lung carcinoma, pancreatic islet cell tumors, thymic tumors, renal cell carcinoma, bronchial carcinoid), Cushing's disease (pituitary adenoma), congenital adrenal hyperplasia (adrenogenital syndrome).

Decreased: Adrenal adenoma or carcinoma, nodular adrenal hyperplasia, pituitary insufficiency, corticosteroid use.

ACTH Stimulation Test (Cortrosyn Stimulation Test)

Used to help diagnose adrenal insufficiency. Cortrosyn (an ACTH analogue) is given at a dose of 0.25 mg IM or IV in adults or 0.125 mg in children younger than 2 years. Collect blood at 0, 30, and 60 min for cortisol and aldosterone.

Normal response: Three criteria are required: (1) basal cortisol of at least 5 μg/dL, (2) an incremental increase after Cortrosyn injection of at least 7 μg/dL and (3) a final serum cortisol of at least 16 μg/dL at 30 min or 18 μg/dL at 60 min or a cortisol increase of > 10 μg/dL. Aldosterone increases > 5 ng/dL over baseline.

Addison's Disease (Primary Adrenal Insufficiency): Neither cortisol nor aldosterone increase over baseline.

Secondary Adrenal Insufficiency: Caused by pituitary insufficiency or suppression by exogenous steroids, cortisol does not increase, but aldosterone increases.

Acetone (Ketone Bodies, Acetoacetate)

(Normal = negative)

Positive: Diabetic ketoacidosis (DKA), starvation, emesis, stress, alcoholism, infantile organic acidemias, isopropanol ingestion

Acid Phosphatase (Prostatic Acid Phosphatase, PAP)

(< 3.0 ng/mL by RIA, or < 0.8 IU/L by enzymatic)

Not a screening test for prostate cancer; most useful as a marker of response to therapy. PSA more sensitive in prostate cancer and largely replacing PAP.

Increased: Carcinoma of the prostate (usually outside of prostate), prostatic surgery or trauma (including prostatic massage), rarely in infiltrative bone disease (Gaucher's disease, myeloid leukemia), prostatitis, or benign prostate hypertrophy.

Albumin

(adult 3.5–5.0 gm/dL [SI: 35–50 g/L]; child 3.8–5.4 gm/dL [SI: 38–54 g/L]).

Follows total protein levels but does not detect gamma globulins.

Decreased: Malnutrition, over hydration, nephrotic syndrome, cystic fibrosis, multiple myeloma, Hodgkin's disease, leukemia, protein-losing enteropathies, chronic glomerulonephritis, alcoholic cirrhosis, inflammatory bowel disease, collagen-vascular diseases, hyperthyroidism.

Albumin/Globulin Ratio (A/G RATIO)

(normal > 1)

A calculated value (total protein minus albumin = globulins. Albumin divided by globulins = A/G ratio). Serum protein electrophoresis is a more informative test.

Decreased: Cirrhosis, liver diseases, nephrotic syndrome, chronic glomerulonephritis, cachexia, burns, chronic infections and inflammatory states, myeloma.

Aldosterone

(Serum: supine 3–10 ng/dL [SI:0.083–0.277 nmol/L] early AM, normal sodium intake [3 g sodium/d]; upright: 5–30 ng/dL [SI:0.138–0.831 nmol/L]; urinary 2–16 μg/d [SI:5.54–44.32 nmol/d]).

Stop antihypertensives and diuretics 2 wk before test. Upright samples should be drawn after 2 h. Primarily used to screen hypertensive patients for possible Conn's syndrome (adrenal adenoma producing excess aldosterone). Urinary studies are of limited utility. Should be done along with a plasma renin.

Increased: Primary hyperaldosteronism (Conn's syndrome), idiopathic hypertrophy bilateral hyperplasia of zona glomerulosa), secondary hyperaldosteronism is more common (CHF, sodium depletion, nephrotic syndrome, cirrhosis with ascites, others), upright posture, very low sodium diet.

Decreased: Adrenal insufficiency (Addison's disease), panhypopituitarism, supine posture.

Alkaline Phosphatase

(adult: 20–70 U/L, child: 20–150 U/L)

A fractionated alkaline phosphatase differentiates the bone or liver origin of the enzyme: heat-stable fraction from liver; heat-labile fraction from bone ("bone burns"). If heat-stable fraction is < 20%, c/w bone origin; if < 25–55%, c/w liver) Largely replaced by the gamma-glutamyl transpeptidase (GGT) and 5' nucleotidase, both increased in liver disease.

Increased: Increased calcium deposition in bone (hyperparathyroidism), Paget's disease, osteoblastic bone tumors (metastatic or osteogenic sarcoma), osteomalacia, rickets, pregnancy, childhood (especially in periods of active growth), healing fracture, liver disease such as biliary obstruction (masses, drug therapy), hyperthyroidism.

Decreased: Malnutrition, excess vitamin D ingestion.

Alpha-Fetoprotein (AFP)

(<16 ng/mL [SI: <16 μL]; third trimester of pregnancy, maximum 550 ng/ml [SI:550 μL]).

Increased: Hepatoma (hepatocellular carcinoma), testicular tumor (embryonal carcinoma, malignant teratoma, yolk sac tumor), neural tube defects (in mother's serum [spina bifida, anencephaly, myelomeningocele]), fetal death, multiple gestations, ataxia-telangiectasia, some cases of benign hepatic diseases (alcoholic cirrhosis, hepatitis).

Decreased: Trisomy 21 (Down's syndrome) in maternal serum.

ALT (Alanine Aminotransferase, ALAT) (see SGPT)

Ammonia

(adult: 10–80 μg/dL [SI:5–50 μmol/L]) (to convert μg/dL to μmol/L, multiply by 0.5872).

Increased: Liver failure, Reye's syndrome, portocaval shunt, medications (5-FU), TPN, inborn errors of metabolism, normal neonates (normalizes within 48 h of birth).

Amylase

(50–150 Somogyi units/dL [SI: 100–300 U/L])

Increased: Acute pancreatitis, pancreatic duct obstruction (stones, stricture, tumor, sphincter spasm secondary to drugs), pancreatic pseudocyst or abscess, alcohol ingestion, mumps, parotiditis, renal disease, macroamylasemia, cholecystitis, peptic ulcers, intestinal obstruction, mesenteric thrombosis, after surgery.

Decreased: Pancreatic destruction (pancreatitis, cystic fibrosis), liver damage (hepatitis, cirrhosis), normal newborns in the first year of life.

Anion Gap (See Blood Gases, page 284)

Apolipoprotein A & B

(APO-A: male, 80–151 mg/dL; female, 80–170 mg/dL; APO-B: male, 49–123 mg/dL; female, 26–119 mg/dL).

Used to assess risk of CAD. Ratio of Apo-A/Apo-B greater indicator of CAD than LDL/HDL cholesterol.

Autoantibodies

(Normal = negative)

Antinuclear Antibody (ANA, FANA): (Normal = negative)

A useful screening test in patients with symptoms suggesting collagen-vascular disease, especially if titer is ≥1:160.

Positive: Systemic lupus erythematosus (SLE), drug-induced lupus-like syndromes (procainamide, hydralazine, isoniazid, etc.), scleroderma, mixed connective tissue disease (MCTD), rheumatoid arthritis, polymyositis, juvenile rheumatoid arthritis (5% to 20%). Low titers are also seen in non-collagen-vascular disease.

Anti-DNA (Anti–double-stranded DNA): SLE, chronic active hepatitis, mononucleosis.

Antimitochondrial: Primary biliary cirrhosis, autoimmune diseases such as SLE.

Anti-Smooth Muscle: Low titers are seen in a variety of illnesses; high titers (> 1:100) are suggestive of chronic active hepatitis.

Antimicrosomal: Hashimoto's thyroiditis.

ASO (Antistreptolysin O) Titer (Streptozyme)

(<166 Todd units)

Increased: Streptococcal infections (pharyngitis, scarlet fever, rheumatic fever, poststreptococcal glomerulonephritis), rheumatoid arthritis, and other collagen diseases.

AST (Aspartate Aminotransferase, ASAT) (see SGOT)

Base Excess/Deficit

(–2–+3 mEq/L [SI: –2–+3 mmol/L) (see Blood gases, page 283).

Increased: Metabolic alkalosis.

Decreased: Metabolic acidosis.

Bicarbonate (or "Total CO_2")

(23–29 mmol/L) (See Carbon Dioxide, page 294)

Bilirubin

(Total, 0.3–1.0 mg/dL [SI: 5.1–17.1 μmol/L]; direct, < 0.2 mg/dL [SI: < 3.4 μmol/L]; indirect, < 0.8 mg/dL [SI: < 13.7 μmol/L]). To convert mg/dL to μmol/L, multiply by 17.10.

Increased Total: Hepatic damage (hepatitis, toxins [including many commonly used medications], cirrhosis), biliary obstruction (stone or tumor), hemolysis, congenital liver enzyme anomalies, fasting.

Increased Direct (Conjugated): (NOTE: determination of the direct bilirubin is usually unnecessary with total bilirubin levels of < 1.2 mg/dL [SI:20.5 μmol/L]; this is the form of bilirubin seen in urine). Biliary obstruction/cholestasis (gallstone, tumor, stricture), drug-induced cholestasis, Dubin-Johnson and Rotor's syndromes.

Increased Indirect (Unconjugated): (NOTE: This is calculated as total minus direct bilirubin) So-called hemolytic jaundice caused by any type of hemolytic anemia (transfusion reaction, sickle cell, etc.), Gilbert's disease, physiological jaundice of the newborn, Crigler-Najjar syndrome.

Bilirubin, Neonatal ("Baby Bilirubin")

(Normal levels dependent on prematurity and age in days; "panic levels" usually > 15–20 mg/dL (SI: >257–342 μmol/L in term infants).

Increased: Erythroblastosis fetalis, physiologic jaundice (may be due to breastfeeding), resorption of hematoma or hemorrhage, obstructive jaundice, others.

Bleeding Time

(Duke, Ivy < 6 min; Template < 10 min)
Tests only platelet function, not coagulation factors.

Increased: Thrombocytopenia (disseminated intravascular coagulation [DIC], thrombotic thrombocytopenic purpura [TTP], idiopathic thrombocytopenic purpura [ITP]), von Willebrand's disease, defective platelet function including aspirin therapy.

Blood Gases, Capillary

When interpreting a CBG, apply the following rules:

pH: Same as arterial blood gas or slightly lower (N = 7.35–7.40).

Pco_2: Same as arterial blood gas or slightly higher (N = 40–45).

Po_2: Lower than arterial blood gas (N = 45–60).

O_2 Saturation: > 70% is acceptable. Saturation is probably more useful than the Po_2 itself when interpreting a CBG.

Blood Gases, Arterial & Venous

There is little difference between arterial and venous pH and bicarbonate (except with congestive heart failure and shock); therefore, the venous blood gas may be occasionally used to assess acid-base status, but venous oxygen levels (Po_2) are significantly less than arterial levels (See Table II–1, page 284).)

TABLE II–1. NORMAL BLOOD GAS VALUES.

Measurement	Arterial Blood	Mixed Venous[1]	Venous
ph (range)	7.40 (7.36–7.44)	7.36 (7.31–7.41)	7.36 (7.31–7.41)
Po_2 (decreases with age)	80–100 mm Hg	35–40 mm Hg	30–50 mm Hg
Pco_2	35–45 mm Hg	41–51 mm Hg	40–52 mm Hg
O_2 saturation (%) (decreases with age)	>95%	60–80%	60–85%
$\{HCO_3^-\}$	22–26 mEq/L (mmol/L)	22–26 mEq/L (mmol/L)	22–28 mEq/L (mmol/L)
Base deficit (deficit excess)	–2– +3	–2– +3	–2–+3

[1]Obtained from right atrium, usually through a pulmonary artery catheter.

See individual component for differential diagnosis. For acid-base disorders, see the section below and On Call Problems "Acidosis" (Problem 3, page 15) and Alkalosis (Problem 4, page 20).

Metabolic Acidosis: A fall in plasma HCO_3 followed by a compensatory fall in Pco_2. Use the Anion Gap to help establish the diagnosis.(Table II–2)

Anion Gap = (Na – (Cl + HCO_3)

Normal Gap = 8 – 12 mEq/L

Differential Diagnosis: (See also On Call Problem 3 "Acidosis").

Anion gap acidosis ("normochloremic acidosis": gap >12 mEq/L; caused by a decrease in bicarbonate balanced by an increase in unmeasured acids. Lactic acidosis, ketoacidosis (diabetic, alcoholic, starvation), uremia, intoxication (salicylate, methanol, paraldehyde, ethylene glycol), hyperalimentation.

Non-anion gap acidosis ("hyperchloremic acidosis": Gap between 8–12 mEq/liter; caused by a decrease in Hco_3 balanced by an increase in chloride. Renal bicarbonate losses (renal tubular acidosis, spironolactone, carbonic anhydrase inhibitors), GI tract bicarbonate losses (diarrhea, pancreatic fistulas, biliary tract fistulas, ileal loop, ureterosigmoidostomy.

Low Anion Gap: Gap < 8: Not seen with acidosis, but can be seen with bromide ingestion, hyponatremia and multiple myeloma.

Metabolic Alkalosis: A rise in plasma Hco_3 followed by a compensatory rise in the Pco_2. Spot urine for chloride helps establish the diagnosis (Table II–2) (next page).

TABLE II–2. SIMPLE ACID-BASE DISTURBANCES.

Acid-Base Disorder	Primary Abnormality	Secondary Abnormality	Expected Degree of Compensatory Response
Metabolic acidosis	$\downarrow\downarrow\downarrow[HCO_3^-]$	$\downarrow\downarrow Pco_2$	$Pco_2 = (1.5 \times [HCO_3^-]) + 8$
Metabolic alkalosis	$\uparrow\uparrow\uparrow[HCO_3^-]$	$\uparrow\uparrow Pco_2$	$\uparrow$ in $Pco_2 = \Delta\ HCO_3^- \times 0.6$
Acute respiratory acidosis	$\uparrow\uparrow\uparrow Pco_2$	$\uparrow[HCO_3^-]$	$\uparrow$ in $HCO_3^- = \Delta\ Pco_2/10$
Chronic respiratory acidosis	$\uparrow\uparrow\uparrow Pco_2$	$\uparrow\uparrow[HCO_3^-]$	$\uparrow$ in $HCO_3^- = 4 \times \Delta\ Pco_2/10$
Acute respiratory alkalosis	$\downarrow\downarrow\downarrow Pco_2$	$\downarrow[HCO_3^-]$	$\downarrow$ in $HCO_3^- = 2 \times \Delta\ Pco_2/10$
Chronic respiratory alkalosis	$\downarrow\downarrow\downarrow Pco_2$	$\downarrow\downarrow[HCO_3^-]$	$\downarrow$ in $HCO_3^- = 5 \times \Delta\ Pco_2/10$

Differential Diagnosis: (See also "Alkalosis" page 20)

Urine Chloride < 10 mEq/L ("chloride responsive"): Diuretics, GI tract losses (NG suction, vomiting, diarrhea [villous adenoma, congenital chloride wasting diarrhea in children]), iatrogenic (inadequate chloride intake).

Urine Chloride > 10 mEq/L ("chloride resistant"): Adrenal diseases (Cushing's syndrome, hyperaldosteronism), exogenous steroid use, Bartter's syndrome, licorice ingestion.

Respiratory Acidosis: A primary rise in Pco_2 with a compensatory rise in plasma Hco_3 not higher than 30 meq/L if acute. (Table II–2)

Differential Diagnosis: (See also "Acidosis" page 15)

Acute: CNS depression (oversedation, narcotics, anesthetic), CNS trauma (CVA, head injury, spinal cord trauma), neuromuscular diseases (myasthenia gravis, Guillain-Barré disease), airway obstruction, laryngospasm, iatrogenic mechanical underventilation, pulmonary lesions (acute pulmonary edema, severe pneumonia), chest trauma (hemothorax, pneumothorax, flail chest).

Chronic: Chronic asthma, emphysema or bronchitis, Pickwickian syndrome

Respiratory Alkalosis: A primary fall in Pco_2. (Table II–2)

Differential Diagnosis: (See also "Alkalosis" page 20)

Central nervous system causes: Anxiety, hyperventilation syndrome, pain, head trauma, CVA, encephalitis, CHS tumors, salicylates (early toxicity), fever, early sepsis

Peripheral stimulation: Pulmonary embolus, CHF, Interstitial lung disease, pneumonia, altitude, hypoxemia of any cause
Miscellaneous: Delirium tremens, cirrhosis, thyrotoxicosis, pregnancy, pregnancy, iatrogenic overventilation

Blood Urea Nitrogen (BUN)

(Birth–1 year: 4–16 mg/dL [SI: 1.4–5.7 mmol/L]; 1–40 years 5–20 mg/dL [SI: 1.8–7.1 mmol/L]; gradual slight increase with increasing age). To convert mg/dL to mmol/L, multiply by 0.3570.

Increased: Renal failure, prerenal azotemia (decreased renal perfusion secondary to congestive heart failure [CHF], shock, volume depletion), postrenal (obstruction), gastrointestinal (GI) bleeding, stress, drugs (especially aminoglycosides).

Decreased: Starvation, liver failure (hepatitis, drugs), pregnancy, infancy, nephrotic syndrome, overhydration.

BUN/Creatinine Ratio (BUN/Cr)

(mean 10, range 6–20)

Increased: Prerenal azotemia (renal hypoperfusion), GI bleeding, high protein diet, ileal conduit, drugs (steroids, tetracycline).

Decreased: Malnutrition, pregnancy, low protein diet, ketoacidosis, hemodialysis, SIADH, drugs (cimetidine).

CBC Differential Diagnosis (See also Tables II–3 and II–4, pages 287–288, for normal ranges).

Basophils: (0–1%)

Increased: Chronic myeloid leukemia, rarely in recovery from infection and from hypothyroidism.

Decreased: Acute rheumatic fever, lobar pneumonia, after steroid therapy, thyrotoxicosis, stress.

Eosinophils: (1–3%)

Increased: Allergy, parasites, skin diseases, malignancy, drugs, asthma, Addison's disease, collagen-vascular diseases (handy mnemonic NAACP: Neoplasm, Allergy, Addison's disease, Collagen-vascular diseases, Parasites), pulmonary diseases including Löffler's syndrome and PIE (pulmonary infiltrates with eosinophilia).

TABLE II–3. NORMAL COMPLETE BLOOD COUNT FOR SELECTED AGE RANGES.

Age	WBC Count (cells/cu mm) [SI: 10^9/L]	RBC Count 10^6/µL [SI: 10^{12}/L]	Hemoglobin (gm/dL) [SI: g/L]	Hematocrit (%)	MHC (pg) [SI: pg]	MCHC (g/dL) [SI: g/L][1]	MCV (cu µm) [SI: fl]	RDW
Adult male	4500–11,000	4.73–5.49	14.40–16.60	42.9–49.1	27–31	33–37	76–100	11.5–14.5
	[4.5–11.0]	[4.73–5.49]	[144–166]					
Adult female	As above	4.15–4.87	12.2–14.7	37.9–43.9	As above	As above	As above	As above
		[4.15–5.49]	[122–147]					
11–15 years	4500–13,500	4.8	13.4	39	28	34	82	—
6–10 years	5000–14,500	4.7	12.9	37.5	27	34	80	—
4–6 years	5500–15,500	4.6	12.6	37.0	27	34	80	—
2–4 years	6000–17,000	4.5	12.5	35.5	25	32	77	—
4 months–2 years	6000–17,500	4.6	11.2	35.0	25	33	77	—
1 week–4 mo	5500–18,000	4.7 ± 0.9	14.0 ± 3.3	42.0 ± 7.0	30	33	90	—
24 hr–1 week	5000–21,000	5.1	18.3 ± 4.0	52.5	36	35	103	—
First day	9400–34,000	5.1 ± 1.0	19.5 ± 5.0	54.0 ± 10.0	38	36	106	—

[1]To convert from standard reference value to SI units, multiply by 10.

TABLE II–4. NORMAL PLATELET AND WHITE BLOOD CELL DIFFERENTIAL FOR SELECTED AGES

Age	Platelet Count (103μL) [SI: 10^9/L]	Lymphocytes Total (% WBC Count)	Neutrophils, Band (% WBC Count)	Neutrophils, Segmented (% WBC Count)	Eosinophils (% WBC Count)	Basophils (% WBC Count)	Monocytes (% WBC Count)
Adult male	238 ± 49	34%	3.0%	56%	2.7%	0.5%	4.0%
Adult female	270 ± 58	As above	As above	As above	As above	As above	As above
11–15 years	282 ± 63	38%	3.0%	51%	2.4%	0.5%	4.3%
6–10 years	351 ± 85	39%	3.0%	50%	2.4%	0.6%	4.2%
4–6 years	357 ± 70	42%	3.0%	39%	2.8%	0.6%	5.0%
2–4 years	357 ± 70	59%	3.0%	30%	2.6%	0.5%	5.0%
4 months–2 years	As above	61%	3.1%	28%	2.6%	0.4%	4.8%
1 week–4 mo	As above	56%	4.5%	30%	2.8%	0.5%	6.5%
24 hr–1 week	240–380	24–41%	6.8–9.2%	39–52%	2.4–4.1%	0.5%	5.8–9.1%
First day	As above	24%	10.2%	58%	2.0%	0.6%	5.8%

Decreased: After steroids, adrenocorticotropic hormone (ACTH), after stress (infection, trauma, burns), Cushing's syndrome.

Hematocrit: (male 40–54%; female 37–47%).

Decreased: Megaloblastic anemia (folate or B_{12} deficiency), iron deficiency anemia, sickle cell anemia, etc.), acute or chronic blood loss, hemolysis, dilutional, alcohol, drugs.

Increased: Primary polycythemia (polycythemia vera), secondary polycythemia (reduced fluid intake or excess fluid loss, congenital and acquired heart disease, lung disease, high altitudes, heavy smokers, tumors [renal cell carcinoma, hepatoma], renal cysts).

Hemoglobin: (see Table II–3, page 287 for normal values). See Problem 6 "Anemia".

Increased: Polycythemia vera, secondary polycythemia, high altitude, vigorous exercise.

Decreased: see Hematocrit

Lymphocytes: (24–44%)

Increased: Virtually any viral infection (AIDS, measles, German measles, mumps, whooping cough, smallpox, chickenpox, influenza, hepatitis, infectious mononucleosis), acute infectious lymphocytosis in children, acute and chronic lymphocytic leukemias.

Decreased: (Normal finding in 22% of population), stress, burns, trauma, uremia, some viral infections, AIDS, AIDS-related complex, bone marrow suppression after chemotherapy, steroids.

Lymphocytes, Atypical

>20%: Infectious mononucleosis, cytomegalovirus (CMV) infection, infectious hepatitis, toxoplasmosis.

<20%: Viral infections (mumps, rubeola, varicella), rickettsial infections, TB.

MCH (Mean Cellular (Corpuscular) Hemoglobin): (27–31 pg [SI: 27–31 pg])

The weight of hemoglobin of the average red cell. Calculated by

$$MCH = \frac{\text{Hemoglobin (g/L)}}{\text{RBC } (10^6/\mu L)}$$

Increased: Macrocytosis (megaloblastic anemias, high reticulocyte counts).

Decreased: Microcytosis (iron deficiency, sideroblastic anemia, thalassemia).

MCHC (Mean Cellular [Corpuscular] Hemoglobin Concentration): (33–37 g/dL [SI:330–370 g/L]).

The average concentration of hemoglobin in a given volume of red cells. Calculated by the following formula:

$$\text{MCHC} = \frac{\text{Hemoglobin (g / dL)}}{\text{Hematocrit}}$$

Increased: Very severe, prolonged dehydration; spherocytosis.

Decreased: Iron deficiency anemia, overhydration, thalassemia, sideroblastic anemia.

MCV (Mean Cell [Corpuscular] Volume): (76–100 μm^3 [SI: 76-100 fL]). The average volume of red blood cells. Calculated by the following formula:

$$\text{MCHC} = \frac{\text{Hematocrit} \times 1000}{\text{RBC } (10^6 / \mu L)}$$

Increased: Megaloblastic anemia (B_{12}, folate deficiency), macrocytic (normoblastic) anemia, reticulocytosis, Down's syndrome, chronic liver disease.

Decreased: Iron deficiency, thalassemia, some cases of lead poisoning.

Monocytes: (3–7%)

Increased: Bacterial infection (TB, subacute bacterial endocarditis [SBE], brucellosis, typhoid, recovery from an acute infection), protozoal infections, infectious mononucleosis, leukemia, Hodgkin's disease, ulcerative colitis, regional enteritis.

Platelets: (150–450,000 μL)

Platelet counts may be normal in number, but abnormal in function as occurs in aspirin therapy. Abnormalities of platelet function are assessed by bleeding time.

Increased: Sudden exercise, after trauma, bone fracture, after asphyxia, after surgery (especially splenectomy), acute hemorrhage, polycythemia vera, primary thrombocythemia, leukemias, after childbirth, carcinoma, myeloproliferative disorders.

Decreased: Disseminated intravascular coagulation (DIC), idiopathic thrombocytopenic purpura (ITP), thrombotic thrombocytopenic purpura, congenital disease, marrow suppressants (chemotherapy, thiazide diuretics, alcohol, estrogens, x-rays), burns, snake and insect bites, leukemias, aplastic anemias, hypersplenism, infectious mononucleosis, viral infections, cirrhosis, massive transfusions, eclampsia and pre-eclampsia, more than 30 different drugs.

PMNs (Polymorphonuclear Neutrophils): (40–76%)

Increased:

- Physiologic (normal): Severe exercise, last months of pregnancy, labor, surgery, newborns, steroid therapy.
- Pathologic: Bacterial infections, noninfective tissue damage (myocardial infarction, pulmonary infarction, crush injury, burn injury), metabolic disorders (eclampsia, diabetic ketoacidosis, uremia, acute gout).

Decreased: Pancytopenia, aplastic anemia, PMN depression (a mild decrease is referred to as neutropenia, severe is called agranulocytosis), marrow damage (radiographs, poisoning with benzene or antitumor drugs), severe overwhelming infections (disseminated TB, septicemia), acute malaria, severe osteomyelitis, infectious mononucleosis, atypical pneumonias, some viral infections, marrow obliteration (osteosclerosis, myelofibrosis, malignant infiltrate), drugs (more than 70, including chloramphenicol, phenylbutazone, chlorpromazine, quinine), B_{12} and folate deficiencies, hypoadrenalism, hypopituitarism, dialysis, familial decrease, idiopathic causes.

RDW (Red Cell Distribution Width): (11.5–14.5).
A measure of the degree of anisocytosis (variation in RBC size) and measured by the automated hematology counters (eg, Coulter Counter).

Increased: Many anemias (concomitant macrocytic and microcytic anemia).

White Blood Cell Count: (see Table II–3 and II–4, pages 287–288)

Increased: Infections (especially bacterial), leukemia, leukemoid reactions, tissue necrosis, postsplenectomy, exercise, fever, pain, anesthesia, labor.

Decreased: Sepsis, overwhelming bacterial infections, certain nonbacterial infections (influenza, hepatitis, mononucleosis), aplastic anemia, pernicious anemia, hypersplenism, cachexia, chemotherapeutic agents, ionizing radiation.

C-PEPTIDE

(Fasting, < 4.0 ng/mL [SI: < 4.0 μg/L]; male > 60 years, 1.5–5.0 ng/mL [SI: 1.5–5.0 [μg/L]; female 1.4–5.5 ng/mL [SI: 1.4–5.5 μg/L]).

Differentiates between exogenous and endogenous insulin production/administration.

Increased: Insulinoma, pancreas transplant, oral hypoglycemic agents (sulfonylureas).

Decreased: Diabetes (decreased endogenous insulin), insulin administration (factitious or therapeutic), hypoglycemia.

Captopril Test

Used in the evaluation of renovascular hypotension, captopril is an angiotensin converting enzyme (ACE) inhibitor that blocks angiotensin II. Captopril is administered (25 mg IV at 8 AM). Aldosterone decreases 2 h later from baseline in normal or essential hypertension, but it is not suppressed in patients with aldosterpnism. For renovascular hypertension, the plasma renin activity (PRA) increases > 12 ng/mL/h. An absolute increase of 10 ng/mL/h plus a 400% increase in PRA is noted when the pretest level is < 3 ng/mL/h, and the PRA is more than 150% over baseline when the pretest PRA is > 3 ng/mL/h. The test is now also combined with a nuclear renal scan to identify renal artery stenosis.

CA 15–3

Used to detect breast cancer recurrence in asymptomatic patients and monitor therapy. Levels related to stage of disease.

Increased: Progressive breast cancer, benign breast disease and liver disease.

Decreased: Response to therapy (25% change considered significant).

CA 19–9 (< 37 U/mL [SI: < 37 kU/L]).

Primarily used to determine resectability of pancreatic cancers (ie, >1000U/mL, 95% unresectable).

Increased: Gastrointestinal cancers such as pancreas, stomach, liver, colorectal, hepatobiliary, some cases of lung and prostate, pancreatitis.

CA 125 (<35 U/mL [SI: <35 kU/L])

Not a useful screening test for ovarian cancer when used alone; used in conjunction with ultrasound and physical exam for detection. Rising levels after resection predictive for recurrence.

Increased: Ovarian (serous), cervical adenocarcinoma, endometrial and colon cancer, endometriosis, inflammatory bowel disease, pelvic inflammatory disease, pregnancy, breast lesions and benign abdominal masses (teratomas).

Calcitonin (Thyrocalcitonin)

(<19 pg/mL [SI: <19 ng/L]).

Increased: Medullary carcinoma of the thyroid, C-cell hyperplasia (precursor of medullary carcinoma), oat cell carcinoma of the lung, newborns, pregnancy, chronic renal insufficiency, Zollinger-Ellison syndrome, pernicious anemia.

Calcium, Serum

(infants to 1 month: 7–11.5 mg/dL [SI: 1.75–2.87 mmol/L]; 1 month to 1 year: 8.6–11.2 mg/dl [SI: 2.15–2.79 mmol/L]; > 1 year and adults: 8.2–10.2 mg/dL [SI: 2.05–2.54 mmol/L]; ionized: 4.75–5.2 mg/dL [SI: 1.19–1.30 mmol/L]). To convert mg/dL to mmol/L, multiply by 0.2495).

When interpreting a total calcium value, the total protein and albumin must be known. If these are not within normal limits, a corrected calcium can be roughly calculated by the following formula:

Corrected total Ca = 0.8 (Normal albumin − measured albumin) + reported Ca

Values for ionized calcium need no special corrections.

Increased: (NOTE: levels > 12 mg/dL [2.99 mmol/L] may lead to coma and death). Primary hyperthyroidism, parathyroid hormone (PTH) secreting tumors, vitamin D excess, metastatic bone tumors, osteoporosis, immobilization, milk-alkali syndrome, Paget's disease, idiopathic hypercalcemia of infants, infantile hypophosphatasia, thiazide drugs, chronic renal failure, sarcoidosis, multiple myeloma.

Decreased: (NOTE: levels < 7 mg/dL [< 1.75 mmol/L] may lead to tetany and death). Hypoparathyroidism (surgical, idiopathic), pseudohypoparathyroidism, insufficient vitamin D, calcium and phosphorus ingestion (pregnancy, osteomalacia, rickets), hypomagnesemia, renal tubular acidosis, hypoalbuminemia (cachexia, nephrotic syndrome, cystic fibrosis), chronic renal failure (phosphate retention), acute pancreatitis, factitious decrease because of low protein and albumin.

Calcium, Urine (24-Hour Urine)

On a calcium-free diet (< 150 mg/d [3.7 mmol/d]); average calcium diet (600–800 mg/d) 100–250 mg/24 hr [2.5–6.2 mmol/d].

Increased: Hyperparathyroidism, hyperthyroidism, hypervitaminosis D, distal renal tubular acidosis (type I), sarcoidosis, immobilization, osteolytic lesions (bony metastasis, multiple myeloma), Paget's disease, glucocorticoid excess.

Decreased: Thiazide diuretics, hypothyroidism, renal failure, steatorrhea, rickets, osteomalacia.

Carbon Dioxide ("Total CO_2" or Bicarbonate)

(adult 23–29 mmol/liter, child 20–28 mmol/liter) (See also Pco_2 values).

Increased: Compensation for respiratory acidosis, metabolic alkalosis, emphysema, severe vomiting, primary aldosteronism, volume contraction, Bartter's syndrome.

Decreased: Compensation for respiratory alkalosis, metabolic acidosis, starvation, diabetic ketoacidosis, lactic acidosis, alcoholic ketoacidosis, toxins (methanol, ethylene glycol, paraldehyde), severe diarrhea, renal failure, drugs (salicylates, acetazolamide), dehydration, adrenal insufficiency.

Carbon Dioxide, Arterial (Pco_2)

(see Table II–1 page 284).

Increased: Respiratory acidosis, compensatory increase in metabolic alkalosis.

Decreased: Respiratory alkalosis, compensatory in metabolic alkalosis.

Carboxyhemoglobin (Carbon Monoxide)

(nonsmoker < 2%; smoker < 9%; toxic > 15%).

Increased: Smokers, smoke inhalation, automobile exhaust inhalation, normal newborns.

Carcinoembryonic Antigen (CEA)

(nonsmoker < 3.0 ng/mL [SI: < 3.0 μg/L], smoker < 5.0 ng/mL [SI: < 5.0 μg).

Not a screening test; useful for monitoring response to treatment and tumor recurrence of adenocarcinomas of the gastrointestinal tract.

Increased: Carcinoma (colon, pancreas, lung, stomach), smokers, nonneoplastic liver disease, Crohn's disease, ulcerative colitis.

Catecholamines, Fractionated, Serum

(Values are variable and depend on the lab and method of assay used. Normal levels below are based on an HPLC technique.)

Catecholamine	Plasma (supine) levels
Norepinephrine	70–750 pg/mL [SI: 414–4435 pmol/L]
Epinephrine	0–100 pg/mL [SI: 0–546 pmol/L]
Dopamine	< 30 pg/mL [SI: 196 pmol/L]

Increased: Pheochromocytoma, neural crest tumors (neuroblastoma), with extra-adrenal pheochromocytoma; norepinephrine may be markedly elevated compared with epinephrine.

Catecholamines, Fractionated (24-h Urine)

(Values are variable and dependent on the assay method used). Norepinephrine: 15–80 μg/d [SI: 89–473 nmol/d]; epinephrine: 0–20 μg/d [0–118 nmol/d]; dopamine: 65–400 μg/d [SI: 384–2364 nmol/d].

Used to evaluate neuroendocrine tumors including pheochromocytoma and neuroblastoma. Avoid caffeine, and methyldopa (Aldomet) prior to test.

Increased: Pheochromocytoma, neuroblastoma, epinephrine administration, drugs (methyldopa, tetracyclines are false increases).

Chloride, Serum

(97–107 mEq/L [SI: 97–107 mmol/L]).

Increased: Diarrhea, renal failure, nephrotic syndrome, renal tubular acidosis, mineralocorticoid deficiency, hyperalimentation, medications (acetazolamide, ammonium chloride, hydrochlorothiazide).

Decreased: Vomiting (includes NG suction), diarrhea, diabetes mellitus with ketoacidosis, mineralocorticoid excess, (SIADH), excessive diuretic use, chronic respiratory acidosis, renal disease with sodium loss.

Cholesterol (Total)

(normal, see Table II–5 below); to convert mg/dL to mmol/L, multiply by 0.02586. Fasting specimen recommended because triglyceride levels may be affected.

Increased: Idiopathic hypercholesterolemia, secondary hyperlipoproteinemias (nephrotic syndrome, biliary cirrhosis, nephrosis, hypothyroidism), pancreatic disease (diabetes), pregnancy, oral contraceptives, steroid administration, hyperlipoproteinemia (types IIb, III, V).

Decreased: Liver disease (hepatitis, malignancy, etc.), hyperthyroidism, malnutrition (cancer, starvation), chronic anemias, burns, lipoproteinemias.

High Density Lipoprotein-Cholesterol (HDL, HDL-C)

(fasting: 30–70 mg/dL [SI: 0.8–1.80 mmol/L]; female 30–90 mg/dL [SI: 0.80–2.35 mmol/L]).

HDL-C has the best correlation with the development of coronary artery disease; decreased HDL-C in males leads to an increased risk. Levels < 45 mg/dl are associated with increased risk of coronary artery disease.

Increased: Estrogen (females), exercise, ethanol.

Decreased: Males, uremia, obesity, diabetes, liver disease, Tangier's disease.

Low Density Lipoprotein-Cholesterol (LDL, LDL-C)

(50–190 mg/dL [SI: 1.30–4.90 mmol/L]).

TABLE II–5. NORMAL TOTAL CHOLESTEROL LEVELS BY AGE.

Age	Standard Units	SI Units
Infant	<65–175 mg/dL	<1.68–4.52 mmol/L
1–19	<120–220 mg/dL	<3.10–5.68 mmol/L
20–29	<200 mg/dL	<5.20 mmol/L
30–39	<225 mg/dL	<5.85 mmol/L
40–49	<245 mg/dL	<6.35 mmol/L
>50	<265 mg/dL	<6.85 mmol/L

Increased: Excess dietary saturated fats, myocardial infarction (MI), hyperlipoproteinemia, biliary cirrhosis, endocrine disease (diabetes, hypothyroidism).

Decreased: Malabsorption, severe liver disease, abetalipoproteinemia, nicotinic acid.

Clostridium Difficile Toxin Assay

Fecal (normal = negative)

Majority of patients with pseudomembranous colitis have positive *C difficile* assay; use endoscopy to confirm plaques. Often positive in antibiotic-associated diarrhea and colitis. Can be seen in some normals and neonates.

Clotting Time, Activated (ACT)

(5–15 minutes).

Most often used in the OR or dialysis unit to monitor acute anticoagulation status.

Increased: Heparin therapy, plasma-clotting factor deficiency (except Factors VII and XIII). (NOTE: This is not a sensitive test, therefore it is not considered a good screening test.)

Cold Agglutinins

(< 1:32)

Increased: Atypical pneumonia (mycoplasmal pneumonia), other viral infections (especially mononucleosis, measles, mumps), cirrhosis, parasitic infections.

Complement C3

(85–155 mg/dL, [SI: 800–1500 ng/L]).

Increased: Rheumatoid arthritis (variable finding), rheumatic fever, various neoplasms (gastrointestinal, prostate, others).

Decreased: Erythematosus, glomerulonephritis (poststreptococcal and membranoproliferative), sepsis, subacute bacterial endocarditis (SBE), chronic active hepatitis.

Complement C4

(20–50 mg/dL [SI: 200–500 ng/L]).

Increased: Rheumatoid arthritis (variable finding), neoplasia (gastrointestinal, lung, others).

Decreased: SLE, chronic active hepatitis, cirrhosis, glomerulonephritis, hereditary angioedema.

Complement CH50 (Total)

(33–61 mg/ml [SI: 330–610 ng/L]).
Tests for complement deficiency in the classic pathway.

Increased: Acute phase reactants (tissue injury, infections, etc.).

Decreased: Hereditary complement deficiencies.

Coombs' Test, Direct (Direct Antiglobulin Test)

(Normal = negative).
Uses patient's erythrocytes; tests for the presence of antibody on the patient's cells.

Positive: Autoimmune hemolytic anemia (leukemia, lymphoma, collagen-vascular diseases), hemolytic transfusion reaction, some drug sensitizations (methyldopa, levodopa, cephalothin), hemolytic disease of the newborn (erythroblastosis fetalis).

Coombs' Test, Indirect (Antibody Screening Test)

(Normal = negative).
Uses serum that contains antibody, usually from the patient.

Positive: Isoimmunization from previous transfusion, incompatible blood because of improper cross-matching.

Cortisol, Serum

(8 AM, 5.0–23.0 μg/dL [SI: 138–365 nmol/L]; 4 pm, 3.0–15.0 μg/dL [SI: 83–414 nmol/L]).
Most useful when used with ACTH stimulation test (page 278) or dexamethasone suppression test (page 301).

Increased: Adrenal adenoma, adrenal carcinoma, Cushing's disease, nonpituitary adrenocorticotropic hormone (ACTH)-producing tumor, steroid therapy, oral contraceptives.

Decreased: Primary adrenal insufficiency (Addison's disease), congenital adrenal hyperplasia, Waterhouse-Friderichsen syndrome, ACTH deficiency.

Cortisol, Free (24-h Urine)

(30–100 μg/d.)
Used to evaluate adrenal cortical function, screening test of choice for Cushing's Syndrome.

Increased: Cushing's syndrome (adrenal hyperfunction), stress during collection, oral contraceptives, pregnancy.

Counterimmunoelectrophoresis (CIEP, CEP)

(Normal = negative).

An immunologic technique that allows rapid identification of infecting organisms from fluids including serum, urine, cerebrospinal fluid (CSF), and other body fluids. Organisms identified include *Neisseria meningitidis, Streptococcus pneumoniae, Haemophilus influenzae,* and group B *Streptococcus.*

Creatine Phosphokinase (CPK)

(25–145 mU/mL [SI: 25–145 U/L]).

Increased: Muscle damage (acute myocardial infarction, myocarditis, muscular dystrophy, muscle trauma [injection], after surgery), brain infarction, defibrillation, cardiac catheterization and surgery, rhabdomyolysis, polymyositis, hypothyroidism.

CPK Isoenzymes

MB: (normal < 6%, heart origin), increased in acute myocardial infarction (begins in 2–12 h, peaks at 12–40 h, returns to normal in 24–72 h), pericarditis with myocarditis, rhabdomyolysis, crush injury, Duchenne's muscular dystrophy, polymyositis, malignancy hyperthermia, and cardiac surgery.

MM: (normal 94–100%, skeletal muscle origin) increased in crush injury, malignant hyperthermia, seizures, IM injections.

BB: (normal 0%, brain origin) brain injury (cerebrovascular accident [CVA], trauma), metastatic neoplasms (prostate), malignant hyperthermia, colonic infarction.

Creatinine, Serum

(adult male: < 1.2 mg/dL [SI: 106 μmol/L], adult female: < 1.1 mg/dL [SI: 97 μmol/L], child: 0.5–0.8 mg/dL [SI: 44–71 μmol/L]).To convert mg/dL to μmol/L, multiply by 88.40.

Increased: Renal failure (prerenal, renal, or postrenal obstruction), gigantism, acromegaly, ingestion of roasted meat, aminoglycosides and other drugs (cimetidine, some cephalosporins, ascorbic acid, others), false positive with DKA.

Decreased: Pregnancy, decreased muscle mass, severe liver disease.

Creatinine (Urine) & Creatinine Clearance

(Adult Male: total creatinine, 1–2 g/d [8.8–17.7 mmol/d]; clearance, 85–125 mL/min per 1.73 m^2; adult female: total creatinine, 0.8–1.8g/d [7.1–15.9 mmol/d]; clearance, 75–115 mL/min per 1.73 m^2 [1.25–1.92 mL/s per 1.73 m^2]); child: total creatinine, (> 3 years) 12–30 mg/kg/d; clearance 70–140 mL/min per 1.73 m^2 [1.17–2.33 mL/s per 1.73 m^2]).

Decreased: A decreased creatinine clearance results in an increase in serum creatinine usually secondary to renal insufficiency.

Increased: Early diabetes mellitus, pregnancy.

Calculation of Creatinine Clearance: Order a concurrent serum creatinine and a 24-h urine creatinine. A shorter time interval can be used; for example, 12 h, but remember that the formula must be corrected for this change and that a 24-h sample is less prone to collection error.

Example: (A quick formula is also found on page 455 under "Aminoglycoside Dosing.").

Calculation of the creatinine clearance from a 24-h urine sample with a volume of 1000 mL, a urine creatinine of 108 mg/100 mL, and a serum creatinine of 1 mg/100 mL (1 mg/dL):

$$\text{Clearance} = \frac{\text{Urine creatinine} \times \text{total urine volume}}{\text{Plasma creatinine} \times \text{time (1440 min if 24-h collection)}}$$

$$\text{Clearance} = \frac{(108\ \text{mg}/100\ \text{mL})\ (1000\text{mL})}{(1\text{mg}/100\ \text{mL})\ (1440\ \text{min})} = 75\ \text{mL}/\text{min}$$

Some clinicians advocate a preliminary determination to see if the urine sample is valid by determining first if the sample contains at least 18–25 mg/kg/24 h of creatinine for adult males or 12–20 mg/kg/24 h for adult females. This preliminary test is not a requirement, but can help with the determination if a 24-h sample was collected or if some of the sample was lost.

If the patient is an adult (150 lb = body surface area of 1.73 m^2), adjustment of the clearance for body size is not routinely done. Adjustment for pediatric patients is a necessity. If the values in the previous example were for a 10-year-old boy who weighed 70 lb (1.1 m^2; see page 000 for the conversion formula), then the clearance would be

$$\frac{75\text{mL}/\text{min} \times 1.73\ \text{m}^2}{1.1\ \text{m}^2} = 118\ \text{mL}/\text{min}$$

Dehydroepiandrosterone (DHEA)

(male: 2.0–3.4 ng/mL [SI: 5.2–8.7 μmol/L]; female, premenopausal: 0.8–3.4 ng/mL [SI: 2.1–8.8 μmol/L]; postmenopausal: 0.1–0.6 ng/mL [SI: 0.3–1.6 μmol/L]).

Increased: Anovulation, polycystic ovaries, adrenal hyperplasia, adrenal tumors.

Decreased: Menopause

Dehydroepiandrosterone Sulfate (DHEA-S)

(male: 1.7–4.2 ng/mL [SI: 6–15 μmol/L]; female: 2.0–5.2 ng/mL [SI: 7–18 μmol/L]).

Increased: Hyperprolactinemia, adrenal hyperplasia, adrenal tumor, polycystic ovaries, lipoid ovarian tumors.

Decreased: Menopause.

Dexamethasone Suppression Test

Used in the differential diagnosis of Cushing's syndrome(elevated cortisol).

Overnight "Rapid" Test: 1 mg of dexamethasone at 11 PM is given PO, and a fasting 8 AM plasma cortisol is obtained. Normally the cortisol level should be < 5.0 μg/dL [138 nmol/L]. If the value is > 5 μg/dL [138 nmol/L], this usually confirms the diagnosis of Cushing's syndrome; however obesity, alcoholism, or depression may occasionally show the same result. In these patients, the best screening test is a 24-h urine for free cortisol.

Low Dose Test: Can be performed if needed after collection of baseline serum cortisol and 24-h urine free cortisol levels, dexamethasone 0.5 mg PO is administered every 6 h for 8 doses. Serum and urine cortisol are repeated on the second day. Failure to suppress to a serum cortisol of < 5.0 μg/dL [138 nmol/L] and a urine free cortisol of < 30 μg/dL (82 nmol/L) confirms Cushing's syndrome.

High Dose Test: Can be performed if needed after the low-dose test, dexamethasone, 2 mg PO every 6 h for 8 doses will cause a fall in urinary free cortisol to 50% of the baseline value in patients with bilateral adrenal hyperplasia (Cushing's disease), but not in patients with adrenal tumors or ectopic adrenocorticotropic hormone (ACTH) production.

Erythropoetin (EPO)

5–36 mU/L (5–36 IU/L).

Increased: Pregnancy, secondary polycythemia (high altitude, COPD, etc), tumors (renal cell carcinoma, cerebellar hemangioblastoma, hepatoma, others), PCKD, anemias with bone marrow unresponsiveness (aplastic anemia, iron deficiency, etc).

Decreased: Bilateral nephrectomy, anemia of chronic disease (ie, renal failure, nephrotic syndrome), primary polycythemia (Note: the determination of EPO levels before administration of recombinant EPO for renal failure is not usually necessary).

Erythrocyte Sedimentation Rate, (ESR)

(See Sedimentation Rate, page 322)

Estradiol,Serum

Serial measurements useful to assess fetal well being, especially in high risk pregnancy.

Phase	Normal Values(Female)
Follicular Phase	25–75 pg/mL
Midcycle Peak	200–600 pg/mL
Leuteal Phase	100–300 pg/mL
Pregnancy 1st trimester	1–5 ng/mL
2nd trimester	5–15 ng/mL
3rd trimester	10–40 ng/mL
Postmenopause	5–25 pg/mL

Estrogen & Progesterone Receptor Assays

(<3–5 fmol/mg negative, >10 fmol/mg positive, >100 fmol/mg highly positive).

Determined on fresh surgical specimens but also can be determined on fixed specimens. The presence of the receptors is associated with a longer disease-free interval and survival from breast cancer and is more likely to respond to endocrine therapy.

Fecal Fat

(2–6 g/d on a 80–100 g/d fat diet; 72-h collection time).

Increased: Cystic fibrosis, pancreatic insufficiency, Crohn's disease, chronic pancreatitis, sprue, diarrhea states with or without fat malabsorption (Note: barium can interfere).

Ferritin

(male: 15–200 ng/mL [SI: 15–200 μg/L]; female: 12–150 ng/mL [SI: 12–150 μg/L]).

Increased: Hemochromatosis, hemosiderosis, sideroblastic anemia.

Decreased: Iron deficiency (earliest and most sensitive test before red cells show any morphologic change), severe liver disease.

Fibrin D-Dimer (D-DIMER)

(normal = negative).
Useful in screening for DIC.

Increased: DIC, DVT, acute MI, PE, arterial thrombosis.

Fibrin Degradation Products (FDP), Fibrin Split Products (FSP)

(<10 μg/mL)

Increased: Disseminated intravascular coagulation (DIC) (usually > 40 μg/mL), any thromboembolic condition (deep venous thrombosis, myocardial infarction, pulmonary embolus), hepatic dysfunction, fibrinolytic therapy.

Fibrinogen

(200–400 mg/dL [SI: 2.0–4.0 g/L]).

Increased: Inflammatory reactions, oral contraceptives, pregnancy, cancer (kidney, stomach, breast).

Decreased: Disseminated intravascular coagulation (sepsis, amniotic fluid embolism, abruptio placentae), surgery (prostate, open heart), neoplastic and hematologic conditions, acute severe bleeding, burns, venomous snake bite, congenital.

Folic Acid, Serum Folate

(> 2.0 ng/mL [SI: > 5 nmol/L).

Folic Acid, RBC

(125–600 ng/mL [283–1360 nmol/L).
Serum folate can fluctuate with diet. RBC levels are more indicative of tissue stores. B_{12} deficiency can result in the inability of RBC to take up folate in spite of normal serum folate levels.

Increased: Folic acid administration.

Decreased: Malnutrition/malabsorption (folic acid deficiency), massive cellular growth (cancer), medications (trimethoprim, some anticonvulsants, oral contraceptives), vitamin B_{12} deficiency (low RBC levels), pregnancy.

Follicle Stimulating Hormone (FSH)

(males: < 22 IU/L; females:non-midcycle, < 20 IU/L; midcycle surge, < 40 IU/L (midcycle peak should be 2 times basal level; postmenopausal, 40–160 IU/L).

Increased: (Hypergonadotropic > 40 IU/L), postmenopausal, surgical castration, gonadal failure, gonadotropin-secreting pituitary adenoma.

Decreased: (Hypogonadotropic < 5 IU/L prepubertal), hypothalamic and pituitary dysfunction, pregnancy.

FTA-ABS (Fluorescent Treponemal Antibody Absorbed)

(Normal = nonreactive).

Positive: Syphilis (test of choice to confirm diagnosis), other treponemal infections.(Note: may be negative in early primary syphilis and remain positive in spite of adequate treatment).

Fungal Serologies

(negative <1:8)

This is a complement-fixation fungal antibody screen that usually detects antibodies to members of the genera *Histoplasma, Blastomyces, Aspergillus,* and *Coccidioides* spp.

Gastrin, Serum

(fasting: < 100 pg/mL [SI: 47.7 pmol/L], postprandial: 95–140 pg/mL [SI: 45.3–66.7 pmol/L]) Note: patient must be off proton pump inhibitors or H_2 blockers.

Increased: Zollinger-Ellison syndrome, pyloric stenosis, pernicious anemia, atrophic gastritis, ulcerative colitis, renal insufficiency, steroid and calcium administration.

GGT (Gamma-Glutamyl Transpeptidase, SGGT)

(male 9–50 U/L; female 8–40 U/L).

Generally parallels changes in serum alkaline phosphatase and 5′ nucleotidase in liver disease.

Increased: Liver disease (hepatitis, cirrhosis, obstruction, both intrinsic and extrinsic), pancreatitis, primary and metastatic neoplasms, medications (phenytoin, alcohol, barbiturates).

Glucose

(fasting, 70–105 mg/dL [SI: 3.89–5.83 nmol/L]; 2 h postprandial: < 120 mg/dL [SI: < 6.67 nmol/L]). To convert mg/dL to nmol/L, multiply by 0.05551.

Increased: Diabetes mellitus, Cushing's syndrome, acromegaly, increased epinephrine (injection, pheochromocytoma, stress, burns, etc.), acute pancreatitis, adrenocorticotropic hormone (ACTH) administration, spurious increase caused by drawing blood from a site above an IV line containing dextrose, elderly patients, pancreatic glucagonoma, drugs (glucocorticoids, some diuretics).

Decreased: Pancreatic disorders (pancreatitis, islet cell tumors), extrapancreatic tumors (carcinoma of the adrenals, stomach), hepatic disease (hepatitis, cirrhosis, tumors), endocrine disorders (early diabetes, hypothyroidism, hypopituitarism), functional disorders (after gastrectomy), pediatric problems (prematurity, infant of a diabetic mother, ketotic hypoglycemia, enzyme diseases), exogenous insulin, oral hypoglycemic agents, malnutrition, sepsis.

Glucose Tolerance Test, Oral

(***Note:*** If fasting blood glucose is > 140 mg/dL, the GTT is unnecessary.) Used to aid in the diagnosis of diabetes mellitus, especially when diagnosis cannot be made on the basis of fasting blood sugar levels. The test is unreliable in severe infection, prolonged fasting, or after insulin. After an overnight fast, a fasting blood glucose is drawn, and the patient is given a 75-g oral glucose load (100 g for gestational diabetes screening, 1.75 mg-kg ideal body weight in children up to 75 g). Plasma glucose is then drawn at 30, 60, 120, and 180 minutes.

Interpretation:

Adult Onset Diabetes: Any fasting blood sugar >140, or >200 at both 120 min and one other time interval measured.

Gestational Diabetes: At least two of the following: any fasting blood sugar > 105, at 60 min > 190, at 120 min > 165, or at 180 min > 145.

Glycohemoglobin (Hemoglobin A_{1c}, Glycosylated Hemoglobin) (4.6–7.1%)

Increased: Diabetes mellitus (uncontrolled; reflects levels over preceding 3–4 mo).

Decreased: Chronic renal failure, hemolytic anemia, pregnancy, chronic blood loss.

Gram's Stain

Used in the identification of gram-negative and gram-positive bacteria.

Technique

1. Smear the specimen (sputum, peritoneal fluid, etc.) on a glass slide in a fairly thin coat. If time permits, allow the specimen to air dry. The smear may also be fixed under very low heat (excessive heat can cause artifacts). When a Bunsen burner is not available, other heat sources include a hot light bulb, or an alcohol swab set on fire. Heat the slide until it is warm, but not hot when touched to the back of the hand.
2. Timing for the stain is not critical, but at least 10 s should be allowed for each set of reagents.
3. Apply the crystal violet (Gram's stain), rinse the slide with tap water, apply iodine solution, and rinse with water.
4. Decolorize the slide carefully with the acetone-alcohol solution until the blue color is barely visible in the runoff. (This is the step where most Gram's stains are ruined.)
5. Counterstain with a few drops of safranin, rinse the slide with water, and blot it dry with lint-free bibulous or filter paper.
6. Use the high dry and oil immersion lenses on the microscope to examine the slide. If the Gram's stain is satisfactory, any polys on the slide should be pink with light blue nuclei. On a Gram's stain of sputum, an excessive number of epithelial cells means the sample was more saliva than sputum.

Gram's Stain Characteristics Of Common Pathogens

Gram-Positive Cocci: *Staphylococcus, Streptococcus, Diplococcus, Micrococcus, Peptococcus* (anaerobic), and *Peptostreptococcus* (anaerobic) species (If *Staphylococcus* initially is reported as coagulase positive, suspect *S aureus*; if coagulase is negative, suspect *S epidermidis*).

Gram-Positive Rods: *Clostridium* (anaerobic), *Corynebacterium, Listeria,* and *Bacillus* species.

Gram-Negative Cocci: *Neisseria (Branhamella)* species.

Gram-Negative Coccoid Rods: *Haemophilus, Pasteurella, Brucella,* and *Bordetella* species.

Gram-negative Straight Rods: *Escherichia, Salmonella, Shigella, Proteus, Enterobacter, Klebsiella, Serratia, Pseudomonas, Providencia, Yersinia, Acinetobacter (Mima, Herellea), Eikenella, Legionella, Bacteroides* (anaerobic), *Fusobacterium* (anaerobic), and *Campylobacter* (comma-shaped) species.

5-HIAA 5-Hydroxyindoleacetic Acid (24-h Urine)

(2–8 mg [SI: 10.4–41.6] μmol/24-h urine collection).

5-HIAA is a serotonin metabolite and is useful to diagnose carcinoid syndrome.

Increased: Carcinoid tumors (usually metastatic), certain foods (avocado, banana, pineapple, tomato), phenothiazine derivatives.

Haptoglobin

(40–180 mg/dL [SI: 0.4–1.8 g/L])

Increased: Obstructive liver disease, any cause if increased erythrocyte sedimentation rate (ESR) (inflammation, collagen-vascular diseases).

Decreased: Any type of hemolysis (transfusion reaction, etc.), liver disease, anemia, oral contraceptives.

Helicobacter Pylori Serology

(normal = negative)

Most patients with gastritis and ulcer disease (gastric or duodenal) have chronic *H pylori* infection that should be treated. Positive in 35–50% asymptomatic patients (increases with age). Use in dyspepsia controversial.

Hepatitis Testing

Recommended hepatitis panel tests based on clinical settings is shown in Table II–6, page 308. Interpretation of testing patterns is shown in Table II–7, page 309.

Specific Hepatitis Tests

HBsAg	Hepatitis B surface antigen (formerly Australia antigen, HAA). Indicates either chronic or acute infection with hepatitis B. Used by blood banks to screen donors.
Total Anti-HBc	IgG and IgM antibody to hepatitis B core antigen; confirms either previous exposure to hepatitis B virus (HBV) or ongoing infection. Used by blood banks to screen donors.

TABLE II–6. HEPATITIS PANEL TESTING TO GUIDE IN THE ORDERING OF HEPATITIS PROFILES FOR GIVEN CLINICAL SETTINGS.

Medical Setting	Test	Purpose
Screening tests		
Pregnancy	• HBsAg	All expectant mothers should be screened during 3rd trimester.
High risk patients on admission (homosexuals, dialysis patients	• HBsAg	To screen for chronic or active infection
Percutaneous inoculation (donor)	• HBsAg • Anti-HBc IgM • Anti-hepatitis C	To test patients blood (especially dialysis patients and HIV-infected individuals) for infectivity with HBV and HCV if health care worker exposed.
Percutaneous inoculation (victim)	• HBsAg • Anti-HBc • Anti-hepatitis C	To test exposed health care worker for immunity or chronic infection.
Pre-HBV Vaccine	• Anti-HBc • Anti-HBs	To determine if an individual is infected or has antibodies to HBV.
Screening blood donors	• HBsAg • Anti-HBc • Anti-hepatitis C	Used by blood banks to screen donors for hepatitis B and C.
Diagnostic tests		
Differential diagnosis of acute jaundice, hepatitis,or fulminant liver failure	• HBsAg • Anti-HBc IgM • Anti-HAV IgM • Anti-hepatitis C	To differentiate between HBV, HAV, and HCV in acutely jaundiced patient with hepatitis or fulminant liver failure.
Chronic hepatitis	• HBsAg + HBeAg +Anti-HBe +Anti hepatitis D (total +Igm)	To diagnose HBV infection + If positive for HBsAg to determine infectivity + If HBsAg patient worsens or is very ill, to diagnose concomitant infection with hepatitis delta virus.
Monitor		
Infant follow-up	• HBsAg • Anti-HBc • Anti-HBs	To monitor the success of vaccination and passive immunization for perinatal transmission of HBV 12–15 months after birth.
Postvaccination screening	• Anti-HBs	To ensure immunity has been achieved after vaccination (CDC mends titer determination,but usually qualitiative assay adequate).
Sexual contact	• HBsAg • Anti-HBc • Anti-hepatitis C	To monitor sexual partners of patient with chronic HBV or HCV.

(Reproduced, with permission, from Gomella LG (editor): Diagnosis: Chemistry, Immunology, and Serology. *In: Clinician's Pocket Reference, 9/e. Mc Graw Hill, 2000).*

TABLE II–7. INTERPRETATION OF VIRAL HEPATITIS SEROLOGIC TESTING PATTERNS.

Anti-HAV (IgM)	HBsAg	Anti-HBc (Igm)	Anti-HBc (Total)	Anti-HCV (Elisa)	Interpretation
+	—	—	—	—	Acute hepatitis A
+	+	—	+	—	Acute hepatitis A in hepatitis B carrier
—	+	—	+	—	Chronic hepatitis B[1]
—	—	+	+	—	Acute hepatitis B
—	+	+	+	—	Acute hepatitis B
—	—	—	+	—	Past hepatitis B infection
—	—	—	—	+	Hepatitis C[2]
—	—	—	—	—	Early hepatitsis C or other cause (other virus, toxic etc.)

[1]Patients with chronic hepatitis B (either active hepatitis or carrier state) should have HBeAg and Anti-HBe checked to determine activity of infection and relative infectivity. Anti-HBs is used to determine response to hepatitis B vaccination.
[2]Anti-HCV often takes 3–6 months before being posttive. Replaced by more sensitive tests, eg, HCV-RNA PCR.

Anti-HBc IgM IgM antibody to hepatitis B core antigen. Early and best indicator of acute infection with hepatitis B.

HBeAg Hepatitis Be antigen; when present, indicates high degree of infectivity. Order only when evaluating a patient with chronic HBV infection.

Anti-HBe Antibody to hepatitis Be antigen; presence associated with resolution of active inflammation, but often signifies virus is integrated into host DNA, especially if the host remains HBsAg positive.

Anti-HBs Antibody to hepatitis B surface antigen; when present, typically indicates immunity associated with clinical recovery from HBV infection or previous immunization with hepatitis B vaccine. Order only to assess effectiveness of vaccine and request titer levels.

Anti-HAV Total antibody to hepatitis A virus; confirms previous exposure to hepatitis A virus.

Anti-HAV IgM	IgM antibody to hepatitis A virus; indicative of recent infection with hepatitis A virus.
Anti-HDV	Total antibody to delta hepatitis; confirms previous exposure. Order only in patients with known acute or chronic HBV infection.
Anti-HDV IgM	IgM antibody to delta hepatitis; indicates recent infection. Order only in patients with known acute or chronic HBV infection.
Anti-HCV	Antibody against hepatitis C (formerly known as non-A, non-B hepatitis) and is the major cause of post-transfusion hepatitis. Used by blood banks to screen donors. Many false positives.
HCV-RNA PCR	Useful to detect Hepatitis C infection be fore antibodies rise; associated with viremia.

High Density Lipoprotein Cholesterol

(See Cholesterol, Page 296)

HLA (Human Leukocyte Antigens; HLA Typing)

This test identifies a group of antigens on the cell surface that are the primary determinants of histocompatibility and are useful in assessing transplantation compatibility. Some are associated with specific diseases, but are not diagnostic of these diseases.

HLA-B27: Ankylosing spondylitis, psoriatic arthritis, Reiter's syndrome, juvenile rheumatoid arthritis.

HLA-DR4/HLA DR2: Chronic Lyme disease arthritis

HLA-DRw2: Multiple sclerosis.

HLA-B8: Addison's disease, juvenile onset diabetes, Grave's disease, gluten sensitive enteropathy.

Human Immunodeficiency Virus (HIV) Testing

(Normal = negative)

Used in the diagnosis of acquired immunodeficiency syndrome (AIDS) and to screen blood for use in transfusion. Note: CDC guidelines indicate that any HIV-positive person older than 13 years with a CD4+ T-cell level < 200/μL or an HIV-positive person with a series of indicator conditions (such as pulmonary candidiasis, disseminated histoplasmosis, HIV wasting, Kaposi's sarcoma,

TB, various lymphomas, *Pneumocystis carinii,* pneumonia, and others) is considered to have AIDS. If HIV-EIA is positive, confirm with Western blot. Next, confirm with HIV RNA viral load and CD4/CD8 ratio to stage disease.

HIV-EIA: Enzyme-linked immunosorbent assay to detect HIV antibody; a positive test should be confirmed by Western blot.

Positive: AIDS, asymptomatic HIV infection, false-positive (recent administration of flu vaccine, dialysis, alcoholic hepatitis, positive RPR, hypergammaglobulinemia, others).

HIV Western Blot

(normal = negative)

The reference procedure for confirming the presence or absence of HIV antibody, usually after a positive HIV antibody by ELISA determination. Polymerase chain reaction (PCR) may become the confirmatory test for HIV.

Positive: AIDS, asymptomatic HIV infection (If indeterminate, repeat in 1 mo).

HIV RNA ("Viral Load")

Earliest marker of HIV infection, positive within 2 wk of infection. Used to monitor therapy and/or progression.

P24 Antigen Assay: Specific for HIV infection; largely replaced by RNA assay.

HIV CD4 Counts

Widely used predictor of opportunistic infection and HIV progression (likely with counts < 200 cells/μL). Used to guide therapeutic intervention (usually < 500 cells/μL)

Human Chorionic Gonadotropin, Serum (HCG, Beta Subunit)

(Normal, < 3.0 mIU/mL; 7–10 d post-conception, >3 mIU/mL; 30 d, 100–5000 mIU/mL; 10 wk, 50,000–140,000 mIU/mL; >16 weeks, 10,000–50,000 mIU/mL; thereafter, levels slowly decline) [SI units IU/L equivalent to mIU/mL] (See also Urinary HCG)

Increased: Pregnancy, testicular tumors, trophoblastic disease (hydatidiform mole, choriocarcinoma levels usually > 100,000 mIU/mL).

Iron

(Males: 65–175 μg/dL [SI: 11.64–31.33 μmol/L]; females: 50–170 μg/dL [SI: 8.95–30.43 μmol/L]). To convert μg/dL to μmol/L, multiply by 0.1791.

Increased: Hemochromatosis, hemosiderosis caused by excessive iron intake, excess destruction or decreased production of erythrocytes, liver necrosis.

Decreased: Iron deficiency anemia, nephrosis (loss of iron-binding proteins), normochromic anemia of chronic diseases and infections.

Iron-Binding Capacity (Total) (TIBC)

(250–450 μg/dL [SI: 44.75–80.55 μmol/L]).

The normal iron/TIBC ratio is 20–50%; < 15% is almost diagnostic of iron deficiency anemia. Increased ratio is seen with hemochromatosis.

Increased: Acute and chronic blood loss, iron deficiency anemia, hepatitis, oral contraceptives.

Decreased: Anemia of infection and chronic diseases, cirrhosis, nephrosis, hemochromatosis.

17-Ketogenic Steroids (17–KGS, Corticosteroids) (24-h Urine)

Males: 5–24 mg/d [17–83 μmol/d]; females: 4–15 mg/d [14–52 μmol/d]

Overall adrenal function test, largely replaced by serum or urine cortisol levels.

Increased: Adrenal hyperplasia (Cushing's syndrome), adrenogenital syndrome.

Decreased: Panhypopituitarism, Addison's disease, acute steroid withdrawal.

17-Ketosteroids, Total (17-KS) (24-h Urine)

(Adult male: 8–20 mg/d [28–69 μmol/L]; adult female: 6–15 mg/dL [21–52 μmol/L] (Note: lower values in prepubertal children).

Measures dehydroepiandrosterone (DHEA), androstenedione (adrenal androgens); largely replaced by assay of individual elements.

Increased: Adrenal cortex abnormalities (hyperplasia [Cushing's disease], adenoma, carcinoma, adrenogenital syndrome), severe stress, adrenocorticotropic hormone (ACTH) or pituitary tumor, testicular interstitial tumor and arrhenoblastoma (both produce testosterone).

Decreased: Panhypopituitarism, Addison's disease, castration in men.

KOH Preparation (Potassium Hydroxide Wet Mount)

KOH preps are used for diagnosis of fungal infections.

Technique

1. Apply the specimen (vaginal secretion, sputum, skin scrapings) to a slide.
2. Add 1–2 drops of 10% KOH solution and mix. Gentle heating may help.
3. Put a coverslip over the specimen and examine the slide for branching hyphae and blastospores that indicate the presence of a fungus. KOH should destroy most elements other than fungus. If there is dense keratin and debris, allow the slide to sit for several hours and then repeat the microscopic examination. Lowering the substage condenser will give better contrast between organisms and the background.

Positive: filaments, hyphae, spores, budding yeast suggest fungal infection; note that false positives can be seen with cotton or cellulose fibers that may be mistaken for hyphae.

Lactate Dehydrogenase (LDH)

(adults < 200 U/L, higher levels in childhood).

Increased: Acute myocardial infarction, pulmonary embolus, cardiac surgery, pernicious anemia, malignant tumors, AIDS-related lymphoma, *Pneumocystis carinii* pneumonia, hemolysis (prosthetic valve, anemias or factitious), renal infarction, muscle injury, megaloblastic anemia, liver disease (hepatitis, obstructive jaundice, medications).

LDH Isoenzymes (LDH 1 to LDH 5): Normally, the ratio LDH 1/LDH 2 is < 0.6–0.7. If the ratio becomes > 1 (also termed "flipped"), suspect a recent myocardial infarction (change in ratio can also be seen in pernicious or hemolytic anemia). With an acute myocardial infarction, the LDH will begin to rise at 12–48 h, peak at 3–6 d and return to normal at 8–14 d. LDH 5 is > LDH 4 in liver diseases.

Lactic Acid (Lactate)

(4.5–19.8 mg/dL [SI: 0.5–2.2 mmol/L]).

Increased: Lactic acidosis due to hypoxia, hemorrhage, shock, sepsis, cirrhosis, exercise, ethanol, DKA, regional ischemia (extremity, bowel) spurious (prolonged tourniquet).

LE (Lupus Erythematosus) Preparation

(Normal = no cells seen)

Positive: Systemic lupus erythematosus (SLE), scleroderma, rheumatoid arthritis, drug-induced lupus (procainamide, others).

Lipase

(0–1.5 U/mL [SI: 10–150 U/L] by turbidimetric method).

Increased: Acute and chronic pancreatitis, pancreatic pseudocyst, pancreatic duct obstruction (stone, stricture, tumor, drug-induced spasm), gastric malignancy, intestinal perforation, fat embolus syndrome, renal failure, diabetes (usually in DKA only), dialysis (usually normal in mumps).

Low Density Lipoprotein-Cholesterol (LDL, LDL-C)

(See Cholesterol, Page 296)

Luteinizing Hormone, Serum (LH)

(males: 7–24 IU/L; female; 6–30 IU/L, midcycle peak increase 2–3-fold over baseline).

Increased: (Hypergonadotropic > 40 IU/L), postmenopausal, surgical or radiation castration, ovarian or testicular failure, polycystic ovaries.

Decreased: (Hypogonadotropic <40 IU/L prepubertal), hypothalamic, and pituitary dysfunction, Kallman's syndrome, LH–RH analog administration (e.g. Leuprolide)

Lyme Disease Serology

(Normal varies with assay)

Most useful when comparing acute and convalescent serum levels to compare titers. Marked interlaboratory variability is present.

Positive: Infection with *Borrellia burgdorferi* (some cross reactivity with antibodies to Epstein-Barr, syphilis, rickettsia)

Lymphocyte Subsets

Specific monoclonal antibodies are used to identify specific T and B cells. Lymphocyte subsets (also called lymphocyte marker assays, or T- and B-cell assay) are useful in the diagnosis of acquired immune deficiency syndrome (see page 310), and various leukemias and lymphomas. The designation CD ("clusters of differentiation") has largely replaced the older antibody designations (such as Leu 3a, or OKT3). Results are most reliable when reported as an absolute number of cells/µL rather than a percentage of cells. CD4/CD8 ratio < 1 is seen in patients with AIDS. Absolute CD4 count is used to guide HIV therapy

Normal Lymphocyte Subsets

- Total lymphocytes 0.66–4.60 thousand/µL
- T-cell 644–2201 µL (60–88%)
- B-cell 82–392 µL (3–20%)
- T-helper/inducer cell (CD4,Leu 3a,OKT4) 493–1191 µL (34–67%)
- Suppressor/cytotoxic T cell (CD8, Leu 2, OKT8) 182–785 µL (10–42%)
- CD4/CD8 ratio > 1

Magnesium

(1.6–2.6 mg/dL [SI: 0.80–1.30 mmol/L]).

Increased: Renal failure, hypothyroidism, magnesium–containing antacids, Addison's disease, diabetic coma, severe dehydration, lithium intoxication.

Decreased: Malabsorption, steatorrhea, alcoholism and cirrhosis, hyperthyroidism, aldosteronism, diuretics, acute pancreatitis, hyperparathyroidism, hyperalimentation, nasogastric suctioning, chronic dialysis, renal tubular acidosis, drugs (cisplatin, amphotericin B, aminoglycosides), hungry bone syndrome, hypophosphatemia, intracellular shifts with respiratory or metabolic acidosis.

Metanephrines (24-Hour Urine)

< 1.3 mg/d [< 7.1 µmol/d] for adults, but variable in children.

These are metabolic products of epinephrine and norepinephrine, a primary screening test for pheochromocytoma.

Increased: Pheochromocytoma, neuroblastoma (neural crest tumors), false positive with drugs (phenobarbital, guanethidine, hydrocortisone, others).

MHA-TP (Microhemagglutination, *Treponema Pallidum*)

(normal < 1:160)

Confirmatory test for syphilis, similar to FTA-ABS. Once positive, it remains so; therefore, it cannot be used to judge the effect of treatment. False positives with other treponemal infections (pinta, yaws, etc.), mononucleosis, and systemic lupus.

Monospot

(Normal = negative)

Positive: Mononucleosis, rarely in leukemia, serum sickness, Burkitt's lymphoma, viral hepatitis, rheumatoid arthritis.

Nucleotidase

(2–15 U/L)

Used in the workup of increased alkaline phosphatase and biliary obstruction.

Increased: Obstructive/cholestatic liver disease, liver metastasis, biliary cirrhosis.

Osmolality, Serum

(278–298 mOsm/kg [SI: 278–298 mmol/kg])

A rough estimation of osmolality is [2(sodium) + BUN/2.8 + glucose/18]. Measured value is usually greater than calculated value. If measured is 15 mOsm/kg > than calculated, consider methanol, ethanol or ethylene glycol ingestion.

Increased: Hyperglycemia, alcohol ingestion, increased sodium because of water loss (diabetes, hypercalcemia, diuresis), ethylene glycol ingestion, mannitol.

Decreased: Low serum sodium, diuretics, Addison's disease, inappropriate antidiuretic hormone (ADH) (syndrome of inappropriate ADH [SIADH], seen in bronchogenic carcinoma, hypothyroidism), iatrogenic causes (poor fluid balance).

Osmolality, Urine (See Urine, Spot)

Oxygen, Arterial (Po_2) (see Table II–1)

See On-Call Problems 48 "Hypoxia," page 190 and 74 "Ventilator Management: Low Po_2/High Pco_2," page 265.

Decreased: Ventilation–perfusion ($\dot{V}/\dot{Q}$) abnormalities, COPD (asthma, emphysema), atelectasis, pneumonia, pulmonary embolus, respiratory distress syndrome, pneumothorax, TB, cystic fibrosis, obstructed airway.

Alveolar hypoventilation: Skeletal abnormalities, neuromuscular disorders, Pickwickian syndrome.

Decreased pulmonary diffusing capacity: Pneumoconiosis, pulmonary edema, pulmonary fibrosis (Bleomycin).

Right to left shunt: Congenital heart disease (Tetralogy of Fallot, transposition, etc.).

pH, Arterial

(see Table II–1, page 284)

Increased: Metabolic and respiratory alkalosis (See also On Call Problem "Acidosis," page 15).

Decreased: Metabolic and respiratory acidosis (See also On Call Problem "Alkalosis," page 20).

P-24 Antigen (HIV Core Antigen)

(normal = negative)

Used to diagnose recent acute HIV infection; can be positive as early as 2–4 wk but becomes undetectable during antibody seroconversion (periods of latency). With progression of disease, P-24 usually becomes evident again.

Parathyroid Hormone (PTH)

(normal based on serum calcium provided on the lab report; values vary depending on whether the n-terminal, c-terminal or mid-molecule is measured. PTH mid molecule, 0.29–0.85 ng/mL [SI: 29–85 pmol/L]; with calcium, 8.4–10.2 mg/dL [SI: 2.1–2.55 mmol/L])

Increased: Primary hyperparathyroidism, secondary hyperparathyroidism (hypocalcemic states such as chronic renal failure, others), drugs (furosemide, lithium).

Decreased: Hypercalcemia not due to hyperparathyroidism (ie, malignancy), hypoparathyroidism, hyperthyroidism.

Partial Thromboplastin Time (Activated Partial Thromboplastin Time, PTT, APTT)

(27–38 s)

Increased: Heparin and any defect in the intrinsic coagulation system (includes Factors I, II, V, VIII, IX, X, XI, and XII), prolonged use of a tourniquet before drawing a blood sample, hemophilia A and B.

Decreased: DIC

Phosphorus

(adult: 2.5–4.5 mg/dL [SI: 0.81–1.45 mmol/L], child: 4.0–6.0 mg/dL [SI: 1.29–1.94 mmol/L]). To convert mg/dL to mmol/L, multiply by 0.3229.

Increased: Hypoparathyroidism (surgical, pseudohypoparathyroidism), excess vitamin D, secondary hyperparathyroidism, renal failure, bone disease (healing fractures), Addison's disease, childhood, factitious increase (hemolysis of specimen).

Decreased: Hyperparathyroidism, alcoholism, diabetes, hyperalimentation, acidosis, alkalosis, gout, salicylate poisoning, IV steroid, glucose and/or insulin administration, hyperparathyroidism, hypokalemia, hypomagnesemia, diuretics, vitamin D deficiency, phosphate-binding antacids.

Potassium, Serum

(3.5–5 mEq/L [SI: 3.5–5 mmol/L]).

Increased: Factitious increase (hemolysis of specimen, thrombocytosis), renal failure, Addison's disease, acidosis, dehydration, hemolysis, massive tissue damage, excess intake (oral or IV), potassium–containing medications, drugs (spironolactone, triamterene, pentamidine, NSAIDs).

Decreased: Diuretics, decreased intake, vomiting, nasogastric suctioning, villous adenoma, diarrhea, Zollinger-Ellison syndrome, chronic pyelonephritis, renal tubular acidosis (I and II), metabolic alkalosis (primary aldosteronism, Cushing's syndrome).

Potassium, Urine

(see Urine, Spot, page 331)

Progesterone

Used to confirm ovulation and corpus luteum function.

Phase	Normal Values(Female)
Follicular	< 1 ng/mL
Luteal	5–20 ng/mL
Pregnancy 1st trimester	10–30 ng/mL

2nd trimester	50–100 ng/mL
3rd trimester	100–400 ng/mL
Postmenopause	< 1 ng/mL

Prolactin

(males 1–20 ng/mL [SI: 1–20 μg/L]; females 1–25 ng/mL [SI: 1–25 μg/L])

Increased: Pregnancy, nursing after pregnancy, prolactinoma, hypothalamic tumors, sarcoidosis or granulomatous disease of the hypothalamus, hypothyroidism, renal failure, Addison's disease, phenothiazines, haloperidol.

Prostate-Specific Antigen (PSA)

(<4 ng/dL by monoclonal, eg, Hybritech assay)

Most useful as a measure of response to therapy of prostate cancer; approved for screening for prostate cancer. Although any elevation increases suspicion of prostate cancer, levels > 10.0 ng/dL are associated with carcinoma at the 90% confidence level. Age-corrected levels gaining popularity (40–50 y, 2.5 ng/dl; 50–60 y, 3.5 ng/dl; 60–70 y, 4.5 ng/dl; >70 y, 6.5 ng/dl).

Increased: Prostate cancer, acute prostatitis, some cases of benign prostatic hypertrophy (BPH), prostatic infarction, prostate surgery (biopsy, resection), vigorous prostatic massage (routine rectal exam does not elevate levels).

Decreased: Radical prostatectomy, response to therapy of prostatic carcinoma (radiation or hormonal therapy), low testosterone levels.

PSA Density (PSAD): Ratio of prostate specific antigen (PSA) level to prostate size, as measured by transrectal ultrasound (TRUS). Proposed as a method to differentiate an elevated PSA between 4.0 and 10.0 ng/mL, A PSAD of 0.15 or greater would warrant prostate biopsy.

PSA Velocity: A rate of rise in PSA of 0.75 ng/mL or greater per year on the basis of at least three separate assays 6 mo apart is suspicious for prostate cancer.

PSA Free And Total: Patients with prostate cancer tend to have lower free PSA levels in proportion to total PSA. Measurement of the free/total PSA can improve the specificity of PSA as a screening test. In mildly elevated PSA (4.0–10.0 ng/mL), patients should have a prostate biopsy only if the free PSA percentage is low. Threshold for biopsy is controversial, ranging from less than 15% to less than 25%, with a higher threshold having improved sensitivity and a lower threshold having improved specificity.

Protein, Serum

(6.0–8.0 gm/dL)

Increased: Multiple myeloma, Waldenström's macroglobulinemia, benign monoclonal gammopathy, lymphoma, chronic inflammatory disease, sarcoidosis.

Decreased: Malnutrition, inflammatory bowel disease, Hodgkin's disease, leukemias, any cause of decreased albumin.

Protein, Urine

(24-h Urine, < 150 mg/d [< 0.15 g/d]).

Increased: (see Urinalysis Differential Diagnosis, page 327), nephrotic syndrome usually associated with >4 gm/d

Prothrombin Time (PT)

(11.5–13.5 seconds)

(International Normalized Ratio [INR] instead of the Patient/ Control ratio now used to guide anticoagulant [Coumadin] therapy).

PT Patient/Control Ratio		INR
Normal	0.9–1.1	0.75–1.30
Therapeutic	1.5–2.5	2.0–4.5

PT evaluates the extrinsic clotting mechanism that includes Factors I, II, V, VII, and X and not altered by heparin.

Increased: Drugs (sodium warfarin [Coumadin]), vitamin K deficiency, fat malabsorption, liver diseases, prolonged use of a tourniquet before drawing a blood sample, disseminated intravascular coagulation (DIC).

RBC Morphology

The following lists some erythrocyte abnormalities and the associated conditions. General terms include poikilocytosis (irregular RBC shape such as sickle and Burr) and anisocytosis (irregular RBC size such as microcytes and macrocytes).

Basophilic Stippling: Lead or heavy metal poisoning, thalassemia, severe anemia.

Howell-Jolly Bodies: After splenectomy, some severe hemolytic anemias, pernicious anemia, leukemia, thalassemia.

Sickling: Sickle cell disease and trait.

Nucleated RBCs: Severe bone marrow stress (hemorrhage, hemolysis, etc.), marrow replacement by tumor, extramedullary hematopoiesis.

Target Cells (Leptocytes): Thalassemia, hemoglobinopathies, obstructive jaundice, any hypochromic anemia, after splenectomy.

Spherocytes: Hereditary spherocytosis, immune or microangiopathic hemolysis, severe burns, ABO transfusion reactions.

Helmet Cells (Schistocytes): Microangiopathic hemolysis, hemolytic transfusion reaction, transplant rejection, other severe anemias, TTP.

Burr Cells (Acanthocytes): Severe liver disease, high levels of bile, fatty acids, or toxins.

Polychromasia (Basophilia): The appearance of a bluish-gray red cell on routine Wright's stain suggests reticulocytes.

Renin, Plasma (Plasma Renin Activity [PRA])

(Adults: Normal sodium diet, upright 1–6 ng/mL/h [SI: 0.77–4.6 nmol/L/h]. Renal vein renin: L & R should be equal).

Useful in the diagnosis of hypertension associated with hypokalemia. Values highly dependent upon salt intake and position. Stop diuretics, estrogens for 2–4 wk before testing.

Increased: Medications (ACE inhibitors, diuretics, oral contraceptives, estrogens) pregnancy, dehydration, renal artery stenosis, adrenal insufficiency, chronic hypokalemia, upright posture, salt-restricted diet, edematous conditions (CHF, nephrotic syndrome), secondary hyperaldosteronism.

Decreased: Primary aldosteronism (renin will not increase with relative volume depletion, upright posture).

Renin, Renal Vein

(normal L & R should be equal).

A ratio of > 1.5 (affected/non-affected) suggestive of renovascular hypertension.

Reticulocyte Count

(normal corrected reticulocyte count is < 1.5 %).

This is reported as a percentage, and you should calculate the corrected reticulocyte count for interpretation of the results (corrected reticulocyte count = reported count × patient's HCT/normal HCT). This corrected count is an excellent indicator of erythropoietic activity. Normal marrow responds to a decrease in erythrocytes (shown by a decreased hematocrit) with an increase in the production of reticulocytes. Lack of increase in a reticulocyte count in an anemic patient suggests a chronic disease, a deficiency disease, marrow replacement, or marrow failure.

Retinol-Binding Protein (RBP)

(adults: 3–6 mg/dL; children: 1.5–3.0 mg/dL).

Decreased: Malnutrition, vitamin A deficiency, intestinal malabsorption of fats, chronic liver disease.

Rheumatoid Factor (RA Latex Test)

(< 15 IU by Microscan kit or < 1:40)

Increased: Rheumatoid arthritis, systemic lupus erythematosus (SLE), syphilis, chronic inflammation, subacute bacterial endocarditis (SBE), some lung diseases.

Sedimentation Rate (Erthryocyte Sedimentation Rate, ESR)

Wintrobe Scale: Males: 0–9 mm/h, females: 0–20 mm/h.

ZETA Scale: 40–54%, normal; 55–59%, mildly elevated; 60–64%, moderately elevated; > 65%, markedly elevated.

Westergren Scale: Males: < 50 years, 15 mm/h; > 50 years, 20 mm/h; female: < 50 years, 20 mm/h; > 50 years, 30 mm/h.

ESR is a very nonspecific test. ZETA rate is not affected by anemia.

Increased: Any type of infection, inflammation, rheumatic fever, endocarditis, neoplasm, acute myocardial infarction.

Semen Analysis

After 48–72 h of abstinence, semen specimen is collected in a wide mouth polypropylene container with a screw top. The sample is kept as close to body temperature as possible and delivered to the lab within 1½ h. The following are general reference parameters and are typically determined on at least two specimens.

- Volume: 1.5–5.0 mL
- Appearance: white, viscid, opaque
- pH: 7.2–8.0

- Sperm density: > 20 x 10^6/mL
- Total sperm count: > 40 x 10^6/mL
- Motility: > 60%
- Forward Progression: > 50%
  or > 2+ on a scale 0–4 (0, no movement; 4, excellent forward progression)
- Morphology: > 60% normal
- Viability: > 50% (by dye exclusion)
- Fructose, quantitative: > 13 micromol per ejaculate
- Liquification: 10–20 minutes (measured on a scale 0–4)
- Agglutination: Minimal clumping (increased clumping suggests inflammatory/immunologic process)

SGOT (Serum Glutamic-Oxaloacetic Transaminase) or AST (Serum Aspartate Aminotransaminase)

(8–20 U/L)
Generally parallels changes in SGPT in liver disease.

Increased: Acute myocardial infarction, liver disease, Reye's syndrome, muscle trauma and injection, pancreatitis, intestinal injury or surgery, factitious increase (erythromycin, opiates), burns, cardiac catheterization, brain damage, renal infarction.

Decreased: Beriberi, severe diabetes with ketoacidosis, liver disease.

SGPT (Serum Glutamic-Pyruvic Transaminase) or ALT (Alanine Aminotransaminase)

(8–20 U/L)
(Note: SGPT is elevated more than SGOT in viral hepatitis; SGOT is elevated more than SGPT in alcoholic hepatitis).

Increased: Liver disease, liver cancer and metastasis, liver abscess, liver injury (ischemia, hypoxia), biliary obstruction, pancreatitis, liver congestion (CHF), medications.

Sodium, Serum

(136–145 mmol/L)

Increased: Associated with low total body sodium (glycosuria, mannitol, urea, excess sweating), normal total body sodium (diabetes insipidus [central and nephrogenic], respiratory losses, and sweating), and associated with increased total body sodium (administration of hypertonic sodium bicarbonate, Cushing's syndrome, hyperaldosteronism).

Decreased: Associated with excess total body sodium and water (nephrotic syndrome, congestive heart failure [CHF], cirrhosis, renal failure), associated with excess body water (syndrome of inappropriate antidiuretic hormone [SIADH], hypothyroidism, adrenal insufficiency), associated with decreased total body water and sodium (diuretic use, renal tubular acidosis, use of mannitol or urea, mineralocorticoid deficiency, vomiting, diarrhea, pancreatitis) and pseudohyponatremia (hyperlipidemia, hyperglycemia, and multiple myeloma).

Note: In factitious hyponatremia due to hyperglycemia, for every 100 mmol/L blood glucose above normal, serum sodium decreases 1.6. For example, assume a patient with a blood glucose of 800 mmol/L and a serum sodium of 129 mmol/L. This would factitiously lower serum sodium by about (7 x 1.6) or 11.2 mmol/L. Corrected serum sodium would therefore be 129 + 11 = 140 mmol/L.

Sodium, Urine (see Urine, Spot)

Stool, Occult Blood [Fecal Occult Blood] (Hemoccult Test) (negative)

Repeat three times for maximum yield. A positive test more informative than a negative test.

Positive: Swallowed blood, ingestion of rare red meat, any gastrointestinal (GI) tract ulcerated lesion (ulcer, carcinoma, polyp, diverticulosis, inflammatory bowel disease), hemorrhoids, telangiectasias, drugs that cause GI irritation (eg, NSAIDs), false positives (horseradish, large doses of vitamin C (> 500 mg/d) and antacids interfere with test (false negatives).

Stool For White Blood Count (WBC)

(Occasional WBC normal)

Increased: (Usually polymorphonuclear leukocytes), *Shigella, Salmonella* spp, enteropathogenic *Escherichia coli,* ulcerative colitis, pseudomembranous colitis.

T_3 RIA (Triiodothyronine)

(120–195 ng/dL [SI: 1.85–3.00 nmol/L])

Increased: Hyperthyroidism, T_3 thyrotoxicosis, oral estrogen, pregnancy, exogenous T_4.

Decreased: Hypothyroidism and euthyroid sick state, any cause of decreased thyroid-binding globulin.

T_3 RU (Resin Uptake)

(24–34%)

Increased: Hyperthyroidism, medications (phenytoin [Dilantin], steroids, heparin, aspirin, others), nephrotic syndrome.

Decreased: Hypothyroidism, pregnancy, medications (estrogens, iodine, propylthiouracil, others).

T_4 Total (Thyroxine)

(5–12 μg/dL [SI: 65–155 nmol/L]; males: >60 years, 5–10 μg/dL [SI: 65–129 nmol]; females: 5.5–10.5 μg/dL [SI: 71–135 nmol/L]).
Good screening test for hyperthyroidism.

Increased: Hyperthyroidism, exogenous thyroid hormone, estrogens, pregnancy, severe illness, euthyroid sick syndrome.

Decreased: Euthyroid sick syndrome.

Testosterone

(male free: 9–30 ng/dL, total, 300–1200 ng/dL; female, see below)

Phase	Normal Values (Female)
Follicular	20–80 ng/dL
Midcycle Peak	20–80 ng/dL
Luteal	20–80 ng/dL
Postmenopause	10–40 ng/dL

Increased: Adrenogenital syndrome, ovarian stromal hyperthecosis, polycystic ovaries, menopause, ovarian tumors, hyperthyroidism, cirrhosis, adrenocortical tumors, trophoblastic disease during pregnancy, medications (oral contraceptives, anticonvulsants).

Decreased: Hypogonadism (primary and secondary testicular failure), LH-RH agonists, orchiectomy, uremia, hepatic failure, hypopituitarism, Klinefelter's syndrome, spironolactone, digoxin.

Thrombin Time

(10–14 s)
Elevation caused by failure of conversion of fibrinogen to fibrin.

Increased: Systemic heparin, disseminated intravascular coagulation (DIC), fibrinogen deficiency, congenitally abnormal fibrinogen molecules, systemic amyloidosis, fibrinolytic therapy.

Thyroxine Binding Globulin (TBG)

(21–52 μg/dL [SI: 270–669 nmol/L]).

Increased: Hypothyroidism, pregnancy, oral contraceptives, estrogens, hepatic disease, acute porphyria.

Decreased: Hyperthyroidism, androgens, anabolic steroids, prednisone, nephrotic syndrome, severe illness, surgical stress, phenytoin, hepatic disease.

Thyroglobulin

(1–20 ng/mL)

Increased: Differentiated thyroid carcinomas (papillary, follicular), Graves' disease, nontoxic goiter.

Decreased: Hypothyroidism, total thyroidectomy, testosterone, steroids, phenytoin.

Thyroid-Stimulating Hormone (TSH)

(0.7–5.3 mU/mL)

Newer sensitive assay is an excellent screening test for hyperthyroidism as well as hypothyroidism. Allows differentiation between a low normal and a decreased TSH.

Increased: Hypothyroidism.

Decreased: Hyperthyroidism. Less than 1% of hypothyroidism is from pituitary or hypothalamic disease resulting in a decreased TSH.

Transferrin

(220–400 mg/dL [SI: 2.20–4.0 g/L)

Increased: Acute and chronic blood loss, iron deficiency.

Decreased: Anemia of chronic disease, cirrhosis, nephrosis, hemochromatosis.

Triglycerides

(Recommended values: Males: 40–160 mg/dL [SI: 0.45–1.81 mmol/L]; females: 35–135 mg/dL [SI: 0.40–1.53 mmol/L]). Can vary with age.

Increased: Hyperlipoproteinemias (types I, IIb, III, IV, V), hypothyroidism, liver diseases, alcoholism, pancreatitis, acute myocardial infarction, nephrotic syndrome, familial increase.

Decreased: Malnutrition, congenital abetalipoproteinemia.

Troponin

(Troponin I < 0.35 ng/mL; Troponin T < 0.2 μg/L)

Used to diagnose acute MI; increases rapidly and may stay elevated for 5–7 d. More cardiac specific than CK-MB.

Uric Acid

(Males: 3.4–7 mg/dL [SI: 202–416 μmol/L]; females: 2.4–6 mg/dL [SI: 143–357 μmol/L]). To convert mg/dL to μmol/L multiply by 59.58.

Increased: Gout, renal failure, destruction of massive amounts of nucleoproteins (leukemia, anemia, chemotherapy, toxemia of pregnancy), drugs (especially diuretics), lactic acidosis, hypothyroidism, polycystic kidney disease, parathyroid diseases.

Decreased: Uricosuric drugs (salicylates, probenecid, allopurinol), Wilson's disease, Fanconi's syndrome.

Urinalysis

Normal Values

1. Appearance: "yellow, clear," or "straw colored, clear."
2. Specific gravity: Neonate: 1.012; Infant: 1.002–1.006; child and adult: 1.001–1.035 (with normal fluid intake 1.016–1.022).
3. pH: Newborn/neonate: 5–7; child and adult: 4.6–8.0.
4. Negative for: Bilirubin, blood, acetone, glucose, protein, nitrite, leukocyte esterase, reducing substances.
5. Trace: urobilinogen.
6. Sediment:
   Red Blood Count (RBC): male, 0–3/high power field (HPF); female 0–5/HPF
   White Blood Count (WBC): 0–4/HPF
   Epithelial cells: Occasional.
   Hyaline casts: Occasional.
   Bacteria: None.
   Crystals: Warm, fresh urine none (Note: refrigeration or urine left standing at room temperature may precipitate various crystals).

Differential Diagnosis For Routine Urinalysis

A. Appearance

1. Colorless: Diabetes insipidus, diuretics, excess fluid intake.
2. Dark: Acute intermittent porphyria, malignant melanoma.
3. Cloudy: Urinary tract infection (pyuria), amorphous phosphate salts (normal in alkaline urine), blood, mucus, bilirubin.
4. Pink/red: Blood, hemoglobin, myoglobin, food coloring, beets, ibuprofen.
5. Orange/Yellow: Phenazopyridine (Pyridium), bile pigments.
6. Brown/black: Myoglobin, bile pigments, melanin, cascara, iron, Macrodantin, alkaptonuria.
7. Green: Urinary bile pigments, indigo carmine, methylene blue, Urised.
8. Foamy: Proteinuria, bile salts.
9. pH
10. Acid: High protein (meat) diet, ammonium chloride, mandelic acid and other medications, acidosis, ketoacidosis (starvation, diabetic), chronic obstructive pulmonary disease (COPD).
11. Basic: Urinary tract infections (UTI), renal tubular acidosis, diet (high vegetable, milk, immediately after meals), sodium bicarbonate therapy, vomiting, metabolic alkalosis.

B. Specific Gravity

Usually corresponds with osmolarity except with osmotic diuresis. Value > 1.023 indicates normal renal concentrating ability.

Increased: Volume depletion; congestive heart failure (CHF); adrenal insufficiency; diabetes mellitus; inappropriate antidiuretic hormone (ADH); increased proteins (nephrosis); if markedly increased (1.040–1.050), suspect artifact or excretion of radiographic contrast media.

Decreased: Diabetes insipidus, pyelonephritis, glomerulonephritis, waterload with normal renal function.

C. Bilirubin

Positive: Obstructive jaundice (intra- and extrahepatic), hepatitis.

D. Blood

Positive: Stones, trauma, tumors (benign and malignant, anywhere in the urinary tract), urethral strictures, coagulopathy, infection, menses (contamination), polycystic kidneys, interstitial ne- phritis, hemolytic anemia, transfusion reaction, instrumentation (Foley catheter, etc).

Note: If the dipstick is positive for blood, but no red cells are seen, there may be free hemoglobin from trauma or a transfusion reaction or from lysis of RBCs (RBCs will lyse if the pH is < 5 or > 8), or there is myoglobin present because of a crush injury, burn, or tissue ischemia.

E. Glucose

Positive: Diabetes mellitus, pancreatitis, pancreatic carcinoma, pheochromocytoma, Cushing's disease, shock, burns, pain, steroids, hyperthyroidism, renal tubular disease, iatrogenic causes.(NOTE: glucose oxidase technique in many kits is specific for glucose and will not react with lactose, fructose or galactose.)

F. Ketones Detects primarily acetone and acetoacetic acid and not beta-hydroxybutyric acid.

Positive: Starvation, high fat diet, diabetic ketoacidosis, vomiting, diarrhea, hyperthyroidism, pregnancy, febrile states (especially in children).

G. Nitrite Many bacteria will convert nitrates to nitrite. (See also Leukocyte Esterase, below.)

Positive: Infection (A negative test does not rule out infection since some organisms such as *Streptococcus faecalis* and other gram-positive cocci will not produce nitrite, and the urine must also be retained in the bladder for several hours to allow the reaction to take place).

H. Protein Persistent proteinuria by dipstick should be quantified by 24-h urine studies.

Positive: Pyelonephritis, glomerulonephritis, Kimmelstiel-Wilson syndrome (diabetes), nephrotic syndrome, myeloma, postural causes, pre-eclampsia, inflammation and malignancies of the lower tract, functional causes (fever, stress, heavy exercise), malignant hypertension, congestive heart failure (CHF).

I. Leukocyte Esterase

Positive: Infection (false positive with vaginal contamination).

J. Reducing Substance

Positive: Glucose, fructose, galactose, false positives (vitamin C, salicylates, antibiotics, etc.).

K. Urobilinogen

Positive: Cirrhosis, congestive heart failure (CHF) with hepatic congestion, hepatitis, hyperthyroidism, suppression of gut flora with antibiotics.

Urine Sediment

Red Blood Cells (RBCs): Trauma, pyelonephritis, genitourinary TB, cystitis, prostatitis, stones, tumors (malignant and benign), coagulopathy, and any cause of blood on dipstick (see above).

White Blood Cells (WBCs): Infection anywhere in the urinary tract, TB, renal tumors, acute glomerulonephritis, radiation, interstitial nephritis (analgesic abuse).

Epithelial Cells: Acute tubular necrosis, necrotizing papillitis (most epithelial cells are from an otherwise unremarkable urethra).

Parasites: *Trichomonas vaginalis, Schistosoma haematobium.*

Yeast: *Candida albicans* (especially in diabetics, immunosuppressed patients, or if a vaginal yeast infection is present).

Spermatozoa: Normal in males immediately after intercourse or nocturnal emission.

Crystals:

Abnormal: Cystine, sulfonamide, leucine, tyrosine, cholesterol.

Normal (in small numbers)

Acid urine: Oxalate (small square crystals with a central cross), uric acid.

Alkaline urine: Calcium carbonate, triple phosphate (resemble coffin lids).

Contaminants: Cotton threads, hair, wood fibers, amorphous substances (all usually unimportant).

Mucus: Large amounts suggest urethral disease (normal from ileal conduit or other forms of urinary diversion).

Glitter Cells: White blood cells (WBCs) lysed in hypotonic solution.

Casts: The presence of casts in a urine localizes some or all of the disease process to the kidney itself.

Hyaline Cast: (Acceptable unless they are "numerous"), benign hypertension, nephrotic syndrome, after exercise.

Red Blood Cell (RBC) Cast: Acute glomerulonephritis, lupus nephritis, subacute bacterial endocarditis (SBE), Goodpasture's disease, after a streptococcal infection, vasculitis, malignant hypertension.

White Blood Cell (WBC) Cast: Pyelonephritis.

Epithelial (tubular) Cast: Tubular damage, nephrotoxin, virus.

Granular Cast: Breakdown of cellular casts, lead to waxy casts. "Dirty brown granular casts" typical for acute tubular necrosis.

TABLE II–8. URINARY INDICES.

Index	Prerenal	Renal (ATN)[1]
Urine Osmolality (mOsm/kg)	> 500	< 350
Urinary Sodium (mEq/L)	< 20	> 40
Urine/Serum Creatinine	> 40	> 20
Urine/Serum Osmolarity	> 1.2	< 1.2
Fractional Excreted Sodium (%)[2]	< 1	< 1.2
Renal Failure Index (RFI)(%)[3]	> 1	> 1

[1]*Acute tubular necrosis (intrinsic renal failure)*
[2]*Fractional excreted sodium(%)*

$$= \frac{\text{Urine Sodium / Serum Sodium}}{\text{Urine Creatinine / Serum Creatinine}} \times 100$$

[3] *Renal Failure Index (%)*

$$= \frac{\text{Urine Sodium}}{\text{Urine Creatinine / Serum Creatinine}} \times 100$$

Waxy Cast: (End-stage of granular cast). Severe chronic renal disease, amyloidosis.
Fatty Cast: Nephrotic syndrome, diabetes mellitus, damaged renal tubular epithelial cells.
Broad Cast: Chronic renal disease.

Urine, Human Chorionic Gonadotropin (HCG)

(negative)
See also Serum HCG

Positive: Pregnancy (may be positive by day 4, most positive by 14 d after expected menstrual date), testicular carcinoma (choriocarcinoma) hydatidiform mole.

Urine, Indices

Urinary indices are useful in the differential diagnosis of oliguria. They help differentiate prerenal from intrinsic renal causes (See Table II–8).

Urine, Spot (Random) Studies

The so-called spot urine is often ordered to aid in diagnosing various conditions, relying on only a small sample (10–20 mL) of urine.

Spot Urine for Electrolytes

The usefulness of this assay is limited because of large variations in daily fluid and salt intake, and the results are usually indeterminate if a diuretic has been given.

1. **Sodium < 10 mEq/L [mmol/L]:** Volume depletion, hyponatremic states, prerenal azotemia (congestive heart failure [CHF], shock, etc.), hepatorenal syndrome.
2. **Sodium > 20 mEq/L [mmol/L]:** SIADH, acute tubular necrosis (usually > 40 mEq/L).
3. **Chloride < 10 mEq/L [mmol/L]:** Chloride-sensitive metabolic alkalosis (vomiting, excessive diuretic use), volume depletion.
4. **Potassium < 10 mEq/L [mmol/L]:** Hypokalemia, potassium depletion, extrarenal loss.

Spot Urine for Protein

(Normal < 10 mg/dL [0.1 g/L] or < 20 mg/dL [0.2 g/L] for a sample taken in the early AM) (See page 328 for the differential diagnosis of protein in the urine.).

Spot Urine for Osmolality/Osmolarity

250–900 mOsm/kg [mmol/kg] (varies with water intake). Patients with normal renal function should concentrate > 800 mOsm/kg [mmol/kg] after a 14-h fluid restriction; < 400 mOsm/kg [mmol/kg] is a sign of renal impairment.

Increased: Dehydration, syndrome of inappropriate antidiuretic hormone (SIADH), adrenal insufficiency, glycosuria, high-protein diet, intraoperatively, hypovolemia, medications (cyclophosphamide, vincristine).

Decreased: Excessive fluid intake, diabetes insipidus, acute renal failure, medications (acetohexamide, lithium, others).

Spot Urine for Myoglobin

(Qualitative negative)

Positive: Skeletal muscle conditions (crush injury, electrical burns, carbon monoxide poisoning, delirium tremens, surgical procedures, malignant hyperthermia), polymyositis.

Vanillylmandelic Acid (VMA) (24-H Urine)

(< 7–9 mg/d [SI: 35–45 μmol/L])

VMA is the urinary product of both epinephrine and norepinephrine; good screening test for pheochromocytoma; also used to diagnose and follow-up neuroblastoma and ganglioneuroma.

Increased: Pheochromocytoma, other neural crest tumors (ganglioneuroma), factitious (chocolate, coffee, tea, monoamine oxidase [MAO] inhibitors, methyldopa).

VDRL Test (Venereal Disease Research Laboratory) or Rapid Plasma Reagin (RPR)

(Normal = nonreactive)

Good for screening syphilis. Almost always positive in secondary syphilis but frequently becomes negative in late syphilis. Also, in some patients with HIV infection, the VDRL can be negative in primary and secondary syphilis.

Positive (Reactive): Syphilis, systemic lupus erythematosus, pregnancy and drug addicts. If reactive, confirm with FTA-ABS (false positives with bacterial or viral illnesses).

Vitamin B_{12} (Extrinsic Factor, Cyanocobalamin)

(>100–700 pg/mL [SI: 74–516 pmol/L])

Increased: Excessive intake, myeloproliferative disorders.

Decreased: Inadequate intake (especially strict vegetarians), malabsorption, hyperthyroidism, pregnancy.

WBC (White Blood Cell Count)

(See CBC, page 286)

WBC (White Blood Cell) Morphology

The following gives conditions associated with certain changes in the normal morphology of WBCs.

- Auer Rods: Acute myelogenous leukemias.
- Döhle's Inclusion Bodies: Severe infection, burns, malignancy, pregnancy.
- Hypersegmentation: Megaloblastic anemias.
- Toxic Granulation: Severe illness (sepsis, burn, high temperature).

Zinc

(60–130 μg/dL [SI: 9–20 μmol/L]).

Increased: Atherosclerosis, coronary artery disease.

Decreased: Inadequate dietary intake (parenteral nutrition, alcoholism), malabsorption, increased needs such as pregnancy or wound healing, acrodermatitis enteropathica.

III. Bedside Procedures

Universal precautions should be used for any invasive procedure during which the operator can be exposed to potentially infectious body fluids. Not all patients infected with transmissible pathogens can be identified at the time of hospital admission or even later in their course. Because blood and body fluid-transmissible pathogens are hazardous to personnel caring for these patients (primarily at the time of invasive procedures), certain precautions are now **required for routine** care of all patients regardless of whether they have been placed on isolation precautions of any type. The CDC defines universal precautions as follows:

1. Hands must be washed before and after all patient contact.
2. Hands must be washed before and after all invasive procedures.
3. Gloves must be worn in every instance in which contact with blood is certain or likely. For example, gloves must be worn for all venipunctures, IV starts, IV manipulation, wound care, etc.
4. Gloves must be worn once and discarded. They may not be worn to perform tasks on two different patients or two different tasks at different sites on the same patient.
5. Gloves must be worn in every instance in which contact with any body fluid is likely, including urine, feces, wound secretions, respiratory tract care, thoracenteses, paracenteses, etc.
6. A gown must be worn when splattering of blood or of body fluids on clothing seems likely.
7. Additional barrier precautions may be necessary for certain invasive procedures in which significant splatter or aerosol generation seems likely. This should not occur during most routine patient care activities. It may occur in certain instances in the operating room, emergency room, the ICUs, and during invasive procedures or cardiopulmonary resuscitation. Masks should always be worn when goggles are worn and vice versa.
8. Patients should be counseled before any procedure concerning its necessity as well as its potential risks and benefits. Explaining the various steps makes the patient more cooperative and the procedure easier for both the patient and the physician. Many procedures (eg, bladder catheterization, nasogastric intubation, or venipuncture) do not require a written informed consent beyond the normal hospital sign-in protocols. Invasive procedures (eg, thoracentesis or lumbar puncture) absolutely require the patient's specific written consent for that procedure. You should check your institution's practice guidelines for more information.

9. All tubes should be clearly labeled after placement with tape and a bold marking pen to prevent inadvertent use of the tube (eg, administering tube feeds through a central venous catheter).

1. Arterial Line

(See also Section I, Problem 7, page 30)

Indications:

1. Frequent sampling of arterial blood.
2. Hemodynamic monitoring when continuous blood pressure readings are needed (eg, patient on pressors).

Materials: Prepackaged arterial line set (eg, Arrow[R]) or 20 gauge (or smaller) 1–2 in IV catheter over needle assembly (Angiocath™ or other), arterial line setup per ICU routine (transducer, tubing and pressure bag with heparinized saline), armboard, sterile dressing, povidone-iodine, 3–0 suture and instruments, lidocaine, 25 gauge needle and syringe).

Procedure:

1. The radial artery is most frequently used. Other sites, in decreasing order of preference, are the dorsalis pedis, femoral, axillary, and brachial arteries; these are used infrequently. Never puncture the radial and ulnar arteries in the same hand because this may compromise blood supply to the hand and fingers.
2. Verify the patency of the radial artery using the Allen test (see page 337) or ultrasound when concern warrants such a procedure.
3. Place the extremity on an armboard with a gauze roll behind the wrist to hyperextend the joint. Prepare the skin with povidone-iodine and drape the extremity with towels. The operator should wear gloves and a mask.
4. Raise a very small skin wheal at the puncture site with 1% lidocaine using a 25-gauge needle. Carefully palpate the artery and choose the puncture site where it appears most superficial.
5. **Standard technique:** See Figure III–1, page 336. While palpating the path of the artery with the left hand, advance the 20-gauge (preferably 2–in long) catheter over the needle assembly into the artery at a 30-degree angle to the skin. Once a "flash" of blood is seen in the hub, advance the entire unit 1–2 mm, so that the needle and catheter are in the artery. If blood flow in the hub stops, carefully pull the entire unit back until the flow is reestablished. Once the catheter is in the

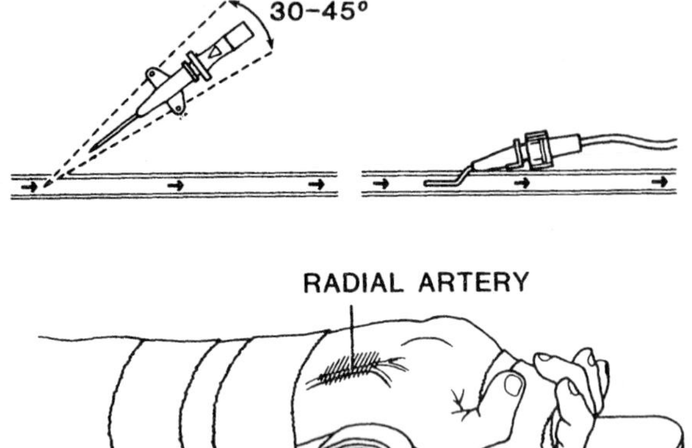

Figure III–1. Technique of radial artery catheterization. (Reproduced, with permission, from Gomella TL (editor): Arterial Access. In: *Neonatology,* 4th ed. Originally published by Appleton & Lange. Copyright © 1999 by The McGraw-Hill companies, Inc.)

artery, hold the needle steady and advance the catheter over the needle into the artery. The catheter should slide smoothly into the artery. Withdraw the needle completely and check for arterial blood flow from the catheter. Briefly occlude the artery with manual pressure while the pressure tubing is being connected.

Note: the pressure tubing system must be preflushed to clear all air bubbles before connection.

6. **Prepackaged technique:** Kits are available with a needle and guidewire that allow the Seldinger technique to be used. The entry needle is placed at a 30-degree angle to the skin site and is inserted until there is a flash of blood that rises in the catheter. The guidewire (orange handle in some kits) is inserted in the vessel, and the catheter is advanced (Seldinger technique). The wire is removed and connected to the pressure tubing.
7. **Alternative procedure ("through and through" technique):** The approach to the artery is the same as in step no. 5, however, the artery is now purposely punctured through the anterior and the posterior walls. This method is probably most useful in children and infants. Once a flash of blood is seen in the hub, the entire unit is advanced together until blood no longer fills the hub. (This can be done in a single motion). The

entire unit is then withdrawn s-l-o-w-l-y until blood starts to fill the hub. The catheter is then advanced as the needle is withdrawn. The tubing is then connected as in step no. 5.

8. Suture in place with 3–0 silk and apply a sterile dressing. Flush systems as necessary to ensure patency and also transducers to allow continuous blood pressure monitoring.

Complications: Infection, hemorrhage, thrombosis of the artery, emboli, pseudoaneurysm formation.

2. Arterial Puncture

Indications:

1. For blood gas determinations.
2. When arterial blood is needed for chemistry determinations (eg, ammonia levels).

Materials: A blood gas sampling kit or 3–5 mL syringe, 23–25-gauge needle (20–22 if femoral artery is involved), 1 mL heparin (1000 U/mL), alcohol or povidone-iodine swabs, and a cup of ice.

Procedure:

1. Use a "heparinized" syringe for blood gas and a nonheparinized syringe for chemistry determinations. "Heparinize" the syringe by drawing up about 0.5–1 mL of heparin, pulling the plunger all the way back, and then discarding the heparin. Obtain a blood gas kit (contains a pre-heparinized syringe) or a small syringe (3–5 mL) with a small-gauge needle (23–25-gauge for radial, 20–22–gauge acceptable for femoral artery).
2. Arteries in the order of preference are radial, femoral, and brachial. If using the radial artery, perform the modified **Allen test** to verify collateral flow in the ulnar artery. Have the patient make a tight fist with the hand slightly flexed. Occlude both the radial and ulnar arteries at the wrist and have the patient open his hand. While maintaining pressure on the radial artery, release the ulnar artery. If the ulnar artery is patent, the hand should flush red within 6 s. If the Allen test is positive (no radial flow), the artery should probably not be used.
3. If using the femoral artery, the mnemonic **NAVEL** aids in locating the important structures in the groin. Palpate the femoral artery just below the inguinal ligament. From lateral to medial the structures are Nerve, Artery, Vein, Empty space, Lymphatic. The clinician may inject 1% lidocaine subcutaneously for anesthesia. Palpate the artery proximally and distally with two fingers or trap the artery between two fingers placed on either side of the vessel. If using the upper extremity, hyperextension of the joint will often bring the radial and brachial arteries closer to the surface.

4. Prepare the area with either a povidone-iodine solution or alcohol swab. Hold the syringe like a pencil with the needle bevel up and enter the skin at a 60–90-degree angle. Maintain a slight negative pressure on the syringe.
5. Obtain blood on the downstroke or upon slow withdrawal. Aspirate very slowly. A good arterial sample should require only minimal backpressure. If a glass or special blood-gas syringe is used, the barrel may rise spontaneously.
6. When the vessel cannot be located, redirect the needle without its coming out of the skin. A portable Doppler probe can also be used to help locate the vessel.
7. Withdraw the needle quickly and apply firm pressure at the site for at least 5 min, even if the sample was not obtained to avoid a hematoma. Longer time may be needed for patients with elevated coagulation parameters.
8. If the sample is for a blood gas, expel any air from the syringe, mix the contents thoroughly by twirling the syringe between your fingers and make the syringe airtight with a cap. Place the syringe in an ice bath if more than a few minutes will pass before the sample is processed. Deliver promptly to the lab.

Complications: Infection, hemorrhage, thrombosis of the artery, emboli, and pseudoaneurysm formation.

3. Bladder Catheterization

(See also Section I, Problem 32, (page 132).

Indications:
1. Relieve urinary retention.
2. Collect an uncontaminated urine sample.
3. Monitor urinary output accurately.
4. Perform bladder tests (cystogram, cystometrogram).

Contraindications: Urethral disruption associated with pelvic fracture, or acute prostatitis (relative).

Materials: A prepackaged Foley catheter tray (may need to add a catheter), a drainage bag (often not part of the kit), a catheter of choice (16–20 Fr Foley in adults, 8–15 Fr in children; elbowed [coudé] catheters have a bend to allow easier passage in males; three-way catheters are usually larger 22–30 Fr to allow irrigation of fluid and clots.) See Figure III–2, page 339 for catheter description.

Procedure:
1. Place the patient in a supine position in a well-lighted area. With females, the knees are flexed wide and the heels are placed together to get adequate exposure of the meatus.

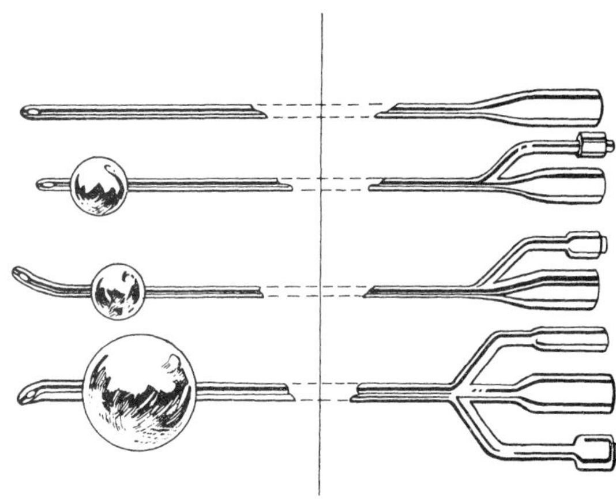

Figure III–2. Types of urethral/bladder catheters (from the top): straight Robinson catheter ("red rubber"), Foley catheter with standard 5 mL balloon, coudé ("elbow") catheter, and irrigating ("three-way") Foley catheter with 30 mL balloon. (Reproduced, with permission,m from Gomella LG (editor): *Clinician's Pocket Reference,* 9th ed., McGraw Hill. Copright © 2001.)

2. Open the kit and put on the gloves. Get all the materials ready before attempting to insert the catheter. Open the prep solution and soak the applicator balls. Apply the sterile drapes.
3. Inflate and deflate the balloon of the Foley catheter with 5–10 mL of sterile water to ensure its proper function. Coat the end of the catheter with lubricant jelly.
4. For females, use one gloved hand to prep the urethral meatus in a pubis-toward-anus direction; hold the labia apart with the other gloved hand. With uncircumcised males, retract the foreskin to prep the glands; use a gloved hand to hold the penis still.
5. Do not touch or insert the catheter with the hand used to hold the penis or labia. Disposable forceps in the kit can be used to insert the catheter, or the forceps can be used to prep, then the gloved hand can insert the catheter.
6. In the male, stretch the penis upward perpendicular to the body to eliminate any folds in the urethra that might lead to the creation of a false passage. Gentle and steady pressure should be used to advance the catheter. A slight resistance may be felt as the catheter passes the external sphincter and prostate gland. Encourage the patient to take slow deep breaths and not "bear down." Any significant resistance that

is encountered may represent a stricture or false passage and requires urologic consultation. In males with benign prostatic hypertrophy (BPH), a coudé tip catheter may facilitate the passage. Other helpful tricks to get a catheter to pass in a male are to make sure that the penis is well stretched and to instill 30–50 mL of sterile surgical lubricant into the urethra with a catheter-tipped syringe or 2% lidocaine jelly with a urethral instillation nozzle.

7. In both males and females, insert the catheter to the hilt of the drainage end. Compress the penis toward the pubis. These maneuvers help ensure that the balloon will be inflated in the bladder and not in the urethra. The balloon is inflated with 5–10 mL of sterile water or, occasionally, air (avoid using saline to fill the balloon). After inflation, pull the catheter back until the balloon rests on the bladder neck. There should be good urine return when the catheter is in place. Note: In an uncircumcised male, after the catheter is inserted, the clinician must reposition the foreskin to prevent paraphimosis and massive edema of the glans penis.
8. If no urine returns, attempt to irrigate with sterile saline and a catheter-tipped syringe. A catheter that will not irrigate may have its tip in the urethra, rather than the bladder.
9. Catheters in females can be taped to the leg. In males, the catheter should be taped to the abdominal wall to decrease urethral stricture formation.
10. If blood or clots are present, the bladder should be gently irrigated with a catheter-tipped syringe and normal saline. The Urology service should be consulted because there may have been insertion trauma (false passage) or the patient may need a three-way catheter placed to allow continuous bladder irrigation.
11. For sample collection or determination of residual urine, a straight red rubber catheter without a balloon (Robinson catheter) can be used according to the previously noted technique.

Complications: Infection, bleeding, false passage.

4. Central Venous Catheterization

(See also Section I, Problem 20, page 90 and Peripherally Inserted Central Catheters, page 367)

Indications:

1. For the administration of fluids and medications, especially when there is no peripheral access.
2. For the administration of hyperalimentation solutions.
3. For the measurement of central venous pressure (CVP).

4. As an adjunct to the placement of a pulmonary artery catheter or a transvenous pacemaker.
5. For performing acute dialysis or plasmapheresis (eg, Shiley catheter).

Materials: Minor procedure tray and instrument tray (see Table III–8, page 337), gloves, hat, mask, gown (essential for hyperalimentation lines), central venous catheter of choice (Intracath, Cordis or Swan-Ganz introducer, subclavian line, triple lumen catheters, Shiley for dialysis), IV fluid, and tubing.

Procedures: Written consent is usually necessary for this procedure, if elective. There are several different sites for inserting a "deep line," including the subclavian, internal jugular, supraclavicular, external jugular, antecubital, and femoral. The first two are those most commonly used. The subclavian site is better tolerated by conscious patients and is generally easier to maintain. Shiley catheters for dialysis are typically placed in the subclavian or femoral veins. Additional hints for catheter insertion can be found on page 134. Informed consent is usually needed for elective line placement. Coagulation studies should be available for review.

A. Subclavian Technique (Figure III–3, page 342):

1. Use sterile technique (povidone-iodine prep, gloves, mask, and a sterile field) whenever possible.
2. Place the patient flat or head down in the Trendelenburg position with the head in the center or turned to the opposite side (the "ideal" position is somewhat controversial, and is left up to the individual clinician's preference). The left subclavian vein provides a gentle curve into the superior vena cava and therefore is often the vein of choice for long lines. However, you should remember that the thoracic duct is on the left side, and the dome of the pleura rises higher on the left. It may be helpful (again a controversial point) to place a towel roll along the patient's spine.
3. Use a 25-gauge needle to make a small skin wheal with 1% lidocaine (mixed 1:1 with sodium bicarbonate 1 mEq/L helps removes the sting) 2 cm below the mid-clavicle. At this point, a larger needle (eg, 22 gauge) can be used to anesthetize the deeper tissues as well as to locate the vein.
4. Attach a large-bore, deep-line needle (a 14-gauge needle with a 16-gauge catheter at least 8–12 in long) to a 10–20-mL syringe and introduce it into the site of the skin wheal.
5. Advance the needle under the clavicle, aiming for a location halfway between the suprasternal notch and the base of the thyroid cartilage. The vein will be encountered under the clavicle, just medial to the lateral border of the clavicular head of the sternocleidomastoid muscle. In most patients

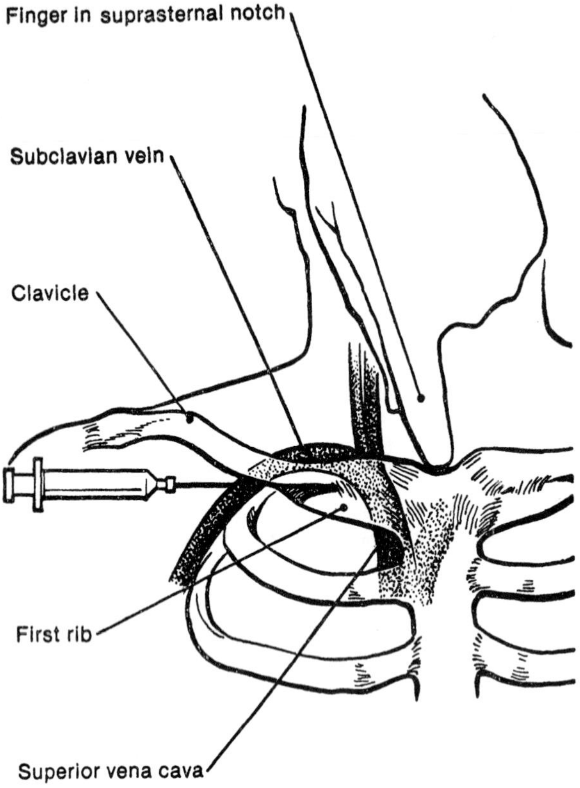

Figure III–3. The technique for subclavian vein catheterization. (Reproduced, with permission, from Gomella LG (editor): *Clinician's Pocket Reference,* 9th ed., McGraw Hill. Copyright © 2001.)

this is roughly two finger-breadths lateral to the sternal notch. Gentle pressure on the needle at the skin entrance site will assist in lowering the needle under the clavicle.

6. Apply backpressure as the needle is advanced deep to the clavicle, but above the first rib and watch for a "flash" of blood.
7. Free return of blood indicates entry into the subclavian vein. Remember that occasionally the vein is punctured through both walls, and a flash of blood may not appear as the nee-

dle is advanced. Therefore, if a free return of blood does not occur on needle advancement, the needle should be withdrawn slowly with intermittent pressure. A free return of blood will indicate the entry of the end of the needle into the lumen. Bright red blood that forcibly enters the syringe indicates that the subclavian artery has been entered. If arterial entry occurs, remove the needle. In most patients, the surrounding tissues will tamponade any bleeding from the arterial puncture. Since the artery is under the clavicle, holding pressure has little effect on bleeding.

8a. When an Intracath is being used, remove the syringe, place a finger over the needle hub, and advance the catheter an appropriate distance through the needle. Then withdraw the needle to just outside the skin and snap the protective cap over the tip of the needle.

8b. When the Seldinger wire technique is to be used, advance the wire through the needle and then withdraw the needle. The pulse rate or the ECG should be monitored during the wire passage as the wire can induce ventricular arrhythmias. You can resolve arrhythmias, should they occur, by calmly pulling the wire out several centimeters. Nick the skin with a no. 11 blade and advance the dilator approximately 5 cm; remove the dilator and advance the catheter in over the guidewire (use the brown port on the triple lumen catheter). While advancing either the dilator or the catheter over the wire, you should periodically ensure that the wire can move freely in and out. When placing a cordis introducer, the catheter and dilator are advanced over the guide wire as one unit (see page 368 under Pulmonary Artery Catheter Insertion for more details). If the wire does not move freely, it usually has kinked, and the catheter or dilator should be removed and repositioned. Maintain a firm grip on the guidewire at all times. Remove the wire and attach the IV tubing. Note that the wire used to insert a single lumen catheter is shorter than the wire supplied with the triple lumen catheter. This is most critical when exchanging a triple lumen for a single lumen catheter; the clinician must use the longer triple lumen wire and insert the wire into the brown port. Shiley catheters are placed using the Seldinger wire technique.

9. Attach the catheter to the appropriate IV solution and place the IV bottle below the level of the deep-line site to ensure a good backflow of blood into the tubing. If there is no backflow, the catheter may be kinked or is not in the proper position.

10. Securely suture the assembly in place with 2–0 or 3–0 silk. Apply an occlusive dressing with povidone-iodine ointment.

11. Obtain a chest radiograph immediately to verify placement of the catheter tip and to rule out pneumothorax. The catheter tip will ideally lie in the superior vena cava at its junction with the right atrium, at about the fifth thoracic vertebra. Catheters that go superiorly into the neck may be used only for saline infusion and not for monitoring or TPN infusion. Catheters that cannot be manipulated at the bedside into the chest usually can be repositioned properly with the aid of fluoroscopy.

B. Internal Jugular Technique (Central Approach) (Figure III–4):

1. & 2. Follow steps 1 and 2 for the subclavian technique.

3. Locate the triangle formed by the clavicle and the two heads of the sternocleidomastoid muscle. Use a 25-gauge needle and 1% lidocaine (mixed 1:1 with sodium bicarbonate 1 mEq/L removes the sting) to raise a small skin wheal at the

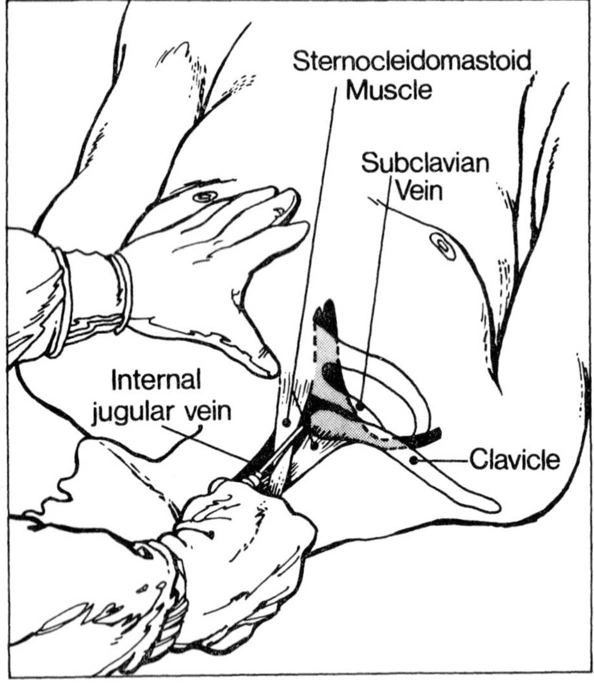

Figure III–4. The technique for internal jugular vein catheterization, central approach. (Reproduced, with permission, from Gomella LG (editor): *Clinician's Pocket Reference*, 9th ed., McGraw-Hill. Copyright © 2001.)

apex of this triangle. Change to a 22-gauge needle to anesthetize the deeper layers, and then use gentle aspiration, with the same needle, to initially locate the internal jugular vein. Some prefer to leave this needle and syringe in the vein and place the large-bore needle directly over the smaller needle, into the vein. This is commonly called the "seeker needle" technique.

4. Attach a large-bore, deep-line needle (14-gauge needle with a 16-gauge catheter at least 12 in long) to a 10–20-mL syringe. Direct the needle through the skin wheal caudally, directed toward the ipsilateral nipple and at a 30-degree angle to the frontal plane. If the vein is not entered, withdraw the needle slightly and redirect it 5–10 degrees more laterally. Apply intermittent backpressure.
5. If bright red blood forcibly fills the syringe, the carotid artery has been punctured. Remove the needle and apply firm pressure for 10 min.
6. Follow steps 8 through 11 as described for the subclavian technique.

C. Femoral Vein Approach: There are several advantages to this procedure: it is safer because arterial and venous sites are easily compressible and it is impossible to cause pneumothorax from this site. Placement can be accomplished without interrupting cardiopulmonary resuscitation. This site can be used to place a variety of intravascular appliances, including temporary pacemakers, pulmonary artery catheters (expertise with fluoroscopy is needed), and triple-lumen catheters. The major disadvantage is the high risk of sepsis and the immobilization it causes. In addition, fluoroscopy is usually required for placement of pulmonary artery catheters or transvenous pacemakers.

1. Place the patient in the supine position.
2. Use sterile preparation and appropriate draping. Administer local anesthesia in the area to be explored.
3. Palpate the femoral artery. Use the NAVEL technique (see page337) to locate the vein.
4. Guard the artery with the fingers of one hand.
5. Explore for the vein just medial to the operator's fingers with a needle and syringe.
6. It may be helpful to have a small amount of anesthetic in the syringe ready for injection during the exploration.
7. The needle is directed cephalad at about a 30-degree angle and should be inserted below the femoral crease.
8. Puncture is indicated by the return of venous, non-pulsatile blood on the application of negative pressure to the syringe.
9. Advance the guidewire through the needle.
10. The guidewire should pass with ease into the vein to a depth at which the distal tip of the guidewire is always under the op-

erator's control even when the sheath/dilator or catheter is placed over the guidewire.

11. Remove the needle once the guidewire has advanced into the femoral vein.
12. If the catheter is 6 Fr or larger, a skin incision with a scalpel blade generally is needed. The catheter can then be advanced in unison with the guidewire into the femoral vein. Be sure always to control the distal end of the guidewire.
13. Follow steps 1 through 6 for the internal jugular technique.

Complications: Pneumothorax, hemothorax, hydrothorax, arterial puncture with hematoma, catheter tip embolus, air embolus. When you suspect an air embolus, place the patient head down and turned on the left side to keep the air in the right atrium; attempt to aspirate the air through the catheter. Obtain an immediate portable chest radiograph to see if air is present in the heart.

5. Chest Tube Insertion

(See also Section I, Problem 13, page 66)

Indications:

1. Pneumothorax (simple or tension).
2. Hemothorax.
3. Hydrothorax.
4. Empyema.

Materials: Chest tube (28–36 Fr for adults; 18–28 Fr for children), water-seal drainage system (Pleurevac™, etc) with connecting tubing, minor procedure tray and instrument tray (see page 337), silk suture (0 or 2–0), Vaseline gauze.

Procedure:

1. For a pneumothorax, choose a high anterior site, such as the second or third intercostal space, midclavicular line, or subaxillary position (more cosmetic). Place a low lateral chest tube in the fifth or sixth intercostal space in the midaxillary line and directed posteriorly for fluid removal. In most patients, this location corresponds to the inframammary crease. For a traumatic pneumothorax, use a low lateral tube because this condition usually is associated with bleeding. Use a 24–28 Fr tube for pneumothorax and a 36 Fr tube for fluid removal.
2. If the procedure is elective, sedation may be helpful. Prep the area with antiseptic and drape it with towels. Use 1% lidocaine (with or without epinephrine) to anesthetize the skin and periosteum of the rib; start at the center of the rib and gently

work over the top. Remember, the neurovascular bundle runs under the rib (Figure III–5).

3. Make a 2–3-cm transverse incision over the center of the rib. Use a hemostat to bluntly dissect over the top of the rib and create a subcutaneous tunnel. Injection of additional lidocaine into the muscle will help ease the discomfort.
4. Puncture the parietal pleura with the hemostat and spread the opening. Insert a gloved finger into the pleural cavity to gently clear any clots or adhesions and to make certain the lung is not accidentally punctured by the tube.
5. Carefully insert the tube superiorly into the desired position with a hemostat or gloved finger. Make sure all the holes in the tube are in the chest cavity. Rotating the tube away from the patient's body while it is being inserted will assist in posterior placement. Attach the end of the tube to a water-seal or Pleurevac™ suction system.
6. Suture the tube in place. Place a heavy silk (0 or 2–0) suture through the incision next to the tube. Tie the incision together, then tie the ends around the chest tube. Alternatively, a purse string suture can be placed. Make sure all of the suction holes are beneath the skin before the tube is secured. An alternative technique is to secure the tube with tape and suture the tape to the skin. This is most useful for smaller chest tubes used in infants and children (Figure III–5).

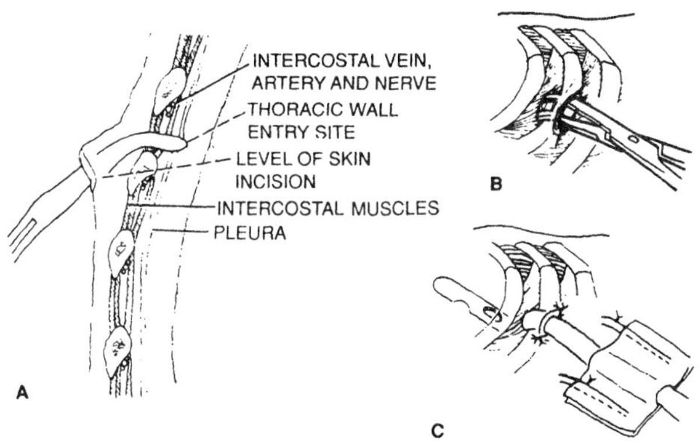

Figure III–5. Chest tube technique, demonstrating the location of the neurovascular bundle and the creation of the subcutaneous tunnel. (Reproduced, with permission, from Gomella LG (editor): Chest Tube Placement. In: *Neonatology,* 4th ed. Originally published by Appleton & Lange. Copyright © 1999 by The McGraw-Hill Companies, Inc.).

7. Wrap the tube with Vaseline gauze and cover with plain gauze. Make the dressing as airtight as possible with tape.
8. Start suction (usually –20 cm in adult; –16 cm in children) and take a chest radiograph immediately to check the placement of the tube and to evaluate for residual pneumothorax or fluid. Exercise great caution in patients with large pleural fluid collections. Rapid evacuation of large amounts of fluid can be fatal because of hypotension caused by volume shifts.
9. When a patient manifests signs of a tension pneumothorax (acute shortness of breath, hypotension, distended neck veins, tachypnea, tracheal deviation) before a chest tube is placed, urgent treatment is needed. Insert a 14-gauge needle into the chest in the second intercostal space in the midclavicular line to rapidly decompress the tension pneumothorax and proceed with chest tube insertion.
10. To remove a chest tube, make sure the pneumothorax or hemothorax is cleared. Check for an air leak by having the patient cough; observe the water-seal system for bubbling that indicates either a system (tubing leak) or a persistent pleural air leak.
11. Take the tube off suction **but not off water seal** and cut the retention suture. Have the patient perform the Valsalva maneuver while the clinician applies pressure with Vaseline gauze and 4 x 4 gauze squares or Tegaderm. Pull the tube rapidly and make an airtight seal with tape. Check an upright chest radiograph for pneumothorax.

Complications: Infection, bleeding, lung damage, subcutaneous emphysema, persistent pneumothorax or fluid collection, poor tube placement, liver injury, splenic injury, post-procedure shock.

6. Cricothyrotomy (Needle and Surgical)

Indications: Mechanical ventilation is indicated, but an endotracheal tube cannot be placed (eg, severe maxillofacial trauma, excessive oropharyngeal hemorrhage).

Contraindications: Surgical cricothyrotomy is contraindicated in children younger than 12 years.

Materials:

Needle Cricothyrotomy: 12–14-gauge catheter over needle (Angiocath or Jelco), 6–12-mL syringe, 3-mm pediatric endotracheal tube adapter, oxygen connecting tubing, high-flow oxygen source (tank or wall).

Surgical Cricothyrotomy (Minimum Requirements): Povidone-iodine solution, sterile gauze pads, scalpel handle and blade (No. 10 preferred), hemostat (optional), No. 5 to No. 7 tracheostomy tube, tracheostomy tube adapter to connect to bag-mask ventilator. (Often it is easier to place a 5–7-mm endotracheal tube rather than a tracheostomy tube.)

Procedures:

A. Needle Cricothyrotomy:

1. Palpate the cricothyroid membrane, which resembles a notch located between the caudal end of the thyroid cartilage and the first tracheal ring (also called the cricoid cartilage).
2. Prep the area with povidone-iodine solution. Local anesthesia can be used if the patient is awake.
3. Mount the syringe on the 12 or 14-gauge catheter over the needle assembly, and advance through the cricothyroid membrane at a 45-degree angle, applying backpressure on the syringe until air is aspirated.
4. Advance the catheter and remove the needle. Attach the hub to a 3-mm endotracheal tube adapter, which is connected to the oxygen tubing. Allow the oxygen to flow at 15 L/min for 1–2 s on, then 4 s off by using a "Y-connector" or a hole in the side of the tubing to turn the flow on and off.
5. The needle technique is only useful for about 45 min because the exhalation of CO_2 is suboptimal.

B. Surgical Cricothyrotomy:

1. **& 2.** Follow steps 1 and 2 for needle cricothyrotomy.
3. While stabilizing the trachea with the nondominant hand by holding the thyroid cartilage, a no. 11-blade scalpel is used to penetrate the skin and membrane in one move. Care should be taken not to injure the posterior wall of the trachea with the blade. The blade is then moved horizontally, incising the skin and membrane simultaneously for 2 cm. The handle of the knife can then be placed into the wound and turned 90 degrees to dilate the opening.
4. Insert a small (5–7 mm) tracheostomy tube or a 5–7-mm endotracheal tube, inflate the balloon (if present), and secure it in position with the attached cotton tapes.
5. A surgical cricothyrotomy may be left in place for up to 1 wk with minimal complications. When a long-term intubation is contemplated, it may be converted to a formal tracheostomy in the operating room.

Complications: Bleeding, esophageal perforation, subcutaneous emphysema, pneumomediastinum and thorax, CO_2 retention (especially with the needle procedure).

7. Endotracheal Intubation

Indications:

1. For airway management during cardiopulmonary resuscitation.
2. When there is any indication for using mechanical ventilation (coma, surgery, etc).
3. When "better to intubate 24 h too early than 5 min too late" applies to the situation.

Contraindications: Massive maxillofacial trauma, fractured larynx, suspected cervical spinal cord injury.

Materials: Endotracheal tube (see Table III–1, page 351), laryngoscope handle and blade (straight or curved, No. 3 for adults, No. 1–1.5 for small children), 10-mL syringe, adhesive tape, suction equipment, malleable stylet (optional).

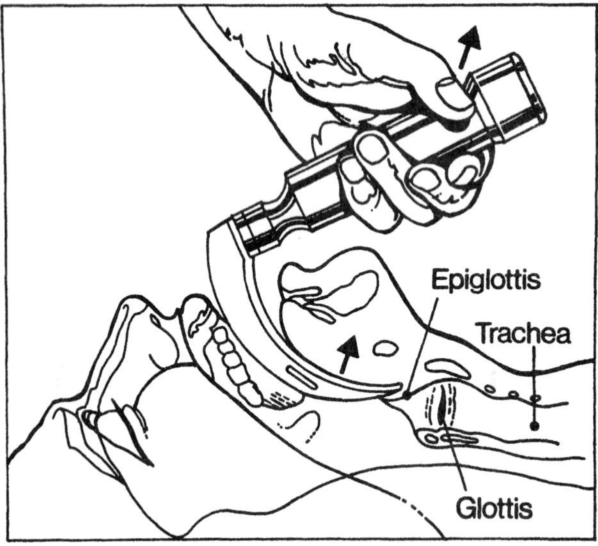

Figure III–6. Endotracheal intubation using a curved laryngoscope blade. (Reproduced, with permission, from Gomella LG (editor): *Clinician's Pocket Reference,* 8th ed., Appleton & Lange. Copright © 1997.)

TABLE III–1. RECOMMENDED ENDOTRACHEAL TUBE SIZES.

Patient	Internal Diameter (mm)
Premature infant	2.5–3.0 (uncuffed)
Newborn infant	3.5 (uncuffed)
3–12 months	4.0 (uncuffed)
1–8 years	4.0–6.0 (uncuffed)[1]
8–16 years	6.0–7.0 (cuffed)
Adult	7.0–9.0 (cuffed)

[1]Rough estimate is to measure the patient's little finger.

Procedure:

1. Orotracheal intubation is most commonly used. The use of orotracheal intubation should be done with great care in any patient with possible cervical spine trauma. Two people are required, one to intubate, and one to hold constant in-line traction. Some clinicians opt for nasotracheal intubation in such instances.
2. Any patient who is hypoxic or apneic must be ventilated before attempting endotracheal intubation (bag-mask or mouth-to-mask). Remember to avoid prolonged periods of no ventilation if the intubation is difficult.
3. Extend the laryngoscope blade to 90 degrees to verify the light is working and check the balloon on the tube (if present) for leaks.
4. Place the patient's head in the "sniffing position" (neck extended anteriorly and the head extended posteriorly). Use suction to clear the upper airway if needed.
5. Hold the laryngoscope in the left hand, hold the mouth open with the right hand, and use the blade to push the tongue to the patient's left, and make certain the tongue remains anterior to the blade. Advance carefully toward the midline until the epiglottis is seen.
6. If a straight laryngoscope blade is passed under the epiglottis, the blade can then be lifted upward, and the vocal cords visualized. If a curved blade is used, it is placed anterior to the epiglottis and gently lifted anteriorly. The handle should not be used to pry the epiglottis open, but rather gently lifted in both cases (Figure III–6).
7. While maintaining visualization of the cords, the tube is grasped in the right hand and passed through the cords. With more difficult intubations, the malleable stylet can be used to direct the tube.

8. When using a cuffed tube (adult and older children), gently inflate with a 10-m L syringe until there is an adequate seal (about 5 mL). Ventilate the patient while auscultating and visualizing both sides of the chest to verify positioning. If the left side does not seem to be ventilating, it may signify that the tube has been advanced down the right mainstem bronchus. Withdraw the tube 1–2 cm and recheck the breath sounds. An end-tidal CO_2 detector may be attached to the endotracheal tube to further confirm tracheal intubation. Verify positioning with an immediate chest radiograph. The end of the endotracheal tube should lie approximately 3 cm below the cords and 3 cm above the carina.
9. Tape the tube in position and insert an oropharyngeal airway to prevent the patient from biting the tube.

Complications: Bleeding, oral or pharyngeal trauma, improper tube positioning (esophageal intubation, right mainstem bronchus), aspiration, tube obstruction or kinking.

8. Gastrointestinal Tubes

(See also Section I, Problems 54 and 55, pages 209, 211, respectively).

Indications:

1. For gastrointestinal decompression (ileus, obstruction, pancreatitis, postoperatively).
2. For lavage of the stomach with gastrointestinal bleeding or drug overdose.
3. For prevention of aspiration in an obtunded patient.
4. For feeding a patient who is unable to swallow.

Materials: Gastrointestinal tube of choice (see below), lubricant jelly, catheter tip syringe, glass of water with a straw, stethoscope.

Types of Gastrointestinal Tubes:

A. Nasogastric Tubes:

1. **Levin tube:** Single lumen tube that must be placed on intermittent suction to evacuate gastric contents.
2. **Salem-sump tube:** A double lumen tube, with the smaller tube acting as an air intake vent. Use 14–18 Fr size in adults-the best tube for continuous suction.
3. **Ewald tube:** Large (18–36 Fr) double lumen tube, especially suited for gastric lavage of drug overdose, more often inserted by the orogastric route.

B. Intestinal Tubes: These tubes are mentioned mainly for historical interest. No study has shown these types of tubes to be superior to dual-lumen sump tubes in the treatment of small-bowel obstruction, even for distal obstructions. In addition, they require the instillation of mercury, which can be difficult to handle; mercury spills are hazardous and require special measures to clean.

1. **Cantor tube:** A long single lumen tube with a rubber balloon at the tip. The balloon is partially filled with mercury (3–5 mL), which allows it to gravitate into the small bowel with the aid of peristalsis.
2. **Miller-Abbott tube:** A long double lumen tube with a rubber balloon at the tip. One lumen is used for aspiration; the other is connected to the balloon. After the tube is in the stomach, it is inflated with 5–10 mL of air, 2–3 mL of mercury is injected, and then the air is aspirated.
3. **Dennis, Baker, Leonard tubes:** These are used for intraoperative decompression of the bowel and are manually passed into the bowel at the time of laparotomy.

C. Feeding Tubes: Although any small bore nasogastric tube can be used as a feeding tube, certain weighted tubes are designed to pass into the duodenum and decrease the risk of aspiration of gastric contents.

1. **Dobbhoff, Entriflex, Keogh tubes:** Weighted mercury tip with stylet.
2. **Vivonex:** Tungsten tipped.

D. Sengstaken-Blakemore tube: A triple lumen tube used exclusively for the control of bleeding esophageal varices by tamponade. One lumen is for aspiration, one is for the gastric balloon, and the third is for the esophageal balloon. Be sure to read the accompanying instruction manual before placing the tube!

Procedure (General outline for most nasogastric tubes):

1. Inform the patient about the procedure and encourage cooperation, when the patient is able to do so. Choose the nasal passage that appears to be most open.
2. Lubricate the distal 3–4 in of the tube with a water-soluble jelly (K-Y jelly or viscous 2% lidocaine) and insert the tube gently along the floor of the nasal passageway. Maintain gentle pressure that will allow the tube to pass into the nasopharynx.
3. When the patient can feel the tube in the back of the throat, ask the patient to swallow small amounts of water (if PO fluids are allowed) through a straw as you advance the tube 2–3 in at a time.
4. To be sure that the tube is in the stomach, aspirate gastric contents or blow air into the tube and listen over the stomach with a stethoscope for a "pop" or "gurgle."

5. Attach one lumen of the dual-lumen sump tube (eg, Salem-sump) to continuous low wall suction and the single lumen tube (Levin) to intermittent suction.
6. Feeding tubes and pediatric feeding tubes in adults are more difficult to insert because they are more flexible. Many are provided with stylets that make their passage easier. Feeding tubes are best placed into the duodenum or jejunum to decrease the risk of aspiration. Administering 10 mg of metoclopramide intravenously 10 min before insertion of the tube will assist in placing the tube into the duodenum.
7. Once the feeding tube is in the stomach, the bell of the stethoscope can be placed on the right side of the patient's mid-abdomen. As the tube is advanced, air can be injected to confirm progression of the tube to the right, toward the duodenum. If the sound of the air becomes more faint, the tube is probably curling in the stomach. Pass the tube until a slight resistance is felt, indicating the presence of the tip of the tube at the pylorus. Holding constant pressure and slowly injecting water through the tube is often rewarded with a "give" that signifies its passage through the pylorus. The tube often can be advanced far into the duodenum with this method. The duodenum usually provides constant resistance which will "give" with a slow injection of water. Placing the patient in the right lateral decubitus position may help the tube enter the duodenum. Always confirm the location of the tube with an abdominal radiograph.
8. Tape the tube securely in place but do not allow it to apply pressure to the ala of the nose. Patients have been disfigured because of ischemic necrosis of the nose caused by a poorly positioned tube.
9. A chest radiograph must be obtained before starting any feeding through a tube to verify its placement in the stomach.

Complications: Inadvertent passage into the trachea (life-threatening if feedings are administered into the lung), coiling of the tube in the mouth or pharynx, bleeding in the mucosa of the nose, pharynx, or stomach.

9. IV Techniques, Peripheral

(See Section I, Problem 52, page 203)

Indications: To establish a routine IV access for the administration of fluids, blood, or medications.

Materials: IV fluid, connecting tubing, a tourniquet, an alcohol swab, intravenous cannulas (a catheter over a needle, such as

Angiocath, Jelco, or a butterfly needle), antiseptic ointment, dressing, and tape. Note: It helps to rip the tape into strips and to flush the air out of the tubing before beginning.

Procedure:

1. Verify before starting that there are no relative contraindications for using an extremity for an IV. Contraindications include a recent axillary node dissection and a planned or recently placed AV-fistula or graft. The upper, nondominant extremity is usually the site of choice for an IV. Choose a distal vein so that if the vein is lost, you can reposition the IV more proximally. Avoid veins that cross a joint space. Also avoid inserting an IV into the leg, because of the high incidence of thrombophlebitis. If no extremity vein can be found, try the external jugular. If all these fail, the only alternatives are a deep line or a venous cutdown (see page 377).
2. Apply a tourniquet above the proposed IV site. Techniques to help expose veins that are difficult to locate include (1) wrapping the extremity in a warm towel, (2) leaving the arm in a dependent position for a few minutes after the tourniquet is applied, or (3) using a blood pressure cuff as a tourniquet inflated as much as possible without obstructing arterial inflow. (See Section I, Problem 20 for a more complete discussion of the patient with a difficult IV access.). Carefully clean the site with an alcohol or povidone-iodine swab. If a large-bore IV is to be used (16 or 14 Fr), local anesthesia with 1% lidocaine is helpful.
3. Stabilize the vein distally with the thumb of your free hand. Using the catheter over the needle assembly (Intracath or Angiocath), either enter the vein directly or enter the skin alongside the vein first, and then stick the vein along the side at about a 20-degree angle. Once the vein is punctured, blood should appear in the "flash chamber." Advance a few more millimeters to be sure that both the needle and the tip of the catheter have entered the vein. Carefully withdraw the needle as you advance the catheter into the vein. **Caution: Never withdraw the catheter over the needle because the plastic tip can be sheared off and cause a catheter embolus.** Apply pressure with your thumb over the vein just proximal to the site to prevent significant blood loss while you connect the IV line to the catheter.
4. Observe the site with the IV fluid running for signs of induration or swelling that indicate improper placement or damage to the vein.
5. Tape the IV securely in place, apply a drop of povidone-iodine or antibiotic ointment, and a sterile dressing. Ideally, the dressing should be changed every 24–48 h to help reduce in-

fections. Armboards are also useful to help maintain an IV site.

6. When the veins are deep and difficult to locate, a small 3–5-mL syringe can be mounted on the catheter assembly. The proper position inside the vein is determined by the aspiration of blood.
7. If venous access is limited, a "butterfly" needle can sometimes be used, or the external jugular may be considered as a site for catheter placement.

10. Joint Aspiration (Arthrocentesis)

Indications:

1. **Diagnostic:** Arthrocentesis is helpful in the diagnosis of new-onset arthritis; it also may be useful to rule out infection in acute or chronic, unremitting joint effusion.
2. **Therapeutic:** Arthrocentesis can be useful to instill steroids and maintain drainage of septic arthritis.

Materials: A minor procedure tray (Table III–8, page 377) 18 or 20-gauge needle (smaller for a finger or toe); ethyl chloride spray can be substituted for lidocaine; two heparinized tubes for cell count and crystal examination; colleagues in your microbiology lab can be consulted to determine their preference for transporting fluid for bacterial, fungal, acid-fast bacillus (AFB) culture, and Gram's stain. A Thayer-Martin plate is needed when *Neisseria gonorrhoeae* is suspected. A small syringe containing a long-acting corticosteroid, eg, Depo-Medrol or triamcinolone, is optional for therapeutic arthrocentesis.

Procedures:

A. General:

1. Obtain a consent form describing the procedure and review the possible complications.
2. Determine the optimal site for aspiration and mark the site with indelible ink.
3. When aspiration is to be followed by corticosteroid injection, maintain a sterile field with sterile implements to minimize the risk of infection to the patient.
4. Clean the area with Betadine, dry, and wipe over the aspiration site with alcohol. Betadine can render cultures negative. Let the alcohol dry before beginning the procedure.
5. Anesthetize the area with lidocaine using a 25-gauge needle, taking care not to inject into the joint space. Lidocaine is bactericidal. Avoid preparations containing epinephrine, especially in a small digit. Alternatively, spray the area with ethyl chloride just before needle aspiration.

6. Insert the aspirating needle, applying a small amount of vacuum to the syringe. Remove as much fluid as possible, repositioning the syringe if necessary.
7. When a corticosteroid is to be injected, remove the aspirating syringe from the needle that is still in the joint space. It is helpful to ensure that the syringe can be removed easily from the needle before performing the previous step
8. Attach the syringe containing the corticosteroid, pull back on the plunger to ensure the syringe is not in a vein and inject the contents. **Never inject steroids when there is any possibility of an infected joint.** Remove the needle and apply pressure to the area. Generally, the equivalent of 40 mg of methylprednisolone is injected into large joints, such as the knee, and 20 mg into medium-sized joints, such as the ankle or wrist.
9. Send the joint fluid for cell count and differential, crystal exam, Gram's stain, and cultures for bacteria, fungi and AFB, as indicated.

B. Specific Sites:

1. **Arthrocentesis of the knee:**
   a. The knee should be fully extended with the patient supine. Wait until the patient has a relaxed quadriceps muscle, because its contraction plants the patella against the femur, making aspiration painful.
   b. Insert the needle posterior to the medial portion of the patella into the patellar-femoral groove. Direct the advancing needle slightly posteriorly and inferiorly (Figure III–7A).
2. **Arthrocentesis of the wrist:**
   a. The easiest site for aspiration is between the navicular bone and the radius on the dorsal wrist. Locate the distal radius between the tendons of the extensor pollicus longus and the extensor carpi radialis longus to the second finger. This site is just ulnar to the anatomic snuff box. Mark the site, and direct the needle perpendicular to the mark (Figure III–7B).
3. **Arthrocentesis of the ankle:**
   a. The most accessible site is between the tibia and the talus. The angle of the foot to the leg is positioned at 90 degrees. Make a mark lateral and anterior to the medial malleolus and medial and posterior to the tibialis anterior tendon. The advancing needle is directed posteriorly toward the heel.
   b. The subtalar ankle joint does not communicate with the ankle joint and is difficult to aspirate even by an expert. You should be aware that "ankle pain" may originate in the subtalar joint rather than in the ankle (Figure III–7C).

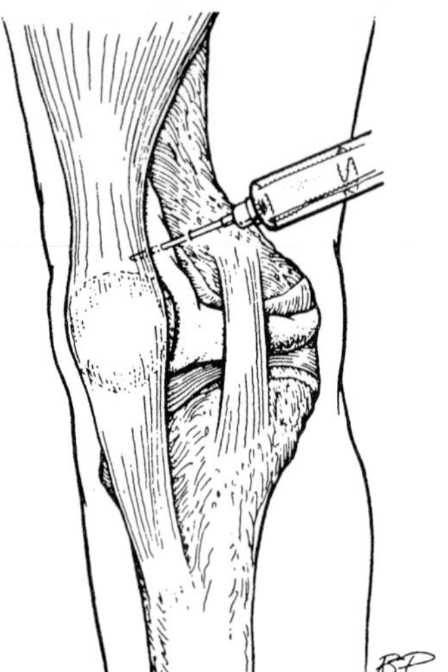

A

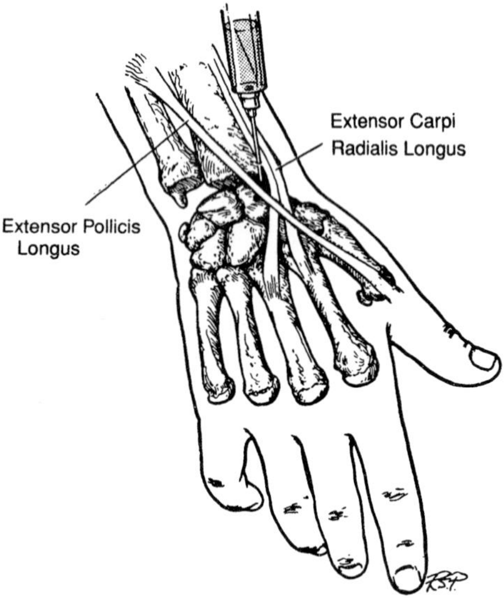

Extensor Carpi Radialis Longus

Extensor Pollicis Longus

B

Figure III–7A: Arthrocentesis of the knee. **7B:** Arthrocentesis of the wrist. **7C:** Arthrocentesis of the ankle. (Reproduced, with permission, from Haist SA et al editors): Internal Medicine On-Call, 2nd ed. Originally published by Appleton & Lange. Copyright © 1997 by the McGraw-Hill Companies, Inc.)

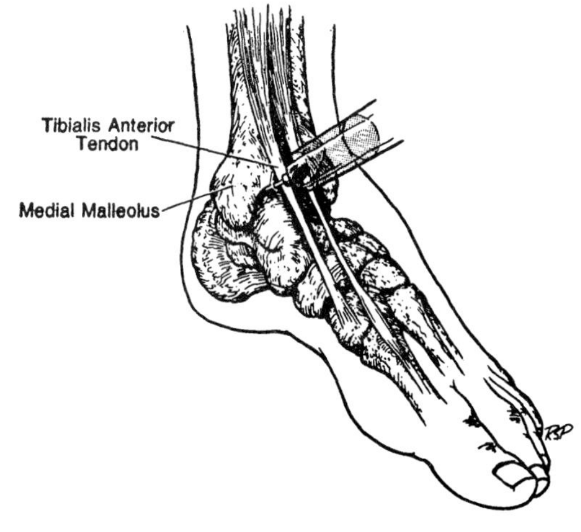

Figure III–7. *(continued)*

Synovial Fluid Interpretation

A. Differential Diagnosis:

1. Noninflammatory Arthritis: Traumatic tap, lupus, rheumatic fever.
2. Inflammatory Arthritis: Osteoarthritis, gout, pseudogout, rheumatoid arthritis.
3. Septic Arthritis: *Staphylococcus aureus* and *Neisseria gonorrhoeae* are most common.

B. Laboratory Data from Joint Fluid:

1. Total WBC: Normal, 0–300/μL; 300–2000, noninflammatory; 2000–75,000, inflammatory; > 100,000, septic arthritis.
2. WBC Differential: Normal, < 25% neutrophils; > 50% neutrophils, inflammatory; > 90% neutrophils, septic; > 2% eosinophils suggests Lyme disease.
3. Uric Acid: Normal, < 8 mg/dL.
4. Microscopic: Normal, no debris, crystals or bacteria; urate, gout; calcium pyrophosphate, pseudogout; bacteria, septic (33% of cases of septic arthritis may be initially negative).

Complications: Infection, bleeding, pain. Post-injection flare of joint pain and swelling can occur after steroid injection and persist up to 24 h. This complication is believed to be a crystal-induced synovitis, resulting from the crystalline suspension used in long-acting steroids.

11. Lumbar Puncture

Indications:

1. For diagnostic purposes (analysis of cerebrospinal fluid [CSF]).
2. For measurement of CSF pressure.
3. For injection of various agents (contrast media, chemotherapy).

Contraindications: Increased intracranial pressure, (papilledema, mass lesion), infection near the puncture site, planned myelography or pneumoencephalography, coagulopathy.

Materials: A sterile, disposable LP kit or minor procedure tray (see Table III–8, page 377), spinal needles (20–21 gauge for adults, 22 gauge for children), and sterile specimen tubes.

Procedure:

1. Examine the visual fields for evidence of papilledema, and review the CT scan of the head, if available. Discuss the procedure with the patient to dispel any myths. Some prefer to call the procedure a "subarachnoid analysis" rather than a spinal tap. Obtain informed consent from the patient or legal representative.
2. Place the patient in the lateral decubitus position close to the edge of the bed or table. The patient (held by an assistant, if possible) should be positioned with the knees pulled up toward the abdomen and the head flexed onto the chest. This enhances flexion of the vertebral spine and widens the interspaces between the spinous processes. Place a pillow beneath the patient's side to prevent sagging and ensure alignment of the spinal column. In an obese patient or a patient with arthritis or scoliosis, the sitting position or leaning forward may be preferred.
3. Draw an imaginary line between the iliac crests. This should cross the spine at the L4 vertebral body and assist in locating the L4–L5 interspace.
4. Open the kit, put on sterile gloves, and prep the area with povidone-iodine solution in a circular fashion, covering several interspaces. Next, drape the patient.
5. Using a 25-gauge needle and 1% lidocaine, raise a skin wheal over the L4–L5 interspace. Anesthetize the deeper structures with a 22-gauge needle.

6. Examine the spinal needle with stylet for defects and then insert it into the skin wheal and into the spinous ligament. Hold the needle between your index and middle fingers, with your thumb holding the stylet in place. Direct the needle cephalad at a 30–45-degree angle in the midline and parallel to the bed.
7. Advance through the major structures and "pop" into the subarachnoid space through the dura. An experienced operator can feel these layers, but an inexperienced one may need to periodically remove the obturator to look for the return of fluid. Direct the bevel of the needle parallel to the long axis of the body so that the dural fibers are separated rather than sheared; this method helps cut down on "spinal headaches."
8. If no fluid returns, it is sometimes helpful to rotate the needle slightly. When still no fluid appears, and you think that you are within the subarachnoid space, 1 mL of air can be injected, because it is not uncommon for a piece of tissue to clog the needle. **Never inject saline or distilled water.** If no air returns and if spinal fluid cannot be aspirated, the bevel of the needle probably lies in the epidural space; advance it with the stylet into place.
9. When fluid returns, attach a manometer and stopcock and measure the pressure. Normal opening pressure is 70–180 mm water. Increased pressure may be the result of a tense patient, CHF, ascites, subarachnoid hemorrhage, infection, or a space-occupying lesion. Decreased pressure may result from needle position or obstructed flow (you may need to leave the needle in for a myelogram, because if it is moved, the subarachnoid space may be lost).
10. Collect 0.5–2.0 mL samples in serial, labeled containers. Send them to the lab in the following order:

    1st tube for bacteriology: Gram's stain, routine culture and sensitivity (C&S), acid-fast bacilli (AFB), and fungal cultures and stains.

    2nd tube for glucose and protein.

    3rd tube for cell count: CBC with differential.

    4th tube for special studies: VDRL test, etc.

    Note: Some prefer to send the first and last tubes for CBC because this procedure permits a better differentiation between a subarachnoid hemorrhage and a traumatic tap. In a traumatic tap, the number of red blood cells in the first tube should be much higher than in the last tube. In a subarachnoid hemorrhage, the cell counts should be equal, and xanthochromia of the fluid should be present, indicating the presence of old blood.
11. Withdraw the needle and place a sterile dressing over the site.

12. Instruct the patient to remain recumbent for 6–12 h and encourage an increased fluid intake to help prevent spinal head-aches. Interpret the results on the basis of Table III–2.

Complications: Spinal headache is the most common complication and is seen about 20% of the time. It typically goes away when the patient is lying down and is aggravated when sitting up. To help prevent spinal headaches, keep the patient recumbent for 6–12 h, encourage the intake of fluids, use the smallest needle possible, and keep the bevel of the needle parallel to the long axis of the body to help prevent a persistent CSF leak. Other complications include trauma to nerve roots, herniation of either the cerebellum or the medulla, and meningitis.

12. Nasal Packing

(See page 119).

TABLE III–2. DIFFERENTIAL DIAGNOSIS OF CEREBROSPINAL FLUID.

Condition	Color	Opening Pressure (mmH_2O)	Protein (mg/100mL)	Glucose (mg/100mL)	Cells (#/mL)
Adult (normal)	Clear	70–180	15–45	45–80	0–5 lymphs
Newborn (normal)	Clear	70–180	20–120	2/3 serum Glucose	40–60 lymphs
Viral infection	Clear or opalescent	Normal or slightly increased	Normal or slightly increased	Normal	10–500 lymphs (polys early)
Bacterial infection	Opalescent or yellow, may clot	Increased	50–1500	<, usually <20	25–10,000 polys
Granulomatous (TB, fungal)	Clear or opalescent	Often >	>, but usually <500	<, usually 20–40	10–500 lymphs
Subarachnoid hemorrhage	Bloody or xanthochromic after 2–8 hr	Usually>	>	Normal	WBC/RBC[1] ratio same as blood

[1]WBC = white blood cell; RBC = red blood cell.

13. Paracentesis (Peritoneal)

Indications:

1. To determine the cause of ascites.
2. To determine if intra-abdominal bleeding is present, or if a viscus has ruptured. Diagnostic peritoneal lavage is considered a more accurate test.
3. Therapeutic removal of fluid (eg, respiratory distress).

Contraindications: Abnormal coagulation factors, uncertainty whether distention is due to peritoneal fluid or to a cystic structure (ultrasound can often differentiate these).

Materials: A minor procedure tray (see Table III–8, page 377), a catheter over needle IV needle (18–20 gauge with a 1½-in needle), a 20–60 mL syringe, sterile specimen containers.

Procedure:

1. Obtain an informed consent. Have the patient empty the bladder.
2. The entry site is usually the midline 3–4 cm below the umbilicus. Avoid old surgical scars, because the bowel may be clinging to the abdominal wall. Alternatively, the entry site can be in the left or right lower quadrant midway between the umbilicus and the anterior superior iliac spine or in the patient's flank, ultrasound may help to identify a "safe" spot..
3. Prep and drape the patient. Raise a skin wheal with 1% lidocaine over the proposed entry site.
4. With the Angiocath mounted on the syringe, go through the anesthetized area carefully while gently aspirating. You will meet some resistance as you enter the fascia. When you get free return of fluid, leave the catheter in place, remove the needle, and begin to aspirate. Sometimes it is necessary to reposition the catheter because of an abutting bowel.
5. Aspirate the amount needed for tests (20–30 mL). For a therapeutic tap, do not remove more than 500 mL in 10 min. One liter is the maximum that should be removed at one time.
6. Quickly remove the needle, apply a sterile 4 x 4 gauze square, and apply pressure with tape.
7. Depending on the clinical picture of the patient, send samples for total protein, specific gravity, lactate dehydrogenase (LDH), amylase, cytology, culture, stains, CBC, or food fibers. See Table III–3 for the differential diagnosis of the fluid obtained.

Complications: Peritonitis, perforated viscus, hemorrhage, precipitation of hepatic coma if patient has severe liver disease, oliguria, hypotension.

TABLE III–3. DIFFERENTIAL DIAGNOSIS OF ASCITIC FLUID. TRANSUDATIVE ASCITES: CIRRHOSIS, NEPHROSIS, CONGESTIVE HEART FAILURE. **EXUDATIVE ASCITES:** MALIGNANCY, PERITONITIS (TB, PERFORATED VISCUS), HYPOALBUMINEMIA.

Lab Value	Transudate	Exudate
Specific gravity	<1.016	>1.016
Protein (Ascitic fluid)	<3 gm/100 mL	> 3 gm/100 mL
Protein (Ascitic to serum ratio)	<0.5	>0.5
LDH (Ascitic to serum ration)	<0.6	>0.6
Ascitic fluid LDH	<200 IU	>200 IU
Glucose (Serum to ascitic ratio)	<1	>1
Fibrinogen (Clot)	No	Yes
White blood cells	<500/μL	>1000/μ
Red blood cells		>100 RBC/μL

Food fibers: [Found in most causes of a perforated viscus.]
Cytology: [Bizarre cells with large nuclei may represent reactive mesothelial cells and not a malignancy; malignant cells suggest a tumor.]

14. Pericardiocentesis

Indications: For emergency treatment of cardiac tamponade (see Figure III–8, pages 365), to diagnose pericardial effusion.

Materials: Electrocardiogram machine, procedure and instrument tray (see Table III–8, page 377), a pericardiocentesis needle or a 16–18-gauge needle 10 cm long.

Procedure:

1. If time permits, use sterile prep and drape with gown, mask, and gloves.
2. The approach to drainage of pericardiocentesis can be either left paraxiphoid or through a left parasternal fourth intercostal approach. The paraxiphoid is more commonly used (see Figure III–8).
3. Anesthetize the insertion site with lidocaine. Connect the needle with an alligator clip to lead V on the ECG machine. Attach the limb leads and monitor the machine.
4. Insert the pericardiocentesis needle just to the left of the xiphoid and direct it upward 45 degrees toward the left shoulder.
5. Aspirate while advancing the needle until the pericardium is punctured and the effusion is tapped. If the ventricular wall is felt, withdraw the needle slightly. Additionally, if the needle contacts the myocardium, pronounced ST segment elevation will be noted on the ECG.

6. When the procedure is performed for cardiac tamponade, the removal of as little as 50 mL of fluid may dramatically improve blood pressure.
7. Blood from a bloody pericardial effusion is usually defibrinated and will not clot, whereas blood from the ventricle will clot.
8. Send fluid to the lab for hematocrit, cell count, or cytology, if indicated. Serous fluid is consistent with CHF, bacterial, tuberculous, hypoalbuminemia or viral pericarditis. Bloody fluid (Hct > 10%) may be traumatic or iatrogenic, or can be the result of an MI, uremia, coagulopathy, or a malignancy (lymphoma, leukemia, breast, and lung are most common).

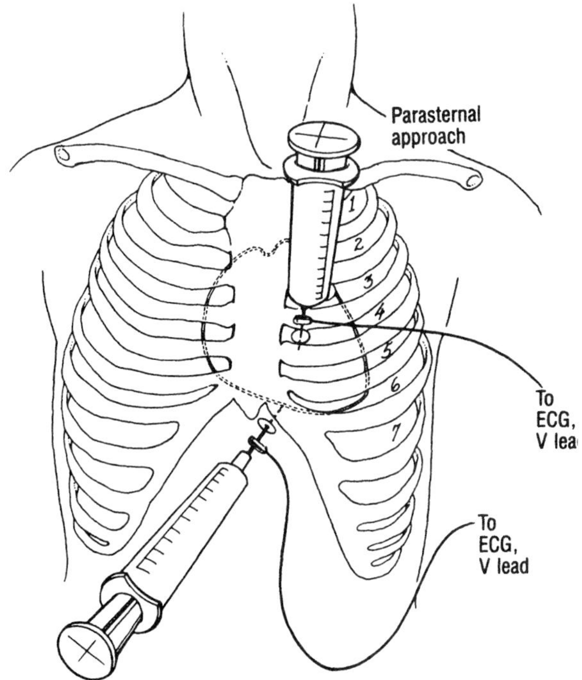

Figure III–8. Techniques for pericardiocentesis. The paraxiphoid approach is the most popular. (Reproduced, with permission, from Stillman RM (editor): *Surgery, Diagnosis, and Therapy*. Originally published by Appleton & Lange. Copyright © 1989 by The McGraw-Hill Companies, Inc.)

Complications: Arrhythmia, ventricular puncture, lung injury.

15. Peritoneal Lavage (Diagnostic Peritoneal Lavage)

Indications:

1. Evaluation of intra-abdominal trauma (bleeding, perforation).
2. Acute peritoneal dialysis.

Contraindications: None are absolute. Relative contraindications include multiple abdominal procedures, pregnancy, and any coagulopathy.

Materials: Prepackaged diagnostic peritoneal lavage or peritoneal dialysis tray.

Procedure:

1. For a diagnostic peritoneal lavage (DPL), a Foley catheter and an NG tube must be in place. Prep the abdomen from above the umbilicus to the pubis. Wear gloves and mask.
2. The site of choice is in the midline 1–2 cm below the umbilicus. Avoid the site of old surgical scars (danger of adherent bowel). When a subumbilical scar or pelvic fracture is present, a supraumbilical approach is preferred.
3. Infiltrate the skin with 1% lidocaine with epinephrine. Incise the skin in the midline vertically and expose the fascia.
4. Pick up the fascia and either incise it or puncture it with the trocar and peritoneal catheter. Caution is needed to avoid puncturing any viscera. Use one hand to hold the catheter near the skin and to control the insertion while the other hand applies pressure to the end of the catheter. After entering the peritoneal cavity, remove the trocar and direct the catheter inferiorly into the pelvis.
5. For a diagnostic lavage, gross blood indicates a positive tap. If no blood is encountered, instill 10 mL/kg (about 1 L in adults) of lactated Ringer's solution or normal saline into the abdominal cavity.
6. Gently agitate the abdomen to distribute the fluid and after 5 min, drain off as much fluid as possible into a bag on the floor (minimum fluid for a valid analysis is 200 mL in an adult). Send the fluid for analysis (amylase, bile, bacteria, food fibers, hematocrit, cell count). See Table III–4, page 367 for the diagnosis of the fluid.
7. Remove the catheter and suture the skin. When the catheter is inserted for pancreatitis or peritoneal dialysis, suture it in place.
8. A negative DPL does not rule out retroperitoneal trauma. A false-positive DPL can be caused by a pelvic fracture.

TABLE III–4. DIAGNOSTIC PERITONEAL LAVAGE FINDINGS THAT SUGGEST INTRA-ABDOMINAL TRAUMA.

Positive	20 mL gross blood on free aspiration (10 mL in children)
	>100,000 RBC/μL
	>500 WBC/μL (if obtained > 3 hours after the injury)
	>175 units amylase/dL
	Bacteria on Gram stain
	Bile (by inspection or chemical determination of billrubin contents)
	Food particles (microscopic analysis of strained or spun specimen)
Intermediate	Pink fluid on free aspiration
	50,000–100,000 RBC/μL
	in blunt trauma
	100–500 WBC/μL
	75–175 units amylase/dL
Negative	Clear aspirate
	<100 WBC/μL
	<75 units amylase/dL

(Reproduced, with permission, from Macho JR, Lewis FR Jr, Krupski WC: Management of the Injured Patient. In: Current Surigical Diagnosis & Treatment, *10/e Way LW (editor). Appleton & Lange, 1994.)*

Complications: Infection, bleeding, perforated viscus.

16. Peripherally Inserted Central Catheters (PICC).

Indications:

1. Home infusion of hypertonic or irritating solutions and drugs.
2. Infusion of a short course of intravenous antibiotics.
3. Total parenteral nutrition.
4. Repetitive venous blood sampling. (Note: not for CVP measurements).

Contraindications: Inadequate upper-extremity veins, infection near placement site.

Materials: A PICC catheter kit, a tourniquet, sterile gauze, a dressing, sterile gloves, a mask, a sterile gown, sterile towels, Betadine, alcohol, 1% lidocaine with epinephrine, heparin flush, 10-ml syringes.

Procedure:

1. Using a measuring tape, determine the length of the catheter required. Measure the distance from the proposed insertion site to the superior vena cava (ie, sternal notch). Follow the manufacturer's instructions for trimming the catheter.
2. Wear mask, gown, protective eyewear, and sterile gloves. Carefully wipe any powder off the gloves. Prep and drape the

skin in the standard fashion. Set up an adjacent sterile working area. Anesthetize the skin at the proposed area of insertion. Apply a tourniquet above the proposed IV site. Insert the catheter and introducer needle into the antecubital vein as detailed in the section on IV techniques. Once the catheter is in the vein, remove the introducer needle.

3. Flush the PICC and then insert the catheter into the vein. Advance it gradually until the catheter has been inserted to the requisite length. Remove the inner stiffening wire slowly, once the catheter has been adequately advanced. Flush the catheter with heparin solution. Set up a Luer-Lok syringe. Apply a sterile dressing over the IV site.
4. Confirm the catheter placement in the central circulation with a chest radiograph. Always document the type of PICC, the length inserted and the site of its radiologically confirmed placement.
5. When vein cannulation is difficult, a surgical cutdown may be necessary to cannulate the vein.
6. Instruct the patient on the maintenance of the PICC. The PICC should be flushed with heparinized saline after each use. Dressing changes should be performed at least every 7 d under sterile conditions. The patient must be instructed to evaluate his PICC site for signs and symptoms of infection. The patient must also be instructed to come to the emergency room for evaluation of any fevers.
7. For venous samples, a specimen with a volume at least $1\frac{1}{2}$ times the catheter volume (1–3 cc) must first be withdrawn and then discarded. The PICC must always be flushed with heparinized saline after each blood draw.

PICC removal: Position the patient's arm at a 90-degree angle to the body. Remove the dressing and gently pull the PICC out. Apply pressure to the site for 2–3 min. Always measure the length of the catheter and check prior documentation to ensure that the PICC line has been removed in its entirety. If a piece of a catheter is left behind, an emergency interventional radiology consult may be necessary.

Complications: Subclavian thrombosis, bleeding, clotted catheter, infection, broken catheter, embolization.

17. Pulmonary Artery Catheterization

(See also Section I, Problem 61, page 226)

Indications:

1. Acute heart failure.
2. Complex circulatory and fluid conditions (burn patients, patients in shock).

3. Diagnosis of cardiac tamponade.
4. Perioperative management (elderly or debilitated patients, patients with severe cardiac or pulmonary diseases).

Materials: Central venous catheter equipment (see page 340); a flow-directed balloon-tipped catheter (aka Swan-Ganz catheter); a 7 Fr catheter with thermistor or pulse oximetry port is most frequently used in adults (Figure III–9A); a sheath, a dilator, a No.11 blade, and guide wires for catheter insertion (usually supplied as a kit, such as Cordis or Arrow Introducer Kit); connecting tubing; a transducer and oscilloscope; heparin flush solution (1 U heparin/mL normal saline); pressure bags; an ECG monitor; a crash cart; and rapid access to 100-mg lidocaine bolus for IV use.

Procedure:

1. Informed consent is needed. The patient must be on an ECG monitor, have a working IV in place, and the crash cart should be nearby, because arrhythmias are a frequent complication. Coagulation profile should ideally be normal. Placement may be contraindicated for patients with second-degree heart block.
2. Gown, gloves, mask, and a cap along with a wide sterile field are needed.
3. Remove the pulmonary artery catheter from the package, place it on a sterile field and flush all the lumens with heparinized saline. Balance the transducer at the reference point of the midaxillary line with the patient supine. Connect all ports to the monitoring lines. Check the function of the transducer by gently flicking the tip and observing oscillation on the monitor.
4. Check the flow balloon at the end of the catheter by gently inflating with 1.5 mL of air (for a 7 Fr catheter). Some operators check the balloon in a cup of sterile water for leaks. If there is the possibility of a left-right shunt, carbon dioxide is suggested for inflation. Liquid should not be used to inflate the balloon.
5. Obtain access to a central vein as described in "Central venous catheter placement," page 340 using a guide wire technique. The subclavian access is usually preferred because of the ease of securing the catheter to the relatively flat upper chest wall. The internal jugular, antecubital routes are also acceptable. Avoid the femoral vein, if possible, because of the increased risk of infection and an embolism.
6. Place the guide wire in the introducer set at least halfway into the vein. The patient must be monitored continuously during the procedure, because arrhythmia, most frequently ventricular, may occur.
7. Mount the dilator inside the introducer, nick the skin with a No. 11 blade, and advance the assembly slowly over the guide wire.

8. Flush the pulmonary artery catheter ports with heparinized saline one more time to remove air bubbles. Remove the guide wire and dilator, and leave the introducer in position. Place a finger over the end of the introducer to prevent excessive bleeding or an air embolus. Mount a telescoping clear plastic contamination guard, if necessary, to the hub of the introducer. A rubber gasket assembly usually prevents excessive bleeding before the time the catheter is threaded into the introducer. This guard allows the catheter to be adjusted over a range of approximately 20 cm under sterile conditions after the catheter has been positioned.
9. Slowly advance the catheter to approximately the right atrium. Follow the characteristic patterns as the catheter is advanced (Figure III–9B). Most catheters have markings every 10 cm.

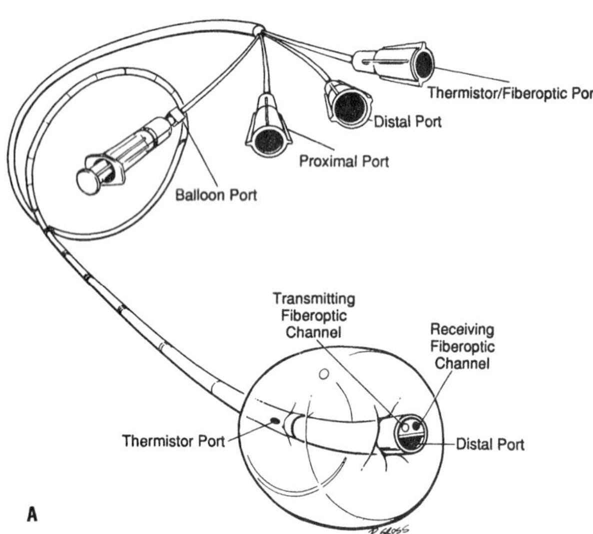

Figure III–9 A: An example of a pulmonary artery catheter. This one has an oximetric measuring feature. (Reproduced, with permission, from Gomella LG (editor): Clinician's Pocket Reference, 8th ed., Appleton & Lange. Copyright © 1997). **B:** Positioning and pressure wave forms seen as the pulmonary artery catheter is advanced. (Reproduced, with permission, from Stillman RM (editor): *Surgery, Diagnosis, and Therapy.* Originally published by Appleton & Lange. Copyright © 1989 by The McGraw–Hill Companies, Inc.)

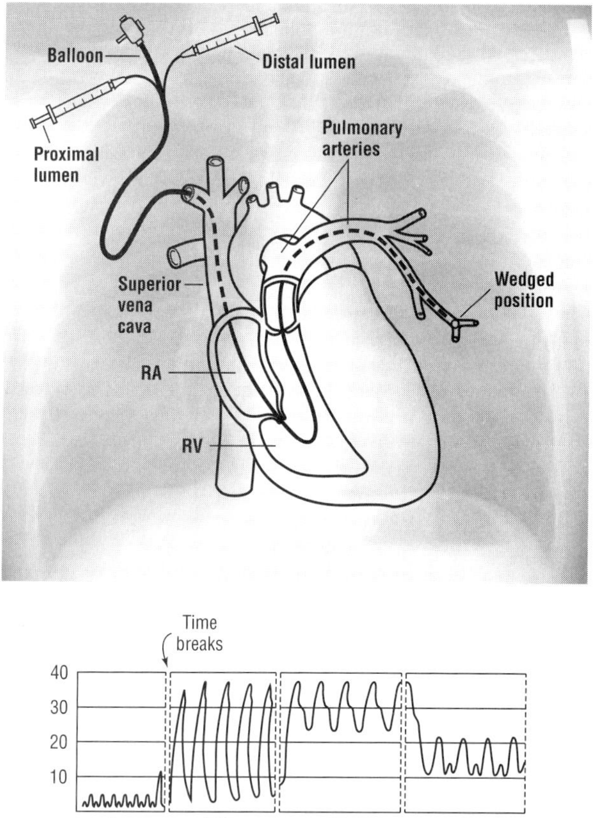

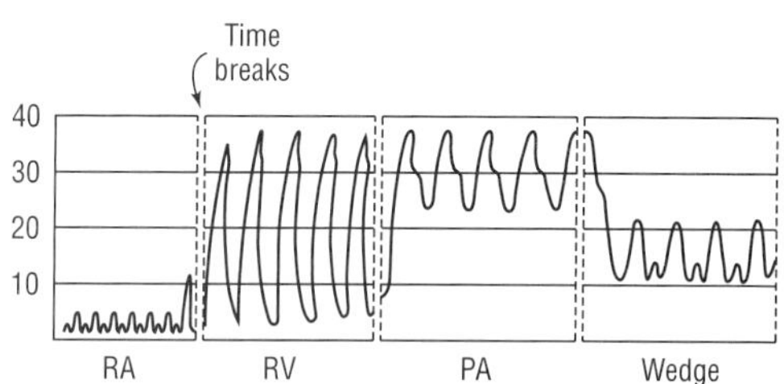

B

Figure III–9. (continued)

The reference lengths to the right atrium are as follows: right internal jugular or subclavian, 10–20 cm; left internal jugular or subclavian, 20–30 cm; left or right antecubital vein, 40–50 cm; left or right femoral vein, 30 cm.

10. While at the approximate level of the right atrium, slowly inflate the balloon of the 7 Fr catheter with 1.5 mL air (0.8 mL for the 5 Fr catheter). Advance the catheter and observe the pressure tracing (Figure III–9B) on the oscilloscope from the distal port to follow the catheter tip as it flows through the right ventricle and out the pulmonary artery. Do not hesitate if ventricular ectopy is seen. Rapidly pass the catheter through the ventricle and use IV lidocaine (50–100-mg IV bolus) if the ectopy persists. Once at the pulmonary artery, advance the catheter 10–20 cm farther to obtain the wedge pressure. If multiple attempts fail to successfully pass the catheter out of the pulmonary artery, fluoroscopy may be needed.

11. Deflate the balloon and the pulmonary artery tracing should reappear. Adjust the catheter as needed so that this pattern is reproduced. **Never** leave the balloon inflated continuously, as pulmonary infarction or an arterial rupture may occur. **Never** leave the balloon inflated while pulling the catheter back. The pulmonary artery tracing should be observed at all times unless the balloon is inflated.
12. Suture the introducer and pulmonary artery catheter in position with 2–0 silk. If there is a contamination shield, extend it about halfway to allow the catheter to be moved, should repositioning be needed.
13. Dress the site with povidone-iodine and gauze or transparent shield dressing (eg, Op-Site).
14. Obtain an immediate portable chest radiograph to verify the proper catheter position and to rule out a pneumothorax. A properly positioned pulmonary artery catheter should follow a smooth curve and the tip of the catheter should not be further than 5 cm from the midline, and most often in the right pulmonary artery.

TABLE III–5. NORMAL PULMONARY ARTERY CATHETER MEASUREMENTS.

Parameter	Range
Right atrial pressure	1–7 mm Hg
Right ventricular systolic pressure	15–25 mm Hg
Right ventricular diastolic pressure	0–8 mm Hg
Pulmonary artery systolic pressure	15–25 mm Hg
Pulmonary artery diastolic pressure	8–15 mm Hg
Pulmonary artery mean pressure	10–20 mm Hg
Pulmonary capillary wedge pressure	6–12 mm Hg
SVR (systemic vascular resistance)[1]	900–1200 dynes/sec/cm^5
Cardiac output	3.5–5.5 L/min
Cardiac index	2.8–3.2L/min

[1] $SVR = \frac{\text{(mean arterial pressure} - \text{central venous pressure)} \times 80}{\text{Cardiac output}}$

TABLE III–6. DIFFERENTIAL DIAGNOSIS OF COMMON PULMONARY ARTERY CATHETER READINGS.

Low right atrial pressure: Volume depletion
High right artial pressure: Volume overload, congestive heart failure, cardiogenic shock, increased pulmonary vascular resistance (hypoxia, ventilator effects of PEEP, pulmonary disease, primary pulmonary hypertension)
Low right ventricular pressures: Volume depletion
High right ventricular pressures: Volume overload, congestive heart failure, cardiogenic shock, increased pulmonary vascular resistance (see above)
High pulmonary artery pressure: Congestive heart failure, increased pulmonary vascular resistance (hypoxia, ventilator effect of PEEP, pulmonary disease), cardiac tamponade
Low wedge pressure: Volume depletion
High wedge pressure: Cardiogenic shock, left ventricular failure, ventricular septal defect, mitral regurgitation and stenosis, severe hypertension, volume overload, cardiac tamponade

15. Normal pulmonary artery parameters are listed in Table III–5, and diagnosis of conditions associated with certain readings are listed in Table III–6.

Complications: All complications associated with central venous catheter placement (see page 346), arrhythmia, pulmonary artery rupture or pulmonary infarction, knotting of catheter or rupture of the balloon, sepsis, complete heart block.

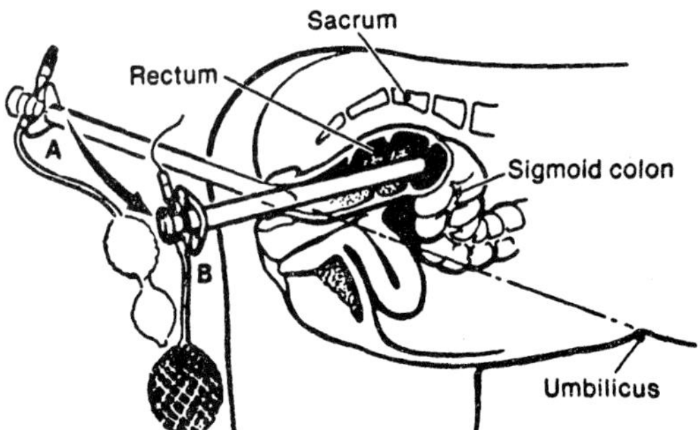

Figure III–10. The sigmoidoscope is advanced under direct vision as shown. (Reproduced, with permission, from Gomella LG (editor): *Clinician's Pocket Reference,* 8th ed., Appleton & Lange. Copyright © 1997.)

18. Sigmoidoscopy

Indications:

1. Workup of gastrointestinal tract bleeding or lower gastrointestinal tract symptoms.
2. Evaluation of trauma.

Materials: Gloves, lubricant, hemoccult paper and developer, sigmoidoscope and light source, an insufflation bag, tissues, long (rectal) swabs and a suction catheter, a proctologic examination table (not essential).

Procedure:

1. Enemas and cathartics are not given routinely before sigmoidoscopy, although some clinicians prefer to give a mild prep, such as a Fleet's Enema, just before the exam. Explain the procedure and have the patient sign an informed consent form.
2. Sigmoidoscopy can be performed with the patient in bed lying on his side in the knee-chest position, but the best results are obtained with the patient in the "jackknife" position on the proctologic table. Do not position the patient until all materials are at hand and you are ready to start.
3. Converse with the patient to create distraction and to relieve apprehension. Announce each maneuver in advance. Put on gloves before proceeding.
4. Observe the anal region for skin tags, hemorrhoids, fissures, etc. Do a careful rectal exam and a Hemoccult test with a gloved finger using plenty of lubricant.
5. Lubricate the sigmoidoscope well and insert it with the obturator in place. Aim towards the patient's umbilicus initially. Advance 2–3 cm past the internal sphincter and remove the obturator.
6. Always advance under direct vision and make sure that the lumen is always visible (Figure III–10). Insufflation (introducing air) may be used to help visualize the lumen, but remember this may be painful to the patient. It is necessary to follow the curve of the sigmoid toward the sacrum by directing the scope more posteriorly toward the back. A change from a smooth mucosa to concentric rings indicates entry into the sigmoid colon. The scope should reach 15 cm with ease. Use suction and the rectal swabs as needed to clear the way.
7. At this point, the sigmoid curves to the patient's left. Warn the patient that a cramping sensation may be felt. If you ever have difficulty negotiating a curve, **do not force the scope**.
8. After advancing as far as possible, slowly remove the scope; use a small rotary motion to view all surfaces. Observation here is critical. Remember to release the air from the colon before withdrawing the scope.

9. Inform the patient that mild cramping may be experienced after the procedure.

Complications: Bleeding, perforation, abdominal cramping.

19. Thoracentesis

Indications:

1. For the diagnosis of pleural effusion.
2. For the therapeutic removal of pleural fluid.
3. For the instillation of sclerosing compounds (such as tetracycline) to obliterate the pleural space

Contraindications: Pneumothorax, hemothorax, or respiratory impairment in the contralateral side, coagulopathy (relative).

Materials: A prepackaged thoracentesis kit or minor procedure tray (see page 377) plus a 20–60-mL syringe, 20- or 22-gauge needle 1½-inch needle, three-way stopcock, and specimen containers.

Procedure:

1. It takes at least 300 mL of fluid to visualize a pleural effusion on a standard chest radiograph.
2. Discuss the procedure with the patient and obtain an informed consent. Teach the patient the Valsalva maneuver or make sure the patient can hum. Some recommend oxygen supplementation by mask while performing thoracentesis.
3. The usual site for the thoracentesis is the posterolateral back over the diaphragm but under the fluid level. Percuss out the fluid level or use the chest radiograph and count out the ribs. The site will be above the rib to avoid the neurovascular bundle that travels below the rib.
4. Prep the area with povidone-iodine and drape. The patient should be sitting up comfortably, leaning slightly forward. The bed stand is helpful for this.
5. Make a skin wheal over the proposed site with a 25-gauge needle and 1% lidocaine. Change to a 22-gauge, 1½-inch needle and infiltrate up and over the rib; try to anesthetize the deeper structures and the pleura. During this time you should be aspirating back for pleural fluid. Once fluid returns, note the depth of the needle and mark it with a hemostat. This gives you an approximate depth. Remove the needle.
6. Measure the 15–18-gauge thoracentesis needle to the same depth as the first needle with a hemostat. Penetrate through the anesthetized area with the thoracentesis needle. You may also use a catheter over needle assembly (Angiocath) and leave the plastic catheter in position to remove the fluid. Always go over the top of the rib to avoid the neurovascular

bundle that runs below the rib. Never pull the catheter back over the needle to prevent shearing. Attach the three-way stopcock and tubing and aspirate the amount needed. Turn the stopcock and evacuate the fluid through the tubing. **Never** remove more than 1000 mL per tap!

7. Have the patient hum or do the Valsalva maneuver as you withdraw the needle. This maneuver increases intrathoracic pressure and decreases the chances of a pneumothorax. Bandage the site.
8. Obtain a chest radiograph to evaluate the fluid level and to rule out a pneumothorax. An expiratory film may be best, because it helps reveal a small pneumothorax.
9. Distribute specimens in containers, label slips, and send them to the lab. Always order pH, specific gravity, protein, LDH, cell count and differential, glucose, Gram's stain and cultures, acid-fast and fungal cultures, and smears. Optional lab studies are cytology if you suspect a malignancy, amylase if you suspect an effusion secondary to pancreatitis (usually on the left), and a Sudan stain and triglycerides if a chylothorax is suspected. See Table III–7 for the differential diagnosis.

TABLE III–7. DIFFERENTIAL DIAGNOSIS OF PLEURAL FLUID.
TRANSUDATE: NEPHROSIS, CONGESTIVE HEART FAILURE (CHF), CIRRHOSIS.
EXUDATE: INFECTION (PNEUMONIA, TB), MALIGNANCY, EMPYEMA, PERITONEAL DIALYSIS, PANCREATITIS, CHYLOTHORAX.

Lab Value	Transudate	Exudate
Specific gravity	<1.016	>1.016
Protein (Pleural fluid)	<2.5 gm/100 mL	> 3 gm/100 mL
Protein ration (Pleural fluid to serum ratio)	<0.5	>0.5
LDH ratio (Pleural fluid to serum ratio)	<0.5	>0.6
Pleural fluid LDH	<200 IU	>200 IU
Fibrinogen (Clot)	No	Yes
Cell count and differential	Very low WBC	Suspect an inflammatory Exudate (early polys, later monos)

Grossly bloddy tap: Trauma, pulmonary infarction, tumor, and iatrogenic causes.

pH: The pH of pleural fluid is usually > 7.3. If between 7.2 and 7.3, suspect TB or malignancy or both. if < 7.2, suspect an empyema.

Glucose: Normal pleural fluid glucose is 2/3 serum glucose pleural fluid glucose is much lower than serum glucose in effusions due to rheumatoid arthritis (0–16 mg/100 mL).

Triglycerides and positive sudan stain: Chylothorax.

Complications: Pneumothorax, hemothorax, infection, pulmonary laceration, and hypotension.

20. Venous Cutdown

Indication: Venous access when percutaneous puncture is not practical.

Materials: A prepackaged cut down tray or minor procedure tray and instrument tray (Table III–8) (below) with silk suture (3–0, 4–0), and a catheter of choice (eg, Medicut, Angiocath).

Procedure (Figure III–11):

1. The most common site for a cut down is the greater saphenous vein. The best location for a cut down is approximately one finger breadth anterior and superior to the medial malleolus. Other sites on the foot, hand, or arm can be used.
2. Apply a tourniquet proximal to the site. Children may need to be restrained. Prep the skin with antiseptic solution, drape the patient, and put on sterile gloves.
3. Infiltrate the skin over the vein with 1% lidocaine. Incise the skin transversely.
4. Spread the incision in the direction of the vein with a hemostat until the excess tissue is cleaned off. Lift the vein off the posterior tissues.

TABLE III–8. MOST PROCEDURES CAN BE ACCOMPLISHED WITH COMMERICALLY AVAILABLE KITS, IN THE EVENT THESE KITS ARE NOT AVAILABLE, THE FOLLOWING GUIDELINES ARE PROVIDED AND REFERRED TO IN EACH PROCEDURE SECTION WHERE APPROPRIATE. A USEFUL NEEDLE GAUGE AND FRENCH CATHETER GUIDE CAN BE FOUND IN FIGURE III–12, PAGE 380.

Minor Procedure tray

* Sterile gloves
* Sterile towels/drapes
* 4 × 4 gauze sponges
* Povidone–iodine (Betadine) prep solution
* Syringes 5, 10, 20 mL
* Needles 18, 20, 22, 25 guage
* 1% lidocaine (with or without epinephrine)
* Adhesive tape

Instrument tray

* Scissors
* Needle holder
* Hemostat
* Scalpel and blade (No.10 for adult, No. 15 for children or delicate work)
* Suture of choice

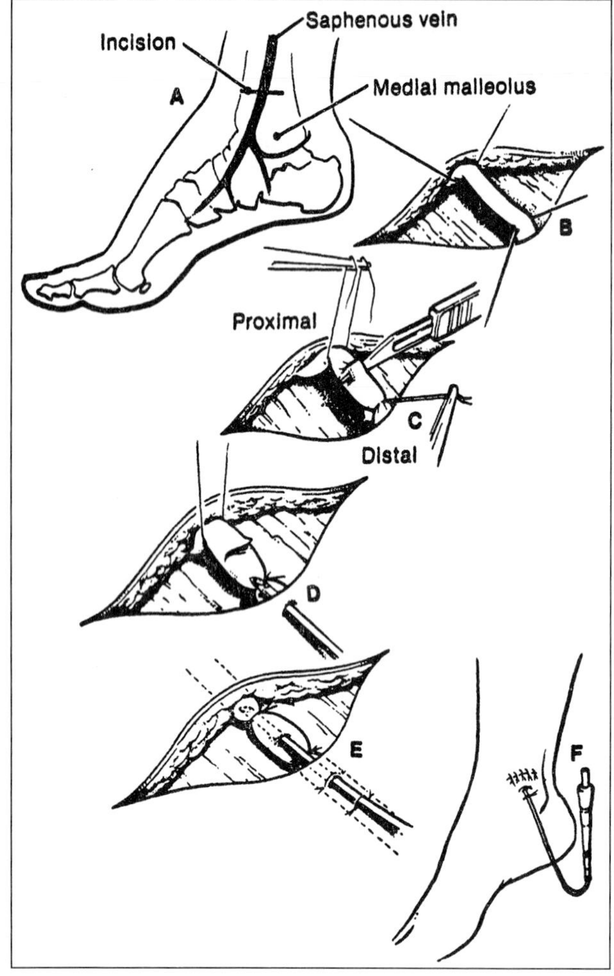

Figure III–11. Venous cutdown using the saphenous vein. Here the catheter is inserted through a separate stab wound. (Reproduced with permission from Gomella L G, ed.: *Clinician's Pocket Reference,* 5th ed. Appleton-Century-Crofts, 1986)

5. Pass two chromic or silk ties (3–0 or 4–0) behind the vein. Tie off the distal vein. The upper tie is used for traction.
6. Make a transverse nick in the vein. You may need a catheter introducer ("banana") to hold open the lumen of the vein.
7. Insert the plastic catheter or IV cannula into the vein and tie the proximal suture to secure it in place. The catheter may also be inserted through a separate stab wound and then passed into the vein.
8. Attach the fluid, release the tourniquet, and close the skin with a silk or nylon suture. Apply a sterile dressing.

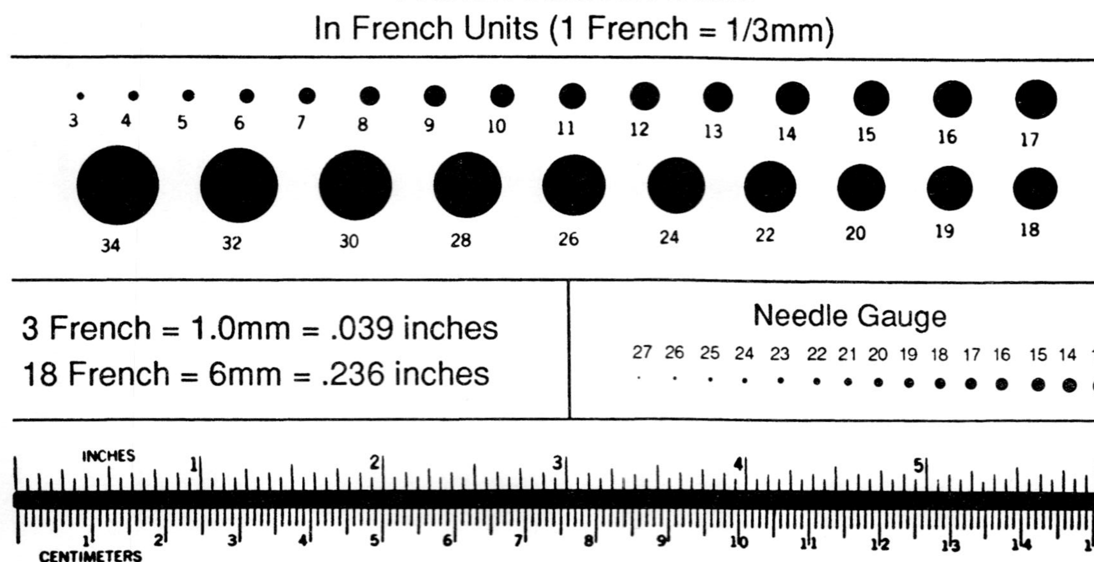

Figure III–12. French catheter guide and needle gauge reference. (Courtesy Cook Urological, Spencer, Indiana).

IV. Fluids & Electrolytes

INTRAVENOUS FLUIDS

Knowledge of basic principles governing internal and external exchanges of water and salt is mandatory for proper care of the surgical patient. The daily water losses in a normal 70-kg male include approximately 250 mL as stool, 800 to 1500 mL as urine, and approximately 600 to 900 mL as insensible losses per day. The urine output must exceed 500 to 800 mL/d to excrete the products of catabolism (> 20 to 30 mL/h). Daily sodium requirements vary between 50 and 90 mEq/d, and potassium requirements are about 50 mEq/d in a 70-kg male. The following are general guidelines to ordering maintenance and replacement fluids for patients. Clinical judgment is needed to modify these appropriately.

A. **Maintenance Fluids.** In the perioperative period, D5 1/4 NS with 20 mEq KCl/L at 125 cc/h is a good choice to provide adequate water to meet daily fluid requirements, to replace losses, and to supply sufficient sodium and potassium to meet daily requirements. Routine administration of potassium is not recommended for posttraumatic patients and for patients when renal failure is suspected. The use of albumin solutions, in addition to balanced salt solutions, to replace extracellular fluid perioperatively, is not necessary and may be harmful. The use of D5 1/2 NS is usually acceptable with normal renal function, although the patient is given more sodium than needed.
   1. **70-kg male.** D5 1/4 NS with 20 mEq KCl/L at 125 mL/h.
   2. **Other patients.** Also use D5 1/4 NS with 20 mEq KCl/L. Determine their 24-h water requirement by the following formula, called the "Kg Method":

      •For the first 10 kg body weight: 100 mL/kg/d plus
      •For the second 10 kg body weight: 50 mL/kg/d plus
      •For weight above 20 kg: 20 ml/kg/d

      Divide by 24 h to determine the hourly rate.

      Remember that the rate of fluid administration depends on the severity and type of fluid disturbance and may vary considerably according to the presence of fluid sequestration ("third-space" losses), fluid losses, and cardiac status.
   3. **Pediatric patients.** Use the same solution, but determine the daily fluid requirements by either of the following:
      a. **Body weight method:** As previously outlined.
      b. **Body surface area method:** Maintenance fluids are 2000 mL/m^2/d. Divide by 24 to get the flow rate

per hour (not accurate for infants < 10-kg body weight). To calculate the surface area, use the body surface area charts in the Appendix.

B. Specific Replacement Fluids. Table IV–1 gives general guidelines for the daily production and composition of various body fluids. Replacement of these losses is recommended as follows:

1. **Gastric (NG tube, emesis).** D5 1/2 NS with 20 mEq/L KCl.
2. **Diarrhea.** D5 1/2 NS with 15 mEq/L KCl. Use body weight as a replacement guide (about 1 L for each 1 kg or 2.2 lb lost).
3. **Small bowel.** D5LR with 25 mEq/L (1/2 ampule) of HCO_3.
4. **Bile.** D5LR with 25 mEq/L (1/2 ampule) of HCO_3.
5. **Pancreatic fluid.** D5LR with 50 mEq/L (1 ampule) HCO_3.
6. **Burn patients.** See Figure IV–1. Use the "Parkland Formula":

   Total fluid required during the first 24 h =
   (Percentage of body burn) × (body weight in kg) × 4 mL

Replace with lactated Ringer's solution over 24 h:

- 1/2 total during first 8 h (from time of burn)
- 1/4 total during second 8 h
- 1/4 total during third 8 h

TABLE IV–1. COMPOSITION AND DAILY PRODUCTION OF BODY FLUIDS

Fluid	Electrolytes Na	Cl	K	HCO	Average Daily Production[1] (mL)
		(mEq/L)			
Sweet	50	40	5	0	Varies
Saliva	10	15	26	50	1500
Gastric juice	60–100	100	10	0	1500–2000
Duodenum	130	90	5	0–10	300–2000
Bile	145	100	5	15–35	100–800
Pancreatic juice	140	75	5	70–115	100–800
Ileum	140	100	5	15–30	2000–3000
Diarrhea	50	40	35	45	—

[1]In adults

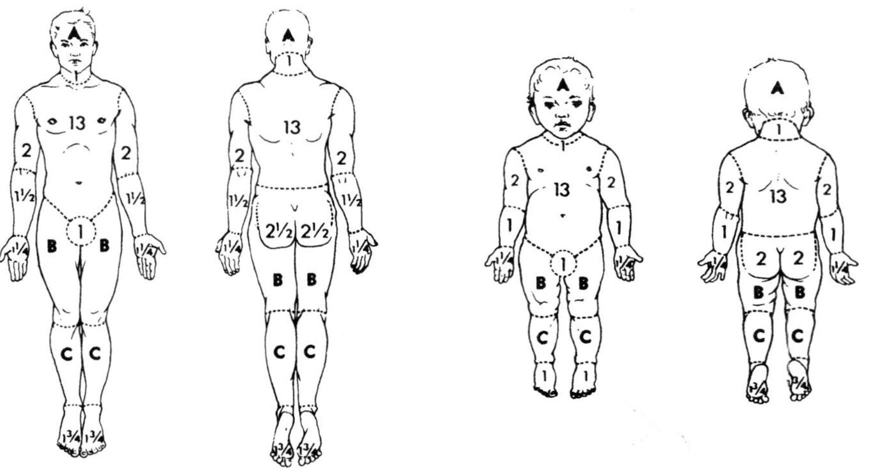

Figure IV-1. Tables for estimating the extent of burns in adults and children. In adults, a reasonable system for calculating the percentage of body burned is the "Rule of nines": Each arm equals 9%; the head equals 9%; the anterior and posterior trunk each equal 18%; each leg equals 18%; and the perineum equals 1%. (Reproduced, with permission, from Demling RH, Way LW: Burns & other thermal injuries. In Way LW (editor): *Current Surgical Treatment & Diagnosis,* 10th ed. Originally published by Appleton & Lange. Copyright © 1994 by The McGraw-Hill Companies, Inc.)

There is considerable variability among institutions regarding the exact composition of fluid used in resuscitation of the burn patient. One should be sure to use the appropriate fluid.

COMPOSITION OF PARENTERAL FLUIDS

Parenteral fluids are generally classified on the basis of molecular mass and oncotic pressure. Colloids are generally >8000 Dalton molecular mass and have high oncotic pressure (albumin, blood, dextran, hetastarch, plasma protein fraction). Crystalloids are <8000 Dalton molecular mass and have low oncotic pressure (most IV fluids). See Table IV–2 below for the composition of commonly used crystalloid solutions.

TABLE IV–2. COMPOSITION OF COMMONLY USED CRYSTALLOIDS.

Fluid	Glucose (gm/L)	Na	Cl (mEq.L)	K	Ca	HCO_3[1]	Mg	HPO4	KCal/L
D5W (Dextrose 5% in water)	50	—	—	—	—	—	—	—	170
D10W (Dextrose 10% in water)	100	—	—	—	—	—	—	—	340
D20W (Dextrose 20% in water)	200	—	—	—	—	—	—	—	680
D50W (Dextrose 50% in water)	500	—	—	—	—	—	—	—	1700
1/2 NS[2] (0.45% NaCl)	—	77	77	—	—	—	—	—	0
3% NS[2]	513	513	—	—	—	—	—	—	0
NS[2] (0.9% NaCl	—	154	154	—	—	—	—	—	0
D 5% 1/4 NS[2]	50	38	38	—	—	—	—	—	17
D 5% 1/2 NS[2] (0.45% NaCl)	50	77	77	—	—	—	—	—	17
D 5% NS[2] (0.9% NaCl	50	154	154	—	—	—	—	—	17
D 5% Lactated Ringer's (D5LR)	50	130	110	4	3	27	—	—	18
Lactated Ringer's	—	130	110	4	3	27	—	—	<1
Ionosol MB	50	25	22	20	—	23	3	3	17
Normosol M	50	40	40	13	—	16	3	—	17

[1]HCO^3 is administered in these solutions as Lactate that is converted to bicarbonate.
[2]NS = normal saline

V. Nutritional Management of the Surgical Patient

Adequate nutritional support is of paramount importance in the care of the surgical patient. Suboptimal responses to therapeutic modalities occur in the malnourished patient, and complications, such as poor wound healing, impaired organ function, and compromised immunity may be observed. Therefore, when adequate nutritional support of the patient is not addressed, clinical management of the patient is often more complex, and patient outcome may be compromised. Specialized nutritional support, whether enteral or parenteral, when used appropriately, can help to prevent the nutrition-related morbidities in the surgical patient. However, the approach to specialized nutritional support may not always be clear. There are no data supporting the use of routine nutritional support in the preoperative period except in the severely malnourished patient.

Assessment (Table V–1)

Differentiation of acute and chronic malnutrition is helpful in the decision of when to initiate specialized nutritional support. Acute malnutrition, also called **kwashiorkor** or **acute hypoalbuminemia**, is defined as starvation occurring during a catabolic stress, such as surgery, infection, burn, or trauma, and is a more aggressive nutritional insult than simple starvation for a brief period. Chronic malnutrition, also called **marasmus,** is characterized by growth retardation and wasting of muscle and subcutaneous fat while maintaining an appetite. Frequently in the surgical patient, these two nutritional insults may be superimposed. The most recent guidelines from the American Society for Parenteral and Enteral Nutrition state, "patients should be considered malnourished or at risk of developing malnutrition if they have inadequate nutrient intake for 7 d or more or if they have a weight loss of 10% or more of their pre-illness body weight." The formula for determination of percentage weight loss is:

$$\%\text{ weight loss} = \frac{(\text{usual weight} - \text{present weight})}{\text{usual weight}} \times 100$$

Formal evaluation is important to identify patients at nutritional risk and to provide a baseline to assess the achievement of therapeutic goals with the specialized nutritional support. The patient's history is useful to evaluate weight loss and dietary intolerance (eg, glucose or lactose and disease states that may influence nu-

TABLE V–1. PARAMETERS OF NUTRITIONAL ASSESSMENT.

Parameter	Type of Malnutrition	Comment
Weight loss	Chronic	Affected by volume status
Anthropometric measurements (MAMC, TSF[1])	Chronic	Interobserver variability
Lymphocyte count	Acute or chronic	Reflects immune function
Anergy testing	Acute or chronic	Reflects immune function
Albumin	Acute	Affected by hydration status
Prealbumin	Acute	More sensitive visceral protein marker of nutritional status than albumin
Retinol binding protein	Acute	Limited availability
Transferrin	Acute	Affected by iron status
Urinary urea nitrogen	Acute or chronic	Indicates nitrogen balance and efficacy of nutritional regimen. Potential for collection problems

[1]MAMC = midarm muscle circumference: TSF = triceps skin fold.

tritional tolerance). Anthropometric evaluations such as midarm muscle circumference (MAMC) and triceps skin fold (TSF) have much interobserver variability and are generally not useful unless performed by an experienced evaluator. Absolute lymphocyte count and response to skin test antigens provide insight to the patient's immune function. Visceral protein markers, such as prealbumin and transferrin, may be helpful in evaluating nutritional insult and catabolic stress. Although the most commonly quoted laboratory parameter of nutritional status is serum albumin, its concentration often reflects hydration status and metabolic response to injury (ie, the acute phase response) more than the nutritional state of the patient. This is true particularly in the patient with intravascular volume deficits. Because of its long half-life, serum albumin level may be normal in the malnourished patient. Prealbumin is superior as an indicator of malnutrition only because of its shorter half-life. However, these serum proteins as indicators of malnutrition are subject to the same limitations, because they are affected by catabolic stress.

Urinary urea nitrogen collected during a 24-h period is an important tool to evaluate nitrogen balance and the adequacy of the patient's nutritional regimen if the specimen is collected accurately.

- Nitrogen balance = Nitrogen input – nitrogen output
- Nitrogen input = Protein in grams / 6.25 (6.25g protein contains 1g nitrogen)

- Nitrogen output = 24-h urinary urea nitrogen (UUN) + 4 g/d (nonurinary loss).

Certain disease states, including high output fistulas or massive diarrhea, will increase the amount of nonurinary losses for nitrogen. Fecal nitrogen measurements are difficult to obtain, but are most useful in the patient's assessment.

Example of Nitrogen Balance Calculation

A patient receives 2 L TPN per 24 h with 27.5 g synthetic amino acid (protein) solution per liter.

1. 27.5 g protein per L x 2 L = 55 g protein per 24 h.
2. Recall that 1 g of nitrogen = 6.25 g of protein.
3. Nitrogen input = 55 g protein at 6.25 g protein per gram N = 8.8 g N.
4. Patient voided 22.5 dL urine per 24 h with UUN 66 mg/dL
5. Nitrogen lost in urine = 22.5 dL x 66 mg/dL = 1485 mg or about 1.5 g
6. Add 4.0 g for nonurine nitrogen loss
7. Nitrogen output = 1.5 g + 4.0 = 5.5 g
8. Nitrogen balance = input – output = 8.8 – 5.5 = positive 3.3 g nitrogen.

A positive nitrogen balance ensures that the amount of protein being administered is sufficient to cover the losses of endogenous protein, which occur secondary to catabolism. Once positive balance has been achieved, protein replacement has been optimized. This may not be possible in the acute phase of injury, in severe trauma or burn patients. Thus a minimization of loss (between 2 and 4 g/d) may be the goal during this period. A negative nitrogen balance indicates insufficient protein replacement for the degree of skeletal muscle loss. Under most circumstances, an attempt to achieve positive balance should be made. Patients with renal dysfunction or severe stress may not be able to achieve a positive balance because of safety concerns.

A number of considerations including preexisting illnesses and coexisting metabolic abnormalities are commonly present in the critically ill patient. Preexisting conditions, such as hepatic insufficiency, congestive heart failure, and renal impairment must be taken into consideration when instituting nutritional support. For example, a high carbohydrate load for patients with respiratory failure can lead to a significant increase in CO_2 production. In general, it is important to correct coexisting metabolic abnormalities, such as hypophosphatemia or hyperglycemia, before instituting nutritional support, particularly parenteral nutrition. It is not usually critically important to correct other metabolic abnormalities before instituting TPN.

The decision to begin nutritional support is not an "On-Call Problem" in the literal sense. It is never a decision that must be made late at night by the house officer. Rather, it should be a considered decision made by the team responsible for the care of the patient. Clear indications for nutritional support include

- Weight loss > 12% or more of body weight (or weight < 85% of ideal body weight).
- Expected > 5–7 d of no oral intake.
- Inadequate nutrient intake for 7 or more days.
- Albumin < 3.5 g/dL, transferrin < 200 mg/dL.

Hospital Diets

There are a number of standard dietary formulations available in the hospital. Most hospitals have a manual available for reference that provides details of the available diets. In addition, registered dieticians are available for consultation. This service should be used when questions arise about the use of specialized diets and dietary supplements in the care of individual patients.

Regular. Used for adult patients without dietary restrictions. The composition is based on Recommended Dietary Allowances.

Soft. Calorically and nutritionally similar to a regular diet, but tender foods are used (this is not a ground/pureed diet). Useful in patients with oral problems preventing the chewing of food.

Mechanical Soft. Uses ground foods, also useful for those with chewing difficulties (eg, edentulous patients).

Pureed. Foods are ground finely, also useful in patients with difficulty chewing or swallowing.

Clear Liquids. Usually used in the immediate preoperative or postoperative period, particularly in the transition from NPO to starting oral feedings. This diet leaves little residue and requires minimal digestive activity for absorption. In general, this diet should not be used for more than 3 d without supplementation.

Full Liquids. Includes foods that are liquid at room temperature, such as, milk or milk-products (eg, puddings, ice cream, etc). In the past, this diet was used widely as a transition diet from clear liquids to regular, but it is used less often now. This diet can be difficult for many patients because it contains high-fat, lactose-containing ingredients.

Low Fiber (Residue). Indicated for patients with colitis, ileitis, or diarrhea. Decreases fecal volume.

High Fiber. Useful for atonic constipation, diverticular disease, irritable bowel syndrome, and diabetes.

Diabetic (ADA). Used for patients with IDDM or NIDDM. These diets are prescribed at a specified number of calories per day (eg, 2000 calories ADA, 2400 calories ADA, etc). Assessment by a clinical dietician helps to determine the appropriate calorie level, as well as help the patient maintain the correct diet after leaving the hospital.

Reduction. Used to assist in weight loss to achieve ideal body weight. Assessment by a clinical dietician is helpful in determining the appropriate calorie level.

Pediatric. Usually ordered as "Diet for age."

Hyperlipidemia. Used for patients with lipid abnormalities. Diet is written as type I, IIa, IIb, III, IV, or V depending on the diagnosis of each individual patient.

Low Fat. Designed to limit fat intake to approximately 50 g/d. Indicated for some diseases of the gallbladder, liver, or pancreas.

Protein Restricted. Useful in patients with renal failure or hepatic disorders. Specify number of grams of protein to be given.

Sodium Restricted. Used for the management of patients with congestive heart failure (CHF), hypertension, or other diseases resulting in fluid retention. Specify amount of sodium in milligrams or grams. Sodium restriction at levels < 1000 mg/d is not recommended because of the poor palatability of such diets. Average person in the United States consumes 12.5–15 g salt per day.

5–6 g sodium	Regular diet includes table salt.
4 g sodium	Regular diet without added salt, approx 180 mEq = 10 g salt.
2 g sodium	Restricted sodium diet, no sodium in food preparation, avoids processed meats. Practical for home use with a cooperative patient, approx. 87 mEq sodium or 5 g salt.
1 g sodium	Limitations of most foods including breads. Practical for home use only with an exceptionally cooperative patient, approx 2.5 g salt.

Potassium Restricted. Used mostly for patients with renal failure. Specify in grams or milliequivalents. A typical renal diet is limited to 40 mEq of potassium daily.

Nutritional Requirements

Overall, nutritional requirements are the same whether feeding the patient enterally or parenterally. Appropriate calculations of calories and protein are important to achieve optimal anabolism while avoiding the metabolic complications associated with overfeeding.

Caloric Requirements. Caloric requirements are dictated by the patient's needs for energy to support metabolic processes and activity. Catabolic patients with stresses from infections, burns, surgery, or trauma require additional energy to allow for the increased basal metabolic rate and increased metabolic demands associated with these conditions. Using the appropriate weight to predict energy needs is important for the patient who is not at ideal body weight. For an underweight patient, it is important to use the actual weight to avoid the complications associated with overfeeding. Similarly, for the overweight patient, it is important to estimate the amount of mass that is metabolically active to avoid unnecessary metabolic stress. This weight is 25% of the difference between the ideal weight and the actual weight added to the ideal weight.

Ideal body weight:

Males: 50 kg + 2.3 kg/in > 5 feet.
Females: 45.5 kg + 2.3 kg/in > 5 feet.

Metabolically active weight for obese patients = (Actual weight − ideal body weight × 0.25 + ideal body weight.

The amount of energy to support the metabolic process can be estimated from a number of equations or a nomogram. The Harris-Benedict equation is frequently used to provide an estimation of basal energy expenditure (see below). The predicted basal energy expenditure should be approximately 22 kcal/kg when calculated correctly. To estimate a patient's caloric requirement, the basal energy expenditure is multiplied by a factor for activity and injury.

Factors used to adjust the basal energy expenditure are less than originally published as the risks of overfeeding became apparent. Modified factors can be seen in Table V–2. Overall, total caloric provision (protein + nonprotein calories) should not exceed 25–30 kcal/kg for the nonstressed patient and 30–35 kcal/kg for the catabolically stressed patient. The burn victim will have higher requirements based on the amount of body surface area involved. In general, target nutritional support can be estimated to be:

TABLE V–2. CALCULATION OF CALORIC REQUIREMENTS. THE CALCULATION RELIES ON THE HARRIS-BENEDICT EQUATION FOR MEN AND WOMEN AND IS ADJUSTED FOR ACTIVITY LEVEL OR INJURY FACTORS.

Caloric requirement (men) = 66.47 + (13.75 × wgt [kg]) + (5.0 × hgt (cm]) − (6.76 × age [yrs]) × (activity factor) × (injury factor)

Caloric requirement (women) = 655.10 + (9.56 × wgt[kg]) + (1.65 × hgt [cm]) − (4.68 × age [yrs]) × (activity factor) × (injury factor)

Activity	**Factor**
Paralyzed	1.1
Confined to bed	1.2
Out of bed	1.3
Normal activity	1.5
Injury (choose highest factors)	
Surgery	
Minor	1.1
Major	1.1–1.3
Infection	
Minor	1.1
Severe	1.1–1.3
Trauma	
Skeletal	1.2–1.3
Head injury with steroids	1.6
Burns	
Up to 20% BSA[1]	1–1.5
20–40% BSA	1.5–1.85
>40% BSA	1.85–1.95

[1]BSa = % body surface area.

Nonstressed: 25–30 kcals/kg/d.
Stressed: 30–35 kcals/kg/d.

Protein Requirements. Protein is required to minimize endogenous net catabolism by supporting anabolic processes. Daily maintenance protein requirements are 0.8–1 g/kg. Patients with mild to moderate physiologic stress require 1.2–1.5 g/kg/d. Those with severe injuries may require as much as 2.5 g/kg/d. Protein administration may be limited by relative hepatic or renal insufficiency. For patients with a history of hepatic encephalopathy, protein doses > 0.8 g/kg are rarely tolerated. Such patients may benefit from amino acid formulations with higher concentrations of branched chain amino acids.

Carbohydrates & Fat. Generally, the caloric goal is achieved using carbohydrate and fat when feeding a patient parenterally. The protein is not counted as calories in the acutely stressed patient. Conceptually, this is to provide adequate calories for nitrogen incorporation and to allow adequate protein for tissue anabolism, although this practice differs in various medical centers. Optimal calorie to nitrogen ratios to achieve nutritional anabolism are estimated to be 150:1 for the nonstressed patient and 100:1 in the catabolic patient. On the average, protein consists of 16% nitrogen.

The majority of calories are provided as carbohydrate. This is consistent with the typical diet. Carbohydrate administration, either enterally or parenterally may be limited owing to hyperglycemia, increased CO_2 production, or fatty liver infiltration. Generally, the maximal glucose administration tolerated is 4–5 mg/kg/min or 20–25 kcal/kg/d.

A minimum amount of fat must be given to the parenterally fed patient to prevent the development of essential fatty acid deficiency (EFAD). This minimum is 4% of the total calories in the form of linoleic acid. However, additional fat calories are used to provide energy and to decrease the metabolic stress of glucose in the intolerant patient. Maximal intravenous fat administration is between 1 and 2.5 g/kg/d. Fat emulsions should not be infused in patients with triglyceride values >300–400 mg/dL. Although at one time, practitioners considered intravenous fat emulsion contraindicated in pancreatitis, IV fat may be a better tolerated fuel source for patients with pancreatitis without hypertriglyceridemia. Intravenous fat emulsion has been associated with impaired immune function in animal studies. For this reason, IV fat emulsion should not be administered to acutely septic patients or to patients during the immediate perioperative period.

Determining the Route of Nutritional Support

Having determined that nutritional support is indicated, select the route to be used. Clinical and laboratory studies demonstrate that the intestinal tract plays a critical role in the progress of numerous disease states. Enteral nutrition helps to preserve gut morphology, is better tolerated metabolically, and is less expensive. In addition, in animal studies, enteral nutrition has been shown to prevent translocation of bacteria across the gut mucosa; therefore, enteral nutrition may have a role in preventing septicemia. Furthermore, there is no advantage to parenteral nutrition in the patient with a functioning gastrointestinal tract. Parenteral nutrition does not achieve greater anabolism nor provide greater control over a patient's nutritional regimen. Thus, parenteral nutrition is indicated **only** when the enteral route is not usable. In other words: **"If the gut works, use it."**

The factors involved in choosing the route for enteral nutrition include the duration, gastrointestinal tract pathophysiology, and risk for aspiration. Nasally placed tubes are the most frequently used.

Patient comfort is maximized when a small-bore flexible tube is used. However, such tubes do not allow monitoring of residual volumes that may be significant when gastric emptying is questionable. Patients at risk for aspiration require longer tubes into the jejunum or duodenum. When long-term feeding is anticipated, a tube enterostomy is required. Percutaneous endoscopic gastrostomy tubes (PEG) are usually placed without general anesthesia. However, patients with tumors, gastrointestinal obstruction, adhesions from prior upper-abdominal surgery, or abnormal anatomy may require open surgical placement. A jejunal feeding tube may be threaded through a PEG for small bowel feeding. The placement of a needle catheter or Witzel jejunostomy during surgery generally allows earlier postoperative feeding with an elemental formulation than if one had to wait for the return of gastric emptying and colonic function (see page 352 for enteral tube placement procedures).

Some patients, because of their disease states, cannot be fed enterally and require parenteral feedings. Enteral nutrition is avoided for patients with active, massive gastrointestinal bleeding, obstruction, high-output fistulas, or short-gut syndrome. Other contraindications for enteral feeding include severe diarrhea of small bowel origin, peritonitis, severe acute pancreatitis, shock, or intestinal hypomotility.

1. ENTERAL NUTRITION: Enteral nutrition is best tolerated when instilled into the stomach, because there are less problems with osmolarity or feeding volumes. Remember that the stomach serves as a barrier to hyperosmolarity, thus the use of isotonic feedings is mandated only when instilling nutrients directly into the small intestine. The use of gastric feedings is thus preferable and should be used whenever appropriate. Patients at risk for aspiration or with impaired gastric emptying may need to be fed past the pylorus into the jejunum or the duodenum. Feedings via a jejunostomy placed at the time of surgery can often be initiated on the first postoperative day obviating the need for parenteral nutrition.

Although enteral nutrition is generally safer than parenteral nutrition, aspiration can be a significant morbid event in the care of a patient. Appropriate monitoring for residual volumes in addition to keeping the head of the bed elevated can help prevent this complication. A significant residual may be defined as 2 times the instillation rate. This can be treated by a number of methods. There may be a transient postoperative ileus best treated by waiting. Metoclopramide, erythromycin, or cisapride may be useful pharmacologic therapy. Patients who have been tolerating feedings and who develop a new high residual should be carefully assessed for the cause, concentrating on intra-abdominal infections.

The question of when to start enteral feedings in the postoperative patient must be clarified. Often, the presence of bowel sounds is used as the single criterion. It is important to realize that the presence of bowel sounds may not be a reliable indicator of gastrointestinal motility. The passage of flatus indicates colonic motility, and because the colon is the last part of the gastrointestinal tract to regain motility after laparotomy in most cases, this may be a more useful indicator.

However, a more global approach to assessment of the gastrointestinal tract is warranted. If feeding into the stomach, gastric emptying should be evaluated. Generally, when an adult patient drains 600 mL per 24-h shift on nasogastric suction, the pylorus is functioning appropriately. Clamping of the nasogastric tube to evaluate gastric emptying is contraindicated, as it exposes the patient to the risk of aspiration unnecessarily. Tolerance to enteral feeding can be assessed with the instillation of an isotonic diet given for 24 h at 30 mL/h as a trial. Feeding intolerance is characterized by vomiting, abdominal distention, diarrhea, or high gastric residual volumes.

The nutritional components and osmolality of the enteral product help classify the formulations to simplify selection. The protein component can be supplied as intact proteins, partially digested hydrolyzed proteins, or crystalline amino acids. Each gram of protein provides 4 calories when oxidized. The carbohydrate source may be intact complex starches, glucose polymers, or simpler disaccharides, such as sucrose. Carbohydrates provide 4 calories/g. Fat in enteral products usually is supplied as long-chain fatty acids. However, some enteral products contain medium-chain triglycerides (MCT), which are transported directly in the portal circulation rather than via chyle production. Because MCT oil does not contain essential fatty acids, it cannot be used as the sole fat source. Long-chain fatty acids provide 9 calories/g and MCT oil provides 8 calories/g.

The osmolality of an enteral product is determined primarily by the concentration of carbohydrates, electrolytes, amino acids, or small peptides. The clinical importance of osmolality is often debated. Hyperosmolal formulations with osmolalities exceeding 450 mosm/L may contribute to diarrhea by acting in a manner similar to osmotic cathartics. Hyperosmolal feedings are well tolerated when delivered into the stomach (as opposed to the small bowel), because gastric secretions dilute the feeding before it leaves the pylorus to traverse the small bowel. Thus, feedings administered directly to the small bowel (eg, via feeding jejunostomy) should not exceed 450 mosm/L.

On the basis of osmolality and macronutrient content, the clinician can classify enteral products into several categories. Low osmolality formulas are isotonic and contain intact macronutrients. They usually provide 1 calorie/mL and require approximately 2 L to provide the RDA for vitamins. These products are appropriate for the general patient population. Two examples are Ensure and Isocal.

High-density formulas may provide up to 2 calories/mL. These concentrated solutions are hyperosmolar and also contain intact nutrients. The RDA for vitamins can be met with volumes of 1500 mL or less. These products are used for volume-restricted patients. Examples are Nutren 2.0 and Ensure Plus HN Liquid.

Chemically defined or elemental formulas provide the macronutrients in the predigested state. These formulations are usually hyperosmolar and have poor palatability. Patients with compromised nutrient absorptive abilities or gastrointestinal function may benefit from elemental type feedings. Vivonex TEN and Peptamen are two such products.

Several enteral formulas have been developed that have been altered for various disease states. Products for pulmonary patients, such as Pulmocare, contain a higher percentage of calories from fat to decrease the carbon dioxide load from the metabolism of excess glucose. A low carbohydrate, high-fat product for persons with diabetes is available that also contains fiber that may help regulate glucose control. Other fiber-containing enteral feedings are available to help regulate bowel function, for example, Enrich. Patients with hepatic insufficiency may benefit from formulations containing a higher concentration of the branched chain amino acids and less aromatic amino acids in an attempt to correct their altered serum amino acid profile, for example, Hepatic-Aid II. Formulas containing only essential amino acids have been marketed for the renal failure patient. The clinical usefulness of many specialty products remains controversial.

Oral supplements differ from other enteral feedings by design so that they are more palatable to improve compliance. Furthermore, oral supplements contain lactose, which is inappropriate for patients with lactase deficiency; whereas, most enteral products do not contain lactose.

Guidelines for ordering enteral feedings are outlined in Table V–3. page 396 In summary, when using enteral feedings

- Determine nutritional needs.
- Assess gastrointestinal tract function and appropriateness of enteral feedings.
- Determine fluid requirements and volume tolerance on the basis of overall status and concurrent disease states.
- Select an appropriate enteral feeding product.
- Verify that the regimen selected satisfies micronutrient requirements.
- Monitor and assess nutritional status to evaluate the need for changes in the selected regimen.

Complications of Enteral Nutrition

A. Diarrhea: A common complication of enteral feeding is diarrhea. It occurs in about 10–60% of patients receiving enteral feed-

TABLE V–3. ROUTINE ORDERS FOR ENTERAL NUTRITION.

1. Confirm tube placement.
2. Elevate head of bed to 45 degrees.
3. Check gastric residuals in patients receiving gastric feedings. Hold feeding is >1.5– 2 × infusion rate. Significant residuals should be reinstilled and rechecked in 1 hour. If continues to be elevated, hold tubefeeding and begin NG suction.
4. Check patient's weight 3 times per week.
5. Record strict input and output (I&O).
6. Routine laboratory studies.

ings. The clinician must be certain to evaluate the patient for other causes of diarrhea (see Section I, Problem 22, page 98). Formula-related causes include contamination, excessive cold temperature, lactose intolerance, osmolality, and the method and/or route of delivery. Eliminate potential causes before using antidiarrheal medications:

- Check medication profile for possible drug-induced cause.
- Rule out *C difficile* colitis for patients receiving antibiotics.
- Attempt to decrease rate.
- Change formulation: Limit lactose, reduce osmolality.
- Use pharmacologic therapy only after eliminating treatable causes.

B. Constipation: Although less common than diarrhea, constipation can occur in the enterally fed patient. Check to be sure that adequate fluid volume is being given. Patients with additional requirements may benefit from water boluses or dilution of the enteral formulation. Fiber can be added to help regulate bowel function.

C. Aspiration: Aspiration is a serious complication of enteral feedings and is more likely to occur in the patient with diminished mental status. The best approach here is prevention, accomplished by elevating the patient's head and carefully monitoring residual fluid volume. Before instituting enteral feedings, one should further evaluate any patient suspected of possible aspiration or assessed to be at increased risk of aspiration. Such a patient may not be a candidate for gastric feedings and may require small bowel feedings (see Section I, Problem 8, page 32).

D. Drug Interactions: The vitamin K content of various enteral products varies from 22 mg to 156 mg per 1000 calories. This can significantly affect the anticoagulation profile of a patient receiving warfarin. Tetracycline products should not be administered 1 h before or 2 h after enteral feedings to avoid the inhibition of absorption. Similarly, enteral feedings should be stopped 2 h before and after the administration of phenytoin.

2. Parenteral Nutrition:

Peripheral Versus Central Parenteral Nutrition. The use of **total parenteral nutrition (TPN)** necessitates a central venous catheter with its concomitant risks. Although some patients require total parenteral nutrition, others have nutritional needs that can be met better with the use of **peripherally administered parenteral nutrition (PPN).**

The limiting factor in the use of PPN is the osmolality of the solution. Because centrally administered fluids are rapidly diluted at the catheter tip, osmolality is not a concern, whereas peripherally administered fluids of high osmolality rapidly result in venous sclerosis owing to the relatively low flow and slow dilution of these fluids. Thus, only patients with modest nutritional requirements will be able to meet these criteria for the necessarily low-calorie-containing solutions that can be administered peripherally.

PPN can be up to 900 mosm/kg and can be prepared from amino acid mixtures (5%), dextrose solutions (10%), and fat emulsions (20%). They have a low caloric density (0.3–0.6 kcal/mL) compared to TPN solutions and can thus only provide 1200–2300 kcal/d in 2000–3500 mL of solution. Thus, with PPN, the ability to provide caloric needs in relatively small volumes is lost; this may be clinically significant for patients requiring fluid restriction.

In general, the largest bore intravenous catheter should be used. The site should be changed frequently, usually every 72 h. Fat emulsion can be given through a Y-connector or using a three-in-one bag as is commonly used for centrally administered parenteral nutrition. Septic complications are uncommon, but thrombophlebitis can occur at the infusion site.

Although peripherally administered parenteral nutrition alleviates some of the complications associated with central TPN, its use is limited by the inability to provide the level of nutritional support frequently needed in the surgical patient. Patients with large nutritional requirements owing to stress or chronic malnutrition, high electrolyte needs, fluid restrictions, or prolonged intravenous feeding are inappropriate candidates for PPN.

Prescribing Total Parenteral Nutrition (Central TPN). Central vein infusions allow greater concentrations of both macronutrients and electrolytes. Therefore, central TPN is much more flexible in meeting a patient's nutritional requirements. With the use of permanent types of catheters (eg, the tunneled subclavian catheter, the implantable port, or a peripherally inserted central line), TPN can be administered in the hospital or home setting, depending on the patient's overall clinical condition.

When calculating caloric provision of parenteral nutrition, intravenous fat emulsion 10% provides 1.1 kcal/mL, and 20% provides 2 kcal/mL. Intravenous dextrose provides 3.4 kcal/g rather than 4 kcal/g because it is a monohydrate and therefore less calorically dense.

Centrally administered TPN is given through a central venous catheter (placed percutaneously or an operatively placed tunneled catheter) (see Section III, page 340). The solutions are usually >1900 mosm/kg and contain at least 1 kcal/mL. Thus the usual infusion of 2000–2500 L/d provides at least 2000–2500 kcal/d. This is sufficient to meet the nutritional needs of most surgical patients.

The solutions are formulated in the hospital pharmacy and are typically ordered using a standard "checklist" available in most hospitals. A commonly used method uses a single infusion bag containing all components to be infused over a 24-h period. A typical 24-h single bag will contain

Amino acids (10%)	1000 mL
Dextrose (50%)	500 mL
Fat emulsion (20%)	500 mL
Total	2000 mL

Electrolytes and vitamins to create a solution containing all nutrient requirements:

Sodium	30 mEq/L
Potassium	30 mEq/L
Phosphate	15 mmol/L
Magnesium	8 mEq/L
Calcium gluconate	4.7 mEq/L
Chloride	50 mEq/L
Acetate	70 mEq/L

The values given here represent commonly used amounts, but must be adapted to the nutritional and electrolyte needs of individual patients, and must consider concurrent disease states, such as renal or hepatic failure.

Electrolyte administration must also be changed to reflect losses. Salts are usually administered as chloride or acetate, usually in similar amounts. However, patients losing fluid by nasogastric suction require increased amounts of chloride. Similarly, patients with high-output pancreatic or small bowel fistulae will require more acetate.

Trace elements are added daily. Commercially available mixtures are usually adequate to provide needed amounts. Similarly, vitamins are usually added as premade mixtures. In addition to these mixtures (eg, MVI-12 Table V–4), the clinician must administer vitamin K, 5–10 mg IM weekly. Increased amounts of zinc are necessary with small bowel losses.

TABLE V–4. VITAMINS PROVIDED BY TWO VIALS OF MVI–12.

Ascorbic acid	100 mg
Vitamin A	1 mg
Vitamin D	5 μg
Biotin	60 μg
Folic acid	40 μg
Vitamin B_{12}	5 μg
Pyridoxine (B_6)	4 mg
Dexpanthenol	15 mg
Vitamin E	10 mg
Thiamine (B_1)	3 mg
Riboflavin (B_2)	3.6 mg

Trace element	Parenteral daily dose
Zinc	2.5–6 mg
Copper	0.3–0.5 mg
Selenium	20–50 mg
Chromium	10–15 mg
Manganese	0.4–8 mg

Starting TPN (Table V–5). TPN is usually begun at 25–50 mL/h, with increases of 25 mL/h until the precalculated final rate is

TABLE V–5. SAMPLE ORDERS FOR PATIENTS ON CENTRAL TOTAL PARENTERAL NUTRITION (TPM)

Routine orders on starting TPN

- Specify infusion (typically start 25–50 mL/hr for 24 hours: if tolerating well, especially sugars, can increase up to 2 L/d)
- Daily electrolytes
- Liver funtions test twice weekly
- CBC daily
- Vital signs qshift
- Fingerstick blood sugar qshift
- Strict intake and output
- Prealbumin

Routine orders once stabilzed on TPN

- Electrolytes and liver function tests twice weekly
- Weight weekly
- Prsalbumin (weekly)
- Urinary nitrogen (weekly)

achieved. Glucose is carefully monitored, especially in the early phase of TPN administration because glucose intolerance is very common. Be sure to check serum electrolytes (especially PO4) and glucose before starting TPN. Remember that glucose intolerance in a patient who had normal glucose levels while on TPN may be an early sign of sepsis. If a patient is undergoing surgery, the TPN usually is tapered to help prevent stress-related hyperglycemia and assist in fluid administration.

Stopping TPN. Although commonly practiced, weaning is generally not necessary. Most patients tolerate cessation of TPN, especially if they are taking oral nutrition at the time TPN is stopped. If there are concerns about hypoglycemia, the TPN rate can be halved for 1 h and then stopped completely. When TPN solution is stopped in a patient who is not on another form of feeding, then peripherally infused 10% Dextrose solution is used to avoid hypoglycemia.

Complications. Complications associated with parenteral nutrition are generally divided into mechanical, infectious, and metabolic problems.

A. *Mechanical Complications:* Following placement of the central venous catheter, a chest radiograph is obtained to evaluate the catheter tip position and the presence of a pneumothorax. The tip should be at the atrial-caval junction. A catheter tip well into the right ventricle can cause arrhythmias and may damage the tricuspid valve. Pneumo- and hydrothorax should be treated with appropriate chest tube drainage.

B. *Infectious Complications:* The use of central lines always has the potential for infectious problems. Always consider infection in a patient with new glucose intolerance on TPN. The line is usually the source of infection. Once suspected, the line should be removed. If TPN is still necessary, then a new site should be used. The catheter tip should be carefully removed and cultured. Secondary infection of the catheter, seeding from another septic site is also possible and also may necessitate catheter removal.

C. *Hyperglycemia:* The most frequently occurring metabolic complication is hyperglycemia. Hyperglycemia for the patient receiving TPN is defined as a glucose > 200 mg/dL. The approach to hyperglycemia should be dictated by first determining its cause. The initial step in this process is to assess the appropriateness of overall caloric provisions and to clarify the fuel sources. Carbohydrate calories in excess of 30–35 kcal/kg should be decreased. For patients who are diabetic, are on steroids, or are otherwise glucose intolerant, glucose in excess of 150–200 g/d may be tolerated poorly. Fat calories should be increased to approximately 30% of the nonprotein calories in the nonseptic patient. If, after adjustments, hyperglycemia should persist, a review of the patient's clinical condition and medications would be warranted.

Patients with new onset hyperglycemia should always be evaluated for an infection. Corticosteroids are the leading culprit in hyperglycemia. For patients with infections or changing steroid doses, management of hyperglycemia can be achieved with sliding scale insulin or insulin infusions when the patient is in the ICU. Insulin should not be incorporated in the TPN of patients with new onset hyperglycemia, because their hyperglycemia is due to increased hepatic gluconeogenesis and a relative insulin resistance, not to a lack of endogenously released insulin. Hyperglycemia associated with parenteral nutrition generally requires aggressive sliding scale coverage (Table V–6.) Only regular insulin should be used to manage hyperglycemia in TPN patients. Patients who are stable on a given amount of insulin may have the insulin placed in the TPN bag.

Insulin infusions are typically compounded by adding 150 units of regular insulin to 150 mL of 0.9% sodium chloride solution. The infusion is started at 1–2 U/h and titrated upward to control the glucose at 200 mg/dL. When insulin infusions exceed 8–10 U/h, insulin resistance is occurring. At this point, it is often best to discontinue the TPN and to correct the hyperglycemia.

D. *Refeeding Syndrome:* Often when malnutrition is recognized, the inclination is to rapidly and aggressively initiate specialized nutritional support. Unfortunately, this approach is associated with more hazards than the underlying malnutrition. The refeeding syndrome and morbidity associated with overfeeding are real clinical hazards associated with both parenteral and enteral nutrition. The refeeding syndrome is a constellation of severe fluid and electrolyte shifts associated with initiating nutrition in the chronically malnourished individual.

Typically, hypophosphatemia, hypomagnesemia, and hypokalemia are the electrolyte abnormalities that can result in cardiac and respiratory dysfunction and failure. Thiamine deficiency, hyper-

TABLE V–6. SLIDING SCALE DOSAGE FOR SUBCUTANEOUS INSULIN ADMINSTRATION.

	Dose of Regular Insulin (in units)	
Blood Sugar (mg/dl)	**Adequate Renal Function**	**Renal Failure**
200–250	5	2
251–300	10	4
301–350	15	6
351–400	20	8

glycemia, and volume overload have also occurred. The best approach to the refeeding syndrome is prevention. TPN should be started at no more than 1000 kilocalories or 20 kcal/kg on the first day and titrated according to patient tolerance, as defined by glucose monitoring and electrolyte values. Empiric replacement of vitamins, phosphorous, magnesium, and potassium is appropriate in the patient at risk.

E. *Electrolyte Abnormalities:* In general, when electrolyte deficiencies are present in the patient before initiating TPN, it is best to correct the problems and delay intravenous feeding. Electrolyte deficiencies that occur once the patient is receiving parenteral nutrition should be corrected with runs outside of the parenteral nutrition. If the patient has increased maintenance requirements because of chronic gastrointestinal losses or other reasons, the maintenance requirements should be incorporated into the parenteral nutrition mixture. The use of inadequate or excessive amounts of any additive results in the corresponding electrolyte abnormality. The amount of the corresponding electrolyte must be adjusted to correct the abnormality.

F. *Acid-Base Disturbances:* Hyperchloremic metabolic acidosis is fairly common in patients receiving TPN and may result from bicarbonate loss, which can be caused by severe diarrhea, pancreatic fistulae, or small bowel losses. The treatment is to administer more Na and K as acetate salts (instead of the Cl salt).

G. *Impaired Liver Function Tests:* Hepatic and biliary complications associated with parenteral nutrition are generally characterized by the duration of parenteral nutrition. Abnormal liver function tests are common in both short-term and long-term patient populations. The most common hepatic complication associated with short-term TPN administration is hepatic steatosis. This fatty liver infiltration is thought to be a result of overfeeding, especially of carbohydrate calories. The incidence of hepatic steatosis has decreased with the introduction of IV fat emulsion and the growing consideration of conservative caloric feeding. Biliary sludge formation and cholelithiasis with its associated complications have been noted in patients receiving TPN for 3 weeks or longer. Biliary stasis caused by the lack of stimulation resulting from bowel rest or short-gut is thought to be the primary mechanism. Long-term TPN administration is associated with hepatic steatonecrosis. Its pathogenesis is unclear at this time.

The diagnosis of TPN-associated hepatotoxicity is a diagnosis of exclusion. Once other causes have been ruled out, management of hepatotoxicity includes reformulation of the caloric regimen, cyclic administration of TPN, and metronidazole.

H. *Prerenal Azotemia:* Excessive amino acid infusion with inadequate calorie administration can result in prerenal azotemia. A rising BUN should be monitored, but probably not treated until it is >100 mg/dL. This is treated by reducing the amino acid intake and increasing calories administered as glucose. Prerenal azotemia resulting from intravascular volume depletion should be ruled out.

I. *Bleeding Abnormalities:* These can be caused by inadequate amounts of vitamin K, iron deficiency, folate deficiency, or vitamin B12 deficiency. Adjust the nutrient administration to the required amount.

J. *Overfeeding:* It is imperative to nutritionally support a patient on a rational and quantitative basis. To do this, the clinician must know the requirements for each nutritional component. Energy requirements are dependent on gender, weight, height, age, energy expenditure, and seriousness of the injury. Overfeeding places patients at risk for hepatic complications, increased carbon dioxide production, and hyperglycemia.

3. TPN in Specific Disease States: The administration of TPN must be changed for patients with certain diseases including.

Cardiac Failure. Fluid administration is limited in these patients. Instead of the usual 1-mL water per calorie (as in tube feedings), water is given at 0.5 mL/calorie. Alternatively, water can be given at a rate equal to 500 mL (insensible losses) plus measured losses. Protein can be limited to 0.8–1 g/kg, and sodium limited to 0.5–1.5 g/d.

Diabetes. Use increased calories from fat in these patients to limit the carbohydrate calories while providing sufficient calories for protein anabolism. Insulin can be added to the bag in a patient with stable insulin requirements. In general, fat should provide no more than 50% of total caloric intake and no more than 2.5 g/kg/d.

Hepatic Dysfunction. Patients with hepatic dysfunction usually benefit from increased amounts of branched-chain amino acids (leucine, valine, and isoleucine) and reduced amounts of aromatic amino acids, which are precursors to centrally active amines and thus contribute to hepatic encephalopathy. Specialized mixtures of amino acids are available and should be used only for patients with hepatic encephalopathy. Lipid emulsions should be limited in those patients with severe hepatic dysfunction.

Renal Disease. These patients have a number of specific restrictions that must be carefully accounted for in the administration of TPN including fluid, protein, potassium, magnesium, and sodium. Protein must be restricted to 0.6–0.8 g/kg/d for patients not undergoing dialysis. Patients receiving hemodialysis generally require 1.2 g/kg of protein per day, and patients undergoing peritoneal dialysis need 1.5 g/kg. The latter patient also absorbs approximately 500 kcals/d of dextrose from the dialysate, which must be considered when designing their nutritional regimen. Patients on hemodialysis may receive the usual protein load of 1–1.5 g/kg/d. For these patients, specially formulated amino acid mixtures are used that contain higher amounts of essential amino acids. In general, TPN should not contain potassium or magnesium in renal failure patients. Reduced sodium may also be necessary.

Pulmonary Dysfunction. Carbohydrate metabolism (including overfeeding) results in production of CO_2. Thus, patients with impaired ventilation, who already may retain CO_2, are further stressed when high carbohydrate loads are administered. This problem may be treated by increasing the percentage of calories provided by fat (up to 50%). Overall, calories should not exceed 30–35 kcal/kg. These patients also may be sensitive to phosphate depletion and should be monitored carefully for the development of hypophosphatemia. Once identified, this is treated with phosphate supplementation.

REFERENCES

ASPEN Board of Directors. Guidelines for the use of parenteral and enteral nutrition in adult and pediatric patients. *J Parenter Enteral Nutr* 1993;17:6SA.

Gomella LG (editor): Total parenteral nutrition. In *Clinician's Pocket Reference,* 9th ed. Copyright © 2001 by The McGraw-Hill Companies Inc.

VI. Blood Component Therapy

APPROACH TO THE BLEEDING PATIENT

When called to evaluate a patient for a low hemoglobin/hematocrit level (Hgb/Hct) or for active bleeding, as in all such situations, start with the ABCs (Airway, Breathing, Circulation). Once the airway and breathing issues are controlled, the HR, BP, and the need for blood components/transfusions or just IV fluid should be assessed. First, obtain good IV access with 2 large-bore IVs, 16-gauge FR or larger, and order a CBC and coagulation studies (PT, PTT, platelet count). A Type & Screen (T & S) or Type & Cross (T & C) should also be ordered, depending on the clinical situation.

Questions to ask:

- What is the current Hgb/Hct level?
- What is the last Hgb/Hct level?
- Is the patient on any anticoagulants?

An attempt should be made to assess the location and amount of the patient's bleeding, and the patient's vital signs should be monitored very closely. "Transfusion triggers" have changed during the past several years, and it is no longer mandatory to maintain a hemoglobin > 10g/dL in all patients. Considerations include a patient's age; comorbid conditions, including risk factors for coronary artery disease (HTN, DM, smoking, age over 50 years in men, hypercholesterolemia); and rapidity of the bleeding and the fall in Hgb/Hct level. In young healthy patients, the Hgb, in certain clinical situations, has been allowed to fall as low as 6g/dL, (note females have a lower baseline Htc than males of the same age). Oxygen delivery is partially dependent on the hemoglobin/hematocrit levels. Several studies suggest that for noncritically ill patients, the threshold for transfusion is 7–8 g/dL. However this level does not appear acceptable for patients with significant risk factors for CAD, or for patients with symptomatic anemia, tachycardia, and so forth. Having a hemoglobin of 8g/dL or even 10g/dL in light of ongoing active bleeding (eg, lower/upper GIB) may also be an indication for transfusion, because the hemoglobin takes time to equilibrate. Continued blood loss may cause the next hemoglobin measurement to be only 6g/dL when one does not consider ongoing blood loss. It should be remembered that a fall in the hemoglobin may be a **late** sign of active bleeding.

BLOOD BANKING PROCEDURES

Type & Screen (T & S): The blood bank will type the patient's blood and screen it for antibodies. If a rare antibody is found, the physician will usually be notified. When there is any chance the patient may need blood in the immediate future, it is advisable to type and crossmatch a bleeding patient. When one waits until the laboratory test indicates the Hct level is low and a transfusion is immediately required, a waiting period of another hour is necessary for a crossmatch to be ready. Remember when seeing patients in regular floor care rooms that most ICUs can do a rapid spun hematocrit and while a laboratory Hgb/Hct measurement is pending, a specimen can be sent to the ICU to check a spun hematocrit. Once a T & S has been sent, blood usually can be crossmatched within an hour by most blood bank facilities.

Type & Cross (T & C): The blood bank will type and screen the patient's blood and match the patient with specific donor units. The number of units to be crossed and held must be specified. If the request is made "stat," the bank will set up blood immediately and usually hold it for 12 h. For routine requests, the blood is set up at a date and time that the physician specifies, and the blood is usually held for 36–48 h.

PREOPERATIVE BLOOD SET UP

Many institutions have established parameters for setting up blood before procedures (Table VI–1). Depending on the institution and the operating surgeon, various procedures require T & S and/or T & C; -the use of one or both may change as clinical experience with a given procedure increases (eg, liver transplant). Therefore, instead of supplying specific numbers for specific procedures, residents who are more senior or the attending physician should be asked for their advice before ordering preoperative T & C or T & S.

BLOOD BANK PRODUCTS & BLOOD COMPONENT THERAPY

Table VI–2 and Table VI–3 describe products used in blood component therapy and give some common indications for their use.

TRANSFUSION PROCEDURE

1. Draw a clot tube ("red top") and sign the lab slips to verify it is the sample from the correct patient. The patient should be identified by the identification (ID) bracelet. If the patient can speak, ask the patient's name. The name, hospital number, date, and physician's signature should be placed on the test tube label.
2. When the blood products become available, make sure that the patient has good venous access for the transfusion (18 gauge or larger is preferred in an adult).
3. Remember to verify the information with another person, such as a nurse, on the request slip, blood bag, and with the

TABLE VI–1. TYPICAL PARAMETERS FOR SETTING UP BLOOD BEFORE PROCEDURES.

Procedure	Guidelines
Amputation (lower extremity)	2 units
Cardiac procedure (CABG, valve)	4 units
Cholecystectomy (open and laparoscopic)	T & S
Colostomy	T & S
Colon resection	2 units
Cystectomy (radical with diversion)	4 units
Esophageal resection	2 units
Exploratory laparotomy	2 units
Gastrectomy	2 units
Gastrostomy	T & S
Hemorrhoidectomy	T & S
Hernia	T & S
Hysterectomy	2 units
Liver resection	6 units
Liver transplant	6 units
Mastectomy	T & S
Nephrectomy	2 units
Pancreatectomy	4 units
Parathyroidectomy	T & S
Pulmonary resection	2 units
Radical neck dissection	2 units
Radical prostatectomy	2–4 units
Renal transplant	2 units
Small bowel resection	2 units
Splenectomy	2 units
Thyroidectomy	T & S
Tracheostomy	2 units
Total hip	2 units
Transurethral resection of prostate (TURP)	2 units
Vascular procedures	
Abdominal aortic aneurysm	6 units
Carotid endarterectomy	T & S
Aortofemoral bypass	4 units
Aortoiliac bypass	4 units
Femoral popliteal bypass	4 units
Iliofemoral bypass	4 units
Portacaval shunt	6 units
Splenorenal shunt	6 units
Vein stripping	T & S

TABLE VI–2. BLOOD BANK PRODUCTS THAT USUALLY REQUIRE A "CLOT TUBE" TO BE SENT FOR TYPING.

Product	Description	Common Indications
Whole blood	No elements removed; 1 unit = 450 mL ; contains red cells, white cells, plasma and platelets (platelets may be nonfunctional)	Not for routine use; acute massive bleeding:open heart surger; neonatal total exchange
Packed red blood cells (PRBC) (also see page 363)	Most plasma removed; unit = 250–300 mL: 1 unit should raise Hct 3 %	Replacement in chronic and acute (PRBC) blood loss, GI bleeding, trauma
Universal pedi-packs	250–300 mL divided into 3 bags; contains red cells, some white cells, some plasma and platelets	Transfusion for infants
Platelets (also see page 363)	1 "pack" should raise count by 5–8000; "6–pack" means a pool of platelets from 6 units of blood; 1 pack = about 50 mL	Decreased production or destruction (ie, aplastic anemia, acute leukemia, postchemo, etc); counts <5000 (risk of spontaneous hemorrhage); counts 5–30,000 if risk of bleeding (headache, GI losses, contiguous petechiae) or active bleeding; counts <50,000 if life-threatening bleed or preop; counts <100,000 in some case of post-CABG bleeding or with neuro- or ophthalmic. surgery; usually not indicated in idiopathic throm–bocytopenic purpura [ITP] or thrombotic thrombocy-topenic purpura [ITP] unless life-threatening bleed or preoperatively
Leukocyte poor red cells	Most WBC removed less antigenic; 1 unit = 200–250 mL	Previous fabrile transfusion reactions; patients requiring multiple transfusions (eg, leukemia)
Washed RBCs	Like leukocyte poor red cells but WBC almost completely removed; 1 unit = 300 mL	As for leukocyte poor red cells, but very expensive and much more purified

(continued)

TABLE VI–2. BLOOD BANK PRODUCTS THAT USUALLY REQUIRE A "CLOT TUBE" TO BE SENT FOR TYPING. (*continued*).

Product	Description	Common Indications
Cryoprecipitated antihemophilic factor ("cryo")	Contains factor VIII, factor XIII, von Willebrand's factor, and fibrinogen; 1 unit = 10 mL	Hemophilia A (factor VIII deficiency), when safer factor VIII concentrate not available; von Willebrand's disease; fibrinogen deficiency, fibrin surgical glue
Fresh frozen plasma (FFP)	Contains factors II, VII, IX, X, XI, XII, XIII and heat labile V and VII; about 1 hr to thaw; 150–250 mL (400–600 mL if single donor pheresis)	Emergency reversal of Coumadin; massive transfusion (>5 L in adults); Hypoglobunemia (IV immune globulin preferred); suspected or documented coagulopathy (congenital or acquired) with active bleeding or before surgery; clotting factor replacement when concentrate unavailable; no longer' recommended for volume replacement
Single donor plasma	Like FFP, but lacks factors V and VIII; about 1 hr to thaw; 150–200 mL	No longer routinely used for plasma replacement; stable clotting factor replacement; Coumadin reversal, Hemophilia B (Christmas disease)
RhoGam (RhoD immune globulin)	Antibody against Rh factor	Rh^- mother with Rh^+ baby within 72-hr of delivery

patient's identification (ID) bracelet. Note: Nearly all hospitals have defined protocols for this procedure; check guidelines for specific institution.

4. Blood products to be transfused may be mixed with only isotonic normal saline. Using hypotonic products, such as D5W, may result in hemolysis of the blood in the tubing. Lactated Ringer's should not be used because the calcium could chelate the anticoagulant citrate.
5. When transfusing large volumes of packed red cells (0.6–8 units), it is necessary to also transfuse platelets and fresh frozen plasma (FFP) periodically (dilutional thrombocytopenia is the most common complication of multiple transfusions). Studies demonstrate higher mortality rates for patients not given platelets and factors early during a massive

TABLE VI–3. BLOOD BANK PRODUCTS THAT ARE DISPENSED BY MOST HOSPITAL PHARMACIES AND ARE ORDERED AS MEDICATION.

Product	Description	Common Indications
Factor VIII (purified antihemophilic factor)	From pooled plasma, pure factor VIII	Routine for hemophilia A (factor VII deficiency); increased hepatitis risk
Factor IX concentrate (prothrombin complex	Increased hepatitis risk; factors II, VII, IX, and X equivalent to 2 units of plasma	Active bleeding in Christmas disease (Hemophilia B or factor IX deficiency)
Immune serum globulin	Precipitate from plasma; gamma globulin	Immune globulin deficiency: disease prophylaxis (eg. hepatitis A, measles)
5% albumin or 5% plasma protein fraction	Precipitate from plasma (see Section IX)	Plasma volume expanders in acute blood loss
25% albumin	Precipitate from plasma	Hypoalbuminemia, volume expander, burns; draws extravascular fluid into circulation

resuscitation. Also, a calcium replacement is sometimes needed, because the preservative used in the blood (citrate) is a calcium binder, and hypocalcemia can result after large amounts of blood are transfused. Also, the blood should be warmed, if at all possible, in all transfusions. In cases where massive resuscitation efforts are necessary, warming is essential to prevent hypothermia, coagulopathy, and cardiac arrhythmias. Massive blood transfusions are associated with acute lung injury (ARDS) and possibly disseminated intravascular coagulation (DIC).

BLOOD GROUPS

Table VI–4 gives information on the major blood groups and their relative occurrences. O– is the universal donor and AB+ is the universal recipient.

TRANSFUSION FORMULA

Red Blood Cells

As a rule of thumb, 1 unit of packed red cells raises the hematocrit by 3% (hemoglobin 1 g/dL) in the average adult. To roughly determine the volume of whole blood or packed red cells needed to raise a hematocrit to a specific amount, use the following formula:

TABLE VI–4. BLOOD GROUPS

Type (ABO/Rh)	Occurrences	Can Usually Receive Blood From
0^+	1 in 3	0 ($^{+/-}$)
0^-	1 in 15	0 ($^-$)
A^+	1 in 3	A ($^{+/-}$) or 0 ($^{+/-}$)
A^-	1 in 16	A ($^-$) or 0 ($^-$)
B^+	1 in 12	B ($^{+/-}$) or 0 ($^{+/-}$)
B^-	1 in 67	B ($^-$) or 0 ($^-$)
AB^+	1 in 29	AB, A, B or 0 (all $^+$ or $^-$)
AB-	1 in 167	AB, A, B or 0 (all $^-$)

$$\text{Volume of cells} = \frac{\text{Total blood volume of patient x (desired Hct } - \text{ actual Hct)}}{\text{Hct of transfusion product}}$$

where total blood volume = 70 mL/kg in adults, 80 mL/kg in children; Hct, packed cells = approximately 70%; Hct, whole blood = approximately 40%.

Platelets

Before a major surgical procedure, some clinicians seek a platelet count of > 100,000 and for minor surgery > 50,000. The occurrence of spontaneous hemorrhage is thought to occur with platelet counts < 20,000. However, the experience of many surgeons treating patients with ITP is that patients with splenic abnormalities, hematologic cancers, or other disorders causing thrombocytopenia often do not bleed even with platelet counts as low as 5,000. The exact platelet count needed to avoid the morbidity of bleeding in a thrombocytopenic patient is undefined at the present time.

Platelets are often transfused at a dose of 1 U per 10 kg body weight. After administration of 1 unit of multiple donor platelets, the count should rise 5–8,000/mL within 1 h of transfusion and 4,500 mL within 24 h. Normally, stored platelets that are transfused should survive in vivo 6–8 d after infusion. Clinical factors (DIC, alloimmunization) can significantly shorten these intervals. To standardize the corrected platelet count to an individual patient, use the corrected count increment (CCI). Measure the platelet count immediately before and 1 h after the platelet infusion. If the correction is less than expected, workup of platelet refractoriness (antibodies, splenomegaly, etc) should be performed. ABO type is not as much of a concern with platelet transfusions; blood group A can receive A,

AB, and O. Group B can receive B, AB, and O; AB can receive- AB, A, and O; and O can receive any O. Rh antigens are not expressed on platelets; however, women of child-bearing age should be given Rh-negative platelets to prevent the formation of antibodies when they are Rh negative.

$$CCI = \frac{(\text{Posttransfusion count} - \text{Pretransfusion count}) \times \text{Body surface area } (m^2)}{\text{Platelets given} \times 10^{11}}$$

EMERGENCY TRANSFUSIONS

The transfusion of non-crossmatched blood is occasionally necessary in cases of trauma and/or massive hemorrhage. Type-specific blood (ABO and Rh-matched only), is usually available in 10 min and can be used. If even this time is too long, type O, Rh negative, packed red cell blood can be used. Most blood banks can do a complete crossmatch within 1 h. As per advanced trauma life support (ATLS) protocol, a 2-liter challenge of crystalloid is used to support BP; however, when hypotension persists or there are massive ongoing blood losses, transfusion of blood may be warranted.

TRANSFUSION REACTIONS

See Section I, Problem 68, page 247. More than 85% of adverse hemolytic transfusion reactions relate to clerical error.

AUTOLOGOUS BLOOD TRANSFUSIONS

Because of concerns over the transmission of disease by blood transfusion therapy, prehospital autologous blood banking (predeposit phlebotomy) has become popular in the elective surgery patient. General guidelines for autologous banking include good overall health status, an Htc > 34% and arm veins that can accommodate a 16-gauge needle. Patients can usually donate up to 1 unit every 3–7 d, until 3–7 d before surgery (individual blood banks have their own specifications), depending on the needs of the planned surgery. Iron supplements (such as ferrous gluconate 325 mg PO tid) are usually given before and several months after the donation. Units of whole blood can be held for up to 35 d.

DIRECTED DONOR BLOOD PRODUCTS

Because of concerns over disease transmission, this form of donation is becoming more widely used, although this varies by region. This involves a person, often a relative, donating blood for a specific patient. This cannot be used in the emergency setting because it takes up to 48 h to process the blood for transfusion.

There are some drawbacks to this system: relatives may be unduly pressured to give blood, risk factors that would normally exclude the use of the blood (eg, hepatitis or HIV positivity) become problematic, and ultimately the routine donation of blood for emergency transfusion may be adversely affected. These units are usually stored as packed red cells and released into the general transfusion pool 8 h after surgery unless otherwise requested.

APHERESIS

Apheresis procedures are used to collect single donor platelets (platelet pheresis) or white blood cells (leukapheresis); the remaining components are returned to the donor. Therapeutic apheresis is the separation and removal of a particular component to achieve a therapeutic effect (eg, erythrocytapheresis to treat polycythemia).

HEPATITIS & AIDS RISKS

Before administering a transfusion, the risks of the procedure should be explained to the patient and/or the patient's family, and an informed consent should be obtained. An exception to this practice is in emergency/trauma cases where this is not practical. Statistics published in 1999 estimate the current risk of contracting HIV nationally from a blood transfusion is 1/200,000–1/2,000,000. The risk of hepatitis B is estimated to be 1/30,000–1/250,000; hepatitis C, 1/30,000–1/150,000; hepatitis A, 1/1,000,000; acute hemolytic reaction, 1/250,000–1/1,000,000. As can be seen, hepatitis C is the most common form of hepatitis transmitted via transfusions. The most common infectious agent transmitted is CMV, which is a concern in immunocompromised patients.

The greatest risk is with pooled factor products, such as concentrates of factor VIII. Use of albumin and globulins, and the new genetically engineered factor VIII concentrates involves no risk of hepatitis or HIV.

OTHER OPTIONS

Blood Product Substitutes

Research to find a suitable blood product alternative that could bind oxygen and deliver the oxygen to the tissues has thus far not met with much success. Potential advantages would include eliminating the risk of passing on HIV and hepatitis and using these products for patients who refuse blood transfusions.

Erythropoietin: Current studies are underway to answer the question of whether the administration of erythropoietin could potentially decrease the number of transfusions necessary for a patient who is admitted to the hospital with a low hematocrit.

VII. Ventilator Management

INDICATIONS & SET-UP

I. Indications for Ventilatory Support

A. Hypoxemic Respiratory Failure. The inability to oxygenate is an important indication for ventilatory support. A PaO_2 < 60 mm Hg on > 50% inspired fraction of oxygen (FIO_2) constitutes hypoxemic respiratory failure. Although these patients can sometimes be managed with higher FIO_2 delivery systems (eg, partial or nonrebreather masks or continuous positive airway pressure (CPAP) delivered by mask), they are at high risk for respiratory arrest and should be closely monitored in an intensive care unit (ICU). These delivery systems are at a significant disadvantage compared with mechanical ventilation, because it is difficult to continuously maintain and guarantee a high FIO_2 delivery. Worsening of the respiratory status necessitates prompt intubation and ventilatory support. The most common cause for pure hypoxemic respiratory failure is adult respiratory distress syndrome (ARDS) in which the high shunt fraction leads to refractory hypoxemia.

B. Ventilatory Failure. Rigid criteria for defining ventilatory failure are found in Table VII–1. In general, ventilatory failure is based on the degree of hypercarbia. A $PaCO_2$ > 50 mm Hg indicates ventilatory failure; however, many patients with chronic pulmonary conditions, such as COPD, will have chronic ventilatory failure with renal compensation (retaining HCO_3–) to adjust the pH toward normal. Thus, absolute pH is often a better guide than $PaCO_2$ in determining the need for ventilatory assistance. A respiratory acidosis with a rapidly falling pH or an absolute pH ≤ 7.24 is an indication for ventilatory support. The typical example of pure ventilatory failure is the drug overdose patient in whom there is a sudden loss of central respiratory drive with uncontrolled hypercarbia. Patients with sepsis, neuromuscular disease, and chronic obstructive pulmonary disease (COPD) may also have hypercarbic ventilatory failure.

C. Mixed Respiratory Failure. Most patients have failure of both ventilation and oxygenation (eg, COPD with acute bronchitis). The indications for ventilatory support remain the same as listed earlier. The threshold for initiating ventilatory support will be even lower for patients with ventilation and oxygenation failure, because oxygen management may

TABLE VII–1. CRITERIA FOR DIAGNOSIS OF ACUTE RESPIRATORY FAILURE.[1]

Parameter	Normal	Respiratory Failure
Respiratory rate	12–20	>35
Vital capacity (mL/kg body wt)[2]	65–75	<15
FEV_1 (mL/Kg body wt)[2]	50–60	≤10
Inspiratory force (cm H_2O)	⁻(75–100)	≥25
Compliance (mL/cm H_2O)	100	<20
P_aO_2 (mm/cm H_2O)	80–95 room air	<70
A-aDo_2 (mm Hg) (Fio_2 = 1.0)	25–65	>450
Os/Ot (%)	5–8	>20
$Paco_2$	35–45	>55[3]
VD/VT	0.2–0.3	>0.60

[1]*(Reproduced, with permission, from Demling RH, Goodwin CW: Pulmonary Dysfunction. In:* Care of the Surgical Patient. *Willmore DW (editor). Scientific American, 1989.)*
[2]Ideal body weight should be used.
[3]Chronic lung disease constitutes the exception.
FEV_1–Forced expiratory volume in 1 second; P_aO_2–Partial pressure of oxgen in arterial blood;A-aDo_2–Aveolar-arterial oxygen gradient; Fio_2–Fraction of inspired oxygen Qs/Qt–shunt fraction; P_aCO_2–Partial pressure of carbon dioxide in arterial blood; VD/VT–Ratio of dead space to tidal volume.

further compound hypercarbia. Bronchospasm alters the ventilation-perfusion ratio ($\dot{V}/\dot{Q}$) relationships leading to worsening hypoxemia. Bronchospasm and accumulated secretions lead to a high work of breathing and consequent hypercarbia.

D. Neuromuscular Failure. This is a category of ventilatory failure but deserves special mention because the management is different. Hypercarbia occurs just before arrest, and thus, criteria other than arterial blood gases (ABGs) are needed.

1. In progressive tachypnea, breathing rates > 24/min are an early sign of respiratory failure. A progressive rise in the respiratory rate or sustained breathing rates > 35/min are an indication for ventilatory support.
2. Abdominal paradox indicates dyssynergy of chest wall muscles and hemidiaphragms with impending respiratory failure. It is manifested by inward movement of the abdominal wall during inspiration rather than the normal outward motion.
3. A vital capacity < 15 mL/kg (1000 mL for a normal body-sized person) is associated with acute respiratory arrest

and an inability to clear secretions. Similarly, a negative inspiratory force less negative than –25 cm H_2O implies impending respiratory arrest. Guillain-Barré syndrome is the typical example of a neuromuscular disease in which the preceding criteria merit strict attention. A patient with Guillain-Barré syndrome should be observed closely and followed up with frequent vital capacity (VC) determinations. A rapidly falling VC or VC < 1000 mL requires initiation of respirator support.

II. Endotracheal Intubation.(see Section III, page 350).

Endotracheal intubation is often the most difficult and potentially hazardous part of ventilator initiation. Skill and experience are required for correct placement. Aspiration, esophageal intubation, and right main stem bronchus intubation are common complications. Bilateral breath sounds always need to be confirmed by chest auscultation in each axilla. The most accurate method of confirming proper placement is by measuring expired CO_2. Many hospitals have monitoring devices that can detect the presence of CO_2 by color change. An immediate postintubation portable chest radiograph should be obtained. Intubation can be accomplished by 3 routes: nasotracheal intubation, orotracheal intubation, or tracheostomy. When an intubation is difficult or complicated, one should not hesitate in finding another physician with more experience.

A. Nasotracheal Intubation. This can be accomplished blindly and in an awake patient. It requires experience and adequate local anesthesia. Complications include esophageal intubation, nosebleeds, kinking of the endotracheal tube (ETT), and postobstructive sinusitis. A smaller ETT is usually required for nasotracheal versus orotracheal intubation; this leads to a higher work of breathing because of increased resistance, difficulties with adequate suctioning, and higher ventilation pressures. Nasotracheal ETTs are more comfortable than orotracheal ETTs and are less damaging to the larynx because of better stabilization in the airway. Nasotracheal intubation should not be attempted by those without experience in an emergency setting.

B. Orotracheal Intubation. Placement of orotracheal tubes requires normal neck mobility to allow hyperextension of the neck for direct visualization of the vocal cords. Larger ETTs can be placed by this route. Adequate local anesthesia or sedation is necessary for safe placement without aspiration. Performing the intubation without the use of paralytics allows inexperienced physicians additional safety as the patient can continue to breathe. Key factors in successful intubation are complete preparation of all supplies before attempting intubation, proper hand placement, and use of the laryngoscope.

C. Tracheostomy. Cricothyroidotomy is the surgical procedure most often done in acute cases for upper-airway obstruction; however, in patients who require more than 14–21 days of ventilatory support, a formal surgical tracheostomy is recommended to prevent tracheal stenosis and vocal cord damage. Tracheostomy tubes facilitate the weaning process by decreasing tube resistance as the tube is shorter and of greater radius. Patients are able to eat and find the tubes more comfortable

III. Ventilator Set-up

A. The Ventilator. Almost all modern adult ventilators are time- and flow (volume)-cycled and can be used in adults and in children older than 2 years. Children younger than 2 years and infants are usually managed on pressure-limited continuous flow. Pressure-controlled ventilation is an alternate mode of support most frequently used for patients with ARDS. High frequency or "jet" ventilators are only indicated for use in patients with tracheobronchial fistulas and are not used commonly. Elaborate alarm systems are present to alert personnel to inadequate ventilation, high pressure, disconnection of the ETT, and so forth. Effective ventilation is measured by changes in $Paco_2$. Minute ventilation (V^e) is tidal volume × respiratory rate. Thus, ventilation may be adjusted by changing the respiratory rate, the tidal volume, or both. Tidal volumes above 12 mL/kg may cause overdistention of alveoli and increase the risk of pneumothorax. Most initial tidal volumes are therefore set at 10–12 mL/kg. Oxygenation is adjusted by changing Fio_2 and positive end expiratory pressure (PEEP). There is a current trend toward reducing tidal volume to decrease the effects of barotrauma. Some clinicians are using 5–8 mL/kg as a guideline for tidal volumes. Prolonged Fio_2 > 60% may cause pulmonary fibrosis. Thus, down-adjustment to "safe levels" sufficient to maintain O_2 saturation > 90% should be attempted if indicated by ABGs. If an O_2 saturation > 90% cannot be maintained when decreasing the Fio_2 < 60%, other means, eg, increasing positive end-expiratory pressure (PEEP), can be used. The mode of ventilation should be specified.

1. Control mode delivers a set rate and tidal volume irrespective of patient efforts and is used for patients who are paralyzed or unable to initiate a breath. (Rarely, if ever, used.)

2. Assist control (AC) mode allows patient triggering of machine breaths once a threshold of inspiratory flow or effort is made. It also supplies a back-up rate in case of apnea or paralysis. This mode provides the full specified tidal volume each time the threshold effort is achieved, and it should be considered the primary mode of ventilation in all patients who require higher F_{IO_2} or remain hemodynamically unstable. This mode removes the slight work of breathing required to initiate breaths in intermittent mandatory ventilation modes.
3. Intermittent mandatory ventilation (IMV) provides a set number of machine breaths per minute and also allows the patient to make spontaneous breaths. Synchronized intermittent mandatory ventilation (SIMV) allows synchronization of the IMV breaths with patient efforts and is the generally preferred method. As the rate is decreased, the patient assumes more and more of the work of breathing. This mode can be used in conjunction with pressure support ventilation (PSV). All efforts by the patient between synchronized breaths are against the resistance of the tubing or with the assistance of a specified pressure support. This mode is well tolerated by patients who continue to require mechanical ventilation but are awake and otherwise stable.
4. Pressure support ventilation is used to help decrease the inspiratory work of breathing. Pressure support supplies a positive pressure when the patient initiates a breath. The patient sets the flow, respiratory rate, and tidal volume. Used in association with augmented minute ventilation (AMV), this is becoming a popular technique to wean patients from ventilatory support, because both the inspiratory pressure and the minute ventilation backup can be weaned.
5. Continuous positive airway pressure (CPAP) allows completely spontaneous respirations while the patient is still connected to the ventilator. A set amount of continuous pressure is applied during inspiration and expiration (from 0 to 30 cm H_2O). There are no ventilator-delivered breaths. The amount of support provided by the machine during patient inspirations can be specified by increasing the pressure support. Weaning from the ventilator can also be attempted using CPAP. Patients are started with a high-pressure support that is gradually reduced over time.
6. Currently, high frequency (jet) ventilation is not used widely except in specific situations. The process relies on

low airway pressure, low tidal volumes (4 mL/kg), and very high rates (typically 100–400) cycles per minute.

B. Ventilator Settings

1. Initial ventilator settings should be dictated by the underlying condition and previous blood gas results. There are 5 parameters to order when writing initial ventilator orders. The patient's PO_2 is affected by the FIO_2 and the PEEP level. The patient's PCO_2 is affected by the rate and the tidal volume. Lastly, the mode of ventilation should be specified.
   a. **Fraction of inspired oxygen (FIO_2):** There are many approaches to the first orders for oxygen, but the most prudent is to start every patient on 90–100% oxygen. The problem with high oxygen concentrations is toxicity. While oxygen at every amount greater than room air (21%) is toxic, the phenomenon is time-related. Many clinicians recommend 100% until the first blood gas result is available. This should not exceed 1 h, minimizing any toxic effect of 100% oxygen. In general, try to keep FIO_2 < 50% to maintain acceptable oxygenation (generally >90% saturated on ABG).
   b. **Positive-end expiratory pressure (PEEP):** People are subject to about 5 cm H_2O of PEEP in a normal nonintubated condition. Because the normal closing of the glottis at the end of respiration is lost with an intubated patient, PEEP maintains the functional residual capacity above the critical closing volume. Usually start with 3–5 cm H_2O of PEEP. Adjust PEEP higher later to enable adequate oxygenation with lower FIO_2 as needed. High levels of PEEP (> 10–15 cm H_2O) are associated with increased risk of barotrauma and decreased cardiac output; hemodynamic monitoring is usually needed for high levels of PEEP.
   c. **Rate:** Normal respiratory rate is 12–20 per minute. Initially the ventilator should be set at 12 breaths per minute.
   d. **Tidal volume:** Normal tidal volume is 8–10 mL/kg body weight.
   e. **Mode:** There are several modes of operation of most volume-cycled ventilators, including IMV, SIMV, etc, as previously noted. A basic understanding of these modes is important to order the optimum support for a given patient.

   The following list is an example of settings for a patient who is status post respiratory arrest:

- FIO_2 100%
- Assist control mode
- Rate 14
- Tidal volume 800 mL
- PEEP 5 cm H_2O

An attempt should be made to supply the patient with at least as much minute ventilation as was required before intubation. Thus, patients with pulmonary edema, ARDS, or neuromuscular disease may require minute ventilation rates of 14–22 L/min. The AC mode will generally be more comfortable and will alleviate the work of breathing to a large extent. The following list shows sample settings for these patients:

- FIO_2 100%
- Assist control mode
- Rate 18
- Tidal volume 750 mL
- PEEP 5 cm H_2O

The patient with COPD, on the other hand, should not be overventilated initially. Such patients may have a chronically high bicarbonate because of renal compensation, and overventilation could cause a severe alkalosis. The following is a list of sample settings:

- FIO_2 50%
- SIMV mode
- Pressure support 15 cm
- Rate 12
- Tidal volume 800 mL
- PEEP 5 cm H_2O

2. **Secondary ventilator controls.** Most major ventilator controls (inspired oxygen, tidal volume, PEEP, rate, and mode) are ordered by the physician and accomplish the major control of the ventilator's functions. However, there are a series of secondary ventilator controls that can be used to "optimize" or fine-tune the ventilator. Often, secondary controls are determined by local protocol. However, secondary ventilator control settings can be specified including
   a. **Sigh:** During normal breathing, the lungs are inflated to their maximum capacity up to 6 times an hour. The sigh mode delivers a large tidal volume several times an hour to duplicate this normal physiologic breathing pattern. At very high peak inspiratory pressures, the sigh is not needed. To order

sigh, specify the rate, volume delivered, and maximum pressure.

b. **Peak inspiratory pressure (PIP):** This represents the maximum pressure generated and is typically set at 20–30 cm H_20. Pressures above 45 cm are associated with significant barotrauma.

c. **Inspiratory/expiratory ratio (I:E):** Normal is approximately 1:3. Higher ratios favor oxygenation, lower ratios enhance CO_2 removal. Most ventilator alarms sound if the parameters chosen result in an I:E ratio of <1:1.

C. Additional Set-up Requirements

1. Restrain the patient's hands because the natural reaction to the ETT upon awakening is to pull it out.
2. Place a nasogastric tube to decompress the stomach and/or to continue essential oral medications and monitor gastric pH.
3. Consider placement of an arterial catheter. An arterial line provides both a continuous monitor for blood pressure and the ability to easily obtain arterial blood gases. Suitable sites are radial arteries, dorsalis pedis arteries, and femoral arteries.
4. Obtain an immediate portable chest radiograph to confirm ETT placement and to reassess any underlying pulmonary disease. In addition, daily chest radiographs should be obtained to confirm the position of the ETT.
5. Treat any underlying pulmonary disease (maximize bronchodilators in status asthmaticus, frequent chest physiotherapy and suctioning for thick copious secretions associated with a pneumonia or vasodilators and diuretics in pulmonary edema).
6. Consider prophylactic measures such as the administration of Heparin 5000 U or low molecular weight heparin 30 mg subcutaneously every 12 h. These may reduce the incidence of pulmonary embolism while the patient is on bed rest. Stress ulceration bleeding can be prevented by the use of agents such as antacids, ranitidine (Zantac), or sucralfate (Carafate).
7. Order other medications (eg, morphine for pain, lorazepam [Ativan] for restlessness, and haloperidol [Haldol] for agitation) as needed.

ROUTINE MODIFICATION OF SETTINGS

Arterial blood gases should be monitored and adjusted to a normal pH (7.37–7.44) and a $Pao_2 > 60$ mm Hg on $< 60\%$ O_2. Once correlation of the oxygen saturation by pulse oximeter and the blood gas has been established, the arterial blood gases for oxygenation can be minimized. Tachypnea should be investigated for adequacy of ventilation or for any new cause, such as a fever, before sedating the patient.

I. Adjusting Pao_2

A. To Decrease. Fio_2 should be decreased in increments of 10–20% with either ABGs or oximetry checked in between. The "rule of 7s" states that there will be a 7 mm Hg fall in Pao_2 for each 1% decrease in Fio_2.

B. To Increase

1. Ventilation has some effect on Pao_2 (as shown by the alveolar air equation); therefore, correction of the respiratory acidosis will improve oxygenation.
2. Positive-end expiratory pressure (PEEP) can be added in increments from 2 to 4 cm H_2O. PEEP recruits previously collapsed alveoli, holds them open, and restores functional residual capacity (FRC) to a more physiologic level. It counteracts pulmonary shunts and raises Pao_2. PEEP increases intrathoracic pressure and thus may impede venous return and decrease cardiac output. This is particularly true in the presence of volume depletion and shock. If PEEP levels > 10–12 cm water are needed, the placement of a Swan-Ganz catheter is recommended to monitor mixed venous oxygen levels and cardiac output. The effects of PEEP have a slower onset than changes in Fio_2 and require approximately one hour to become apparent in either oximetry or blood gas.
3. Increase I:E ratio, which can be affected even in assist control mode by changing the waveforms in which the specified tidal volume is delivered.

II. Adjusting $Paco_2$

A. To Decrease

1. Increase the rate.
2. Increase the tidal volume.
3. Check for leaks in the system.

B. To Increase

1. Decrease the rate.
2. Decrease the tidal volume.
3. If necessary, switch from AC mode to SIMV mode to eliminate patient-driven central hyperventilation (not recommended). The cause of the hyperventilation should be determined (ie, anxiety, sepsis) and treated appropriately.

Inspect the ventilator for artificial causes of increased respiratory rate, eg, condensation within the tubing can cause water movement that can be mistaken for patient efforts at inspiration. Additionally, adjust the sensitivity of the ventilator to trigger ventilator breaths.

An old but reliable method is to place increased exhalation tubing to increase deadspace and have the patient rebreathe CO_2.

TROUBLESHOOTING

Common problems with intubated patients are discussed in Section I, page xxx. Typical ventilator management problems discussed include

- Agitation, Problem 71, page 255.
- High Inspired Oxygen (F_{IO_2}), Problem 72, page 258.
- High Peak Pressure Problem 73, page 262.
- Low Arterial Oxygen (P_{CO_2})/High Arterial Carbon Dioxide (P_{CO_2}), Problem 74, page 265.

WEANING

I. Requirements. Once the underlying cause of respiratory failure has been corrected, it is time for the most arduous task of all-weaning the patient from the respirator.

A. Stabilization. The underlying disease is under optimum control.

B. Initiation of Weaning. The process is typically begun in the early morning. Patients like to rest rather than work all night. The following is a list of parameters considered minimum by most clinicians:

- $Pa_{O_2} \geq 60$ mm Hg on no PEEP (or <5 cm PEEP) and $F_{IO_2} \leq 0.5$.
- Minute ventilation < 10 L/min.
- Negative inspiratory force more negative than –20 cm water.
- Vital capacity > 800 mL.
- Tidal volume > 300 mL.

II. Techniques

A. T-Piece (or T-tube bypass). The patient is taken off the ventilator for a limited period of time, and the ETT is connected to a constant flow of O_2 (usually 40–50%). If the patient tolerates breathing independently, the length of time off the respirator is progressively increased. This is an extremely effective method. It is particularly easy to use for patients with no underlying lung disease (eg, in a patient recovering from a drug overdose). There are 3 significant drawbacks to this technique: (1) No alarms are available because the patient is totally disconnected from the ventilator; (2) it is time consuming for the respiratory therapists and nurses; and (3) it is much more work than breathing spontaneously without an ETT. This is due to the relatively small diameter of the tube. Remember, resistance increases by the fourth power of the radius. Therefore, patients are usually placed on a T-piece for intervals of < 2 h at a time. This method is commonly used by an anesthesiologist and is safe when used in settings in which T-pieces are commonly used. The same effect can be achieved by placing the patient on CPAP with no pressure support and either no or minimal PEEP. This method provides the safety of continued connection to the alarms of a ventilator.

B. **Synchronized Intermittent Mandatory Ventilation.** In this method, fewer and fewer machine breaths are given as the patient begins taking spontaneous breaths in between. For example, a patient breathing at a rate of 14 in AC mode is switched to SIMV mode, rate 14. The rate is then decreased to 10, 6, 4, and then to 0. Most physicians either place the patient on continuous positive airway pressure mode at this juncture or observe the patient briefly on a T-piece. This method has several theoretical advantages over T-piece weaning: (1) Back-up alarms including automatic rates in case of apnea are in place; (2) a graded assumption of work is done allowing respiratory muscle "retraining"; and (3) there is still a high work of breathing because of the ETT resistance and the inherent resistance of the SIMV circuit valves. However, this method has never been proven clearly superior to T-piece weaning.

One way to decrease the work of breathing with the SIMV weaning technique is to add pressure support (PS) to the system. Pressure support is a positive pressure boost that is initiated when a certain liter flow rate during inspiration is sensed by the respirator. It then supplies a set amount of positive pressure (and by Boyle's law, it also supplies some tidal volume). A PS level of 10–15 cm will overcome the increased work caused by the ETT resistance.

C. **Continuous Positive Airway Pressure and Pressure Support.** In this method, the patient is switched to the spontaneous breathing mode, which, in modern ventilators, is the CPAP mode. In current usage, CPAP is equivalent to PEEP except it is used exclusively in spontaneously breathing mode. Anywhere from 0 to 30 cm pressure may be used, but generally the lowest level possible (usually 0–5 cm) is preferred. Pressure support (PS) may be used concomitantly to augment patient spontaneous breaths. It can then be progressively decreased as the patient increases tidal volumes. For example, PS levels of 25, then 20, then 15, and finally 10 can be used while monitoring the patient's breath rate, tidal volumes, and ABGs. This method requires an alert, cooperative patient who is spontaneously breathing. Machine back-up functions remain in place in case of apnea or other inadequate parameters.

D. Pressure Control Ventilation.

1. **Pressure vs Volume.** This mode of ventilation relies on pressure settings to control gas flow to the patient instead of volume settings. This mode is currently most commonly used for patients with ARDS or other diseases requiring markedly elevated FIO_2 for prolonged periods. The major differences in this mode of ventilation is (1) the ability to deliver inverse ratio ventilation (IRV) without erratic pressure changes and (2) a lack of ability to maintain a constant minute ventilation. Pressure control ventilation should only be implemented when the patient is either chemically paralyzed or deeply sedated. IRV is most effective when patients cannot initiate spontaneous respirations.
2. **Settings.**
   a. **Oxygenation:** Oxygenation is controlled by manipulation of the FIO_2 and the PEEP. Oxygenation can further be increased by extending the time spent in inspiration. The I to E ratio refers to the ratio of time spent in inspiration to time spent in expiration. The I to E ratio (or I time) can directly be regulated in pressure control ventilation.
   b. **Ventilation:** Ventilation is controlled by regulating the respiratory rate and manipulation of the pressure delivered. Pressure delivered is referred to as *delta P. *delta P is the difference between the peak inspiratory pressure (PIP) and the PEEP. This pressure differential affects the volume delivered in the inspiratory time specified.
   c. **Initial Settings:** Initial settings for pressure control ventilation should be performed at the patient's bedside with the respiratory therapist present. The PIP should be determined while still on volume control. Baseline oxygen saturation and hemodynamics should also be obtained. Respiratory rate, PEEP, and FIO_2 should be left unchanged. Initial *delta P should be the PIP minus the PEEP then multiplied by a factor of 0.66. ($0.66 \times [PIP - PEEP]$). Finally, the I to E ratio can generally be started at 1 to 1.5 or

1 to 2. This signifies that for each second spent in inspiration the ventilator allows 1.5 or 2 s for exhalation.

Following conversion to pressure control, several parameters must be observed. Tidal volume must be observed to ensure adequate ventilation. Oxygen saturation and blood pressure must be monitored to ensure continued stability. Finally, the pressure/volume graphs must be inspected. This graph is generated by many modern ventilators and graphically depicts the pressure and volume changes during inspiration and expiration. The graph is important to ensure that the settings allow enough time in expiration to prevent Auto-PEEP. Auto-PEEP occurs when inspirations are initiated by the ventilator prior to complete expiration from the previous cycle. Auto-PEEP can cause an increase in the work of breathing to result in cardiovascular sequelae, such as hypotension.

d. Example of conversion:

Assist Control Mode

F_{IO_2}: 1.00
Rate: 20
PEEP: 10
Observed PIP: 70
PIP – PEEP: 60

Pressure Control Mode (New settings)

F_{IO_2}: 1.00
Rate: 20
Delta P: 40
I to E ratio: 1 to 1.5

3. Special considerations. Several factors should be kept in consideration for patients requiring pressure control ventilation. All changes to rate or I to E ratios should be followed by monitoring the pressure volume cycle graphs. Changes to pressure control ventilation generally require additional time to be reflected in measurements of blood gases. Inspiratory time can be maximized by using the pressure/volume cycle graphs to minimize the portion of time spent in expiration. This can be accomplished by manipulating the I to E ratio such that inspiration occurs immediately after complete exhalation.

Additionally, inspiratory time can be increased if the respiratory rate can be decreased, subsequently increasing the inspiration/expiration cycle time. Finally, I to E ratios can be manipulated to reverse the natural tendency of expiration time to exceed inspiration time. Most clinicians limit the inverse ratio ventilation to 3 to 1.

4. **Common Errors.** There are two common problems that can arise after conversion to pressure control ventilation. The first occurs after ventilator setting changes. In particular, rate changes can be associated with subsequent inappropriate I to E ratios if they have not been specified. Secondly, inverse ratio ventilation becomes ineffective when paralytic agents are allowed to become subtherapeutic, and the patient struggles to breathe against the settings of the ventilator.

III. **Timing.** Deciding when to extubate the patient is part of the art of medicine. Still, fulfilling certain criteria ensures success. The following weaning parameters (as discussed earlier) are acceptable:

- Respiratory rate is < 30/min.
- ABGs show a pH > 7.35 and adequate oxygenation.
- The patient is awake and alert.
- A normal gag reflex is present.
- The stomach is not distended.

IV. **Postextubation.** After extubation, it is important that the patient be encouraged to cough frequently and forcefully. Respiratory therapy treatments should be continued. Incentive spirometry should be used several times an hour while the patient is awake to encourage deep breathing. The patient must be carefully observed for stridor, respiratory muscle fatigue, or other signs of failure. Oxygen should be given at the same level or at a level slightly higher than was given via the respirator before intubation, usually by face mask. The ABGs should be checked 2–4 h after extubation to confirm adequate ventilation and oxygenation.

VIII. Management of Perioperative Complications

This section details specific surgical complications that can occur in the postoperative period and sometimes require action by the house officer while "on call." They are listed by complication, rather than by operation, because they can result from many different operations.

Certain complications occur acutely and initial diagnosis and management may be lifesaving (eg, neck hematoma, bronchial stump leak). Each management section includes a discussion on **Immediate Action** detailing plans for life-threatening problems. (The **Immediate Action** appears in boldface; whereas, other management suggestions appear in regular typeface.)

Other complications discussed here are more subacute, but early recognition and management with an understanding of the differential diagnosis and pathophysiology of the problem lead to optimal outcomes. This section does not provide a comprehensive listing of the various specific complications that can occur following general surgical procedures, because the majority of these problems are fixed or chronic (eg, recurrent laryngeal nerve injury, short-gut syndrome) and have no acute management issues.

Acute Gastric Dilatation

A. Operations: Major thoracic procedures and some abdominal operations (eg, splenectomy) if a nasogastric tube is not functioning or was not placed intraoperatively.

B. Pathophysiology: Acute gastric dilatation is the thoracic equivalent of an ileus limited to the foregut.

C. Diagnosis: Tachypnea, tachycardia, diaphoresis, or hiccups. Often the patients do not highlight abdominal distress. Pay attention to the gastric shadow on a chest radiograph in this postthoracotomy patient population (see Problem 37, page 150).

D. Management:

Immediate Action: Place a nasogastric tube, or make the tube that is in place functional. The problem is rapidly resolved by decompression with a nasogastric tube.

adhesions). The possibility of an internal hernia must be considered on the basis of the initial abdominal procedure the patient underwent.

C. Diagnosis: Abdominal distention, crampy pain, obstipation. Abdominal radiographs will show distended loops of small bowel with air-fluid levels. The main differential diagnosis is between a prolonged postoperative ileus, which is a functional problem, and a true mechanical bowel obstruction, which occurs early in the postoperative course. Radiographic features of an adynamic ileus include a dilated colon primarily indicating no physical obstruction at the level of the small bowel (see Section I, Problem 1, page 1).

D. Management:

Immediate Action: Usually not necessary.

Mechanical bowel obstruction in the early postoperative period (5–20 d) is usually treated in a nonoperative manner in contrast to late postoperative mechanical obstruction, which more commonly requires operative intervention. Decompression with a nasogastric tube and observation usually are indicated. The early adhesions at this time are filmy and unlikely to cause strangulation of the bowel. Also, operative repair at this point is difficult because the bowel is friable and susceptible to intraoperative injury. Although some surgeons advocate the use of a long suction tube often identified by the trade name (Cantor tube, Dennis tube, Baker tube, etc) in this situation, there is no evidence that this use is beneficial.

E. Comments: The primary differential diagnosis for early postoperative bowel obstruction is whether it is a true mechanical problem or a prolonged adynamic ileus, which is a functional problem. If a postoperative ileus resolves and the patient tolerates a diet and then develops signs and symptoms of obstruction it is more obvious but often the problems blend together. Gas patterns on abdominal radiographs help with this diagnosis because in functional ileus the colon is typically most affected, whereas in mechanical obstruction it is the small bowel. Another consideration in a postoperative patient who develops abdominal distention and difficulty tolerating a diet is a focal infectious problem.

Major Lymphatic Leak

A. Operations: Cervical procedures in the left neck, left subclavian line placement, esophagectomy, or retroperitoneal dissection can all lead to thoracic duct or major lymphatic duct injury with subsequent chylothorax or chylous ascites.

B. Pathophysiology: Operative injury to major lymphatic vessel with a large amount of lymph leaking out of neck incision or accumulating in the pleural or peritoneal space.

C. Diagnosis: High output drainage (500 mL/d) from cervical drain or chest tube with high concentration of lymphocytes and high triglyceride content. The fluid is usually grossly chylous after fatty meal ingestion. For chylous ascites, postoperative ascites has the fluid characteristics as described above.

D. Management:

Immediate Action: Usually not necessary.

Restrict fatty foods or make patient NPO with TPN to decrease lymph flow and seal leak. Maintain closed suction drainage system while measuring the volume of output daily. Follow serum albumin and serum total lymphocyte counts, which may be depleted in patients with high output leaks. If there is persistent drainage, then surgical exploration with suture ligature of leaking lymphatic may be indicated. Preoperative ingestion of a fatty meal may help to identify the source of leak intraoperatively.

E. Comments: These major lymphatic leaks are ideally detected as fluid in the surgical field during the initial procedure. Knowledge of the anatomy of the thoracic duct is important to avoid this complication.

Neck Hematoma

A. Operations: Thyroidectomy, parathyroidectomy, carotid artery endarterectomy, cervical esophageal procedures (eg, repair of a Zenker's diverticulum).

B. Pathophysiology: Postoperative bleeding into the closed space under the deep cervical fascia where the trachea lies.

C. Diagnosis: Postoperative swelling in neck with difficulty breathing and stridor. Distortion or deviation of tracheal air column may be seen on radiograph.

D. Management:

Immediate Action: Open the skin and deep cervical fascial closure to release the hematoma.

Patients who are stable should be brought to the operating room for this procedure. For patients in whom the airway is compromised, it may be necessary to perform this procedure at the bedside.

Cover the open wound with a sterile dressing before reclosing the incision in the operating room. Avoid attempts at endotracheal intubation because placement of the tube will be difficult as a result of tracheal compression. It should be noted however, that endotracheal intubation may be required.

E. Comments: Any cervical procedure that closes the deep cervical fascia can lead to a trapped hematoma, which can cause tracheal compression and stridor. Opening the wound quickly solves the problem and can be lifesaving.

Pancreatic Fistula or Fluid Collection

A. Operations: Pancreatic resections or splenectomy where the tail of the pancreas may be injured.

B. Pathophysiology: Any violation of the pancreatic parenchyma transects small pancreatic ducts. The digestive enzymes in exocrine pancreatic juice may prevent normal healing or sealing of minor duct injuries with accumulation of a pancreatic fluid collection high in enzyme content. For this reason it is appropriate to drain any pancreatic resection procedure and high output of fluid from these drains rich in pancreatic juice defines the presence of a pancreatic fistula. Percutaneous drainage of a pancreatic fluid collection postoperatively often leads to continued drainage defining a pancreatic fistula.

C. Diagnosis: High amylase content in fluid from peripancreatic drains placed at the time of pancreatic resection. Pancreatic fluid in a drain has a characteristic "dirty dishwater" brown/gray color. Drain output may increase or change in character with initiation of oral intake.

D. Management:

Immediate Actions: Usually not necessary.

Continued and complete drainage of a pancreatic fistula is an imperative component of treatment, and daily monitoring of drain output in terms of volume with intermittent amylase content checks help assess progress in treatment. Additional measures aimed at decreasing exocrine pancreas stimulation are used to help heal the fistula. Making the patient NPO and using TPN (see Section V, page 385) may be necessary for patients with high-output fistulas. Patients continuing oral intake should be given a nonfat diet to decrease pancreatic stimulation. The somatostatin analogue, octreotide, can be given to decrease exocrine pancreas secretions. In fact, for patients undergoing pancreatic procedures, there is evidence that beginning this agent preoperatively decreases postoperative pancreatic leak. When the drain (or fistula) output decreases to acceptable levels (<50 mL/d) with a low amylase content (<3 times the serum level), then octreotide should be stopped. If output remains low, then the drain can be removed.

E. Comments: Dependent on the caliber and location of the pancreatic duct injury the fistula can be low, mid, or high output. Injuries of the main duct or immediate branches of the main duct and injuries in the pancreatic head, as opposed to the distal pancreas, result in greater problems that are more difficult to heal.

Peripheral Lymphatic Leak

A. Operations: Lymph node dissection, vascular procedure with groin or axillary incision.

B. Pathophysiology: Operative injury to lymphatic vessels with leakage of fluid (usually clear) from the incision.

C. Diagnosis: Persistently high drain output via postoperative closed drains in operative field. Fluid leak from wound onto dressings.

D. Management:

Immediate Actions: Usually not necessary.

If drainage is controlled via closed system alternative management options include:

1. Observation with continued drainage including limiting activity, elevation of extremity, and wrapping extremity to decrease drain output.
2. Surgical exploration with suture ligation of leak sites. Preoperative injection of vital dye (methylene blue, etc) subcutaneously in distal extremity may help identify leak sites. Closed drain placed at this operation and components of treatment option No. 1 instituted.
3. Pull drain and observe wound. Sometimes suction drains may induce leakage and by removing the drain the problem is solved. This plan works best for low-output (75–150 mL/d) lymphatic leaks.

Avoid injecting sclerosing agents (eg, bleomycin, tetracycline) into drains because this treatment causes discomfort, increases risk of infection, and is not effective in a controlled trial.

When lymph leak occurs as open drainage through the wound, surgical exploration as in treatment option No. 2 (above) is usually indicated. Open drainage tends to macerate skin and increase chance of wound infection.

E. Comments: Postoperative lymph leaks are often difficult to resolve quickly even by surgical reexploration. Attention to detail by clipping or ligating lymphatics at the initial procedure to prevent this complication should be emphasized. Lymph leaks in vascular procedures can lead to more serious secondary complications of graft infection when artificial graft material is present.

Postoperative Adrenal Insufficiency

A. Operations: Any major surgical procedure, but especially after adrenalectomy or radical nephrectomy.

B. Pathophysiology: Acute postoperative adrenal insufficiency may occur for one of two general reasons. First, the adrenal glands may not respond appropriately to the stress of the surgical procedure because of unrecognized underlying adrenal pathology or because of iatrogenic adrenal suppression owing to steroid medication. A second cause of acute adrenal insufficiency is bilateral adrenal hemorrhage. Patients who are anticoagulated are more susceptible to this complication, but the majority of patients suffering that have this life-threatening problem are not anticoagulated.

C. Diagnosis: This condition is often very difficult to diagnose other than the fact that patients do very poorly for no obvious reason. This must be remembered as a possible explanation for poor progress in the postoperative period. Symptoms include hypotension, confusion, vomiting with inability to eat; however, the electrolyte manifestations of Addison's disease may not occur. CT scans of the adrenals may show large bilateral hematomas. The diagnosis can be confirmed by failure to have a cortisol response to ACTH injection. (See Section II, ACTH Stimulation Test, page 278)

D. Management:

Immediate Action: Intravenous steroid administration. Hydrocortisone 100 mg IV STAT.

Once the diagnosis is made (and it often is not realized until a postmortem exam), treatment with stress doses of steroids can be lifesaving.

E. Comments: Awareness of this very rare, but very serious problem is the most important factor. For patients who are failing rapidly but have no obvious source of infection, are not bleeding, and have no other explanations for a "downward clinical spiral," acute adrenal insufficiency should be considered.

Postoperative Bleeding

A. Operations: Any surgical procedure.

B. Pathophysiology: Surgical bleeding is usually a technical error with a bleeding vessel that was not controlled satisfactorily intraoperatively. Occasionally, because of the primary disease, patients may have a coagulopathy with medical bleeding from dissection planes, which normally would be hemostatic, oozing blood as a result of the inability to form clot.

C. Diagnosis: Minor wound bleeding typically appears as bloody drainage from the wound or a subcutaneous hematoma. Major postoperative bleeding shows as signs and symptoms of hemorrhagic shock with hypotension, tachycardia, low urine output, and falling hematocrit. (See On Call Problems 23 and 24 relating to drain output and problem 47 "Hypotension")

D. Management:

Immediate Action: Volume resuscitation, obtain cross-matched blood products, identify source of bleeding.

For major postoperative surgical bleeding the principles of care of hemorrhagic shock of any etiology apply. Volume resuscitation making certain adequate venous access lines are available and ordering blood products to treat the bleeding are the cornerstones of therapy. Assessment of ongoing bleeding and response to volume resuscitation in terms of blood pressure, urine output, and serial hematocrits guides the decision whether the bleeding mandates reoperation. Some situations are clinically obvious with dramatic acute bleeding and large transfusion requirements for which reoperation is needed as soon as possible. Other clinical situations are more subacute and may not require reoperation. In all cases, measurement of coagulation parameters (including protime, prothrombin time, and platelet count) is indicated as some cases of bleeding are primarily a result of coagulopathy, which must be treated with the appropriate blood products.

Minor bleeding resulting in a wound hematoma in the subcutaneous location almost never results in hemodynamically significant blood loss. In most locations, this can be treated with observation, possibly with direct pressure to halt the blood loss. In certain locations, even small hematomas can be symptomatic (see previous section, "Neck Hematoma"). When the subcutaneous bleeding is saturating the wound dressings instead of causing a hematoma, direct pressure often will control the bleeding site. Sometimes the offending vessel is a skin vessel that can be identified by inspecting the wound, and a simple nylon stitch under local anesthesia at the bedside can solve the problem.

E. Comments: An understanding of the volume of blood that can hide in the peritoneal or pleural cavities is needed to appreciate the potential problem that can happen with acute postoperative hemorrhage. Serial measurements of abdominal girth (as is often done) is an insensitive assessment of this potentially life-threatening complication.

Postoperative Intra-Abdominal Fluid Collection/Abscess

A. Operations: Any abdominal operation can result in this problem, particularly infected, contaminated, or clean/contaminated procedures.

B. Pathophysiology: Postoperative intra-abdominal fluid serves as a site for infection to develop from organisms typically originating from the bowel, biliary, or genitourinary tract during the surgical procedure. As patients recover in a supine position, the fluid settles in the most dependent areas of the greater peritoneal cavity in the subphrenic spaces, infrahepatic space (Morrison's pouch), paracolic gutters, and pelvis.

C. Diagnosis: This complication may be evident as leukocytosis, fever, increased abdominal pain, referred pain to shoulders or back, or abdominal distention. Often patients who are recovering from an abdominal procedure after making normal progress, begin to feel worse or lose their ability to eat.

D. Management:

Immediate Action: Usually not necessary.

Current management involves imaging fluid collections by CT scan or ultrasound with a radiologically guided aspiration and drainage if possible. Aspirated fluid should be sent to the laboratory for Gram's stain and culture. If the operative procedure involved the pancreas, assay of the fluid for amylase content will indicate a pancreatic source. Checking the creatinine in the fluid may demonstrate that it is urine. Broad-spectrum antibiotics to treat enteric organisms should be initiated as soon as cultures are obtained. For clinically significant fluid collections that cannot be safely approached percutaneously (eg, interloop fluid collections between loops of small bowel), operative drainage may be indicated.

E. Comments: Advancements in radiographic imaging techniques and interventions have revolutionized the management of this postoperative complication.

Postoperative Intestinal Fistula

A. Operations: Abdominal operations where an intestinal anastomosis was created. Reoperative procedures where significant adhesions exist and there is the possibility of an unintentional enterotomy or a leak from a repaired inadvertent enterotomy. Rarely, sutures used for fascial closure may include a bowel segment with subsequent fistula formation.

B. Pathophysiology: Postoperative fistulas require violation of the bowel wall with leakage of intestinal contents, which eventually find a path out of the body to the skin. The most common cause for bowel wall disruption is an anastomotic leak as previously discussed. However, if the bowel wall was injured or made ischemic during the initial procedure, then it may develop into an intestinal leak, not related to an anastomosis, which can progress to a fistula.

C. Diagnosis: This complication is diagnosed by leakage of intestinal contents to the wound or drain sites.

D. Management:

Immediate Action: Usually not necessary.

Similar to the situation with both anatomic leak and intra-abdominal abscess discussed above, the principles of management of an intestinal fistula are bowel rest (use TPN, see Section V, page 385), antibiotics, and control of the leak with drainage of intra-abdominal fluid collections to limit infection. Obtaining radiologic studies, such as a CT scan, to look for undrained fluid collections and possibly a fistulogram by injecting contrast retrograde into the site of the fistula to define the anatomy of the leak are helpful to define the anatomy of the fistula.

Fistulas are usually categorized as low output (< 500 mL/d) or high output (> 500 mL/d). It is critically important to protect the skin at the site of the fistula. A stoma appliance is usually helpful in this matter as well as collecting the effluent. High-output fistulas should be treated as above, but persistent high-output fistulas usually require operative repair; low-output fistulas usually close gradually with nonoperative management as previously outlined (see also Section I, Problem 77, page 274).

E. Comments: The postoperative complications of intra-abdominal fluid collection, anastomotic leak, and intestinal fistula are all interrelated problems that can occur together in patients undergoing major abdominal procedures.

Seroma

A. Operations: Lymph node dissection, mastectomy, any soft tissue resection.

B. Pathophysiology: Accumulation of lymph or serous fluid in deep wound space with normal healing of skin.

C. Diagnosis: This problem shows as a nontender swelling in the wound that is usually fluctuant. A needle aspirate (performed using sterile technique) reveals serous fluid.

D. Management:

Immediate Actions: Usually not necessary.

Observation for signs of infection or enlargement. Repeated complete aspiration of fluid using sterile technique. Avoid placing an indwelling drain.

E. Comments: Seromas are more of a nuisance than a symptomatic complication. Secondary problems, such as infection or open lymphatic leak, are more worrisome.

Skin Flap Necrosis

A. Operations: Mastectomy, lymph node dissection, soft tissue tumor resection, neck dissection.

B. Pathophysiology: Ischemic necrosis of skin and subcutaneous tissue resulting from inappropriate construction of flap or closure of incision under tension stretching tissues and restricting blood flow.

C. Diagnosis: This is a clinical diagnosis with a variable area of skin along an incision that demarcates and appears various shades of gray or purple, has little or no capillary refill, and eventually becomes black and necrotic.

D. Management:

Immediate Actions: Usually not necessary.

When flap necrosis is initially suspected several maneuvers can be done to minimize skin and soft tissue loss. The patient should be well hydrated to ensure adequate tissue perfusion and placed on oxygen to maximize oxygen tension in the area at risk. Nitropaste may be applied to the endangered area to cause vasodilatation and increased blood flow. When the flap becomes a black eschar, the damage is irreversible, and debridement of the dead tissue with subsequent skin graft or flap coverage should be done as quickly as possible.

E. Comments: Flap necrosis is a vascular problem at the outset-not an infectious one. However, early recognition of this complication and prompt action to increase oxygen delivery to the tissue may salvage some of the ischemic skin flap.

Wound Infection

A. Operations: Any surgical procedure. More common in dirty, contaminated, or clean-contaminated cases.

B. Pathophysiology: The subcutaneous tissue between the skin and fascia is the most susceptible to infection because it is the least vascularized.

C. Diagnosis: Erythema, pain, and warmth at the wound characterize superficial infections. Purulent drainage from a wound in which there is a thick layer of subcutaneous tissue may be the only symptom. Systemic signs, such as fever or leukocytosis, may be present. Inspection of the wound, including palpation to identify and express trapped purulent fluid confirms the diagnosis.

D. Management:

Immediate Actions: Usually not necessary.

After diagnosing a wound infection, treatment of superficial cellulitis involves antibiotics. Parenteral antibiotics are indicated for patients with acute surgical wound infections. Antibiotic coverage for enteric organisms is recommended for dirty cases, that is, when the subcutaneous tissue comes into contact with intestinal contents. For most wound infections, the causative organism is a gram-positive bacteria from the skin (*Staphylococcus* species or *Streptococcus* species), and treatment should be directed toward these organisms. If there is suspicion of an abscess or known drainage of pus from the wound, then the wound needs to be opened widely to achieve drainage. The wound is then managed with dressing changes 2–3 times a day and allowed to heal by secondary intention (see also Section I, Problem 77, page 274.

E. Comments: The assessment of postoperative fever includes evaluation and inspection of the surgical incision. Even early postoperative fever mandates inspection of the wound because the source may be an early streptococcal or clostridial infection that can progress rapidly and cause a high morbidity rate.

IX. Commonly Used Medications

This section is a quick reference to commonly used medications. You should be familiar with all of the dosages, indications, contraindications, side effects, and drug interactions of the medications that you prescribe. Such detailed information is beyond the scope of this manual and can be found in the package insert, Physicians' Desk Reference (PDR), or the American Hospital Formulary Service.

Drugs in this section are listed in alphabetic order by generic names. Common uses are listed that include both labeled indications and common off-label uses on the basis of recommendations of our editorial board. Some of the more common trade names are listed for each medication. Where no pediatric dose is provided, the implication is that the use of the agent is not well established in this age group or is infrequently used. Drugs under the control of the Drug Enforcement Agency (Schedule 2–5 controlled substances) are indicated by the symbol [C].

CLASSIFICATION

Allergic Disorders

Antihistamines

Cetirizine
Chlorpheniramine
Clemastine fumarate
Cyproheptadine
Diphenhydramine
Fexofenadine
Hydroxyzine
Loratadine

Miscellanous Agents

Budesonide
Cromolyn

Antidotes

Acetylcysteine
Charcoal
Digoxin immune FAB
Flumazenil
Ipecac syrup
Mesna
Naloxone
Physostigmine

Antimicrobial Agents

Antibiotics

AMINOGLYCOSIDES

Amikacin
Gentamicin
Neomycin
Streptomycin
Tobramycin

CEPHALOSPORINS

Cefaclor
Cefadroxil
Cefazolin
Cefdinir
Cefepime
Cefixime
Cefmetazole
Cefonicid
Cefoperazone
Cefotaxime
Cefotetan
Cefoxitin
Cefpodoxime
Cefprozil
Ceftazidime
Ceftibutin
Ceftizoxime
Ceftriaxone
Cefuroxime
Cephalexin
Cephapirin
Cephradine
Loracarbef

FLUROQUINOLONES

Ciprofloxacin
Ciprofloxacin and hydrocortisone otic
Gatifloxacin
Levofloxacin
Lomefloxacin
Moxifloxacin
Norfloxacin
Ofloxacin

MACROLIDES

Azithromycin
Clarithromycin
Dirithromycin
Erythromycin

PENICILLINS

Amoxicillin
Amoxicillin-Clavulanate
Ampicillin
Ampicillin-Sulbactam
Cloxacillin
Dicloxacillin
Mezlocillin
Nafcillin
Oxacillin
Penicillin G aqueous
Penicillin G benzathine
Penicillin G procaine
Penicillin V
Piperacillin
Piperacillin-Tazobactam
Ticarcillin
Ticarcillin-Clavulanate

TETRACYCLINES

Doxycycline
Tetracycline

MISCELLANEOUS AGENTS

Aztreonam
Clindamycin
Cortisporin, otic
Fosfomycin
Imipenem-Cilastatin
Linezolid
Meropenem
Metronidazole
Mupirocin
Quinupristin/Dalfopristin
Silver nitrate
Trimethoprim-sulfamethoxazole
Vancomycin

Antifungals

Amphotericin B
Amphotericin B Cholesteryl
Amphotericin B Lipid Complex
Amphotericin B Liposomal
Ciclopirox
Clotrimazole
Econazole
Fluconazole
Itraconazole
Ketoconazole
Miconazole
Nystatin

Antimycobacterials

Ethambutol
Isoniazid
Pyrazinamide
Rifampin
Rifapentine

Antiretrovirals

Delavirdine
Didanosine
Indinavir
Lamivudine
Ritonavir
Saquinavir
Zalcitabine
Zidovudine

Antivirals

Acyclovir
Amantadine
Famciclovir
Foscarnet
Ganciclovir
Oseltamivir
Interferon Alfacon-1
Interferon alpha 2B and ribavirin

Ribavirin
Rimantadine
Valacyclovir
Zanamivir

Miscellaneous Agents

Pentamidine
Silver Sulfadiazine

Antineoplastic Agents

Alkylating Agents

Altretamine
Carboplatin
Cisplatin
Triethylene-triphosphamide

NITROGEN MUSTARDS

Chlorambucil
Cyclophosphamide
Ifosfamide
Melphalan

NITROSUREAS

Carmustine

Antibiotics

Bleomycin Sulfate
Dactinomycin
Daunorubicin
Doxorubicin
Idarubicin
Plicamycin

Antimetabolites

Cytarabine
Cytarabine liposomal
Fludarabine
Flurouracil (S–FU)
Mercaptopurine
Methotrexate
6-Thioguanine

Hormones

Anastrozole
Bicalutamide
Goserelin
Leuprolide Acetate
Megestrol Acetate
Nilutamide
Tamoxifen acetate

Mitotic Inhibitors

Etoposide (VP–16)
Teniposide
Vinblastine
Vincristine
Vinorelbine

Miscellaneous

Aldesleukin
Aminogluthemide
BCG
Dacarbazine
Docetaxel
Hydroxyurea
Levamisole
Mitoxantrone
Paclitaxel
Porfimer
Thiotepa

Cardiovascular Agents

Alpha-1 Adrenergic Blockers

Doxazosin
Prazosin
Terazosin

Angiotensin-Converting Enzyme Inhibitors

Benazepril
Captopril
Enalapril and Enalaprilat
Fosinopril
Lisinopril
Moexipril
Perindopril
Quinapril
Ramipril
Trandolapril

Angiotensin II Receptor Antagonist

Candesartan
Eprosartan
Irbesartan
Losartan
Telmisartan
Valsartan

Antiarrhythmic Agents

Adenosine
Amiodarone
Atropine
Digoxin
Disopyramide
Esmolol
Flecainide
Ibutilide
Lidocaine
Mexiletine
Moricizine
Procainamide
Propafenone
Quinidine
Sotalol
Tocainide

Beta-Blockers

Acebutolol
Atenolol
Atenolol and chlorothiazide
Betaxolol
Bisoprolol
Carteolol
Carvedilol
Labetalol
Metoprolol
Nadolol
Penbutolol
Pindolol
Propranolol
Timolol

Calcium Channel Antagonists

Amlodipine
Bepridil
Diltiazem
Felodipine
Isradipine
Nicardipine
Nifedipine
Nimodipine
Nisoldipine
Verapamil

Centrally Acting Antihypertensive Agents

Clonidine
Guanabenz
Guanadrel
Guanethidine
Guanfacine
Methyldopa

Diuretics

Acetazolamide
Amiloride
Bumetanide
Chlorothiazide
Chlorthalidone
Ethacrynic acid
Furosemide
Hydrochlorothiazide
Hydrochlorothiazide and amiloride
Hydrochlorothiazide and spironolactone
Hydrochlorothiazide and triamterene
Indapamide
Mannitol
Metolazone
Spironolactone
Torsemide
Triamterene

Inotropic Agents

Amrinone
Digoxin
Dobutamine
Dopamine
Epinephrine
Isoproterenol
Milrinone
Norepinephrine
Phenylephrine

Lipid-Lowering Agents

Atorvastatin
Cerivastatin
Cholestyramine
Colestipol
Colesevelam
Fenofibrate
Fluvastatin
Gemfibrozil
Lovastatin
Niacin
Pravastatin
Simvastatin

Vasodilators

Epoprostenol
Fenoldopam
Hydralazine
Isosorbide dinitrate
Isosorbide mononitrate
Minoxidil
Nitroglycerin
Nitroprusside
Tolazoline

Central Nervous System

Antianxiety

Alprazolam
Buspirone
Chlordiazepoxide
Clorazepate
Diazepam
Doxepine

Hydroxyzine
Lorazepam
Meprobamate
Oxazepam
Prazepam

Anticonvulsants

Carbamazepine
Clonazepam
Diazepam
Ethosuximide
Fosphenytoin
Gabapentin
Lamotrigine
Levetiracetam
Lorazepam
Oxcarbazepine
Pentobarbital
Phenobarbital
Phenytoin
Tiagabine
Topiramate
Valproic acid
Zonisamide

Antidepressants

Amitriptyline
Amoxapine
Bupropion
Citalopram
Desipramine
Doxepin
Fluoxetine
Fluvoxamine
Imipramine
Maprotiline
Mirtazapine
Nefazodone
Nortriptyline
Paroxetine
Phenelzine
Sertraline
Trazodone
Trimipramine
Venlafaxine

Antiparkinson Agents

Amantadine
Benztropine
Bromocriptine
Carbidopa/levodopa
Entacapone
Pergolide
Pramipexole
Procyclidine
Selegiline
Trihexyphenidyl

Antipsychotics

Chlorpromazine
Clozapine
Fluphenazine
Haloperidol
Lithium carbonate
Mesoridazine
Molindone
Olanzapine
Perphenazine
Prochlorperazine
Risperidone
Thioridazine
Thiothixene
Trifluoperazine

Sedative Hypnotics

Chloral hydrate
Diphenhydramine
Estazolam
Flurazepam
Hydroxyzine
Midazolam
Pentobarbital
Phenobarbital
Propofol
Quazepam
Secobarbital
Temazepam
Triazolam
Zaleplon
Zolpidem

Miscellaneous Agents

Nimodipine
Tacrine

Endocrine System

Antidiabetic Agents

Acarbose
Acetohexamide
Chlorpropamide
Glimepiride
Glipizide
Glyburide
Insulin
Metformin
Miglitol
Pioglitazone
Repaglinide
Rosiglitazone
Tolazamide
Tolbutamide

Hormone & Synthetic Substitutes

Cortisone
Desmopressin
Dexamethasone
Fludrocortisone acetate
Glucagon
Hydrocortisone
Methylprednisolone
Metyrapone
Prednisolone
Prednisone
Vasopressin

Hypercalcemia Agents

Calcitonin
Etidronate
Gallium Nitrate
Plicamycin

Osteoporosis Agents

Alendronate
Calcitonin
Raloxifene
Risedronate

Thyroid/Antithyroid

Levothyroxine
Liothyronine
Methimazole
Potassium Iodide
Propylthiouracil
Thyroid

Miscellanous Agents

Demeclocycline
Diazoxide

Gastrointestinal Tract

Antacids

Alginic Acid
Aluminum carbonate
Aluminum hydroxide
Aluminum hydroxide with magnesium carbonate
Aluminum hydroxide with magnesium hydroxide
Aluminum hydroxide with magnesium hydroxide and simethicone
Calcium carbonate
Magaldrate
Simethicone

Antidiarrheal

Bismuth subsalicylate
Diphenoxylate with atropine
Kaolin/Pectin
Lactobacillus
Loperamide
Octreotide

Antiemetic

Buclizine
Chlorpromazine
Dimenhydrinate
Dolasetron
Dronabinol
Droperidol
Granisetron
Meclizine
Metoclopramide
Ondansetron
Prochlorperazine
Promethazine
Scopolamine
Thiethylperazine
Trimethobenzamide

Antiulcer

Cimetidine
Famotidine
Lansoprazole
Nizatidine
Omeprazole
Pantoprazole
Rabeprazole
Ranitidine
Sucralfate

Cathartics/Laxatives

Bisacodyl
Docusate calcium
Docusate potassium
Docusate sodium
Glycerin suppositories
Lactulose
Magnesium citrate
Magnesium hydroxide
Mineral oil
Polyethylene glycol-electrolyte solution
Psyllium
Sorbitol

Enzymes

Pancreatin
Pancrelipase

Miscellaneous Agents

Alosetron
Dexpanthenol
Dicyclomine
Hyoscyamine
Hyoscyamine, atropine, scopolamine and phenobarbital
Infliximab
Mesalamine
Metoclopramide

Misoprostol
Olsalazine
Propantheline
Sulfasalazine
Vasopressin

Hematologic Modifiers

Anticoagulants

Ardeparin
Dalteparin
Enoxaparin
Heparin
Protamine
Warfarin

Antiplatelet

Abciximab
Aspirin
Clopidogrel
Eptifibatide
Reteplase
Ticlopidine
Tirofiban

Antithrombic Agents

Alteplase, recombinant (TPA)
Aminocaproic acid
Anistreplase
Aprotinin
Dextran 40
Reteplase
Streptokinase
Tenecteplase
Urokinase

Hemopoietic Stimulants

Epoetin alfa (Erythropoietin)
Filgrastim (G-CSF)
Sargramostim (GM-CSF)

Volume Expanders

Albumin
Dextran 40
Hetastarch
Plasma protein fraction

Miscellaneous Agents

Antihemophelic Factor VIII
Desmopressin
Lepirudin
Pentoxifylline

Immune System

Immunomodulators

Interferon alfa
Interferon alfacon

Immunosuppressive Agents

Antithymocyte globulin (ATG)
Azathioprine
Basiliximab
Cyclosporine
Daclizumab
Muromonab-CD3
Mycophenolate mofetil
Sirolimus
Steroids
Tacrolimus

Vaccine/Serums/Toxoids

CMV Immune globulin
Haemophilus B conjugate
Hepatitis A vaccine
Hepatitis B immune globulin
Hepatitis B vaccine
Immune globulin, intravenous
Pneumococcal vaccine, polyvalent
Pneumococcal 7-valent conjugate
Tetanus immune globulin
Tetanus toxoid

Musculoskeletal Disorders

Antigout Agents

Allopurinol
Colchicine
Probenecid
Sulfinpyrazone

Muscle Relaxants

Aspirin and meprobamate
Baclofen
Carisoprodol
Chlorzoxazone
Cyclobenzaprine
Dantrolene
Diazepam
Metaxalone
Methocarbamol
Orphenadrine

Neuromuscular Blockers

Atracurium
Mivacurium
Pancuronium
Pipecuronium
Succinylcholine
Vecuronium

Miscellaneous Agents

Edrophonium
Leflunomide
Methotrexate

OB/GYN

Contraceptives

Levonorgestrel Implants
Norgestrel

Estrogen Supplementation

Esterified estrogens
Esterified estrogens with methyltestosterone
Estradiol
Estradiol transdermal
Estrogen, conjugated
Estrogen, conjugated with methyltestosterone
Ethinyl estradiol

Vaginal Preparations

Amino-Cerv pH 5.5 cream
Miconazole
Nystatin
Terconazole
Tioconazole

Miscellaneous Agents

Gonadorelin
Leuprolide
Magnesium sulfate
Medroxyprogesterone
Methylergonovine
Oxytocin
Terbutaline

Ophthalmic Agents

Acetazolamide
Apraclonidine
Artificial tears
Atropine
Bacitracin and polymyxin B (Polysporin)
Betaxolol
Brimonidine
Brinzolamide
Carteolol
Ciprofloxacin
Cromolyn
Cyclopentolate
Diclofenac
Dorzolamide
Dorzolamide and timolol
Dipivefrin
Echothiophate iodine
Erythromycin
Fomivirsen
Gentamicin
Ketorolac
Latanoprost
Levobunolol
Levocabastine
Lodoxamide
Naphazoline and antazoline
Naphazoline and pheniramine
Neomycin, bacitracin and polymyxin-B
Neomycin, polymyxin-B and dexamethasone,
Neomycin, polymyxin-B and hydrocortisone
Neomycin, polymyxin-B and prednisolone
Norfloxacin
Ofloxacin
Phenylephrine
Pilocarpine
Prednisolone
Rimexolone
Sulfacetamide
Timolol
Tobramycin
Tobramycin and dexamethasone
Tropicamide
Trifluridine
Vidarabine

Otic Agents

Antipyrine and benzocaine
Hydrocortisone otic
Neomycin, polymyxin-B and hydrocortisone
Oflaxocin otic
Profloxin
Triethanolamine polypeptide oleate

Pain

Local Anesthetics

Antipyrine and benzocaine
Anusol
Capsaicin
Cocaine
Bupivacaine
Dibucaine
Lidocaine
Lidocaine/prilocaine

Narcotics

Alfentanil
Buprenorphine
Butalbital and acetaminophen
Butalbital and aspirin
Butalbital, aspirin, and codeine
Butorphanol
Codeine
Codeine with acetaminophen
Dezocine
Fentanyl
Fentanyl transdermal
Fentanyl transmucosal
Hydrocodone
Hydrocodone and acetaminophen
Hydrocodone and aspirin
Levorphanol
Meperidine
Methadone
Morphine
Nalbuphine
Oxycodone and acetaminophen
Oxycodone and aspirin
Oxymorphone
Propoxyphene
Propoxyphene and acetaminophen
Propoxyphene and aspirin
Pentazocine
Sufentanil

Non-narcotic Agents

Acetaminophen
Tramadol

Nonsteroidal Anti-inflammatory Agents

Aspirin
Aspirin with codeine
Celecoxib
Diclofenac
Diflunisal
Etodolac
Fenoprofen
Flurbiprofen
Ibuprofen
Indomethacin
Ketoprofen
Ketorolac
Meloxicam
Nabumetone
Naproxen
Naproxen Sodium
Oxaprozin
Piroxicam
Rofecoxib
Sulindac
Tolmetin

Respiratory Tract

Antitussives & Decongestants

Acetylcysteine
Benzonatate
Codeine
Dextromethorphan
Guaifenesin
Guaifenesin and codeine
Guaifenesin and dextromethorphan
Guaifenesin and pseudoephedrine
Hydromorphone and guaifensin
Hydrocodone and homatropine
Hydrocodone and pseudoephedrine
Pseudoephedrine

Bronchodilators

Albuterol
Albuterol and ipratroprium
Aminophylline
Bitolterol
Ephedrine
Ephinephrine
Isoetharine
Isoproterenol
Levalbuterol
Metaproterenol
Pirbuterol
Salmeterol
Terbutaline
Theophylline

Respiratory Inhalants

Acetylcysteine
Beclomethasone
Cromolyn sodium
Flunisolide
Fluticasone
Ipratropium
Nedocromil

Miscellanous Agents

Beractant
Montelukast
Zafirlukast
Zileuton

Steroids

Systemic

Betamethasone
Cortisone
Dexamethasone
Hydrocortisone
Methylprednisolone acetate
Methylprednisolone succinate
Prednisone
Prednisolone

Topical

Aclometasone dipropionate
Amcinonide
Augmented betamethasone
Betamethasone dipropionate
Betamethasone valerate
Clobetasol propionate
Clocortolone pivalate
Desonide
Desoximetasone
Dexamethasone
Diflorasone diacetate
Fluocinolone acetonide
Fluocinonide
Flurandrenolide
Fluticasone propionate
Halcinonide
Halobetasol
Hydrocortisone
Hydrocortisone acetate
Hydrocortisone butyrate
Hydrocortisone valerate
Mometasone furoate
Prednicarbate
Triamcinolone

Supplements

Calcium chloride
Calcium acetate
Calcitrol
Cholecalciferol
Cyanocobalamin (vitamin B_{12})
Ferrous sulfate
Folic acid
Iron dextran
Leucovorin
Magnesium oxide
Magnesium sulfate
Phytonadione (vitamin K)
Potassium supplements
Pyridoxine (vitamin B_6)
Sodium bicarbonate
Thiamine (vitamin B_1)

Urinary Tract Agents

Ammonium aluminum sulfate
Belladona and opium suppositories
Bethanechol
DMSO
Flavoxate
Hyoscyamine
Methenamine mandelate
Nalidixic acid
Neomycin-polymyxin bladder irrigant
Nitrofurantoin
Oxybutynin
Pentosan polysulfate
Phenazopyridine
Potassium Citrate
Potassium Citrate and citric acid
Sodium citrate
Trimethoprim

Benign Prostatic Hyperplasia

Doxazosin
Finasteride
Tamsulosin
Terazosin

Miscellaneous Agents

Isotretinoin
Lindane
Megestrol acetate
Metyrosine
Naltrexone
Nicotine gum
Nicotine nasal spray
Nicotine transdermal
Sibutramine
Sildenafil
Sodium polystyrene sulfonate
Witch hazel

GENERIC DRUGS

Abciximab (ReoPro)

COMMON USES: Prevention of acute ischemic complications in patients undergoing percutaneous transluminal coronary angioplasty (PTCA).
DOSAGE: 0.25 mg/kg administered 10–60 min prior to PTCA, then 0.125 μg/kg/min (10 mg/min) continuous infusion for 12 h.
NOTES: Used concomitantly with heparin; may cause allergic reactions.

Acarbose (Precose)

COMMON USES: Type 2 diabetes mellitus.
DOSAGE: 25–100 mg PO tid with meals.
NOTES: May be taken concomitantly with sulfonylureas.

Acebutolol (Sectral)

COMMON USES: Hypertension; ventricular arrhythmias, angina.
DOSAGE: 200–400 mg, PO bid.

Acetaminophen (Tylenol, others)

COMMON USES: Mild pain, headache, fever.
DOSAGE: ***Adults:*** 650–1000 mg PO or PR q4–6h. ***Peds:*** 10 mg/kg/dose PO or PR q4–6h.
NOTES: Overdose causes hepatotoxicity and is treated with *N*-acetylcysteine; charcoal is not usually recommended; it has no anti-inflammatory or platelet-inhibiting action.

Acetaminophen With Codeine (Tylenol No. 1, No. 2, No. 3, No. 4; others) [C]

COMMON USES: No. 1, No. 2, No. 3 for mild-to- moderate pain; No. 4 for moderate-to-severe pain; antitussive.
DOSAGE: ***Adults:*** 1–2 tablets q3–4h prn. ***Peds:*** Acetaminophen 10–15 mg/kg/dose; codeine 0.5–1.0 mg/kg/dose q4–6h (useful elixir dosing guide: 3–6 years, 5 mL/dose; 7–12 years, 10 mL/dose).
NOTES: Capsules contain 325-mg acetaminophen, tablets, 300 mg; Codeine in No.1:7.5 mg, No.2:15 mg, No.3: 30 mg, No.4:60 mg; 5-mL elixir contains 120-mg acetaminophen, 12-mg codeine plus alcohol.

Acetazolamide (Diamox)

COMMON USES: Diuresis, glaucoma, alkalinization of urine, refractory epilepsy.
DOSAGE: ***Adults:*** Diuretic: 250–375 mg IV or PO q24h in divided doses. Glaucoma: 250–1000 mg PO qd in divided doses. ***Peds:*** Epilepsy: 8–30 mg/kg/24h PO in 4 divided doses. Diuretic: 5 mg/kg/24h PO or IV. Alkalinization of urine: 5 mg/kg/dose PO bid–tid. Glaucoma: 20–40 mg/kg/24h PO in 4 divided doses.
NOTES: Contraindicated in renal failure, sulfa hypersensitivity; follow Na^+ and K^+; watch for metabolic acidosis.

Acetohexamide (Dymelor)

COMMON USES: Management of non-insulin-dependent diabetes mellitus.
DOSAGE: 250–1500 mg qd.

Acetylcysteine (Mucomyst)

COMMON USES: Mucolytic agent as adjuvant therapy of chronic bronchopulmonary diseases and cystic fibrosis; as antidote to acetaminophen hepatotoxicity within 24 h of ingestion.
DOSAGE: ***Adults*** and ***Peds:*** Nebulizer: 3–5 mL of 20% solution diluted with equal volume of water or normal saline administered tid–qid. Antidote: PO or NG;

140 mg/kg diluted 1:4in carbonated beverage as loading dose, then 70 mg/kg q4h for 17 doses.
NOTES: Watch for bronchospasm when used by inhalation in asthmatics; activated charcoal adsorbs acetylcysteine when given PO for acute APAP ingestion.

Acyclovir (Zovirax)

COMMON USES: Herpes simplex and herpes zoster viral infections.
DOSAGE: ***Adults:*** Topical: Apply 0.5-inch ribbon q3h. Oral: Initial genital herpes: 200 mg PO q4h while awake; 5 caps per day for 10 d. Chronic suppression: 400 mg PO bid–tid. Intermittent therapy: As for initial treatment, except treat for 5 days at the earliest prodrome. Herpes zoster: 800 mg PO 5 times/d. Intravenous: 5–10 mg/kg/dose IV q8h. ***Peds:*** 5–10 mg/kg/dose IV or PO q8h or 750 mg/m^2/24h divided q8h.
NOTES: Adjust dose in renal insufficiency.

Adenosine (Adenocard)

COMMON USES: Paroxysmal supraventricular tachycardia, including that associated with Wolff-Parkinson-White syndrome.
DOSAGE: ***Adults:*** 6 mg rapid IV, repeated in 1–2 min at 12 mg IV if no response. ***Peds:*** 0.03–0.25 mg/kg IV bolus; repeat higher dose in 1–2 min if no response.
NOTES: Doses >12 mg are not recommended; caffeine and theophylline antagonize the effects of adenosine.

Albumin (Albuminar, Buminate, Albutein, others)

COMMON USES: Plasma volume expansion for shock resulting from burns, surgery, hemorrhage, or other trauma.
DOSAGE: ***Adults:*** 25 g IV initially; subsequent infusions should depend on clinical situation and response. ***Peds:*** 0.5–1.0 g/kg/dose; infuse at 0.05–0.1 g/min.
NOTES: Contains 130–160 mEq Na^+/L.

Albuterol (Proventil, Ventolin)

COMMON USES: Treatment of bronchospasm in reversible obstructive airway disease; prevention of exercise-induced bronchospasm.
DOSAGE: ***Adults:*** 2–4 inhalations q4–6h; 1 Rotocap inhaled q4–6h; 2–4 mg PO tid–qid. ***Peds:*** 2 inhalations q4–6h; 0.1–0.2 mg/kg/dose PO, to maximum dose of 2–4 mg PO tid.

Albuterol and Ipratropium (Combivent)

COMMON USES: Management of COPD.
DOSAGE: 2 inhalations qid.

Aldesleukin [IL-2] (Proleukin)

COMMON USES: Treatment of metastatic renal cell carcinoma, melanoma, and colorectal cancer.
DOSAGE: 600,000 IU/kg (0.037 mg/kg) administered every 8 h by a 15-min infusion for 14 doses. After 9 d of rest, repeat schedule for another 14 doses, for a maximum of 28 doses per cycle.
NOTES: Administer only in a hospital with an intensive care unit and an available specialist; may cause severe hypotension and "capillary leak syndrome," resulting in reduced organ perfusion.

Alendronate (Fosamax)

COMMON USES: Treatment and prevention of osteoporosis, and Paget's disease.
DOSAGE: Osteoporosis treatment: 10 mg PO once daily. Prevention: 5 mg PO once daily. Paget's disease: 40 mg PO once daily.
NOTES: Should take 30 min before meals to avoid GI upset.

Alfentanil (Alfenta) [C]

COMMON USES: Adjunct in the maintenance of general anesthesia.
DOSAGE: ***Adults*** and ***Peds > 12 y:*** 8–75 mg/kg IV infusion; total dose depends on the duration of the operative procedure.

Alginic Acid With Aluminum Hydroxide and Magnesium Trisilicate (Gaviscon)

COMMON USES: Symptomatic relief of heartburn; hiatal hernia.
DOSAGE: 2–4 tablets or 15–30 mL PO qid followed by water.

Allopurinol (Zyloprim, Lopurin)

COMMON USES: Gout, treatment of hyperuricemia of malignancy, uric acid urolithiasis.
DOSAGE: ***Adults:*** Initial 100 mg PO qd; usual 300 mg PO qd. ***Peds:*** Use only for treating hyperuricemia of malignancy in children; 10 mg/kg/24h divided q6–8h (maximum 600 mg/24h).
NOTES: Aggravates acute gout episode, do not begin until acute episode resolves.

Alosetron (Lotronex)

COMMON USES: Irritable bowel syndrome.
DOSAGE: 1 mg twice daily.
NOTES: May be taken without regard to food intake.

Alprazolam (Xanax) [C]

COMMON USES: Anxiety and panic disorders; anxiety associated with depression.
DOSAGE: 0.25–2 mg PO tid.
NOTES: Reduce dose in elderly and debilitated patients.

Alteplase, Recombinant [TPA] (Activase)

COMMON USES: Acute MI and pulmonary embolism.
DOSAGE: 100 mg IV over 3 h.
NOTES: May cause bleeding.

Altretamine (Hexalen)

COMMON USES: Palliative treatment of ovarian cancer.
DOSAGE: 260 mg/m^2/d PO divided q6h, for 14–21 consecutive days of a 28-d cycle.
NOTES: May cause neurologic and hematologic toxicity.

Aluminum Carbonate (Basaljel)

COMMON USES: Hyperacidity (peptic ulcer, hiatal hernia, etc); supplement to management of hyperphosphatemia in renal disease.
DOSAGE: ***Adults:*** 2 capsules or tablets or 10 mL (in water) q2h prn. ***Peds:*** 50–150 mg/kg/24h PO divided q4–6h.

Aluminum Hydroxide (Amphojel, ALTernaGEL, Alu-Cap, Alu-Tab)

COMMON USES: See aluminum carbonate.
DOSAGE: ***Adults:*** 10–30 mL or 2 tablets/capsules PO q4–6h. ***Peds:*** 5–15 mL PO q4–6h.
NOTES: Can be used in renal failure; may cause constipation.

Aluminum Hydroxide With Magnesium Carbonate (Gaviscon)

COMMON USES: Hyperacidity (peptic ulcer, hiatal hernia, etc).
DOSAGE: ***Adults:*** 15–30 PO pc and hs. ***Peds:*** 5–15 mL PO qid or prn.

NOTES: Doses qid are best given after meals and at bedtime; may cause hypermagnesemia.

Aluminum Hydroxide With Magnesium Hydroxide (Maalox)

COMMON USES: Hyperacidity (peptic ulcer, hiatal hernia, etc).
DOSAGE: ***Adults:*** 10–60 mL or 2–4. tablets PO qid or prn. ***Peds:*** 5–15 mL PO qid or prn.
NOTES: Doses qid are best given after meals and at bedtime; may cause hypermagnesemia in renal insufficiency.

Aluminum Hydroxide With Magnesium Trisilicate (Gaviscon-2)

COMMON USES: Hyperacidity.
DOSAGE: Chew 2–4 tablets qid and hs.

Aluminum Hydroxide With Magnesium Hydroxide and Simethicone (Mylanta, Mylanta II, Maalox Plus)

COMMON USES: Hyperacidity with bloating.
DOSAGE: ***Adults:*** 10–60 mL or 2–4. tablets PO qid or prn. ***Peds:*** 5–15 mL PO qid or prn.
NOTES: May cause hypermagnesemia in renal insufficiency; Mylanta II contains twice the amount of aluminum and magnesium hydroxide as Mylanta.

Amantadine (Symmetrel)

COMMON USES: Treatment or prophylaxis of influenza A viral infections; Parkinsonism.
DOSAGE: ***Adults:*** Influenza A: 200 mg PO qd or 100 mg PO bid. Parkinsonism: 100 mg PO qd–bid. ***Peds:*** 1–9 y: 4.4–8.8 mg/kg/24h to a maximum of 150 mg/24h divided qd–bid; > 9 y: same as adults.
NOTES: Reduce dose in renal insufficiency.

Amikacin (Amikin)

COMMON USES: Treatment of serious infections caused by gram-negative bacteria.
DOSAGE: ***Adults*** and ***Peds:*** 15 mg/kg/24h divided q8–12h or based on renal function; refer to Aminoglycoside dosing (Table IX–1, page 455).
NOTES: May be effective against gram-negative bacteria resistant to gentamicin and tobramycin; monitor renal function carefully for dose adjustments; monitor serum levels (see Table IX–3, page 457).

Amiloride (Midamor)

COMMON USES: Hypertension and congestive heart failure.
DOSAGE: 5–10 mg PO qd.
NOTES: Hyperkalemia may occur; monitor serum potassium levels.

Aminocaproic Acid (Amicar)

COMMON USES: Excessive bleeding resulting from systemic hyperfibrinolysis and urinary fibrinolysis.
DOSAGE: ***Adults*** and ***Peds:*** 100 mg/kg IV, then 1 g/m^2/h to maximum of 18 g/m^2/d or 100 mg/kg/dose q8h.
NOTES: Administer for 8 hours or until bleeding is controlled; contraindicated in disseminated intravascular coagulation; not for upper urinary tract bleeding; oral form rarely used.

Aminoglutethimide (Cytadren, Elipten, Orimeten)

COMMON USES: Adrenal cortex carcinoma, Cushing's syndrome, and prostate cancer.

TABLE IX–1. AMINOGLYCOSIDE DOSING.

See Table IX–3, page 457, "Common Drug Levels" for the trough and peak levels of the aminoglycosides gentamicin, tobramycin, and amikacin. Peak levels should be drawn 30 min after the dose is completely infused; trough levels should be drawn 30 min before the dose. As a general rule, draw the peak and trough around the fourth maintenance dose.

Therapy can be initiated with the recommended guidelines that follow. The following calculations are not valid for netilmicin.

Procedure (Adult)

1. Calculate the estimated creatinine clearance (CrCl) based on serum creatinine (SCr), age, and body weight, or you can order a formal creatinine clearance, if time permits.

$$\text{CrCl: Male} = \frac{(140 - \text{age [y]}) \times (\text{body wt. [kg]})}{(\text{SCr [mg/dL]}) \times 72}$$

$$\text{CrCl: Female} = 0.85 \times \text{CrCl}$$

2. Select the loading dose:

Gentamicin: 1.5–2.0 mg/kg Tobramycin: 1.5–2.0 mg/kg

Amikacin: 5.0–7.5 mg/kg

3. By using Table IX–2, page 456 you can now select the maintenance dose (as a percentage of the chosen loading dose) most appropriate for the renal function of the patient based on CrCl and dosing interval. Bold numbers are the suggested percentages and intervals for any given creatinine clearance.

DOSAGE: 750–1500 mg/d in divided doses plus dexamethasone 2–5 mg/d or hydrocortisone 20–40 mg/d.
NOTES: Toxicity includes adrenal insufficiency ("medical adrenalectomy"), hypothyroidism, masculinization, hypotension, vomiting, rare hepatotoxicity, rash, myalgia, and fever.

Amino-Cerv pH 5.5 Cream

COMMON USES: Mild cervicitis, postpartum cervicitis/cervical tears, postcauterization, postcryosurgery, and postconization.
DOSAGE: 1 applicator intravaginally qhs for 2–4 wk.
NOTES: Contains 8.34% urea, 0.5% sodium propionate, 0.83% methionine, 0.35% cystine, 0.83% inositol, benzalkonium chloride.

Aminophylline

COMMON USES: Asthma and bronchospasm; apnea of prematurity.
DOSAGE: ***Adults:*** Acute asthma: Load 6 mg/kg IV, then 0.4–0.9 mg/kg/h IV continuous infusion. Chronic asthma: 24 mg/kg/24h PO or PR divided q6h. ***Peds:*** Load 6 mg/kg IV, then 1.0 mg/kg/h IV continuous infusion.
NOTES: Individualize dose; signs of toxicity include nausea, vomiting, irritability, tachycardia, ventricular arrhythmias, and seizures; follow serum levels carefully; aminophylline is about 85% theophylline (see Table IX–3, page 457); erratic absorption with rectal doses.

Amiodarone (Cordarone)

COMMON USES: Recurrent ventricular fibrillation or hemodynamically unstable ventricular tachycardia.

TABLE IX–2. PERCENTAGE OF LOADING DOSE REQUIRED FOR DOSAGE INTERVAL SELECTED.[1]

CrCl (mL/min)	Dosing Interval 8 h	12 h	24 h
90	**90**	–	–
90	**86**	–	–
70	**84**	–	–
60	**79**	91	–
50	**74**	87	–
40	66	**80**	–
30	57	**72**	92
25	51	**66**	88
20	45	**59**	83
15	37	**50**	75
10	29	40	**64**
7	24	33	**55**
5	20	28	**48**
2	14	20	**35**
0	9	13	**25**

[1]Based on data from Hull JH, Sarubbi FA: Gentamicin serum concentrations: Pharmacokinetic predictions. Ann Intern Med 1976;85:183.
Bold numbers indicate suggested dosage intervals.
This is only an empirical dose to begin therapy. Serum levels should be monitored routinely for optimal therapy. Use Table IX–3, "Common Drug Levels," page 457

DOSAGE: ***Adults:*** Load: 800–1600 mg/d PO for 1–3 weeks. Maintenance: 600–800 mg/d PO for 1 mo, then 200–400 mg/d. Intravenous: 15 mg/min for 10 min, then 1 mg/min for 6 h; maintenance dose of 0.5 mg/min continuous infusion. ***Peds:*** 10–15 mg/kg/24h divided q12h PO for 7–10 d, then 5 mg/kg/24h divided q12h or qd (infants and neonates may require a higher loading dose).
NOTES: Average half-life is 53 d; potentially toxic effects leading to pulmonary fibrosis, liver failure, and ocular opacities, as well as exacerbation of arrhythmias; IV concentrations of > 0.2 mg/mL should be administered via a central catheter.

Amitriptyline (Elavil)

COMMON USES: Depression, peripheral neuropathy, chronic pain, cluster and migraine headaches.
DOSAGE: ***Adults:*** Initially, 50–100 mg PO qhs; may increase to 300 mg qhs. ***Peds:*** Not recommended if < 12 y unless for chronic pain: 0.1 mg/kg qhs initially, then advance over 2–3 wk to 0.5–2 mg/kg qhs.
NOTES: Strong anticholinergic side effects; may cause urinary retention and sedation.

Amlodipine (Norvasc)

COMMON USES: Hypertension, chronic stable angina, and vasospastic angina.
DOSAGE: 2.5–10 mg PO qd.

TABLE IX–3. COMMON DRUG LEVELS.[1]

Drug	Therapeutic Level	Toxic Level
Carbamazepine	8.0–12.0 mg/mL	>15.0 mg/mL
Cyclosporine	150–300 ng/mL (variable)	
Digoxin	0.8–2.0 ng/mL	>2.4 ng/mL
Ethanol		100–200 mg/100mL (legally drunk most states, labile behavior
		150–300 mg/100 mL (confusion)
		250–400 mg/100 mL (stupor)
		350–500 mg/100 mL (coma)
		>450 mg/100 mL (death)
Ethosuximide	40.0–100.0 mg/mL	>150.0 mg/mL
Lidocaine	1.5–6.5 mg/mL	>6.0–8.0 mg/mL
Lithium	0.6–1.2 mmol/L	>2.0 mmol/L
Phenobarbital	15.0–40.0 mg/mL	>45.0 mg/mL
Phenytoin	10.0–20.0 mg/mL	>25.0 mg/mL
Procainamide	4.0–10.0 mg/mL	>16.0 mg/mL
Quinidine	3.0–7.0 mg/mL	>7 mg/mL
Theophylline	10.0–20.0 mg/mL	>20.0 mg/mL
Valproic acid	50–100 mg/mL	>150 mg/mL
Antibiotic (maintain below upper limit)		
	Trough <mg/mL)	Peak (mg/mL)
Amikacin	5.0–7.5	25–35
Gentamicin	1.5–2.0	5–8
Tobramycin	1.5–2.0	5–8
Netilmicin	0.5–2.0	6–10
Vancomycin	5.0–10.0	20–40

[1]Each lab may have values that differ slightly from those provided. Therapeutic levels are usually determined as a trough just before next dose.

Ammonium Aluminum Sulfate (Alum)

COMMON USES: Hemorrhagic cystitis.
DOSAGE: 1–2% solution used with constant bladder irrigation with normal saline.
NOTES: Can be used safely without anesthesia and in the presence of vesicoureteral reflux. Encephalopathy has been reported; obtain aluminum levels, especially in patients with renal insufficiency. Alum solution often precipitates and occludes catheters.

Amoxapine (Asendin)

COMMON USES: Depression and anxiety.
DOSAGE: Initially, 150 mg PO qhs or 50 mg PO tid; increase to 300 mg daily.
NOTES: Reduce dose in elderly patients; taper slowly when discontinuing therapy.

Amoxicillin (Amoxil, Larotid, Polymox, others)

COMMON USES: Treatment of susceptible gram-positive bacteria (streptococci), and gram-negative bacteria *(H influenzae, E coli, P mirabilis)*(ie, SBE prophylaxis, otitis media, respiratory, skin and urinary tract infections).
DOSAGE: ***Adults:*** 250–500 mg PO tid. ***Peds:*** 25–100 mg/kg/24h PO divided q8h; 200 mg–400 mg PO bid (equivalent to 125 mg–250 mg tid).
NOTES: Cross-hypersensitivity with penicillin; may cause diarrhea; skin rash is common; many hospital strains of E coli are resistant.

Amoxicillin/Potassium Clavulanate (Augmentin)

COMMON USES: Treatment of infections caused by β-lactamase-producing strains of *H influenzae, S* aureus, and *E coli.*
DOSAGE: ***Adults:*** 250–500 mg as amoxicillin PO q8h or 875 mg q12h. ***Peds:*** 20–40 mg/kg/d as amoxicillin PO divided q8h.
NOTES: Do not substitute two 250–mg tablets for one 500-mg tablet or an overdose of clavulanic acid will occur; may cause diarrhea and gastrointestinal intolerance. This is a combination of a β-lactamase antibiotic and a β-lactamase inhibitor.

Amphotericin B (Fungizone)

COMMON USES: Severe, systemic fungal infections (eg, *Candida* spp,histoplasmosis, etc.); bladder irrigation for fungal infections,
DOSAGE: ***Adults*** and ***Peds:*** Test dose of 1 mg, then 0.25–1.5 mg/kg/24h IV over 4–6 h. Doses often range from 25 to 50 mg qd or every other day. Total dose varies with indication. Bladder Irrigation: 50 mg in 1-L sterile water irrigated over 24 h; used for 2–7 d or until culture is negative.
NOTES: Severe side effects with IV infusion; monitor renal function; hypokalemia and hypomagnesemia may be seen from renal wasting; pretreat with acetaminophen and antihistamines (Benadryl) to help minimize adverse effects such as fever; topical and oral forms are available.

Amphotericin B Cholesteryl (Amphotec)

COMMON USES: Invasive fungal infection in persons refractory or intolerant to conventional amphotericin B.
DOSAGE: ***Adults*** and ***Peds:*** Test dose of 1.6 mg–8.3 mg, over 15 to 20 min, followed by a dose of 3 to 4 mg/kg/d. Infuse at a rate of 1 mg/kg/h.
NOTES: Do NOT use in-line filter, final concentration, 0.6 mg/mL

Amphotericin B Lipid Complex (Abelcet)

COMMON USES: Invasive fungal infection in persons refractory or intolerant to conventional amphotericin B.
DOSAGE: 5 mg/kg/d IV administered as a single daily dose; infuse at a rate of 2.5 mg/kg/h.
NOTES: Filter solution with a 5-mm filter needle; do not mix in electrolyte-containing solutions. If infusion exceeds 2 h, gently mix contents of the bag.

Amphotericin B Liposomal (Ambisome)

COMMON USES: Invasive fungal infection in persons refractory or intolerant to conventional amphotericin B.
DOSAGE: ***Adults*** and ***Peds:*** 3 to 5 mg/kg/d, infused over 60 to 120 min.

Ampicillin (Amcill, Omnipen)

COMMON USES: Treatment of susceptible gram-negative (*Shigella, Salmonella, E coli, H influenzae, P mirabilis*) and gram-positive (streptococci) bacteria.
DOSAGE: ***Adults:*** Between 500 mg and 2 g PO, IM, or IV q6h. ***Peds:*** Neonates < 7 d: 50–100 mg/kg/24h IV divided q8h. Term infants: 75–150 mg/kg/24h divided q6–8h IV or PO. Infants > 1 mo and children: 100–200 mg/kg/24h divided q4–6h IM or IV; 50–100 mg/kg/24h divided q6h PO up to 250 mg/dose. Meningitis: 200–400 mg/kg/24h divided q4–6h IV.

NOTES: Cross-hypersensitivity with penicillin; can cause diarrhea and skin rash; many hospital strains of *E coli* are now resistant.

Ampicillin/Sulbactam (Unasyn)

COMMON USES: Treatment of infections caused by β-lactamase producing organisms of S aureus, Enterococcus spp, H influenzae, P mirabilis, and Bacteroides species.
DOSAGE: ***Adults:*** 1.5–3.0 g IM or IV q6h. ***Peds:*** Dosed by ampicillin content 100–200 mg ampicillin/kg/d 150–300 mg Unasyn) divided q6h; max daily dose, 8 g ampicillin (12 g Unasyn)/d.
NOTES: 2:1 ratio of ampicillin/sulbactam; adjust dose in renal failure; observe for hypersensitivity reactions.

Amrinone (Inocor)

COMMON USES: Short-term management of congestive heart failure.
DOSAGE: ***Adults*** and ***Peds:*** Initially give IV bolus of 0.75 mg/kg over 2–3 min followed by maintenance dose of 5–10 mg/kg/min.
NOTES: Not to exceed 10 mg/kg/d; incompatible with dextrose-containing solutions; monitor for fluid and electrolyte changes and renal function during therapy.

Anastrozole (Arimidex)

COMMON USES: Treatment of breast cancer following tamoxifen.
DOSAGE: 1 mg once daily.
NOTES: No detectable effect on adrenal. corticosteroids or aldosterone; may increase cholesterol levels.

Anistreplase (Eminase)

COMMON USES: Treatment of acute MI.
DOSAGE: 30 units IV over 2–5 min.
NOTES: May not be effective if readministered more than 5 d after anistreplase, streptokinase, or streptococcal infection because of production of antistreptokinase antibody.

Antihemophilic (AHF) Factor [factor VIII] (Monoclate, others)

COMMON USES: Treatment of classic hemophilia A with factor VIII deficiency.
DOSAGE: ***Adults*** and ***Peds:*** 1 AHF U/kg increases factor VIII concentration in the body by approximately 2%. Units required = Body weight (kg) × (desired factor VIII increase as % normal) × (0.5). Prophylaxis of spontaneous hemorrhage: 5% normal. Hemostasis following trauma or surgery: 30% normal. Head injuries, major surgery, or bleeding: 80–100% normal. Patient's percentage of normal level of factor VIII concentration must be ascertained before dosing for these calculations. Typical dosing is 20–50 U/kg/dose given q12–24h.
NOTES: Not effective in controlling bleeding of patients with von Willebrand's disease; derived from pooled human plasma.

Antipyrine and Benzocaine (Auralgan)

COMMON USES: Temporary relief of painful inflammatory conditions of the ear (serous otitis media, swimmers ear, otitis externa); aid to cerumen removal.
DOSAGE: ***Adults*** and ***Peds:*** Fill ear canal and place cotton plug to retain; repeat q1–2 h prn; cerumen apply tid–qid for 2–3 d.

Antithymocyte Globulin [ATG] (Atgam)

COMMON USES: Management of allograft rejection in renal transplant patients.
DOSAGE: ***Adults:*** 10–30 mg/kg/d. ***Peds:*** 5–25 mg/kg/d.
NOTES: Do not administer to a patient with a history of severe systemic reaction to any other equine gamma globulin preparation; discontinue treatment if severe unremitting thrombocytopenia or leukopenia occurs.

Apraclonidine (Lopridine)

COMMON USES: Glaucoma
DOSAGE: 1–2 drops of 0.5% tid.

Aprotinin (Trasylol)

COMMON USES: Reduction or prevention of blood loss in patients undergoing CABG.
DOSAGE: High-dose: 2 million KIU load, 2 million KIU for the pump prime dose, followed by 500,000 KIU/h until surgery ends. Low-dose: 1 million KIU load, 1 million KIU for the pump prime dose, followed by 250,000 KIU/h until surgery ends. Maximum total dose of 7 million KIU.
NOTES: 1 KIU 5 0.14 mg of aprotinin.

Ardeparin (Normiflo)

COMMON USES: Prevention of DVT and PE following knee replacement.
DOSAGE: 35–50 U/kg SC q12h. Begin the day of surgery and continue for <14 d.
NOTES: Laboratory monitoring is not necessary.

Artificial Tears [OTC] (Tears Naturale, others)

COMMON USES: Dry eyes.
DOSAGE: 1–2 drops tid–qid.

Aspirin (Bayer, Ecotrin, St. Joseph, ASA, others)

COMMON USES: Mild pain, headache, fever, inflammation, prevention of emboli, MI and TIA.
DOSAGE: ***Adults:*** Pain, fever: 325–650 mg q4–6h PO or PR. Rheumatoid arthritis: 3–6 g/d PO in divided doses. Platelet inhibitory action: 325 mg PO qd. Prevention of MI: 160–325 mg PO qd. TIA: 1.3 g/d PO divided bid–qid. ***Peds:*** Caution: Use linked to Reye's syndrome; avoid use with viral illness in children. Antipyretic: 10–15 mg/kg/dose PO or PR q4h up to 80 mg/kg/24h. Rheumatoid arthritis: 60–100 mg/kg/24h PO divided q4–6h (monitor serum levels to maintain between 15–30 mg/dL).
NOTES: Gastrointestinal upset and erosion are common adverse reactions; discontinue use 1 wk before surgery to avoid postop bleeding complications.

Aspirin With Codeine (Empirin No. 1, No. 2, No. 3, No. 4) [C]

COMMON USES: Relief of mild to moderate pain.
DOSAGE: ***Adults:*** 1–2 tablets PO q3–4h prn. ***Peds:*** Aspirin 10 mg/kg/dose; codeine 0.5–1.0 mg/kg/dose q4h.
NOTES: Codeine in #1: 7.5 mg, #2: 15 mg, #3 30 mg, #4: 60 mg.

Aspirin With Meprobamate (Equagesic) [C]

COMMON USES: Treatment of musculoskeletal disease in patients with signs of tension or anxiety.
DOSAGE: ***Adults:*** 1 tablet PO tid–id.

Atenolol (Tenormin)

COMMON USES: Hypertension, angina, post MI, antiarrhythmic, acute alcoholic withdrawal.
DOSAGE: ***Adults:*** HTN and angina: 50–100 mg PO qd. AMI: 5 mg IV x 2 doses, then 50 mg PO bid.

Atenolol and Chlorthalidone (Tenoretic)

COMMON USES: Hypertension.
DOSAGE: 50–100 mg PO qd.

Atorvastatin (Lipitor)

COMMON USES: Elevated cholesterol and triglycerides along with dietary modifications.
DOSAGE: Initial dose 10 mg daily, may be increased to 80 mg/d.
NOTES: May cause myopathy, monitor LFT regularly.

Atracurium (Tracrium)

COMMON USES: Adjunct to anesthesia to facilitate endotracheal intubation.

DOSAGE: ***Adults*** and ***Peds:*** 0.4–0.5 mg/kg IV bolus, then 0.08–0.1 mg/kg every 20–45 min prn.
NOTES: Patient must be intubated and on controlled ventilation. Use adequate amounts of sedation and analgesia.

Atropine

COMMON USES: Preanesthetic, symptomatic bradycardia, asystole; organophosphate poisoning, bronchodilator, mydriatic and cycloplegic for eye exam, uveitis, reversal of neuromuscular blockade with neostigmine or edrophonium.
DOSAGE: ***Adults:*** Emergency cardiac care, bradycardia: 0.5 mg IV q5min up to 2.0 mg total. Asystole 1.0 mg IV, repeat in 5 min. Preanesthetic: 0.3–0.6 mg IM/IV/SC. Ophthalmic: 1–2 drops qid or 1/4 inch of 1% ointment; refraction, administer 1 hour before exam. ***Peds:*** Emergency cardiac care: 0.01–0.03 mg/kg IV q2–5 min up to 1.0 mg total dose; minimum dose of 0.1 mg. Preanesthetic: 0.01 mg/kg/dose SC/IM/IV (maximum 0.4 mg).
NOTES: Can cause blurred vision, urinary retention, dry mucous membranes.

Azathioprine (Imuran)

COMMON USES: Adjunct for the prevention of rejection following organ transplantation; rheumatoid arthritis; systemic lupus erythematosus.
DOSAGE: ***Adults*** and ***Peds:*** 1–3 mg/kg IV or PO daily.
NOTES: May cause gastrointestinal intolerance; injection should be handled with appropriate precautions.

Azithromycin (Zithromax)

COMMON USES: Treatment of acute bacterial exacerbations of chronic obstructive pulmonary disease (COPD), mild community-acquired pneumonia, pharyngitis, otitis media, skin and skin structure infections, nongonococcal urethritis, and PID. Treatment and prevention of mycobacterium avium complex (Mac) infections in HIV-infected persons.
DOSAGE: ***Adults:*** PO: Respiratory tract: 500 mg on the first day, followed by 250 mg PO qd for 4 more days. Nongonococcal urethritis: 1 g as a single dose. Prevention of Mac: 1200 mg PO once a week. Intravenous: 500 mg for at least 2 d, followed by 500 mg PO for total of 7–10 d. ***Peds:*** Otitis media: 10 mg/kg PO on day 1, then 5 mg/kg/d on days 2–5. Pharyngitis: 12 mg/kg/d PO for 5 d.
NOTES: Should be taken before meals.

Aztreonam (Azactam)

COMMON USES: Infections caused by aerobic gram-negative bacteria where beta-lactam may not be useful, including *Enterobacter, H influenzae, Pseudomonas* sepsis, UTI, skin infections, intra-abdominal and gynecologic infections
DOSAGE: ***Adults:*** 1–2 g IV/IM q6–12h. ***Peds:*** Premature infants: 30 mg/kg/dose IV q12h. Term infants, children: 30–50 mg/kg/dose q6–8h.
NOTES: Not effective against gram-positive or anaerobic bacteria; may be given to penicillin-allergic patients.

Bacitracin and polymyxin B (Polysporin)

COMMON USES: Blepharitis, conjunctivitis, and prophylactic treatment of corneal abrasions.
DOSAGE: Apply q3–4h.

Baclofen (Lioresal)

COMMON USES: Spasticity secondary to severe chronic disorders such as multiple sclerosis or spinal cord lesions.
DOSAGE: 5 mg PO tid initially, increase every 3 d to maximum effect; maximum 80 mg/d.
NOTES: Caution in patients with seizure disorder and neuropsychiatric disturbances.

BCG (Theracys, Tice, Pacis)

COMMON USES: Treatment and prophylaxis of superficial bladder cancer.
DOSAGE: 1 ampule in 30–50 mL normal saline instilled into bladder by catheter and held for 2 h (standard induction treatment weekly for 6 wk); maintenance schedules recommended include 3 weekly doses 3, 6, 12, 18, 24 or single monthly dose for 12 mo.
NOTES: Do not give within 10 d of bladder biopsy, if catheterization traumatic or if patient is immunosuppressed.

Basiliximab (Simulect)

COMMON USES: Prevention of acute organ transplant rejections.
DOSAGE: ***Adults:*** 20 mg IV 2 h prior to transplant, then 20 mg IV 4 d post transplant. ***Peds:*** 12 mg/m^2 up to a max. of 20 mg 2 h prior to transplant, then the same dose IV 4 d post transplant.
NOTES: Murine/human monoclonal antibody.

Beclomethasone (Beconase, Vancenase Nasal Inhalers)

COMMON USES: Allergic rhinitis refractory to conventional therapy with antihistamines and decongestants.
DOSAGE: ***Adults:*** 1 spray intranasally bid–qid. ***Peds:*** 6–11 y: 1 spray intranasally tid.
NOTES: Nasal spray delivers 42 mg/dose.

Beclomethasone (Beclovent Inhaler, Vanceril Inhaler)

COMMON USES: Chronic asthma.
DOSAGE: ***Adults:*** 2–4 inhalations tid–qid (maximum 20/d). ***Peds:*** 1–2 inhalations tid–qid (maximum 10/d).
NOTES: Not effective for acute asthmatic attacks; may cause oral candidiasis.

Belladonna and Opium Suppositories (B & O Supprettes) [C]

COMMON USES: Treatment of bladder or rectal spasms; moderate to severe pain.
DOSAGE: Insert 1 suppository rectally q4–6h prn. (15A = 30 mg powdered opium; 16.2 mg belladonna extract. 16A = 60 mg powdered opium; 16.2 mg belladonna extract.)
NOTES: Anticholinergic side effects; caution subjects about sedation, urinary retention, constipation.

Benazepril (Lotensin)

COMMON USES: Hypertension.
DOSAGE: 10–40 mg PO qd.
NOTES: May cause symptomatic hypotension in patients taking diuretics; may cause a nonproductive cough.

Benzonatate (Tessalon Perles)

COMMON USES: Symptomatic relief of nonproductive cough.
DOSAGE: 100 mg PO tid.
NOTES: May cause sedation.

Benztropine (Cogentin)

COMMON USES: Treatment of Parkinson's disease and drug-induced extrapyramidal disorders.
DOSAGE: 1–6 mg PO, IM, or IV in divided doses.
NOTES: Anticholinergic side effects.

Bepridil (Vascor)

COMMON USES: Treatment of chronic stable angina, hypertension and CHF.
DOSAGE: 200–400 mg PO daily (adjust dose after 10 d).

NOTES: May cause serious ventricular arrhythmias, including torsade de pointes and agranulocytosis.

Beractant (Survanta)

COMMON USES: Prevention/treatment of respiratory distress syndrome (RDS) in premature infants.
DOSAGE: 4 mL/kg intratracheally; up to 4 doses in the first 48 h of life at least 6 h apart; additional therapy based on clinical response.

Betamethasone and Clotrimazole, Topical (Lotrisone)

COMMON USES: Topical treatment of fungal skin infections.
DOSAGE: Apply bid.
NOTES: Combination antifungal and anti-inflammatory

Betamethasone, systemic (Celestone, others) (Also see Table IX–4, page 475 and 529)

COMMON USES: Steroid replacement, anti-inflammatory, immunosuppressive.
DOSAGE: 0.6–7.2 mg/d PO divided bid–tid; up to 9 mg/d IM; intra-articular 0.5–2.0 mL.

Betamethasone, topical (Diprolene, Diprolene AF, Valisone, others)(Also see Table IX–4, page 475 and 529)

COMMON USES: Topical steroid therapy of dermatosis (psoriasis, seborrhea, atopic, allergic and neuro dermatitis).
DOSAGE: Apply to lesion up to tid.
NOTES: Betamethasone dipropionate and augmented (Diprolene) available in 0.05% gel, ointment or lotion; betamethasone valerate (Valisone) available as cream 0.01,0.1%, lotion and ointment 0.1%.

Betaxolol (Kerlone)

COMMON USES: Hypertenstion, ocular for glaucoma.
DOSAGE: 10–20 mg PO, qd; ophthalmic: 1–2 drops of solution or suspension bid.

Bethanechol (Urecholine, Duvoid, others)

COMMON USES: Neurogenic atony of the bladder with urinary retention, acute postoperative and postpartum functional (nonobstructive) urinary retention.
DOSAGE: ***Adults:*** 10–50 mg PO tid–qid or 5 mg SC tid–qid and prn. ***Peds:*** 0.3–0.6 mg/kg/24h PO divided tid–qid or Z\c the oral dose SC.
NOTES: Contraindicated in bladder outlet obstruction, asthma, coronary artery disease; do not administer IM or IV.

Bicalutamide (Casodex)

COMMON USES: Treatment of advanced prostate cancer in combination with LHRH analogue.
DOSE: 50 mg PO qd.
NOTES: Follow LFTs; can cause gynecomastia.

Bicarbonate, see Sodium bicarbonate

Bisacodyl (Dulcolax, others)

COMMON USES: Constipation, bowel prep.
DOSAGE: ***Adults:*** 5–10 mg PO or 10 mg rectally prn. ***Peds:*** < 2 y: 5 mg rectally prn; > 2 y: 5 mg PO or 10 mg rectally prn.
NOTES: Do not use with an acute abdomen or bowel obstruction; do not chew tablets; do not give within 1 h of antacids or milk.

Bismuth Subsalicylate (Pepto-Bismol, others)

COMMON USES: Indigestion, nausea, and diarrhea.
DOSAGE: ***Adults:*** 2 tablets or 30 mL PO prn. ***Peds:*** 3–6 y: 1/3 tablet or 5 mL PO prn; 6–9 y: 2/3 tablet or 10 mL PO prn; 9–12 y: 1 tablet or 15 mL PO prn.

Bisoprolol (Zebeta)

COMMON USES: Hypertension
DOSAGE: 5–10 mg qd.

Bitolterol (Tornalate)

COMMON USES: Prophylaxis and treatment of asthma and reversible bronchospasm.
DOSAGE: ***Adults:*** and children >12 y: 2 inhalations q8h.

Bleomycin (Blenoxane)

COMMON USES: Treatment of cervical, ovarian, squamous cell, testicular cancer, and lymphoma; sclerotherapy of malignant pleural effusion.
DOSAGE: 0.25–0.5 U/kg/dose IV, IM, or SC once or twice weekly.
NOTES: Pulmonary toxicity is increased with total doses of > 400 U.

Brimonidine (Alphagan)

COMMON USES: Glaucoma.
DOSAGE: 1 drop bid.
NOTES: Do not apply with soft contact lenses in place.

Brinzolamide (Azopt)

COMMON USES: Glaucoma.
DOSAGE: 1 drop in eye(s) tid.

Bromocriptine (Parlodel)

COMMON USES: Parkinsonian syndrome.
DOSAGE: Parkinson's: 1.25 mg PO bid initially, titrated to effect.
NOTES: Nausea and vertigo are common side effects.

Buclizine (Bucladin-S Softabs)

COMMON USES: Control of nausea, vomiting, and dizziness of motion sickness.
DOSAGE: 50 mg dissolved in mouth bid; 50 mg PO prophylactically 30 min before travel.
NOTES: Not safe in pregnancy; contains tartrazine, observe patient for allergic reactions.

Budesonide (Rhinocort, Pulmicort)

COMMON USES: Management of allergic and nonallergic rhinitis, management of asthma.
DOSAGE: ***Intranasal:*** 2 sprays in each nostril bid. ***Oral inhaled:*** 1–4 inhalations twice daily. ***Peds:*** 1–2 inhalations twice daily.

Bumetanide (Bumex)

COMMON USES: Edema from congestive heart failure, hepatic cirrhosis, and renal disease.
DOSAGE: ***Adults:*** 0.5–2.0 mg PO daily; 0.5–1.0 mg IV q8–24h. ***Peds:*** 0.015–0.1 mg/kg/dose PO, IV, IM q6–24h.
NOTES: Monitor fluid and electrolyte status during treatment.

Bupivacaine (Marcaine, Sensorcaine)

COMMON USES: Local infiltration anesthesia, lumbar epidural.
DOSAGE: Dependent on the procedure, vascularity of the tissues, depth of anesthesia, and degree of muscle relaxation required. Maximum infiltration dose in 70–kg adult is 70 mL of 0.25%.

Buprenorphine (Buprenex) [C]

COMMON USES: Relief of moderate to severe pain.
DOSAGE: 0.3 mg IM or slow IV push every 6 h prn.
NOTES: May induce withdrawal syndrome in opioid dependent subjects.

Bupropion (Wellbutrin, Zyban)

COMMON USES: Treatment of depression, adjunct to smoking cessation.
DOSAGE: Depression: 100–450 mg/d divided bid-tid. Smoking: 150 mg daily for 3 d, then 150 mg twice daily.
NOTES: Has been associated with seizures; avoid use of alcohol and other CNS depressants.

Buspirone (BuSpar)

COMMON USES: Short-term relief of anxiety.
DOSAGE: 5–10 mg PO tid.
NOTES: No abuse potential. No physical or psychological dependence.

Butalbital and Acetaminophen (Fioricet, Medigesic, Phrenilin, Phrenilin Forte, Sedapap-10, others)[C]

COMMON USES: Tension headache, pain.
DOSAGE: 1–2 PO q4h prn, max 6 tabs/d.
NOTES: Butalbital habit forming; Medigesic caps: butalbital 50 mg, caffeine 40 mg, and acetaminophen 325 mg; Phrenilin Forte caps: butalbital 50 mg and acetaminophen 650 mg;
Fioricet Tabs: butalbital 50 mg, caffeine 40 mg, and acetaminophen 325 mg; Phrenilin Tabs: butalbital 50 mg and acetaminophen 325 mg; Sedapap-10: butalbital 50 mg and acetaminophen 650 mg.

Butalbital and Aspirin (Fiorinal, Lanorinal, Marnal, others) [C]

COMMON USES: Tension headache, pain
DOSAGE: 1–2 PO q4h prn, max 6 tabs/d.
NOTES: Butalbital habit forming; Fiorinal, Lanorinal, Marnal Caps and Tabs: Butalbital 50 mg, caffeine 40 mg, and aspirin 325 mg.

Butalbital, Aspirin, and Codeine (Fiorinal With Codeine) [C]

COMMON USES: Moderate pain.
DOSAGE: 1–2 PO q4h prn, max 6/d.
NOTES: Butalbital may be habit forming; may cause sedation; contains butalbital 50 mg, caffeine 40 mg, aspirin 325 mg, codeine 30 mg.

Butorphanol (Stadol) [C]

COMMON USES: Analgesic for moderate to severe pain; migraine headache.
DOSAGE: 1–4 mg IM or 0.5–2 mg IV every 3–4 h prn; 1 spray in 1 nostril (1 mg) reevaluate in 60–90 min and repeat if needed; repeat 2-dose sequence prn in 3–4 h.
NOTES: May induce withdrawal syndrome in opioid-dependent patients.

Calcitrol (Rocaltrol)

COMMON USES: Reduction of elevated parathyroid hormone levels, hypocalcemia associated with dialysis.
DOSAGE: ***Adults:*** renal failure 0.25 μg PO, qd increase 0.25 μg/d every 4–6 wk prn; 0.5 μg 3 times a week IV, increase as needed. *Hyperparathyroidism:* 0.5–2.0 μg/d. ***Peds:*** renal failure 15 ng/kg/d, increase prn typical maintenance 30–60 ng/kg/d. *Hyperparathyroidism:* < 5 y, 0.25–0.75 μg/d; > 6 y, 0.5–2.0 μg/d.
NOTES: 1,25 dihydroxycholecalciferol, a vitamin D analogue; monitor dosing to keep calcium levels within normal range.

Calcitonin (Cibacalcin, Miacalcin)

COMMON USES: Paget's disease of bone; hypercalcemia; osteogenesis imperfecta, postmenopausal osteoporosis.
DOSAGE: Paget's salmon form: 100 U/d IM/SC initially, 50 U/d or 50–100 U q1–3d maintenance. Pagets human form: 0.5 mg/d initially; maintenance: 0.5 mg 2–3 times/wk or 0.25 mg/d, max: 0.5 mg bid. Hypercalcemia salmon calcitonin:

4 U/kg IM/SC q12h; increase to 8 U/kg q12h, max: q6h. Osteoporosis salmon calcitonin: 100 U/d IM/SC; Intranasal: 200 U = 1 nasal spray/d.
NOTES: Human (Cibacalcin) and salmon forms; human only approved for Pagets' bone disease.

Calcium Acetate

COMMON USES: ESRD associated hyperphosphatemia.
DOSAGE: 2–4 tabs PO with meals.
NOTES: Can cause hypercalcemia, monitor levels.

Calcium Carbonate (Alka-Mints, Caltrate, Tums, Os-Cal, others)

COMMON USES: Hyperacidity associated with peptic ulcer disease, hiatal hernia, etc.; calcium supplementation.
DOSAGE: From 500 mg to 2.0 g PO prn.

Calcium Salts (Chloride Gluconate)

COMMON USES: Calcium replacement, ventricular fibrillation, electromechanical dissociation, management of hyperphosphatemia in ESRD.
DOSAGE: ***Adults:*** Replacement: 1–2 g PO qd. Cardiac emergencies:) Calcium chloride 0.5–1.0 g IV every 10 min or Calcium gluconate 1–2 g IV every 10 min. ***Peds:*** Replacement: 200–500 mg/kg/24h PO or IV divided qid. Cardiac emergency: 100 mg/kg/dose IV of gluconate salt every 10 min.
NOTES: Calcium chloride contains 270 mg (13.6 mEq) elemental calcium per gram, and calcium gluconate contains 90 mg (4.5 mEq) elemental calcium per gram.

Candesartan (Atacand)

COMMON USES: Treatment of hypertension.
DOSAGE: 2 to 32 mg per day, usual dose is 16 mg once daily.
NOTES: Monitor BP and titrate to effect; maximum BP response within 2 wk.

Capsaicin (Zostrix, others)

COMMON USES: Topical analgesic (post-herpetic neuralgia, arthritis, postop pain).
DOSAGE: OTC form, apply tid–qid.

Captopril (Capoten)

COMMON USES: Treatment of hypertension, congestive heart failure, and diabetic nephropathy.
DOSAGE: ***Adults:*** Hypertension: Initially, 25 mg PO bid–tid; titrate to a maintenance dose every 1–2 wk by 25 mg increments per dose (maximum 450 mg/d) to desired effect. Congestive heart failure: Initially, 6.25–12.5 mg PO tid; titrate to desired effect. ***Peds:*** Infants < 2 mo, 0.05–0.1 mg/kg/dose PO tid–qid. ***Children:*** Initially, 0.15 mg/kg/dose PO; double q2h until blood pressure is controlled, to maximum of 6 mg/kg/d; maintenance: 0.5–0.6 mg/kg/d PO divided bid–qid.
NOTES: Use with caution in renal failure. Give 1 h before meals; can cause rash, proteinuria, and cough.

Carbamazepine (Tegretol)

COMMON USES: Epilepsy; trigeminal neuralgia.
DOSAGE: ***Adults:*** 200 mg PO bid initially; increase by 200 mg/d; usual 800–1200 mg/d. ***Peds:*** 6–12 y: 100 mg/dose PO bid or 10 mg/kg/24h PO divided qd–bid initially; increase to a maintenance dose of 20–30 mg/kg/24h divided tid–qid.
NOTES: Can cause severe hematologic side effects; monitor CBC; monitor serum levels, see Table IX–3 (page 457); generic products are not interchangeable.

Carbidopa/Levodopa (Sinemet)

COMMON USES: Parkinson's disease.
DOSAGE: Start at 10/100 PO bid–tid; titrate as needed.

NOTES: May cause psychiatric disturbances, orthostatic hypotension, dyskinesias, and cardiac arrhythmias.

Carboplatin (Paraplatin)

COMMON USES: Treatment of cervical, ovarian, and lung cancer.
DOSAGE: Varies with treatment protocol; 300–360 mg/m^2 on day 1 every 4 wk.
NOTES: May cause bone marrow suppression, vomiting, and anaphylaxis; follow platelet and neutrophil counts.

Carisoprodol (Soma)

COMMON USES: Adjunct to sleep and physical therapy for the relief of painful musculoskeletal conditions.
DOSAGE: 350 mg PO qid.
NOTES: Avoid alcohol and other CNS depressants; also available with 16–mg codeine/tablet [C].

Carteolol (Cartrol, Ocupress Ophthalmic)

COMMON USES: Treatment of hypertension; opthalmic solution for increased intraocular pressure.
DOSAGE: 2.5–5 mg PO qd; ophthalmic 1 drop eye/eyes bid.

Carvedilol (Coreg)

COMMON USES: Treatment of hypertension and CHF.
DOSAGE: HTN: 6.25–12.5 mg twice daily. CHF: 3.125–25 mg twice daily.
NOTES: Take with food to slow absorption and reduce incidence of orthostatic hypotension.

Cefaclor (Ceclor)

COMMON USES: Treatment of infections caused by susceptible bacteria involving the upper and lower respiratory tract, skin, bone, urinary tract, abdomen and gynecologic system (*S aureus, S pneumoniae, H influenzae).*
DOSAGE: ***Adults:*** 250–500 mg PO tid. ***Peds:*** 20–40 mg/kg/d PO divided tid.
NOTES: Second generation cephalosporin; more gram-negative activity than first generation cephalosporins.

Cefadroxil (Duricef, Ultracef)

COMMON USES: Treatment of infections caused by susceptible strains of *Streptococcus, Staphylococcus, E coli, Proteus* and *Klebsiella* involving the skin, bone, upper and lower respiratory tract, and urinary tract.
DOSAGE: ***Adults:*** 500–1000 mg PO bid–qd. ***Peds:*** 30 mg/kg/d divided bid.
NOTES: First generation cephalosporin.

Cefazolin (Ancef, Kefzol)

COMMON USES: Treatment of infections caused by susceptible strains of *Streptococcus, Staphylococcus, E coli, Proteus* and *Klebsiella* involving the skin, bone, upper and lower respiratory tract, and urinary tract.
DOSAGE: ***Adults:*** 1–2 g IV q8h. ***Peds:*** 50–100 mg/kg/d IV divided q8h.
NOTES: Widely used for surgical prophylaxis; first generation cephalosporin.

Cefdinir (Omnicef)

COMMON USES: Treatment of infections caused by susceptible bacteria involving the respiratory tract, skin, bone, urinary tract, meningitis, and septicemia.
DOSAGE: ***Adults:*** 300 mg PO bid or 600 mg PO qd. ***Peds:*** 7 mg/kg PO bid or 14 mg/kg PO qd
NOTES: Third generation cephalosporin.

Cefepime (Maxipime)

COMMON USES: Treatment of urinary tract infections and pneumonia caused by susceptible *S pneumoniae, S aureus, K pneumoniae, E coli, P aeruginosa,* and *Enterobacter* spp.

DOSAGE: 1–2 g IV q12h for 5–10 d; UTI 500 mg IV q12h
NOTES: Fourth generation cephalosporin; improved gram positive coverage over third generation.

Cefixime (Suprax)

COMMON USES: Treatment of infections caused by susceptible bacteria involving the respiratory tract, skin, bone, urinary tract, meningitis, and septicemia; single dose to treat gonorrhea.
DOSAGE: ***Adults:*** 200–400 mg PO bid–qd. ***Peds:*** 8 mg/kg/d PO divided bid–qd, 400 mg/max/d
NOTES: Third generation cephalosporin; use suspension to treat otitis media.

Cefmetazole (Zefazone)

COMMON USES: Treatment of infections caused by susceptible bacteria involving the upper and lower respiratory tract, skin, bone, urinary tract, abdomen, and gynecologic system.
DOSAGE: ***Adults:*** treatment of infection, 1–2 g IV 8h; surgical prophylaxis, 2 g IV 30–90 min preop.
NOTES: Second generation cephalosporin with more gram-negative activity than first generation cephalosporins; has anaerobic activity.

Cefonicid (Monocid)

COMMON USES: Treatment of infections caused by susceptible bacteria: respiratory, skin, bone and joint, urinary, gynecologic, and septicemia.
DOSAGE: 1 g IM/IV every 24 h.
NOTES: Second generation cephalosporin.

Cefoperazone (Cefobid)

COMMON USES: Treatment of infections caused by susceptible bacteria: respiratory, skin , urinary tract, sepsis; as a third generation cephalosporin, cefoperazone has activity against gram-negative bacilli (eg, *E coli, Klebsiella,* and *Haemophilus*) but variable activity against *Streptococcus* and *Staphylococcus* species; it has activity against *P aeruginosa,* but less than ceftazidime.
DOSAGE: ***Adults:*** 2–4 g/d, divided q12h IM/IV; 12 g/d max. ***Peds:*** 100–150 mg/kg/d divided q8–12h IM/IV.
NOTES: Third generation cephalosporin; active against gram-negatives but variable activity against *Staphylococcus* and *Streptococcus*; some activity against *Pseudomonas.*

Cefotaxime (Claforan)

COMMON USES: Treatment of infections caused by susceptible bacteria involving the respiratory tract, skin, bone, urinary tract, meningitis, and septicemia.
DOSAGE: ***Adults:*** 1–2 g IV q4–12h. ***Peds:*** 100–200 mg/kg/d IV divided q6–8h.
NOTES: Third generation cephalosporin.

Cefotetan (Cefotan)

COMMON USES: Treatment of infections caused by susceptible bacteria involving the upper and lower respiratory tract, skin, bone, urinary tract, abdomen, and gynecologic system.
DOSAGE: ***Adults:*** 1–2 g IV q12h. ***Peds:*** 40–80 mg/kg/d IV divided q12h.
NOTES: Second generation cephalosporin; more gram-negative activity then first generation cephalosporins; has anaerobic activity.

Cefoxitin (Mefoxin)

COMMON USES: Treatment of infections caused by susceptible bacteria involving the upper and lower respiratory tract, skin, bone, urinary tract, abdomen, and gynecologic system.
DOSAGE: ***Adults:*** 1–2 mg IV q6h. ***Peds:*** 80–160 mg/kg/d divided q4–6h.

NOTES: Second generation cephalosporin; more gram-negative activity then first generation cephalosporins; has anaerobic activity.

Cefpodoxime (Vantin)

COMMON USES: Treatment of infections caused by susceptible bacteria involving the respiratory tract (community acquired pneumonia due to *S pneumonia* or non-beta lactamase *H influenzae*, otitis media, pharyngitis, tonsillitis, skin, bone, urinary tract, gonorrhea, meningitis, and septicemia.
DOSAGE: ***Adults:*** 200–400 mg PO q12h. ***Peds:*** > 6 mo, 10 mg/kg/d PO divided bid.
NOTES: Second generation cephalosporin; drug interactions with agents increasing gastric pH.

Cefprozil (Cefzil)

COMMON USES: Treatment of infections caused by susceptible bacteria involving the upper and lower respiratory tract, skin, bone, urinary tract, abdomen, and gynecologic system.
DOSAGE: ***Adults:*** 250–500 mg PO qd–bid. ***Peds:*** >6 mo, 7.5–15 mg/kg/d PO divided bid.
NOTES: Second generation cephalosporin; more gram-negative activity then first generation cephalosporins; use higher doses for otitis and pneumonia.

Ceftazidime (Fortaz, Ceptaz, Tazidime, Tazicef)

COMMON USES: Treatment of infections caused by susceptible bacteria involving the respiratory tract, skin, bone, urinary tract, meningitis, and septicemia.
DOSAGE: ***Adults:*** 1–2 g IV q8h. ***Peds:*** 30–50 mg/kg/d IV divided q8h.
NOTES: Third generation cephalosporin; useful in patients with pseudomonal infections at risk for nephrotoxicity; empiric therapy in febrile granulocytopenic patients.

Ceftibuten (Cedax)

COMMON USES: Treatment of infections caused by susceptible bacteria involving the respiratory tract (bronchitis), skin, bone, urinary tract, meningitis, and septicemia.
DOSAGE: ***Adults:*** 400 mg PO once daily. ***Peds:*** 9 mg/kg PO once daily (400 mg max).
NOTES: Third generation cephalosporin; take before eating; little activity against *Streptococcus.*

Ceftizoxime (Cefizox)

COMMON USES: Treatment of infections caused by susceptible bacteria involving the respiratory tract, skin, bone, urinary tract, meningitis, and septicemia.
DOSAGE: ***Adults:*** 1–2 g IV q12–8h. ***Peds:*** 150–200 mg/kg/d IV divided q6–8h.
NOTES: Third generation cephalosporin

Ceftriaxone (Rocephin)

COMMON USES: Treatment of infections caused by susceptible bacteria involving the respiratory tract, skin, bone, urinary tract, meningitis, chancroid, uncomplicated gonorrhea, and septicemia.
DOSAGE: ***Adults:*** 1–2 g IV q12–24h; GC and chancroid <45kg, 125 mg IM; > 45 kg, 250–mg IM single dose. ***Peds:*** 50–100 mg/kg/d IV divided q12–24h.
NOTES: Third generation cephalosporin.

Cefuroxime (Ceftin [oral], Zinacef [parenteral])

COMMON USES: Treatment of infections caused by susceptible bacteria involving the upper and lower respiratory tract, skin, bone, urinary tract, abdomen, and gynecologic system.
DOSAGE: ***Adults:*** 750 mg–1.5 g IV q8h or 250–500 mg PO bid. ***Peds:*** 100–150 mg/kg/d IV divided q8h or 20–30 mg/kg/d PO divided bid.

NOTES: Second generation cephalosporin; more gram-negative activity then first generation cephalosporins; IV crosses the blood brain barrier.

Celecoxib (Celebrex)

COMMON USES: Osteoarthritis and rheumatoid arthritis.
DOSAGE: 100–200 mg once or twice daily.

Cephalexin (Keflex, Keftab)

COMMON USES: Treatment of infections caused by susceptible strains of *Streptococcus, Staphylococcus, E coli, Proteus* and *Klebsiella* involving the skin, bone, upper and lower respiratory tract, and urinary tract.
DOSAGE: ***Adults:*** 250–500 mg PO qid. ***Peds:*** 25–100 mg/kg/d PO divided qid.
NOTES: First generation cephalosporin.

Cephaprin (Cefadyl)

COMMON USES: Treatment of infections caused by susceptible strains of respiratory tract, skin, urinary tract, bone and joint, endocarditis, and sepsis (but not enterococcus); some gram-negatives.
DOSAGE: ***Adults:*** 1 g IM/IV q6h (12 g/d max). ***Peds:*** 10–20 mg/kg IM/IV q6h (4 g/24 d max).
NOTES: First generation cephalosporin.

Cephradine (Velocef)

COMMON USES: Treatment of susceptible bacterial infections, including group A beta-hemolytic *Streptococcus*.
DOSAGE: ***Adults:*** 2–4 g/d in 4 divided doses (8 g/d max). ***Peds:*** > 9 mo: 25–100 mg/kg/d divided q6–12h (4 g/d max).
NOTES: First generation cephalosporin.

Cerivastatin (Baycol)

COMMON USES: Reduction of cholesterol, triglycerides, and apolipoprotein B.
DOSAGE: 0.4 mg once daily in the evening.
NOTES: May cause myopathy, monitor LFT regularly.

Cetirizine (Zyrtec)

COMMON USES: Allergic rhinitis and chronic urticaria.
DOSAGE: ***Adults:*** and ***Children > 6 y:*** 5–10 mg/d.

Charcoal, Activated (SuperChar, Actidose, Liqui-Char)

COMMON USES: Emergency treatment for poisoning by most drugs and chemicals.
DOSAGE: ***Adults:*** Acute intoxication: 30–100 g/dose. Gastrointestinal dialysis: 25–50 g q4–6h. ***Peds:*** Acute intoxication: 1–2 g/kg/dose. Gastrointestinal dialysis: 5–10 g/dose q4–8h.
NOTES: Administer with a cathartic; liquid dosage forms are in sorbitol base; powder mixed with water; protect airway in lethargic or comatose patient.

Chloral Hydrate (Noctec) [C]

COMMON USES: Nocturnal and preoperative sedation.
DOSAGE: ***Adults:*** Hypnotic: Between 500 mg and 1 g PO or PR 30 min before sleep or procedure. Sedative: 250 mg PO or PR tid. ***Peds:*** Hypnotic: 50 mg/kg/24h PO or PR 30 min before sleep or procedure. Sedative: 25 mg/kg/24h PO or PR tid.
NOTES: Mix syrup in a glass of water or fruit juice.

Chlorambucil (Leukeran)

COMMON USES: Treatment of ovarian cancer, leukemia, and lymphoma.
DOSAGE: Initially, 0.1–0.2 mg/kg/d PO for 3–6 wk; then maintenance therapy with no more than 0.1 mg/kg/d.

Chlordiazepoxide (Librium) [C]

COMMON USES: Anxiety, tension, alcohol withdrawal.
DOSAGE: ***Adults:*** Mild anxiety, tension: 5–10 mg PO tid–qid or prn. Severe anxiety, tension: 25–50 mg IM or IV tid–qid or prn. Alcohol withdrawal: 50–100 mg IM or IV; repeat in 2–4 h if needed, up to 300 mg in 24 h; gradually taper daily. ***Peds:*** 0.5 mg/kg/24h PO or IM divided q6–8h.
NOTES: Reduce dose in elderly patients; absorption of IM doses can be erratic.

Chlorothiazide (Diuril)

COMMON USES: Hypertension, edema, congestive heart failure.
DOSAGE: ***Adults:*** Between 500 mg and 1.0 g PO or IV qd–bid. ***Peds:*** 20–30 mg/kg/24h PO divided bid.
NOTES: Contraindicated in anuria.

Chlorpheniramine (Chlor-Trimeton, others)

COMMON USES: Seasonal rhinitis, allergic reactions.
DOSAGE: ***Adults:*** 4 mg PO or IV q4–6h or 8–12 mg PO bid of sustained release. ***Peds:*** 0.35 mg/kg/24h PO divided q4–6h or 0.2 mg/kg/24h sustained release.
NOTES: Anticholinergic side effects and sedation are common. Available in many OTC combinations (eg, acetaminophen, phenylephrine, pseudoephedrine).

Chlorpromazine (Thorazine)

COMMON USES: Psychotic disorders, apprehension, intractable hiccups, control of nausea and vomiting.
DOSAGE: ***Adults:*** Acute anxiety, agitation: 10–25 mg PO or PR bid–tid. Severe symptoms: 25 mg IM, can repeat in 1 h, then 25–50 mg PO or PR tid. Hiccups: 25–50 mg PO bid–tid. ***Peds:*** 2.5–6.0 mg/kg/24h PO, PR or IM divided q4–8h.
NOTES: Beware of extrapyramidal side effects, sedation, has alpha-adrenergic blocking properties.

Chlorpropamide (Diabinese)

COMMON USES: Management of non-insulin dependent diabetes mellitus.
DOSAGE: 100–500 mg qd.
NOTES: Use with caution in renal insufficiency.

Chlorthalidone (Hygroton)

COMMON USES: Hypertension, edema associated with congestive heart failure, steroid and estrogen therapy.
DOSAGE: ***Adults:*** 50–100 mg PO qd. ***Peds:*** 2 mg/kg/dose PO 3 times weekly or 1–2 mg/kg PO daily.
NOTES: Contraindicated in anuric patients.

Chlorzoxazone (Paraflex, Parafon Forte DSC)

COMMON USES: Adjunct to rest and physical therapy for the relief of discomfort associated with acute, painful musculoskeletal conditions.
DOSAGE: ***Adults:*** 250–500 mg PO tid–qid. ***Peds:*** 20 mg/kg/d or 600 mg/m^2/d divided in 3–4 doses.

Cholecalciferol [Vitamin D3] (Delta D)

COMMON USES: Dietary supplement for treatment of vitamin D deficiency.
DOSAGE: 400–1000 IU PO daily.
NOTES: 1-mg cholecalciferol = 40,000 IU of vitamin D activity.

Cholestyramine (Questran)

COMMON USES: Adjunctive therapy for the reduction of serum cholesterol in patients with primary hypercholesterolemia; relief of pruritus associated with partial biliary obstruction.

DOSAGE: Individualize dose to 4 g 1–6 times a day.
NOTES: Mix 4 g cholestyramine in 2–6 oz of noncarbonated beverages.

Ciclopirox (Loprox)

COMMON USES: Topical fungal infections (tinea curis, capitis, versicolor and candida).
DOSAGE: Apply and massage into area bid.

Cimetidine (Tagamet)

COMMON USES: Duodenal ulcer; ulcer prophylaxis in hypersecretory states, such as trauma, burns, surgery, Zollinger-Ellison syndrome; and gastroesophageal reflux disease (GERD).
DOSAGE: ***Adults:*** Active ulcer: 2400 mg/d IV continuous infusion or 300 mg IV q4–6h; 400 mg PO bid or 800 mg qhs. Maintenance therapy: 400 mg PO qhs. GERD: 800 mg PO bid; maintenance 800 mg PO hs. ***Peds:*** Neonates: 10–20 mg/kg/24h PO or IV divided q4–6h. Children: 20–40 mg/kg/24h PO or IV divided q4–6h.
NOTES: Extend dosing interval with renal insufficiency; decrease dose in elderly patients.

Ciprofloxacin (Cipro, Ciloxan Ophthalmic)

COMMON USES: Broad spectrum activity against a variety of gram-positive and gram-negative aerobic bacteria (urinary tract infection, prostatitis, sinusitis, skin, infectious diarrhea, osteomyelitis, ocular infections).
DOSAGE: ***Adults:*** 250–750 mg PO q12h or 200–400 mg IV q12h. Ophthalmic: 1–2 drops in eye(s) q2h while awake. ***Peds:*** Not recommended for use in children < 18 y, because of cartilage effects.
NOTES: Little activity against streptococci; drug interactions with theophylline, caffeine, sucralfate, and antacids. Nausea, vomiting, and abdominal discomfort are common side effects. Contraindicated in pregnancy.

Ciprofloxacin and Hydorcorisone (Cipro HC Otic)

COMMON USES: Otitis externa (swimmers ear).
DOSAGE: 3 drops in ear bid–tid for 1 wk.

Cisplatin (Platinol)

COMMON USES: Treatment of cervical, ovarian, testicular, and other solid tumors.
DOSAGE: 20–70 mg/m^2 IV. Dosage and duration of therapy is dependent on individual treatment protocols.
NOTES: Agent is nephrotoxic; hydrate patients with 1–2 L of fluid before infusion.

Citalopram (Celexa)

COMMON USES: Treatment of depression.
DOSAGE: Initially, 20 mg per day, may be increased to 40 mg per day.

Clarithromycin (Biaxin)

COMMON USES: Treatment of upper and lower respiratory tract infections, skin, *H pylori* infections, and infections caused by non-tuberculosis (atypical) *Mycobacterium*; prevention of Mac infections in HIV-infected individuals.
DOSAGE: ***Adults:*** 250–500 mg PO bid. *Mycobacterium*: 500–1000 mg PO bid. ***Peds:*** 7.5 mg/kg/dose PO bid.
NOTES: Increases theophylline and carbamazepine levels; avoid concurrent use with cisapride; causes metallic taste.

Clemastine (Tavist [OTC])

COMMON USES: Allergic rhinitis.
DOSAGE: 1.34–2.68 mg (1–2 tabs) tid, maximum 8.04 mg/d.

Clindamycin (Cleocin)

COMMON USES: Susceptible strains of streptococci, pneumococci, staphylococci, and gram-positive and gram-negative anaerobes, no activity against gram-negative aerobes. Topical agent for severe acne, and vaginal infections.
DOSAGE: ***Adults:*** 150–450 mg PO qid; 300–600 mg IV q6h or 900 mg IV q8h. Topical: apply bid. Vaginal: 1 full applicator instilled at bedtime for 1 wk. ***Peds:*** Neonates: 15–20 mg/kg/24h divided q6–8h. Children > 1 mo: 15–40 mg/kg/24h divided q6–8h,(4 g/d).
NOTES: Beware of diarrhea that may represent pseudomembranous colitis caused by *C difficile.*

Clonazepam (Klonopin) [C]

COMMON USES: Lennox-Gastaut syndrome, akinetic and myoclonic seizures, absence seizures.
DOSAGE: ***Adults:*** 1.5 mg/d PO in 3 divided doses; increase by 0.5–1.0 mg/d every 3 d prn up to 20 mg/d. ***Peds:*** 0.01–0.05 mg/kg/24h PO divided tid; increase to 0.1–0.2 mg/kg/24h divided tid.
NOTES: CNS side effects including sedation.

Clonidine (Catapres)

COMMON USES: Hypertension, opioid and tobacco withdrawal.
DOSAGE: ***Adults:*** 0.10 mg PO bid adjusted daily by 0.1–0.2 mg increments (maximum 2.4 mg/d). ***Peds:*** 5–25 mg/kg/24h divided q6h.
NOTES: Dry mouth, drowsiness, sedation occur frequently; more effective for hypertension when combined with diuretics, rebound hypertension can occur with abrupt cessation of doses above 0.2 mg bid.

Clonidine Transdermal (Catapres TTS)

COMMON USES: Hypertension.
DOSAGE: Apply one patch every 7 d to a hairless area on the upper arm or torso; titrate according to individual therapeutic requirements.
NOTES: TTS-1, TTS-2, TTS-3 (delivers 0.1, 0.2, 0.3 mg respectively of clonidine per day, for 1 wk). Doses above two TTS-3 are usually not associated with increased efficacy.

Clopidogrel (Plavix)

COMMON USES: Reduction of atherosclerotic events.
DOSAGE: 75 mg once daily.
NOTES: Prolongs bleeding time, use with caution in persons at risk of bleeding from trauma, etc.

Clorazepate (Tranxene) [C]

COMMON USES: Acute anxiety disorders, acute alcohol withdrawal symptoms, and adjunctive therapy in partial seizures.
DOSAGE: ***Adults:*** 15–60 mg/d PO in single or divided doses. Elderly and debilitated patients: Initiate therapy at 7.5–15 mg/d in divided doses. Alcohol withdrawal: Day 1: Initially, 30 mg; followed by 30–60 mg in divided doses. Day 2: 45–90 mg in divided doses. Day 3: 22.5–45 mg in divided doses. Day 4: 15–30 mg in divided doses. ***Peds:*** 3.75–7.5 mg/dose bid, to a maximum of 60 mg/d divided bid-tid.
NOTES: Monitor patients with renal and hepatic impairment, since drug may accumulate; CNS depressant effects.

Clotrimazole (Lotrimin, Mycelex)

COMMON USES: Treatment of candidiasis and tinea infections.
DOSAGE: Orally: One troche dissolved slowly in mouth 5 times a day for 14 d. Vaginal: Cream: One applicator qhs for 7–14 d; Tablets: 100 mg vaginally qhs for 7 d or 200 mg (2 tablets) vaginally qhs for 3 d or 500-mg tablet vaginally hs for 3 d. Topical: Apply 3–4 times daily for 10–14 d.
NOTES: Oral prophylaxis commonly used in immunosuppressed patients.

Cloxacillin (Cloxapen)

COMMON USES: Treatment of respiratory, skin, bone, joint infections caused by susceptible strains of penicillinase- producing *Staphylococcus.*
DOSAGE: ***Adults:*** 250–500 mg PO qid. ***Peds:*** 50–100 mg/kg/d divided qid.
NOTES: Take on an empty stomach.

Clozapine (Clozaril)

COMMON USES: Severe schizophrenia that does not respond to standard therapy.
DOSAGE: Initially 25 mg qd–bid, increase dose to 300–450 mg/d over 2 wk. Maintain patient at lowest dose possible.
NOTES: Has limited distribution. Contact local pharmacy for drug availability. Monitor blood counts frequently because of the risk of agranulocytosis. May cause drowsiness and seizures.

Cocaine [C]

COMMON USES: Topical anesthetic for mucous membranes.
DOSAGE: Apply topically lowest amount of topical solution that provides relief; 1 mg/kg max.

Codeine [C]

COMMON USES: Mild to moderate pain; symptomatic relief of cough.
DOSAGE: ***Adults:*** Analgesic: 15–60 mg PO, SC/IM qid prn. Antitussive: 5–15 mg PO or SC q4h prn. ***Peds:*** Analgesic: 0.5–1.0 mg/kg/dose PO or SC q4–6h prn. Antitussive: 1.0–1.5 mg/kg/24h divided q4h, max 30 mg/24h.
NOTES: Most often used in combination with acetaminophen for pain or with agents such as terpin hydrate as an antitussive; 120 mg IM equivalent to 10 mg morphine IM.

Colesevelam (Welchol)

COMMON USES: Reduction of LDL cholesterol.
DOSAGE: 3 tablets PO twice daily with meals.

Colchicine

COMMON USES: Acute gout.
DOSAGE: Initially, 0.5–1.2 mg PO or IV, then 0.5–1.2 mg every 1–2 h until gastrointestinal side effects develop (maximum of 8 mg/d).
NOTES: Caution in elderly patients and patients with renal impairment. Colchicine 1–2 mg IV within 24–48 h of an acute attack can be diagnostic and therapeutic in a monoarticular arthritis.

Colestipol (Colestid)

COMMON USES: Adjunctive therapy for the reduction of serum cholesterol in patients with primary hypercholesterolemia.
DOSAGE: 15–30 g/d divided into 2–4 doses.
NOTES: Do not use dry powder; mix with beverages, soups, cereals, etc.

Cortisone

See Table IX–4, page 475 and "Steroids," page 529.

Cromolyn Sodium (Intal, Nasalcrom, Opticrom)

COMMON USES: Adjunct to the prophylaxis of asthma; prevention of exercise-induced asthma; allergic rhinitis; ophthalmic allergic manifestations.
DOSAGE: ***Adults*** and ***Peds:*** > 12 years: Inhalation: 20 mg (as powder in capsule) inhaled qid or metered-dose inhaler 2 puffs qid. Oral: 200 mg 4 times a day 15–20 min before meals, up to 400 mg 4 times a day. Nasal instillation: Spray once in each nostril 2–6 times daily. Ophthalmic: 1–2 drops in each eye 4–6 times daily. ***Peds:*** Inhalation: 2 puffs qid of metered-dose inhaler. Oral: Infants < 2 y: 20 mg/kg/d in 4 divided doses. 2–12 y: 100 mg 4 times per day before meals.

TABLE IX–4. COMPARISON OF SYSTEMIC GLUCOCORTICOIDS (see page 529).

Drug	Relative Equivalent Dose (mg)	Activity	Mineralocorticoid Duration	Route
Betamethasone	0–0.75	0	36–72 h	PO, IM
Cortisone (Cortone)	25.00	2	8–12 h	PO, IM
Dexamethasone (Decadron)	0.75	0	36–72 h	PO, IV
Hydrocortisone (Solu-Cortef, Hydrocortone)	20.00	2	8–12 h	PO, IM, IV
Methylprednisolone acetate (Depo-Medrol)	4.00	0	36–72 h	PO, IM, IV
Methylprednisolone Succinate (Solu-Medrol)	4.00			PO, IM, IV
Prednisone (Deltasone)	5.00	1	12–36 h	PO
Prednisolone (Delt-Cortef)	5.00	1	12–36 h	PO, IM, IV

NOTES: Has no benefit in acute situations; may require 2-4 wk for maximal effect in perennial allergic disorders.

Cyanocobalamin/Vitamin B12

COMMON USES: Pernicious anemia and other vitamin B12 deficiency states.
DOSAGE: ***Adults:*** 100 mg, IM or SC qd for 5–10 d, then 100 mg IM twice a week for 1 mo, then 100 mg IM monthly. ***Peds:*** 100 mg qd IM or SC for 5–10 d, then 30–50 mg IM every 4 wk.
NOTES: Oral absorption highly erratic, altered by many drugs and not recommended; for use with hyperalimentation, see Section V, page 385.

Cyclobenzaprine (Flexeril)

COMMON USES: Adjunct to rest and physical therapy for the relief of muscle spasm associated with acute painful musculoskeletal conditions.
DOSAGE: 10 mg PO tid.
NOTES: Do not use for longer than 2–3 wk; has sedative and anticholinergic properties.

Cyclopentolate (Cyclogyl)

COMMON USES: Mydriasis and cycloplegia; useful before ocular exam; treatment of iritis.
DOSAGE: One drop 1% in eye(s), followed by a second application 5 min later; use 30–45 min before exam; iritis, apply tid.

Cyclophosphamide (Cytoxan, Neosar)

COMMON USES: Hodgkin's and non-Hodgkin's lymphomas, multiple myeloma, breast cancer, ovarian cancer, mycosis fungoides, neuroblastoma, retinoblastoma, acute leukemias, small- cell lung cancer, and allogeneic and autologous transplantation in high doses; severe rheumatologic disorders.

DOSAGE: 500–1500 mg/m^2 as a single dose at 2- to 4-week intervals; 1.8 g/m^2 to 160 mg/kg (or approximately 12 g/m^2 in a 75-kg individual) in the bone marrow transplantation setting.
NOTES: Toxicity includes myelosuppression (leukopenia and thrombocytopenia), sterile hemorrhagic cystitis, SIADH, alopecia, and anorexia; nausea and vomiting are common. Hepatotoxicity and rarely interstitial pneumonitis may occur. Irreversible testicular atrophy may occur. Cardiotoxicity is rare. Second malignancies (bladder cancer and acute leukemias) have been reported; cumulative risk of 3.5% at 8 y, 10.7% at 12 y. Preventive measures to avoid hemorrhagic cystitis: continuous bladder irrigation and MESNA uroprotection.

Cyclosporine (Sandimmune, Neoral)

COMMON USES: Prophylaxis of organ rejection in kidney, liver, heart, and bone marrow transplants in conjunction with adrenal corticosteroids; other auto-immune diseases.
DOSAGE: ***Adults*** and ***Peds:*** Oral: 15 mg/kg/d beginning 12 h prior to transplant; after 2 wk, taper the dose by 5 mg/wk to 5–10 mg/kg/d. IV: 5–6 mg/kg/d divided q12–24h. If the patient is unable to take the drug orally, give 1/2 of the oral dose IV, switch to PO as soon as possible.
NOTES: May elevate blood urea nitrogen and creatinine, which may be confused with renal transplant rejection; should be administered in glass containers; has many drug interactions; Neoral and Sandimmune are not interchangeable. See Table IX–3, page 457 for drug levels.

Cyproheptadine (Periactin)

COMMON USES: Allergic reactions; especially good for itching.
DOSAGE: ***Adults:*** 4 mg PO tid, maximum of 0.5 mg/kg/d. ***Peds:*** 2–6 y, 0.25/kg/24h divided tid–qid (maximum 12 mg/24h); 7–14 y, 0.25 mg/kg/24h divided tid–qid (maximum of 16 mg/24h).
NOTES: Anticholinergic side effects and drowsiness common; may stimulate appetite in some patients.

Cytomegalovirus Immune Globulin [CMV-IVIG] (Cytogam)

COMMON USES: Attenuation of primary CMV disease associated with transplantation.
DOSAGE: Administered for 16 wk posttransplant, see product information for dosing schedule.

Dacarbazine (DTIC-Dome)

COMMON USES: Treatment of soft tissue and uterine sarcoma, melanoma, and Hodgkin's disease.
DOSAGE: Dependent on individual protocol.
NOTES: May cause myelosuppression.

Daclizumab (Zenapax)

COMMON USES: Prevention of acute organ rejection.
DOSAGE: ***Adults*** and ***Peds:*** 1 mg/kg IV per dose; first dose prior to transplant followed by 4 doses 14 d apart posttransplant.

Dactinomycin (Cosmegen)

COMMON USES: Treatment of Wilm's tumor, rhabdomyosarcoma, choriocarcinoma, testicular carcinoma, Ewing's sarcoma, and sarcoma botryoides.
DOSAGE: ***Adults:*** 0.5 mg/d IV for 5 d. ***Peds:*** 0.015 mg/kg/d IV for 5 d.
NOTES: Severe soft tissue damage may occur with extravasation.

Dalteparin (Fragmin)

COMMON USES: Unstable angina, non-Q-wave MI, prevention of ischemic complications because of clot formation in patients on concurrent aspirin, prevention of DVT after surgery.

DOSAGE: Angina/MI: 120 IU/kg (maximum 10,000 IU) SC q12h with aspirin. DVT prophylaxis: 2500–5000 IU SC 1 to 2 h before surgery, then once daily for 5–10 d. Systemic anticoagulation: 200 IU/kg SC once daily or 100 IU/kg SC twice daily.
NOTES: Predictable antithrombotic effects eliminates need for laboratory monitoring.

Dantrolene Sodium (Dantrium)

COMMON USES: Treatment of clinical spasticity resulting from upper motor neuron disorders such as spinal cord injuries, strokes, cerebral palsy, or multiple sclerosis; treatment of malignant hyperthermic crisis.
DOSAGE: ***Adults:*** Spasticity: Initially, 25 mg PO qd, titrate to effect by 25 mg up to max dose of 100 mg PO qid prn. ***Peds:*** Initially, 0.5 mg/kg/dose bid, titrate by 0.5 mg/kg to effectiveness up to max dose of 3 mg/kg/dose qid prn. ***Adults*** and ***Peds:*** Malignant hyperthermia treatment: Continuous rapid IV push beginning at 1 mg/kg until symptoms subside or 10 mg/kg is reached. Postcrisis follow-up: 4–8 mg/kg/d in 3–4 divided doses for 1–3 d to prevent recurrence.
NOTES: Monitor ALT and AST closely.

Daunorubicin (Cerubidine)

COMMON USES: Leukemia.
DOSAGE: Varies with individual protocol.
NOTES: Severe tissue necrosis if extravasation occurs.

Delavirdine (Rescriptor)

COMMON USES: HIV-1 infection in combination therapy.
DOSAGE: ***Adults:*** 400 mg PO tid.

Demeclocycline (Declomycin)

COMMON USES: Treatment of SIADH
DOSAGE: SIADH: 300–600 mg PO q12h; antimicrobial: 150–300 mg PO q12h.
NOTES: Reduce dose in renal failure. May cause diabetes insipidus.

Desipramine (Norpramin)

COMMON USES: Endogenous depression.
DOSAGE: 25–200 mg/d in single or divided doses; usually as a single bedtime dose.
NOTES: Many anticholinergic side effects, including blurred vision, urinary retention, and dry mouth.

Desmopressin (DDAVP, Stimate)

COMMON USES: Diabetes insipidus; bleeding due to hemophilia A and type I von Willebrand's disease (parenteral); nocturnal enuresis.
DOSAGE: Diabetes Insipidus:***Adults:*** intranasal, 0.1–0.4 mL (10–40 μg) daily in 2–3 divided doses. 0.5–1 mL (2–4 μg) IV/SC daily in 2 divided doses. If converting from intranasal to parenteral dosing, use 1/10 of intranasal dose. ***Peds:*** Between 3 mo and 12 y: intranasal 0.05–0.3 mL daily in single or 2 doses. Hemophilia A and von Willebrand's disease (type I): ***Adults*** and ***Peds:*** > 10 kg: 0.3 mg/kg diluted to 50 mL with NSS infuse over 15–30 min. ***Peds:*** < 10 kg: Same as above with dilution to 10 mL with normal saline. Nocturnal enuresis:***Peds:*** > 6 y: 20 μg (0.2 mL) qhs, adjust as needed 10–40 μg.
NOTES: In very young and old patients, adjust fluid intake to avoid water intoxication and hyponatremia.

Dexamethasone, Neomycin, Polymyxin-B (Maxitrol)

See page 511.

Dexamethasone, Systemic (Decadron, Dexasone, others)

See "Steroids," page 529 and Table IX–4, page 475.

Dexpanthenol (Iopan-Choline,Ilopan)

COMMON USES: Minimize paralytic ileus, treat postoperative distention.
DOSAGE: ***Adults:*** Relief of gas: 2–3 tablets PO tid. Prevention of postoperative ileus: 250–500 mg IM stat, repeat in 2 h, then q6h as needed. Ileus: IM: 500 mg stat, repeat in 2 h, followed by doses every 6 h, if needed.
NOTES: Do not use if obstruction is suspected.

Dextran 40 (Macrodex, Rheomacrodex)

COMMON USES: Plasma expander for adjunctive therapy in shock; prophylaxis of DVT and thromboembolism; adjunct in peripheral vascular surgery.
DOSAGE: Shock: 10 mL/kg infused rapidly with maximum dose of 20 mL/kg in the first 24 h; total daily dose beyond 24 h should not exceed 10 mL/kg and should be discontinued after 5 d. Prophylaxis of DVT and Thromboembolism: 10 mL/kg IV on day of surgery followed by 500 mL IV daily for 2–3 d; then 500 mL IV every 2–3 d based on patient's risk factors for up to 2 wk.
NOTES: Observe for hypersensitivity reactions; monitor renal function and electrolytes.

Dextromethorphan (Vicks Formula 44, many others)

COMMON USES: To control nonproductive cough.
DOSAGE: ***Adults:*** 10–20 mg PO q4h prn. ***Peds:*** 1–2 mg/kg/24h divided tid–qid.
NOTES: May be found in many OTC combination products with guaifenesin, acetaminophen and pseudoephedrine.

Dezocine (Dalgan)

COMMON USES: Management of pain.
DOSAGE: 5–20 mg IM or 2.5–10 mg IV q2–4h prn.
NOTES: Narcotic agonist/antagonist; may cause withdrawal in patients dependent on narcotics.

Diazepam (Valium) [C]

COMMON USES: Anxiety, alcohol withdrawal, muscle spasm, status epilepticus, and preoperative sedation.
DOSAGE: ***Adults:*** Status epilepticus: 0.2–0.5 mg/kg/dose IV q15–30 min to 30 mg max. Anxiety, muscle spasm: 2–10 mg PO or IM q3–4h prn. Preoperative: 5–10 mg PO or IM 20–30 min before procedure; can be given IV just before procedure. Alcohol withdrawal: Initially, 2–5 mg IV, may require up to 1000–2000 mg in 24-h period for severe withdrawal symptoms. ***Peds:*** Status epilepticus: < 5 y: 0.2–0.5 mg/kg/dose IV q15–30min up to maximum of 5 mg; > 5 y: may administer up to maximum of 10 mg. Sedation, muscle relaxation: 0.04–0.2 mg/kg/dose q2–4h IM or IV up to maximum of 0.6 mg/kg in 8 h, or 0.12–0.8 mg/kg/24h PO divided tid–qid.
NOTES: Do not exceed 5 mg/min IV in adults as respiratory arrest can occur; absorption of IM dose may be erratic.

Diazoxide (Hyperstat, Proglycem)

COMMON USES: Hypertensive emergencies; management of hypoglycemia owing to hyperinsulinism.
DOSAGE: ***Adults*** and ***Peds:*** Hypertensive crisis: 1–3 mg/kg/dose IV up to maximum of 150 mg IV; may repeat at 15-min intervals until desired effect is achieved. Hypoglycemia: 3–8 mg/kg/24h PO divided q8–12h. Neonates: Hypoglycemia: 10 mg/kg/24h divided in 3 equal doses; maintenance: 3–8 mg/kg/24h PO in 2 or 3 equal doses.
NOTES: Sodium retention and hyperglycemia frequently occur; possible thiazide diuretic cross-hypersensitivity; cannot be titrated.

Dibucaine (Nupercainal, [OTC])

COMMON USES: Hemorrhoids and minor skin conditions.
DOSAGE: Insert into rectum with applicator bid and after each bowel movement.

Diclofenac (Cataflam, Voltaren)

COMMON USES: Treatment of arthritis (rheumatoid, osteoarthritis) and pain; ophthalmic as an adjunct to cataract surgery.
DOSAGE: 50–75 mg PO bid; ophthalmic 1 drop in eye. qid 24 h postop for up to 2 wk.

Dicloxacillin (Dynapen, Dycill)

COMMON USES: Treatment of infections caused by susceptible strains of *S aureus* and *Streptococcus.*
DOSAGE: ***Adults:*** 250–500 mg qid. ***Peds:*** 12.5–25 mg/kg/d divided qid.
NOTES: Take on an empty stomach.

Dicyclomine (Bentyl)

COMMON USES: Treatment of functional irritable bowel syndromes.
DOSAGE: ***Adults:*** 20 mg PO qid titrated to a maximum dose of 160 mg/d or 20 mg IM q6h. ***Peds:*** > 6 mo: 5 mg/dose tid–qid; children: 10 mg per dose tid–qid.
NOTES: Anticholinergic side effects may limit dose.

Didanosine [ddI] (Videx)

COMMON USES: Treatment of HIV infection in patients who are zidovudine intolerant.
DOSAGE: ***Adults:*** >60 kg: 400 mg PO qd or 200 mg PO bid. <60 kg: 250 mg PO qd or 125 mg PO bid. ***Peds:*** Dose by BSA (See package insert).
NOTES: Reconstitute powder with water; side effects include pancreatitis, peripheral neuropathy, diarrhea, and headache; adults should take 2 tablets for each administration.

Diflunisal (Dolobid)

DOSAGE: Pain: 500 mg PO bid. Osteoarthritis: 500–1500 mg PO in 2–3 divided doses. Supplied tablets 250, 500 mg.
NOTES: May prolong prothrombin time.

Digoxin (Lanoxin, Lanoxicaps)

COMMON USES: CHF, atrial fibrillation and flutter, and paroxysmal atrial tachycardia.
DOSAGE: ***Adults:*** PO digitalization: 0.50–0.75 mg PO, then 0.25 mg PO q6–8h to a total dose between 1.0 and 1.5 mg. IV/IM digitalization: 0.25–0.50 mg IM/IV, then 0.25 mg q4–6h, total dose of about 1 mg. Maintenance: 0.125–0.500 mg PO/IM/IV qd (average daily dose 0.125–0.250 mg). ***Peds:*** Preterm infants: Digitalization: 30 mg/kg PO or 25 mg/kg IV; give 1/2 of dose initially, then 1/4 of dose at 8- to 12-h intervals for 2 doses. Maintenance: 10 mg/kg/24h PO or 6–8 mg/kg/24h IV divided q12h. Term infants to 2 y: Digitalization: 65–75 mg/kg PO or 50 mg/kg IV; give 1/2 of the dose initially, then 1/4 of the dose at 8- to 12-h intervals for 2 doses. Maintenance: 15–20 mg/kg/24h PO or 12–15 mg/kg/24h IV divided q12h. 2–10 y: Digitalization: 30–40 mg/kg PO or 25 mg/kg IV; give 1/2 dose initially, then 1/4 of the dose at 8- to 12-h intervals for 2 doses. Maintenance: 8–10 mg/kg/24h PO or 6–8 mg/kg/24h IV divided q12h. >10 y: Same as for adults.
NOTES: Can cause heart block; low potassium can potentiate toxicity; reduce dose in renal failure; symptoms of toxicity include nausea and vomiting, headache, fatigue, visual disturbances (yellow-green halos around lights), and

cardiac arrhythmias (see Table IX–3, page 457); IM injection can be painful and has erratic absorption.

Digoxin Immune FAB (Digibind)

COMMON USES: Treatment of life-threatening digoxin intoxication.
DOSAGE: ***Adults*** and ***Peds:*** Based on serum level and patient's weight. See dosing charts provided with the drug. Empiric where overdose is not known 20 vials (760 mg) IV in adults.
NOTES: Each vial will bind approximately 0.6 mg of digoxin; in renal failure may require redosing in several days because of breakdown of the immune complex.

Diltiazem (Cardizem, Dilacor)

COMMON USES: Treatment of angina pectoris, prevention of reinfarction, hypertension; atrial fibrillation or flutter, and paroxysmal SVT.
DOSAGE: Oral: 30 mg PO qid initially; titrate to 180–360 mg/d in divided doses as needed. Sustained release: 60–120 mg PO bid, titrate to effect, maximum dose 360 mg/d. Continuous dose: 180–300 mg PO qd. Intravenous: 0.25 mg/kg IV bolus over 2 min; may repeat dose in 15 min at 0.35 mg/kg. May begin continuous infusion of 5–15 mg/h.
NOTES: Contraindicated in sick-sinus syndrome, AV block, and hypotension. Cardizem CD and Dilacor XR are not interchangeable.

Dimenhydrinate (Dramamine)

COMMON USES: Prevention and treatment of nausea, vomiting, dizziness or vertigo of motion sickness.
DOSAGE: ***Adults:*** 50–100 mg PO q4–6h, maximum of 400 mg/d;
50 mg IM/IV prn. ***Peds:*** 5 mg/kg/24h PO or IV divided qid.
NOTES: Anticholinergic side effects.

Dimethyl Sulfoxide DMSO (Rimso 50)

COMMON USES: Interstitial cystitis.
DOSAGE: Intravesical, 50 mL, retain for 15 min; repeat q2 wk until relief.

Diphenhydramine (Benadryl, others)

COMMON USES: Allergic reactions, motion sickness, potentiate narcotics, sedation, cough suppression, treatment of extrapyramidal reactions.
DOSAGE: ***Adults:*** 25–50 mg PO, IV or IM bid–tid. ***Peds:*** 5 mg/kg/24h PO or IM divided q6h (maximum of 300 mg/d).
NOTES: Anticholinergic side effects including dry mouth, urinary retention; causes sedation; increase dosing interval in moderate to severe renal failure.

Diphenoxylate With Atropine (Lomotil) [C]

COMMON USES: Diarrhea.
DOSAGE: ***Adults:*** Initially 5 mg PO tid or qid until under control, then 2.5–5.0 mg PO bid. ***Peds:*** > 2 y: 0.3–0.4 mg/kg/24h divided bid–qid.
NOTES: Atropine-type side effects.

Dipivefrin (Propine)

COMMON USES: Open angle glaucoma.
DOSAGE: 1 drop into eye every 12 h.

Dirithromycin (Dynabac)

COMMON USES: Treatment of bronchitis, community-acquired pneumonia, and skin and skin structure infections.
DOSAGE: 500 mg PO qd for 7–14 d.
NOTES: Absorption is enhanced when taken with food.

Disopyramide (Norpace, Napamide)

COMMON USES: Suppression and prevention of premature ventricular contractions.

DOSAGE: ***Adults:*** 400–800 mg/d divided q6h for regular release products and q12h for sustained release products. ***Peds:*** < 1 y: 10–30 mg/kg/24h PO; 1–4 y: 10–20 mg/kg/24h PO; 4–12 y: 10–15 mg/kg/24h PO; 12–18 y: 6–15 mg/kg/24h PO.

NOTES: Has anticholinergic side effects (urinary retention); negative inotropic properties may induce CHF; decrease dose in impaired hepatic function.

Dobutamine (Dobutrex)

COMMON USES: Short-term use in patients with cardiac decompensation secondary to depressed contractility.

DOSAGE: ***Adults*** and ***Peds:*** Continuous IV infusion of 2.5–15 mg/kg/min; rarely 40 mg/kg/min may be required; titrate according to response.

NOTES: Monitor ECG for increase in heart rate, blood pressure, and increased ectopic activity; monitor pulmonary wedge pressure and cardiac output.

Docetaxel (Taxotere)

COMMON USES: Breast and other cancers.

DOSAGE: 60–100 mg/m^2 IV every 3 wk based on protocol.

Docusate Calcium (Surfak, others)

Docusate Potassium (Dialose)

Docusate Sodium (DOSS, Colace, others)

COMMON USES: Constipation-prone patient; adjunct to painful anorectal conditions (hemorrhoids).

DOSAGE: ***Adults:*** 50–500 mg PO qd. ***Peds:*** Infants to 3 y: 10–40 mg/24h divided qd–qid; 3–6 y: 20–60 mg/24h divided qd–qid; 6–12 y: 40–120 mg/24h divided qd–qid.

NOTES: No significant side effects, no laxative action.

Dolasetron (Anzemet)

COMMON USES: Prevention of nausea and vomiting associated with chemotherapy.

DOSAGE: ***Adults*** and ***Peds:*** 1.8 mg/kg IV as a single dose. ***Adults:*** 100 mg PO as a single dose. ***Peds:*** 1.8 mg/kg PO up to 100 mg as a single dose.

NOTES: May cause prolongation of the QT interval.

Dopamine (Intropin, Dopastat)

COMMON USES: Short-term use in patients with cardiac decompensation secondary to decreased contractility; increases organ perfusion.

DOSAGE: ***Adults*** and ***Peds:*** 5 mg/kg/min by continuous infusion titrated by increments of 5 mg/kg/min to maximum of 50 mg/kg/min based on effect.

NOTES: Dose > 10 mg/kg/min may decrease renal perfusion; monitor urinary output; monitor ECG for increase in heart rate, blood pressure, and increased ectopic activity; monitor pcWP and CO if possible.

Dorzolamide (Trusopt)

COMMON USES: Glaucoma.

DOSAGE: 1 drop in eye(s) tid.

Dorzolamide and Timolol (Cosopt)

COMMON USES: Glaucoma.

DOSAGE: 1 drop in eye(s) bid.

Doxazosin (Cardura)

COMMON USES: Treatment of hypertension and benign prostatic hypertrophy.

DOSAGE: Hypertension: Initially 1 mg PO qd; may be increased to 16 mg PO qd. BPH: Initially 1 mg PO qd, may be increased to 8 mg PO qd.

NOTES: Doses > 4 mg increase the likelihood of excessive postural hypotension; use qhs dosing to limit.

Doxepin (Sinequan, Adapin)

COMMON USES: Depression or anxiety.
DOSAGE: 50–150 mg PO qd usually qhs but can be in divided doses.
NOTES: Anticholinergic, central nervous system, and cardiovascular side effects.

Doxorubicin (Adriamycin)

COMMON USES: Treatment of breast, endometrial, and ovarian cancer, and leukemia.
DOSAGE: 60–75 mg/m^2 IV as a single dose, at 21-d intervals.
NOTES: May cause myelosuppression and cardiotoxicity.

Doxycycline (Vibramycin)

COMMON USES: Broad spectrum antibiotic including activity against *Rickettsia, Chlamydia,* and *M pneumoniae.*
DOSAGE: ***Adults:*** 100 mg PO q12h first day, then 100 mg PO qd or bid or 100 mg IV q12h. ***Peds:*** > 8 y: 5 mg/kg/24h PO up to a maximum of 200 mg/d, divided qd or bid.
NOTES: Useful for chronic bronchitis; tetracycline of choice for patients with renal impairment.

Dronabinol (Marinol) [C]

COMMON USES: Nausea and vomiting associated with cancer chemotherapy; appetite stimulation.
DOSAGE: ***Adults*** and ***Peds:*** Antiemetic: 5–15 mg/m^2/dose q4–6h prn. ***Adults:*** Appetite: 2.5 mg PO before lunch and supper.
NOTES: Principal psychoactive substance present in marijuana; many CNS side effects.

Droperidol (Inapsine)

COMMON USES: Nausea and vomiting, premedication for anesthesia.
DOSAGE: ***Adults:*** Nausea: 1.25–2.5 mg IV prn; Premedication: 2.5–10 mg IV. ***Peds:*** 0.1–0.15 mg/kg/dose.
NOTES: May cause drowsiness, moderate hypotension and occasionally tachycardia.

Echothiophate Iodine (Phospholine Ophthalmic)

COMMON USES: Glaucoma.
DOSAGE: 1 drop eye(s) bid with one dose at bed time.

Econazole (Spectazole)

COMMON USES: Treatment of most tinea, cutaneous *Candida*, and tinea versicolor infections.
DOSAGE: Apply to affected areas bid (qd for tinea versicolor) for 2–4 wk.
NOTES: Relief of symptoms and clinical improvement may be seen early in treatment, but course of therapy should be carried out to avoid recurrence.

Edrophonium (Tensilon)

COMMON USES: Diagnosis of myasthenia gravis; acute myasthenic crisis; curare antagonist; paroxysmal atrial tachycardia.
DOSAGE: ***Adults:*** Test for myasthenia gravis: 2 mg IV in 1 min; if tolerated, give 8 mg IV; a positive test is a brief increase in strength. PAT: 10 mg IV to a maximum of 40 mg. ***Peds:*** Test for myasthenia gravis: total dose of 0.2 mg/kg. Give 0.04 mg/kg as a test dose. If no reaction occurs, give the remainder of the dose in 1-mg increments to a maximum of 10 mg.
NOTES: Can cause severe cholinergic effects; keep atropine available.

Efavirenz (Sustiva)

COMMON USES: HIV-1 infections in combination with at least two other agents.
DOSAGE: ***Adults:*** 600 mg qd at bedtime. ***Peds:*** see insert, based on body weight.

Enalapril (Vasotec)

COMMON USES: Hypertension, CHF.
DOSAGE: ***Adults:*** 2.5–5 mg/d PO titrated by effect to 10–40 mg/d as 1–2 divided doses, or 1.25 mg IV q6h. ***Peds:*** 0.05–0.08 mg/kg/dose PO q12–24h.
NOTES: Initial dose can produce symptomatic hypotension, especially with concomitant diuretics; discontinue diuretic for 2–3 d before initiation if possible; monitor closely for increases in serum potassium; may cause a nonproductive cough.

Enoxaparin (Lovenox)

COMMON USES: Prevention of DVT.
DOSAGE: 30 mg SC twice daily.
NOTES: Does not significantly affect bleeding time, platelet function, PT or APTT.

Entacapone (Comtan)

COMMON USES: Treatment of Parkinson disease.
DOSAGE: 200 mg administered concurrently with each levodopa/carbidopa dose to a maximum of 8 times per day.

Ephedrine

COMMON USES: Acute bronchospasm, nasal congestion, hypotension, narcolepsy, enuresis, myasthenia gravis.
DOSAGE: ***Adults:*** 25–50 mg IM/SC or 5–25 mg/dose slow IV every 10 min to maximum of 150 mg/d or 25–50 mg PO q3–4h prn. ***Peds:*** 0.2–0.3 mg/kg/dose IM or IV q4–6h prn.

Epinephrine (Adrenalin, Sus-Phrine, others)

COMMON USES: Cardiac arrest, anaphylactic reactions, acute asthma.
DOSAGE: ***Adults:*** Emergency cardiac care: 0.5–1.0 mg (5–10 mL of 1:10,000) IV every 5 min to response. Anaphylaxis: 0.3–0.5 mL of 1:1000 dilution SC; may repeat q10–15 min to maximum of 1 mg/dose and 5 mg/d. Asthma: 0.3–0.5 mL of 1:1000 dilution SC repeated at 20-min to 4-h intervals or 1 inhalation (metered dose) repeated in 1–2 min or suspension 0.1–0.3 mL SC for extended effect. ***Peds:*** Emergency cardiac care: 0.1 mL/kg of 1:10,000 dilution IV q3–5 min to response.
NOTES: Sus-Phrine offers sustained action; in acute cardiac settings can be given via endotracheal tube if a central line is not available.

Epoetin Alfa (Epogen, Procrit)

COMMON USES: Treatment of anemia associated with chronic renal failure, zidovudine treatment in HIV-infected patients, and patients receiving cancer chemotherapy; reduction in transfusions associated with surgery.
DOSAGE: ***Adults*** and ***Peds:*** 50–150 U/kg 3 times weekly; adjust the dose every 4–6 wk as needed. Surgery: 300 U/kg/d for 10 d before surgery.
NOTES: May cause hypertension, headache, tachycardia, nausea, and vomiting; store in refrigerator.

Epoprostenol (Flolan)

COMMON USES: Treatment of pulmonary hypertension.
DOSAGE: 4 ng/kg/min IV continuous infusion; make adjustments based on clinical status and package insert guidelines.
NOTES: Availability through a pharmacy benefit manager (PBM).

Eprosartan (Teveten)

COMMON USES: Treatment of hypertension.
DOSAGE: 400–800 mg daily as single dose or twice daily.
NOTES: Avoid use during pregnancy.

Eptifibatide (Integrilin)

COMMON USES: Treatment of acute coronary syndrome.
DOSAGE: 180 μg/kg IV bolus, followed by 2 μg/kg/min continuous infusion.

Erythromycin (E-Mycin, Ilosone, Erythrocin, ERYC, others)

COMMON USES: Infections caused by Group A streptococci (*S pyogenes*), alpha-hemolytic streptococci and *N gonorrhoeae* infections in penicillin-allergic patients, *S pneumoniae, M pneumoniae,* and *Legionella.*
DOSAGE: ***Adults:*** 250–500 mg PO qid or between 500 mg and 1 g IV qid. ***Peds:*** 30–50 mg/kg/24h PO or IV divided q6h, to a maximum of 2 g/d.
NOTES: Frequent mild gastrointestinal disturbances; estolate salt is associated with cholestatic jaundice; erythromycin base not well absorbed from the gastrointestinal tract; some forms such as ERYC are better tolerated with respect to gastrointestinal irritation; lactobionate salt contains benzyl alcohol, therefore use with caution in neonates; base formulation not absorbed and used as part of the "Nichols-Condon Bowel Prep."

Erythromycin, ophthalmic (Ilotycin)

COMMON USES: Conjunctival infections.
DOSAGE: 0.5% ointment, apply q6h.

Esmolol (Brevibloc)

COMMON USES: Supraventricular tachycardia, noncompensatory sinus tachycardia.
DOSAGE: Initial 500 mg/kg load over 1 min, then 50 mg/kg/min for 4 min; if inadequate response, repeat loading dose and follow with maintenance infusion of 100 mg/kg/min for 4 min; continue titration process by repeating loading dose followed by incremental increases in the maintenance dose of 50 mg/kg/min for 4 min until desired heart rate is reached or a decrease in blood pressure occurs; average dose is 100 mg/kg/min.
NOTES: Monitor closely for hypotension; decreasing or discontinuing infusion will reverse hypotension in approximately 30 min.

Estazolam (ProSom) [C]

COMMON USES: Insomnia.
DOSAGE: 1–2 mg PO qhs prn.

Esterified Estrogens (Estratab, Menest)

COMMON USES: Vasomotor symptoms, atrophic vaginitis, or kraurosis vulvae associated with menopause, female hypogonadism.
DOSAGE: Menopause: 0.3–1.25 mg daily; hypogonadism: 2.5 mg PO qd–tid.

Esterified Estrogens With Methyltestosterone (Estratest)

COMMON USES: Moderate to severe vasomotor symptoms associated with menopause, postpartum breast engorgement.
DOSAGE: 1 tablet qd for 3 wk, then 1 wk off.

Estradiol Topical (Estrace)

COMMON USES: Atrophic vaginitis and kraurosis vulvae associated with menopause.
DOSAGE: 2–4 g daily 1–2 wk, then 1 g 1–3 times a week.

Estradiol Transdermal (Estraderm)

COMMON USES: Severe vasomotor symptoms associated with menopause; female hypogonadism.

DOSAGE: 0.05 mg system twice weekly, adjust dose as necessary to control symptoms. Transdermal patches 0.05 mg, 0.1 mg (delivers 0.05 mg or 0.1 mg/24h).

Estramustine (Emcyt)

COMMON USES: Advanced prostate cancer.
DOSAGE: 1 capsule/22 lb body weight, divided tid-qid.

Estrogen, Conjugated (Premarin)

COMMON USES: Moderate to severe vasomotor symptoms associated with menopause; atrophic vaginitis; palliative therapy of advanced prostatic carcinoma; prevention of estrogen deficiency induced osteoporosis.
DOSAGE: 0.3–1.25 mg/d PO cyclically; prostatic carcinoma requires 1.25–2.5 mg PO tid.
NOTES: Do not use in pregnancy; associated with an increased risk of endometrial carcinoma, gallbladder disease, thromboembolism, and possibly breast cancer; generic products are not equivalent.

Estrogen, Conjugated With Methylprogesterone (Premarin With Methylprogesterone)

COMMON USES: Vasomotor symptoms associated with menopause.
DOSAGE: 1 tablet daily.

Estrogen, Conjugated With Methyltestosterone (Premarin With Methyltestosterone)

COMMON USES: Moderate-to-severe vasomotor symptoms associated with menopause, postpartum breast engorgement, atrophic vaginitis.
DOSAGE: 1 tablet every day for 3 wk, then 1 wk off.

Ethacrynic Acid (Edecrin)

COMMON USES: Edema, CHF, ascites, any time rapid diuresis is desired.
DOSAGE: ***Adults:*** 50–200 mg PO qd or 50 mg IV prn. ***Peds:*** 1 mg/kg/dose IV. Repeated doses are not recommended.
NOTES: Contraindicated in anuria; many severe side effects.

Ethambutol (Myambutol)

COMMON USES: Pulmonary tuberculosis and other mycobacterial infections.
DOSAGE: ***Adults*** and ***Peds:*** > 12 y: 15–25 mg/kg PO daily as single dose.
NOTES: May cause vision changes and gastrointestinal upset.

Ethinyl Estradiol (Estinyl, Feminone)

COMMON USES: Vasomotor symptoms associated with menopause, female hypogonadism.
DOSAGE: 0.02–1.5 mg/d divided qd–tid.

Ethosuximide (Zarontin)

COMMON USES: Absence seizures.
DOSAGE: ***Adults:*** 500 mg qd PO initially; increase by 250 mg/d every 4–7 d as needed. ***Peds:*** 20–40 mg/kg/24h PO qd to a maximum of 1500 mg/d.
NOTES: Blood dyscrasias, CNS and gastrointestinal side effects may occur; use caution in patients with renal or hepatic impairment. See drug levels page 457.

Etidronate (Didronel)

COMMON USES: Hypercalcemia of malignancy, hypertrophic ossification associated with spinal cord injury, Paget's disease, postmenopausal osteoporosis.
DOSAGE: Hypercalcemia: 7.5 mg/kg IV in NS over 2 h daily for 3 d, then 20 mg/kg/d PO for 1 mo. Ossification: 20 mg/kg/d for 2 wk, then 10 mg/kg/d for 10 wk.

Etodolac (Lodine)

COMMON USES: Treatment of arthritis and pain.
DOSAGE: 200–400 mg PO bid–qid.

Etoposide (VePesid [VP -16])

COMMON USES: Treatment of gestational trophoblastic disease, ovarian, testicular, and lung cancer.
DOSAGE: 35–100 mg/m^2/d IV. Number of doses and duration of therapy is dependent on individual protocols.
NOTES: May cause bone marrow suppression; has low stability in concentrated solutions.

Famciclovir (Famvir)

COMMON USES: Management of acute herpes zoster (shingles) and genital herpes infections.
DOSAGE: Zoster: 500 mg PO q8h. Simplex: 125–250 mg PO bid.

Famotidine (Pepcid)

COMMON USES: Short-term treatment of active duodenal ulcer and benign gastric ulcer; maintenance therapy for duodenal ulcer, hypersecretory conditions, GERD, and heartburn.
DOSAGE: ***Adults:*** Ulcer: 20–40 mg PO hs or 20 mg IV q12h. Hypersecretory: 20–160 mg PO q6h. GERD: 20 mg PO bid; maintenance 20 mg PO hs. Heartburn: 10 mg PO prn heartburn. ***Peds:*** 1–2 mg/kg/d.
NOTES: Decrease dose in severe renal insufficiency.

Felodipine (Plendil)

COMMON USES: Treatment of hypertension.
DOSAGE: 5–20 mg PO qd.
NOTES: Closely monitor blood pressure in elderly patients and patients with impaired hepatic function; doses of > 10 mg should not be used in these patients.

Fenofibrate (Tricor)

COMMON USES: Treatment of hypertriglyceridemia
DOSAGE: Initial dose 67 mg once daily. May be increased to 67 mg 3 times daily.
NOTES: Take with meals to increase bioavailability; May cause pancreatitis

Fenoldopam (Corlopam)

COMMON USES: Treatment of hypertensive emergency.
DOSAGE: Initial dose 0.03–0.1 μg/kg/min IV continuous infusion, titrate to effect every 15 minutes with 0.05–0.1 μg/kg/min increments, max 1.6 μg/kg/min.
NOTES: Avoid concurrent use with beta-blockers

Fenoprofen (Nalfon)

COMMON USES: Treatment of arthritis and pain.
DOSAGE: 200–600 mg q4–8h, to a maximum of 3200 mg/d.

Fentanyl (Sublimaze) [C]

COMMON USES: Short-acting analgesic used in conjunction with anesthesia.
DOSAGE: ***Adults*** and ***Peds:*** 0.025–0.15 mg/kg IV/IM titrated to effect.
NOTES: Causes significant sedation.

Fentanyl Transdermal System (Duragesic) [C]

COMMON USES: Management of chronic pain.
DOSAGE: Apply patch to upper torso every 72 h. Dose is calculated from the narcotic requirements for the previous 24 h. Transdermal patches deliver 25 mg/h, 50 mg/h, 75 mg/h, 100 mg/h.
NOTES: 0.1 mg of fentanyl is equivalent to 10 mg of morphine IM.

Fentanyl Transmucosal System (Actiq, Fentanyl Oralet) [C]

COMMON USES: Induction of anesthesia and breakthrough cancer pain.
DOSAGE: ***Adults*** and ***Peds:*** Anesthesia: 5–15 μg/kg. Pain: 200, 300 or 400 μg consumed over 15 min, titrate to appropriate effect.

Ferrous Sulfate

COMMON USES: Iron deficiency anemia; iron supplementation.
DOSAGE: ***Adults:*** 100–200 mg/d of elemental iron divided tid–qid. ***Peds:*** 1–2 mg/kg/24h divided qd–bid.
NOTES: May turn stools and urine dark; can cause gastrointestinal upset, constipation; vitamin C taken with ferrous sulfate increases the absorption of iron especially in patients with atrophic gastritis.

Fexofenadine (Allegra)

COMMON USES: Relief of allergic rhinitis.
DOSAGE: ***Adults*** and ***Peds > 12 y:*** 60 mg twice daily.

Filgrastim [G-CSF] (Neupogen)

COMMON USES: To decrease the incidence of infection in febrile neutropenic patients and treatment of chronic neutropenia.
DOSAGE: ***Adults*** and ***Peds:*** 5 μg/kg/d SC or IV as a single daily dose.
NOTES: May cause bone pain. Discontinue therapy when ANC > 10,000.

Finasteride (Proscar, Propecia)

COMMON USES: Treatment of benign prostatic hyperplasia and androgenetic alopecia.
DOSAGE: BPH (Proscar): 5 mg PO qd. Alopecia (Propecia): 1 mg PO qd.
NOTES: Will decrease prostate-specific antigen levels; may take 3–6 mo to see effect on urinary symptoms.

Flavoxate (Urispas)

COMMON USES: Symptomatic relief of dysuria, urgency, nocturia, suprapubic pain, urinary frequency, and incontinence.
DOSAGE: 100–200 mg PO tid–qid.
NOTES: May cause drowsiness, blurred vision, and dry mouth.

Flecainide (Tambocor)

COMMON USES: Life-threatening ventricular arrhythmias.
DOSAGE: 100 mg PO q12h; increase in increments of 50 mg q12h every 4 d to maximum of 400 mg/d.
NOTES: May cause new or worsened arrhythmias; therapy should be initiated in the hospital; may dose q8h if patient is intolerant or uncontrolled at q12h interval; drug interactions with propranolol, digoxin, verapamil, and disopyramide; may cause CHF.

Fluconazole (Diflucan)

COMMON USES: Oropharyngeal and esophageal candidiasis; cryptococcal meningitis; *Candida* infections of the lungs, peritoneum, and urinary tract; prevention of candidiasis in bone marrow transplant patients on chemotherapy or radiation; and candidal vaginitis.
DOSAGE: ***Adults:*** 100–400 mg PO or IV qd. Vaginitis: 150 mg PO as a single dose. ***Peds:*** 3–6 mg/kg PO or IV qd.
NOTES: Adjust dose in renal insufficiency; oral dosing produces the same blood levels as IV dosing, so the oral route should be used whenever possible.

Fludarabine Phosphate (Fludara)

COMMON USES: Treatment of leukemia.
DOSAGE: 25 mg/m^2 IV for 5 consecutive days. Give every 28 d.
NOTES: May cause severe bone marrow suppression and neurologic toxicity.

Fludrocortisone Acetate (Florinef)

COMMON USES: Partial treatment for adrenocortical insufficiency.
DOSAGE: ***Adults*** and ***Peds > 1 y:*** 0.05–0.1 mg PO qd. Infants: 0.1–0.2 mg PO qd.

NOTES: For adrenal insufficiency, must be used in conjunction with a glucocorticoid supplement; dosing changes based on plasma renin activity.

Flumazenil (Romazicon)

COMMON USES: For complete or partial reversal of the sedative effects of benzodiazepines.
DOSAGE: 0.2 mg IV over 15 s, dose may be repeated if the desired level of consciousness is not obtained to a maximum dose of 1 mg.

Flunisolide (AeroBid)

COMMON USES: Control of bronchial asthma in patients requiring chronic corticosteroid therapy.
DOSAGE: ***Adults:*** 2–4 inhalations bid. ***Peds:*** 2 inhalations bid.
NOTES: May cause oral candidiasis; not for acute asthma attack.

Fluorouracil (Adrucil)

COMMON USES: Management of carcinoma of the colon, rectum, breast, stomach, and pancreas.
DOSAGE: Varies with individual protocol.

Fluoxetine (Prozac, Sarafem)

COMMON USES: Treatment of depression, obsessive-compulsive disorders, and bulimia, premenstrual dysphoric disorder (PMDD).
DOSAGE: Initially, 20 mg PO qd; titrate to a maximum of 80 mg/24h; doses of > 20 mg/d should be divided. Bulimia: 60 mg once daily in the morning.
NOTES: May cause nausea, nervousness, and weight loss.

Fluphenazine (Prolixin, Permitil)

COMMON USES: Psychotic disorders.
DOSAGE: 0.5–10 mg/d in divided doses PO q6–8h; average maintenance 5.0 mg/d or 1.25 mg IM initially then 2.5–10 mg/d in divided doses q6–8h prn.
NOTES: Reduce dose in elderly patients; monitor liver functions; may cause drowsiness; do not administer concentrate with caffeine, tannic acid, or pectin-containing products.

Flurazepam (Dalmane) [C]

COMMON USES: Insomnia.
DOSAGE: ***Adults*** and ***Peds > 15 y:*** 15–30 mg PO qhs prn.
NOTES: Reduce dose in elderly patients.

Flurbiprofen (Ansaid)

COMMON USES: Treatment of arthritis.
DOSAGE: 50–100 mg bid–qid, to a maximum of 300 mg/d.

Flutamide (Eulexin)

COMMON USES: Prostate cancer in combination with LHRH analogue.
DOSAGE: 3 (125 mg) capsules PO q8h.
NOTES: Monitor LFT's

Fluticasone nasal (Flonase)

COMMON USES: Seasonal allergic rhinitis.
DOSAGE: 2 sprays per nostril qd; may reduce to 1 spray/d; max 4 sprays/d.

Fluticasone oral (Flovent, Flovent Rotadisk)

COMMON USES: Chronic treatment of asthma.
DOSAGE: ***Adults and adolescents:*** 2–4 puffs bid. ***Peds*** 4–11 y: 50 μg twice daily.
NOTES: Counsel patients carefully on use of device multidose inhaler 44, 110, or 220 μg/activation; Rotadisk dry powder 50, 100, and 250 μg/activation; risk of thrush

Fluvastatin (Lescol)

COMMON USES: Adjunct to diet in the treatment of elevated total cholesterol.
DOSAGE: 20–40 mg PO qhs.

Folic Acid

COMMON USES: Macrocytic anemia.
DOSAGE: ***Adults:*** Supplement: 0.4 mg PO qd; pregnancy: 0.8 mg PO qd; folate deficiency: 1.0 mg PO qd–tid. ***Peds:*** Supplement: 0.04–0.4 mg/24h PO, IM, IV, or SC; folate deficiency: 0.5–1.0 mg/24h PO, IM, IV or SC

Fomvirsen (Vitravene)

COMMON USES: CMV retinitis in AIDS patients who do not respond to other therapies.
DOSAGE: 6.6 mg intraocular injection every other week for 2 wk followed by one injection once every 4 wk.

Foscarnet (Foscavir)

COMMON USES: Treatment of cytomegalovirus; acyclovir-resistant herpes infections.
DOSAGE: Induction: 60 mg/kg IV q8h for 14–21 d. Maintenance: 90–120 mg/kg IV qd (Monday-Friday).
NOTES: Dose must be adjusted for renal function; nephrotoxic; monitor ionized calcium closely (causes electrolyte abnormalities); administer through a central venous catheter.

Fosfomycin (Monurol)

COMMON USES: Uncomplicated urinary tract infection in women.
DOSAGE: 3 g in water (one dose).

Fosinopril (Monopril)

COMMON USES: Hypertension.
DOSAGE: Initially, 10 mg PO qd; may be increased to a maximum of 80 mg/d PO divided qd–bid.
NOTES: Decrease dose in elderly patients, unnecessary to adjust dose for renal insufficiency, may cause a nonproductive cough and dizziness.

Fosphenytoin (Cerebyx)

COMMON USES: Treatment of status epilepticus.
DOSAGE: Loading 15 to 20 mg PE/kg, maintenance 4–6 mg PE/kg/d.
NOTES: Dosed as Phenytoin Equivalents (PE); administer at < 150 mg PE/min to prevent hypotension.

Furosemide (Lasix)

COMMON USES: Edema, hypertension, congestive heart failure.
DOSAGE: ***Adults:*** 20–80 mg PO or IV qd or bid. ***Peds:*** 1 mg/kg/dose IV q6–12h; 2 mg/kg/dose PO q12h–24h.
NOTES: Monitor for hypokalemia; use with caution in hepatic disease; high doses of the IV form may cause ototoxicity.

Gabapentin (Neurontin)

COMMON USES: Adjunctive therapy in the treatment of partial seizures, chronic pain.
DOSAGE: 900–1800 mg/d PO in 3 divided doses.
NOTES: It is not necessary to monitor serum gabapentin levels.

Gallium Nitrate (Ganite)

COMMON USES: Treatment of hypercalcemia of malignancy.
DOSAGE: 100–200 mg/m^2/d for 5 d.

NOTES: Can cause renal insufficiency; 1% acute optic neuritis.

Ganciclovir (Cytovene, Vitrasert)

COMMON USES: Treatment and prevention of cytomegalovirus (CMV) retinitis and prevention of CMV disease in transplant recipients.
DOSAGE: ***Adults*** and ***Peds:*** IV: 5 mg/kg IV q12h for 14–21 d, then maintenance of 5 mg/kg IV qd for 7 d/wk or 6 mg/kg IV qd for 5 d/wk. ***Adults:*** PO: Following induction, 1000 mg PO tid. Prevention: 1000 mg PO tid.
NOTES: Not a cure for CMV; granulocytopenia and thrombocytopenia are the major toxicities; injection should be handled with appropriate precautions; take capsules with food.

Gatifloxacin (Tequin)

COMMON USES: Treatment of acute exacerbation of chronic bronchitis, sinusitis, community acquired pneumonia, urinary tract infections.
DOSAGE: 400 mg PO or IV once daily
NOTES: Avoid use with antacids; do NOT use in children < 18 y, pregnant or lactating women; reliable activity against *S pneumoniae.*

Gemfibrozil (Lopid)

COMMON USES: Hypertriglyceridemia (types IV and V hyperlipoproteinemia).
DOSAGE: 1200 mg/d PO in 2 divided doses 30 min before the morning and evening meals.
NOTES: Monitor liver function test and serum lipids during therapy; cholelithiasis may occur secondary to treatment; may enhance the effect of warfarin.

Gentamicin (Garamycin)

COMMON USES: Serious infections caused by susceptible *Pseudomonas, Proteus, E coli, Klebsiella, Enterobacter, Serratia,* and for initial treatment of gram-negative sepsis.
DOSAGE: ***Adults:*** 3–5 mg/kg/24h IV divided q8–24h. ***Peds:*** Infants > 7 d: 2.5 mg/kg/dose IV q12–24h; children: 2.5 mg/kg/d IV q8h. See Table IX–1, page 455.
NOTES: Nephrotoxic and ototoxic; decrease dose with renal insufficiency; monitor creatinine clearance and serum concentration for dosing adjustments; see Table IX–3, page 457.

Gentamicin, Ophthalmic (Garamycin Ophthalmic)

COMMON USES: Conjunctival infections.
DOSAGE: 0.3% ointment apply bid or tid.

Glimepiride (Amaryl)

COMMON USES: Non-insulin-dependent diabetes mellitus
DOSAGE: 1–4 mg once daily.

Glipizide (Glucotrol)

COMMON USES: Non-insulin-dependent diabetes mellitus.
DOSAGE: 5–15 mg qd–bid.

Glucagon

COMMON USES: Treatment of severe hypoglycemia in diabetic patients with sufficient liver glycogen stores.
DOSAGE: ***Adults:*** 0.5–1.0 mg SC, IM, or IV repeated after 20 min as needed. ***Peds:*** Neonates: 0.3 mg/kg/dose SC, IM, or IV q4h prn; children-0.03–0.1 mg/kg/dose SC, IM or IV repeated after 20 min prn.
NOTES: Administration of glucose IV is necessary; ineffective in states of starvation, adrenal insufficiency, or chronic hypoglycemia.

Glyburide (Diabeta, Micronase)

COMMON USES: Management of non-insulin-dependent diabetes mellitus.
DOSAGE: Nonmicronized: 1.25–10 mg qd–bid. Micronized: 1.5–6 mg qd–bid.

Glycerin Suppository

COMMON USES: Constipation.
DOSAGE: ***Adults:*** 1 adult suppository PR, prn. ***Peds:*** 1 infant suppository PR, qd–bid prn.

Gonadorelin (Lutrepulse)

COMMON USES: Primary hypothalamic amenorrhea.
DOSAGE: 5 μg IV q90min for 21 d using a Lutrepulse reservoir and pump.
NOTES: Risk of multiple pregnancies.

Goserelin (Zoladex)

COMMON USES: Treatment of advanced prostate cancer and endometriosis.
DOSAGE: 3.6 mg SC every 28 d into the abdominal wall.

Granisetron (Kytril)

COMMON USES: Prevention of nausea and vomiting associated with emetogenic cancer therapy.
DOSAGE: ***Adults*** and ***Peds:*** 10 mg/kg IV 30 min before initiation of chemotherapy. ***Adults:*** 1 mg PO 1 h before chemotherapy, then q12 h.

Guaifenesin (Robitussin, others)

COMMON USES: Symptomatic relief of dry nonproductive cough; expectorant.
DOSAGE: ***Adults:*** 200–400 mg (10–20 mL) PO q4h. ***Peds:*** 2–5 y: 50–100 mg (2.5–5 mL) PO q4h; 6–11 y: 100–200 mg (5–10 mL) PO q4h.

Guaifenesin and Codeine (Robitussin AC, Brontex, others) [C]

COMMON USES: Antitussive with expectorant.
DOSAGE: ***Adults:*** 10 mL or 1 tab PO q6–8h. ***Peds:*** 2–6 y: 1–1.5 mg/kg codeine per day divided dose q4–6h. 6–12 y: 5 mL q4h. >12 y: 10 mL q4h, max 60 mL/24h.
NOTES: Bontex tab contains 10 mg codeine; Brontex liquid 2.5 mg codeine/5 mL; others 10 mg codeine/5 mL.

Guaifenesin and Dextromethorphan (Many OTC Brands)

COMMON USES: Cough due to upper respiratory irritation.
DOSAGE: ***Adults*** and ***Peds:*** > 12 y: 10 mL PO q6h. 2–6 y: 2.5 mL q6–8h, 10 mL/d max. 6–12 y: 5 mL q6–8h, 20 mL max/d.

Guanabenz (Wytensin)

COMMON USES: Hypertension.
DOSAGE: ***Adults:*** Initially, 4 mg PO bid, increase by 4 mg/d increments at 1–2 wk intervals up to 32 mg bid. ***Peds: > 12 y:*** 0.5–4 mg/d initially, increase by 0.5–2 mg/d at 1-wk intervals up to 24 mg/d divided bid.
NOTES: Sedation, dry mouth, dizziness, and headache common.

Guanadrel (Hylorel)

COMMON USES: Hypertension.
DOSAGE: 5 mg PO bid initially, increase up to 10 mg/d weekly up to 75 mg PO bid.
NOTES: Interactions with tricyclic antidepressants; less orthostatic changes and impotence than guanethidine.

Guanethidine (Ismelin)

COMMON USES: Hypertension.
DOSAGE: ***Adults:*** Initially, 10–25 mg PO qd, increase dose based on response. ***Peds:*** 0.2 mg/kg/24h PO initially, increase by 0.2 mg/kg/24h increments q7–10d up to maximum dose of 3 mg/kg/24h.

NOTES: May produce orthostatic hypotension especially with diuretic use; may potentiate vasopressors; increased frequency of bowel movements and explosive diarrhea possible; interaction with tricyclic antidepressants reduces the effectiveness of guanethidine.

Guanfacine (Tenex)

COMMON USES: Hypertension.
DOSAGE: 1 mg qhs initially, increase by 1 mg/24h to maximum dose of 3 mg/24h; split dose bid if BP increases at the end of the dosing interval.
NOTES: Use with thiazide diuretic is recommended; sedation, drowsiness common; rebound hypertension may occur with abrupt cessation of therapy.

Haemophilus B Conjugate Vaccine (ProHIBiT)

COMMON USES: Routine immunization between the ages of 18 mo and 5 y against diseases caused by *Haemophilus influenzae* type B.
DOSAGE: ***Peds:*** 0.5 mL (25 mg) IM in deltoid or vastus lateralis.
NOTES: Booster not required; observe for anaphylaxis.

Haloperidol (Haldol)

COMMON USES: Management of psychotic disorders; schizophrenia; agitation; Tourette's disorders; hyperactivity in children.
DOSAGE: ***Adults:*** Moderate symptoms: 0.5–2.0 mg PO bid–tid. Severe symptoms or agitation: 3–5 mg PO bid–tid or 1–5 mg IM q4h prn (max 100 mg/d). ***Peds:*** 3–6 y: 0.01–0.03 mg/kg/24h PO qd; 6–12 y: initially, 0.5–1.5 mg/24h PO, increase by 0.5 mg/24h to maintenance of 2–4 mg/24h (0.05–0.1 mg/kg/24h) or 1–3 mg/dose IM q4–8h to a max of 0.1 mg/kg/24h. Tourette's up to 15 mg/24h PO.
NOTES: Can cause extrapyramidal symptoms, hypotension; reduce dose in elderly patients.

Heparin Sodium

COMMON USES: Treatment and prevention of venous thrombosis and pulmonary emboli, atrial fibrillation with emboli formation, acute arterial occlusion.
DOSAGE: ***Adults:*** Prophylaxis: 3000–5000 units SC q8–12h. Treatment of thrombosis: Loading dose of 50–75 units/kg IV, then 10–20 units/kg IV qh (adjust based on PTT). ***Peds:*** Infants: Load 50 U/kg IV bolus, then 20 U/kg/hr IV infusion. Children: Load 50 U/kg IV then 15–25 U/kg/h continuous infusion or 100 U/kg/dose q4h IV intermittent bolus.
NOTES: Follow PTT, thrombin time, or activated clotting time to assess effectiveness; heparin has little effect on the prothrombin time; with proper dose PTT is about 1 1/2–2 times the control; can cause thrombocytopenia, follow platelet counts.

Hepatitis A Vaccine (Havrix)

COMMON USES: High-risk exposure to hepatitis A (travelers, health care workers, etc.).
DOSAGE: ***Adults:*** 1 mL IM ,booster 6–12 mo. ***Peds:*** 0.5 mL IM day 1 and 30, booster 6–12 mo.

Hepatitis B Immune Globulin (HyperHep, H-BIG)

COMMON USES: Exposure to HBsAg-positive materials: blood, plasma, or serum (accidental needle-stick, mucous membrane contact, oral ingestion).
DOSAGE: ***Adults*** and ***Peds:*** 0.06 mL/kg IM,5 mL max; within 24 h of needlestick or percutaneous exposure; within 14 d of sexual contact; repeat at 1 and 6 mo after exposure.
NOTES: Administered in gluteal or deltoid muscle; if exposure continues should receive hepatitis B vaccine.

Hepatitis B Vaccine (Engerix-B, Recombivax HB)

COMMON USES: Prevention of type B hepatitis in high-risk individuals.
DOSAGE: ***Adults:*** 3 IM doses of 1 mL each, the first 2 given 1 mo apart, the third 6 mo after the first. ***Peds:*** 0.5 mL IM dose given on the same schedule as adults.

NOTES: IM injections for adults and older peds to be administered in the deltoid; other peds to be administered in anterolateral thigh; may cause fever, injection site soreness; derived from recombinant DNA technology.

Hetastarch (Hespan)

COMMON USES: Plasma volume expansion as an adjunct in treatment of shock due to hemorrhage, surgery, burns, and other trauma.
DOSAGE: 500–1000 mL (do not exceed 1500 mL/d) IV at a rate not to exceed 20 mL/kg/h.
NOTES: Not a substitute for blood or plasma; contraindicated in patients with severe bleeding disorders, severe CHF, or renal failure with oliguria or anuria.

Hydralazine (Apresoline)

COMMON USES: Moderate to severe hypertension.
DOSAGE: ***Adults:***10 mg PO qid, increase to 25 mg qid to a maximum of 300 mg/d. ***Peds:*** 0.75–3 mg/kg/24h PO divided q12–6h.
NOTES: Caution with impaired hepatic function, coronary artery disease; compensatory sinus tachycardia can be eliminated with the addition of propranolol; chronically high doses can cause SLE-like syndrome; SVT can occur following IM administration.

Hydrochlorothiazide (HydroDIURIL, Esidrix, others)

COMMON USES: Edema, hypertension, CHF.
DOSAGE: ***Adults:*** 25–100 mg PO qd in single or divided doses. ***Peds:*** 2–3 mg/kg/24h PO divided bid.
NOTES: Hypokalemia is frequent; hyperglycemia, hyperuricemia, hyperlipidemia, and hyponatremia are common side effects.

Hydrochlorothiazide and Amiloride (Moduretic)

COMMON USES: Hypertension, adjunctive therapy for congestive heart failure.
DOSAGE: 1–2 tablets PO qd.
NOTES: Should not be given to diabetics or patients with renal failure.

Hydrochlorothiazide and Spironolactone (Aldactazide)

COMMON USES: Edema (CHF, cirrhosis), hypertension.
DOSAGE: 1–8 tablets (25–200 mg each component per day) 1–2 divided doses.

Hydrochlorothiazide and Triamterene (Dyazide, Maxzide)

COMMON USES: Edema, hypertension.
DOSAGE: Dyazide: 1–2 capsules PO qd–bid. Maxzide: 1 tablet PO qd.
NOTES: Can cause hyperkalemia as well as hypokalemia; follow serum potassium.

Hydrocortisone

See "Steroids," page 529.

Hydrocodone and Acetaminophen (Lorcet, Vicodin, others) [C]

COMMON USES: Moderate to severe pain; hydrocodone has antitussive properties.
DOSAGE: 1–2 PO q4–6h prn.
NOTES: Many different combinations; specify hydrocodone/acetaminophen dose: 2.5/500, 5/400, 5/500, 7.5/400, 10/400, 7.5/500, 7.5/650, 7.5/750, 10/325, 10/400, 10/500, 10/650,
Elixir and solution 2.5 mg hydrocodone/167 mg acetaminophen per 5 mL.

Hydrocodone and Aspirin (Lortab ASA, others) [C]

COMMON USES: Moderate-to-severe pain.
DOSAGE: 1–2 PO q4–6h prn.
NOTES: 5 mg hydrocodone/500 mg aspirin per tablet.

Hydrocodone and Guaifenesin (Hycotuss expectorant, others) [C]

COMMON USES: Non-productive cough associated with respiratory infection.
DOSAGE: ***Adults*** and ***Peds:*** > 12 y: 5 mL q4h, pc and hs. <2 y: 0.3 mg/kg/d divided qid. 2–12 y, 2.5 mL q4h pc and hs.

Hydrocodone and Homatropine (Hycodan, others) [C]

COMMON USES: Relief of cough.
DOSAGE: ***Adults:*** 5–10 mg q4–6h. ***Peds:*** 0.6 mg/kg/d divided tid–qid.
NOTES: Dose based on hydrocodone; syrup 5-mg hydrocodone/5 mL; tablet 5-mg hydrocodone.

Hydrocodone and Ibuprofen (Vicoprofen) [C]

COMMON USES: Moderate to severe pain (less than 10 d).
DOSAGE: 1–2 tablets q4–6h prn.
NOTES: 7.5 mg hydrocodone/200 mg ibuprofen/tab

Hydrocodone and Pseudoephedrine (Entuss-D, Histussin-D, others) [C]

COMMON USES: Cough and nasal congestion.
DOSAGE: 5 mL qid, prn
NOTES: 5-mg hydrocodone/5 mL

Hydrocodone, Chlorpheniramine, Phenylephrine, Acetaminophen, and Caffeine (Hycomine)

COMMON USES: Cough and symptoms of upper respiratory infections.
DOSAGE: 1 PO, q4h, prn.
NOTES: 5-mg hydrocodone/tab.

Hydromorphone (Dilaudid) [C]

COMMON USES: Moderate to severe pain.
DOSAGE: 1–4 mg PO, IM, IV, SC or PR q4–6h prn.
NOTES: 1.5 mg IM equivalent to 10-mg morphine IM.

Hydroxyurea (Hydrea)

COMMON USES: Treatment of cervical and ovarian cancer, melanoma, and leukemia adjunct in sickle cell anemia.
DOSAGE: Continuous therapy: 20–30 mg/kg PO qd; intermittent therapy: 80 mg/kg every 3 d.

Hydroxyzine (Atarax, Vistaril)

COMMON USES: Anxiety, tension, sedation, itching.
DOSAGE: ***Adults:*** Anxiety or sedation: 50–100 mg PO or IM qid or prn (maximum of 600 mg/d); itching: 25–50 mg PO or IM tid–qid. ***Peds:*** 0.6–1.0 mg/kg/24h PO or IM q6h.
NOTES: Useful in potentiating the effects of narcotics; not for IV use; drowsiness, anticholinergic effects are common.

Hyoscyamine (Anaspaz, Cystospaz, Levsin, others)

COMMON USES: Spasm associated with GI and bladder disorders.
DOSAGE: ***Adults:*** 0.125–0.25 mg (1–2 tabs) SL 3–4 times a day, pc and hs; 1 capsule q12h (sustained release [Cystospas-M, Levinex]).

Hyoscyamine, Atropine, Scopolamine, and Phenobarbital (Donnatal, others)

COMMON USES: Irritable bowel, spastic colitis, peptic ulcer, spastic bladder.
DOSAGE: 0.125–0.25 mg (1–2 tabs) 3–4 times a day, 1 capsule q12h (sustained release), 5–10 mL elixir 3–4 times a day or q8h.

Ibuprofen (Motrin, Rufen, Advil, others)

COMMON USES: Treatment of inflammatory conditions (rheumatoid arthritis, others) arthritis and pain, fever, gout, dysmenorrhea.
DOSAGE: ***Adults:*** pain, fever, dysmenorrhea 200–400 mg PO q4–6h, max 1.2 g/d; inflammatory conditions 400–800 mg ID–qid, max 3.2 g/d. ***Peds:*** 4–10 mg/kg/dose in 3–4 divided doses; rheumatoid arthritis 30–50 mg/kg/d divided qid, max 2.4 g/d.

Ibutilide (Covert)

COMMON USES: Rapid conversion of atrial fibrillation or flutter.
DOSAGE: <60 kg 0.01 mg/kg (maximum 1 mg); >60 kg 1 mg IV over 10 min. May be repeated once if needed 10 min later.
NOTES: Do not administer Class I or III antiarrhythmics concurrently or within 4 h of ibutilide infusion.

Idarubicin (Idamycin)

COMMON USES: Treatment of leukemia.
DOSAGE: 12 mg/m^2 daily for 3 d.
NOTES: Do not administer if bilirubin is > 5 mg/dL.

Ifosfamide (Ifex)

COMMON USES: Testicular, breast, sarcoma, and ovarian cancer.
DOSAGE: 1.2 $g/m^2/d$ for 5 consecutive days. Repeat course every 3 wk.
NOTES: Causes hemorrhagic cystitis; hydrate patients well and administer with MESNA.

Imipenem/Cilastatin (Primaxin)

COMMON USES: Serious infections caused by a wide variety of susceptible bacteria; multiresistant infections, inactive against *S aureus,* group A and B streptococci, and others; empiric therapy of gram-negative sepsis in immunocompromised host.
DOSAGE: ***Adults:*** 250–500 mg (Imipenem) IV q6h. ***Peds:*** Children < 3 y: 100 mg/kg/24h IV divided q6h; children > 3 y: 60 mg/kg/24h IV divided q6h.
NOTES: Seizures may occur if drug accumulates; adjust dose for renal insufficiency to avoid drug accumulation if creatinine clearance < 70 mL/min.

Imipramine (Tofranil)

COMMON USES: Depression, enuresis.
DOSAGE: ***Adults:*** Hospitalized for severe depression: Start at 100 mg/24h PO or IV in divided doses, increase over several weeks to 250–300 mg/24h. Outpatient: 50–150 mg PO qhs not to exceed 200 mg/24h. ***Peds:*** Antidepressant: 1.5–5.0 mg/kg/24h divided tid; enuresis: 10–25 mg PO qhs; increase by 10–25 mg at 1–2-wk intervals, treat for 2–3 mo, then taper.
NOTES: Do not use with MAO inhibitors; less sedation than amitriptyline.

Immune Globulin Intravenous (Gamimune N, Sandoglobulin, Gammar IV)

COMMON USES: IgG antibody deficiency diseases (congenital agammaglobulinemia, common variable hypogammaglobulinemia; idiopathic thrombocytopenic purpura (ITP).
DOSAGE: ***Adults*** and ***Peds:*** Immunodeficiency: 100–200 mg/kg IV monthly rate of 0.01–0.04 mL/kg/min to a maximum of 400 mg/kg/dose. ITP: 400 mg/kg/dose IV qd for 5 d. BMT: 500 mg/kg/wk.
NOTES: Adverse effects associated mostly with rate of infusion.

Indapamide (Lozol)

COMMON USES: Hypertension, congestive heart failure.
DOSAGE: 2.5–5.0 mg PO qd.

NOTES: Doses > than 5 mg do not have additional effects on lowering blood pressure.

Indinavir (Crixivan)

COMMON USES: HIV infection as part of a two-drug (nucleosidase plus protease inhibitor) or three-drug (two nucleosidases plus protease inhibitor) treatment.
DOSAGE: 800 mg PO q8h

Indomethacin (Indocin)

COMMON USES: Arthritis and closure of the ductus arteriosus.
DOSAGE: *Adults:* 25–50 mg PO bid–tid, 200 mg/d max. Infants: 0.2–0.25 mg/kg/dose IV; may be repeated in 12–24 h for up to 3 doses.
NOTES: Monitor renal function.

Infliximab (Remicade)

COMMON USES: Treatment of moderate-to-severe Crohn's disease.
DOSAGE: 5 mg/kg IV infusion, subsequent doses 2 and 6 weeks after initial infusion.
NOTES: May cause hypersensitivity reaction, made up of human constant and murine variable regions.

Insulins

COMMON USES: Diabetes mellitus that cannot be controlled by diet and/or oral hypoglycemic agents.
DOSAGE: Based on serum glucose levels; usually given SC can also be given IV or IM (only regular insulin can be given IV). See Table IX–5 on page 497. General guidelines: 0.5–1U/kg/d, 2/3 dose before breakfast, 1/3 before supper; adjust based on blood sugars over several days. Regular or rapid insulin should be dosed q4–6h, NPH or intermediate q8–12h. Keto Acidosis: hydrate patient well with normal saline, 10 U regular insulin IV followed by infusion 0.1 U/kg/h; optimum serum glucose decline: 50–100 mg/dL/h.
NOTES: The highly purified insulins provide an increase in free insulin; monitor these patients closely for several weeks when changing doses; most standard insulins 100 U/mL.

Interferon Alpha (Roferon-A, Intron A)

COMMON USES: Hairy cell leukemia, Kaposi's sarcoma, multiple myeloma, chronic myelogenous leukemia, renal cell carcinoma, bladder cancer, melanoma, and chronic hepatitis C.
DOSAGE: Alfa-2a (Roferon): 3 million IU daily for 16–24 wk SQ or IM. Alfa-2b (Intron): 2 million IU/m^2 IM or SQ 3 times a wk for 2–6 mo; intravesical 50–100 million IU in 50 mL normal saline weekly X 6.
NOTES: Systemic use may cause flu-like symptoms; fatigue is common; anorexia occurs in 20–30% of patients; neurotoxicity may occur at high doses; neutralizing antibodies can occur in up to 40% of patients receiving prolonged systemic therapy.

Interferon Alpha and Ribavirin (Roferon-A, Intron A)

COMMON USES: Chronic hepatitis C.
DOSAGE: Intron A: 3 million IU SQ 3 times with rebtrol 1000–1200 mg divided PO bid for 24 wk.
NOTES: Supplied in combination with multidose pen injector for Intron A.

Interferon Alfacon-1 (Infergen)

COMMON USES: Management of chronic hepatitis C.
DOSAGE: 9 µg SC 3 times per wk.
NOTES: At least 48 h should elapse between injections

Ipecac Syrup

COMMON USES: Treatment of drug overdose and certain cases of poisoning.

TABLE IX–5. COMPARISON OF INSULINS.

Type of Insulin	Onset (h)	Peak (h)	Duration (h)
Ultra Rapid			
Humalog (Lispro)	Immediate	0.5–1.5	3–5
Novolog (Insulin aspart)	Immediate	0.5–1.5	3–5
Rapid			
Regular Iletin II	0.25–0.5	2.0–4.0	5–7
Humulin R	0.5	2.0–4.0	6–8
Novolin R	0.5	2.5–5.0	5–8
Velosulin	0.5	2.0–5.0	6–8
Intermediate			
NPH Iletin II	1.0–2.0	6–12	18–24
Lente Iletin II	1.0–2.0	6–12	18–24
Humulin N	1.0–2.0	6–12	14–24
Novulin L	2.5–5.0	7–15	18–24
Novulin 70/30	0.5	7–12	24
Prolonged			
Ultralente	4.0–6.0	14–24	28–36
Humulin U	4.0–6.0	8–20	24–28
Lantus (Insulin glargine)	4.0–6.0	no peak	24
Combination Insulins			
Humalog Mix (Lispro protamine/Lispro)	0.25–0.5	1–4	24

DOSAGE: ***Adults:*** 15–30 mL PO followed by 200–300 mL water; if no emesis occurs in 20 minutes, may repeat X 1. ***Peds:*** 6–12 mo: 5–10 mL PO followed by water. 1–12 y: 15 mL PO followed by water.
NOTES: Do not use for ingestion of petroleum distillates, strong acid, base, or other corrosive or caustic agents; not for use in comatose or unconscious patients; caution in CNS depressant overdose.

Ipratropium Bromide Inhalant (Atrovent)

COMMON USES: Bronchospasm associated with COPD.
DOSAGE: ***Adults*** and ***Children > 12 y:*** 2–4 puffs qid.
NOTES: Not for initial treatment of acute episodes of bronchospasm.

Irbesartan (Avapro)

COMMON USES: Treatment of hypertension.
DOSAGE: 150 mg PO daily, may be increased to 300 mg daily.

Iron Dextran (Dexferrum)

COMMON USES: Iron deficiency when oral supplementation is not possible.
DOSAGE: Based on estimate of iron deficiency (see package insert).
NOTES: Must give a test dose since anaphylaxis is common (adult 0.5 mL, infants 0.25 mL; may be given deep IM using "Z-track" technique although IV route most preferred.

Isoetharine (Bronkosol, Bronkometer)

COMMON USES: Bronchial asthma and reversible bronchospasm.
DOSAGE: ***Adults*** and ***Peds:*** Nebulization: 0.25–1.0 mL diluted 1:3 with saline q4–6h. Metered dose inhaler: 1–2 inhalations q4h.

Isoniazid (INH)

COMMON USES: Treatment of *Mycobacterium* species infections.
DOSAGE: ***Adults:*** Active TB: 5 mg/kg/24h PO or IM qd (usually 300 mg/d). Prophylaxis: 300 mg PO qd for 6–12 mo. ***Peds:*** Active TB: 10–20 mg/kg/24h PO or IM qd to a maximum of 300 mg/d. Prophylaxis: 10 mg/kg/24h PO qd.
NOTES: Can cause severe hepatitis; given with other antituberculous drugs for active tuberculosis; IM route rarely used; to prevent peripheral neuropathy can give pyridoxine 50–100 mg/d.

Isoproterenol (Isuprel, Medihaler-Iso)

COMMON USES: Shock, cardiac arrest, AV nodal block, antiasthmatic.
DOSAGE: ***Adults:*** Emergency cardiac care: 2–20 mg/min IV infusion, titrated to effect. Shock: 1–4 mg/min IV infusion, titrated to effect. AV nodal block: 20–60 mg IV push; may repeat q3–5 min; 1–5 mg/min IV infusion maintenance. Inhalation: 1–2 inhalations 4–6 times daily. ***Peds:*** Emergency cardiac care: 0.1–1.5 mg/kg/min IV infusion, titrated to effect. Inhalation: 1–2 inhalations 4–6 times daily.
NOTES: Contraindications: tachycardia; pulse > 130 bpm may induce ventricular arrhythmias.

Isosorbide Dinitrate (Isordil)

COMMON USES: Angina pectoris.
DOSAGE: Acute angina: 2.5–10.0 mg PO (chewable tablet) or SL prn q5–10 min; >3 doses should not be given in 15–30-min period. Angina prophylaxis: 5–60 mg PO tid.
NOTES: Nitrates should not be given on chronic q6h or qid basis because of development of tolerance; can cause headaches; usually need to give a higher oral dose to achieve same results as with sublingual forms.

Isosorbide Monohydrate (ISMO)

COMMON USES: Prevention of angina pectoris.
DOSAGE: 20 mg PO bid, with the 2 doses given 7 h apart or extended release 30–120 mg PO qd.

Isradipine (DynaCirc)

COMMON USES: Hypertension.
DOSAGE: 2.5–5.0 mg PO bid.

Itraconazole (Sporanox)

COMMON USES: Treatment of systemic fungal infections caused by *Aspergillus, Blastomyces,* and *Histoplasma.*
DOSAGE: 200 mg PO or IV qd-bid.
NOTES: Administer with meals or cola; should not be used concurrently with H_2-antagonist, omeprazole, antacids.

Kaolin-Pectin

COMMON USES: Treatment of diarrhea.
DOSAGE: ***Adults:*** 60–120 mL PO after each loose stool or q3–4h prn. ***Peds:*** 3–6 y: 15–30 mL/dose PO prn. 6–12 y: 30–60 mL/dose PO prn.

Ketoconazole (Nizoral)

COMMON USES: Systemic fungal infections: candidiasis, chronic mucocutaneous candidiasis, blastomycosis, coccidioidomycosis, histoplasmosis, and paracoccidioidomycosis; topical cream for localized fungal infections due to dermatophytes and yeast; rapid short-term treatment of prostate cancer where rapid reduction of testosterone is needed (ie, spinal cord compression).

DOSAGE: ***Adults:*** Oral: 200 mg PO qd; increase to 400 mg PO qd for very serious infections; prostate cancer 400 mg PO tid (short term). Topical: Apply to affected area once daily. ***Peds:*** 3.3–6.6 mg/kg/24h PO qd.

NOTES: Associated with severe hepatotoxicity; monitor LFTs closely throughout course of therapy; drug interaction with any agent increasing gastric pH preventing absorption of ketoconazole; may enhance oral anticoagulants; may react with alcohol to produce disulfiram-like reaction.

Ketoprofen (Orudis)

COMMON USES: Treatment of arthritis and pain.

DOSAGE: 25–75 mg PO tid–qid, to a maximum of 300 mg/d.

Ketorolac (Toradol)

COMMON USES: Treatment of arthritis and pain.

DOSAGE: 15–30 mg IV/IM q6h or 10 mg PO qid.

NOTES: Do NOT use for longer than 5 d.

Ketorolac (Acular Ophthalmic)

COMMON USES: Itching associated with seasonal allergic conjunctivitis.

DOSAGE: 1 drop in eye(s) qid.

Labetalol (Trandate, Normodyne)

COMMON USES: Hypertension, hypertensive emergencies.

DOSAGE: ***Adults:*** Hypertension: Initially, 100 mg PO bid; then 200–400 mg PO bid. Hypertensive emergency: 20–80 mg IV bolus, then 2 mg/min IV infusion, titrated to effect. ***Peds:*** Oral: 3–20 mg/kg/d in divided doses. Hypertensive emergency: 0.4–3 mg/kg/h IV continuous infusion.

Lactobacillus (Lactinex Granules)

COMMON USES: Control of diarrhea, especially after antibiotic therapy.

DOSAGE: ***Adults*** and ***Peds > 3 y:*** 1 packet, 2 capsules, or 4 tablets with meals or liquids tid.

Lactulose (Chronulac, Cephulac)

COMMON USES: Hepatic encephalopathy; laxative; constipation.

DOSAGE: ***Adults:*** Acute hepatic encephalopathy: 30–45 mL PO q1h until soft stools are observed, then tid-qid. Chronic laxative therapy: 30–45 mL PO tid-qid; adjust the dosage every 1–2 d to produce 2–3 soft stools qd. Rectally: 200 g diluted with 700 mL of water instilled into the rectum. ***Peds:*** Infants: 2.5–10 mL/24h divided tid-qid. Children: 40–90 mL/24h divided tid-qid.

NOTES: Can cause severe diarrhea.

Lamivudine (Epivir, Epivir-HBV)

COMMON USES: Treatment of HIV infection when therapy is warranted based on clinical and/or immunologic evidence of disease progression, and chronic hepatitis B.

DOSAGE: HIV:***Adults*** and ***Peds:*** >12 y: 150 mg PO bid. <12 y: 4 mg/kg twice daily. HBV: 100 mg once daily.

NOTES: Used in combination with zidovudine for HIV; use with caution in pediatric patients because of an increased incidence of pancreatitis.

Lamotrigine (Lamictal)

COMMON USES: Treatment of partial seizures.

DOSAGE: ***Adults:*** Initially 50 mg PO qd, then 50 mg PO bid for 2 wk, then maintenance 300–500 mg/d divided bid. ***Peds:*** 0.15 mg/kg in 1–2 divided doses for week 1 and 2, then 0.3 mg/kg for weeks 3 and 4, then maintenance dose of 1 mg/kg/d in 1–2 divided doses.

NOTES: May cause rash and photosensitivity; the value of therapeutic monitoring has not been established.

Lansoprazole (Prevacid)

COMMON USES: Treatment of duodenal ulcers, *H pylori* infection, erosive esophagitis, and hypersecretory conditions.
DOSAGE: 15–30 mg PO once daily.

Lantanoprost (Xalatan)

COMMON USES: Glaucoma that does not respond to standard therapies.
DOSAGE: 1 drop eye(s) qhs.
NOTES: May darken light irides.

Leflunomide (Arava)

COMMON USES: Treatment of active rheumatoid arthritis.
DOSAGE: 100 mg PO once daily for 3 d, followed by 10–20 mg once daily.
NOTES: Pregnancy category X—DO NOT USE; monitor ALT.

Lepirudin (Refludan)

COMMON USES: Management of heparin-induced thrombocytopenia.
DOSAGE: Bolus of 0.4 mg/kg IV, followed by 0.15 mg/kg continuous infusion.
NOTES: Monitor aPTT 4 h into initial infusion and at least daily; adjust dose based on aPTT ratio; maintain aPTT ratio of 1.5–2.0.

Leucovorin Calcium (Wellcovorin)

COMMON USES: Antidote for folic acid antagonist.
DOSAGE: ***Adults*** and ***Peds:*** Methotrexate rescue: 10–100 mg/m^2/dose IV or PO q3–6h. Adjunct to antimicrobials: 5–10 mg PO qd.
NOTES: Many different dosing schedules exist for Leucovorin rescue following methotrexate therapy.

Leuprolide (Lupron Depot)

COMMON USES: Treatment of prostate cancer, endometriosis, and central precocious puberty (CPP).
DOSAGE: ***Adults:*** Prostate: 7.5 mg IM monthly of depot, 22.5 mg 3-month depot or 30 mg 4-month depot. Endometriosis (depot only): 3.75 mg IM as a single monthly dose. ***Peds:*** CPP: 50 mg/kg/d daily SC injection; titrate upward by 10 mg/kg/d until total down regulation is achieved. Depot: <25 kg: 7.5 mg IM every 4 wk. 25 to 37.5 kg: 11.25 mg IM every 4 wk. >37.5 kg: 15 mg IM every 4 wk.

Levalbuterol (Xopenex)

COMMON USES: Treatment and prevention of bronchospasm.
DOSAGE: 0.63 mg nebulized every 6–8 h.
NOTES: Therapeutically active R-isomer of albuterol.

Levamisole (Ergamisol)

COMMON USES: Adjuvant therapy of node-positive colon cancer (in combination with 5-FU).
DOSAGE: 50 mg PO q8h for 3 d every 14 d during 5-FU therapy.
NOTES: Toxicity includes nausea and vomiting, diarrhea, abdominal pain, taste disturbance, anorexia, hyperbilirubinemia, disulfiram-like reaction on alcohol ingestion, minimal bone marrow depression, fatigue, fever, and conjunctivitis.

Levetiracetam (Kappra)

COMMON USES: Treatment of partial onset seizures.
DOSAGE: 500 mg PO bid, may be increased to a maximum of 3000 mg/d.
NOTES: May cause dizziness and somnolence; may impair coordination.

Levobunol (Betagan Liquifilm Ophthalmic, others)

COMMON USES: Glaucoma.

DOSAGE: 1–2 drops in eye(s) bid.

Levocabastine (Livostin)

COMMON USES: Allergic seasonal conjunctivitis.
DOSAGE: 1 drop in eye(s) qid up to 4 wk.

Levofloxacin (Levaquin)

COMMON USES: Treatment of lower respiratory tract infections, sinusitises, and urinary tract infections.
DOSAGE: 250–500 mg PO or IV once daily.
NOTES: Reliable activity against *S pneumoniae,* drug interactions with cation-containing products.

Levonorgestrel Implants (Norplant)

COMMON USES: Prevention of pregnancy.
DOSAGE: Implant 6 capsules in the mid-forearm.
NOTES: Prevents pregnancy for up to 5 y; capsules may be removed if pregnancy is desired.

Levorphanol (Levo-Dromoran) [C]

COMMON USES: Moderate-to-severe pain.
DOSAGE: 2 mg PO or SC prn.

Levothyroxine (Synthroid)

COMMON USES: Hypothyroidism.
DOSAGE: ***Adults:*** 25–50 mg/d PO or IV initially; increase by 25–50 mg/d every month; usual dose 100–200 mg/d. ***Peds:*** 0–1 y: 8–10 mg/kg/24h PO or IV qd. 1–5 y: 4–6 mg/kg/24h PO or IV qd. >5 y: 3–4 mg/kg/24h PO or IV qd.
NOTES: Titrate dosage based on clinical response and thyroid function tests; Dosage can be increased more rapidly in young to middle-aged patients.

Lidocaine (Xylocaine)

COMMON USES: Local anesthesia; treatment of cardiac arrhythmias.
DOSAGE: ***Adults:*** Arrhythmias: 1 mg/kg (50–100 mg) IV bolus, then 2–4 mg/min IV infusion, should repeat bolus after 5 min. Local anesthesia: Infiltrate a few mL of a 0.5–1.0% solution maximum 3 mg/kg/dose. ***Peds:*** Arrhythmias: 1 mg/kg dose IV bolus, then 20–50 mg/kg/min IV infusion. Local anesthetic: Infiltrate a few mL of a 0.5–1.0% solution, with a maximum of 3 mg/kg/dose.
NOTES: Epinephrine may be added for local anesthesia to prolong effect and help decrease bleeding; for IV forms, dose reduction is required with liver disease, CHF; dizziness, paresthesias, and convulsions are associated with toxicity.

Lidocaine/Prilocaine (EMLA)

COMMON USES: Topical anesthetic; adjunct to phlebotomy or invasive dermal procedures.
DOSAGE: ***Adults:*** EMLA Cream and Anesthetic Disc (1 g/10 cm^2): Thick layer of cream 2–2.5 g applied to intact skin and covered with an occlusive dressing (Tegaderm) for at least 1 h. Anesthetic Disc : 1 g per 10 cm^2 for at least 1 h. ***Peds:*** Max dose: up to 3 mo or < 5 kg: 1 g per 10 cm^2 for 1 h. 3–12 mo and > 5 kg: 2 g per 20 cm^2 for 4 h. 1–6 y and > 10 kg: 10 g per 100 cm^2 for 4 h. 7– 12 y and > 20 kg: 20 g per 200 cm^2 for 4 h.
NOTES: Longer contact time gives greater effect.

Lindane (Kwell)

COMMON USES: Head lice, crab lice, scabies.
DOSAGE: ***Adults*** and ***Peds:*** Cream or lotion: Apply thin layer after bathing and leave in place for 24h; pour on laundry. Shampoo: Apply 30 mL and develop lather with warm water for 4 min; comb out nits.
NOTES: Caution with overuse, may be absorbed into blood; wash clothing and bedding as well to clear infestation.

Linezolid (Zyvox)

COMMON USES: Infections caused by gram-positive bacteria, including vancomycin-resistant and methicillin-resistant strains.
DOSAGE: 400–600 mg IV or PO q12h.
NOTES: A reversible, inhibitor of MAO; therefore avoid foods which contain tyramine; avoid cough and cold products containing pseudoephedrine or phenylpropanolamine.

Liothyronine (Cytomel)

COMMON USES: Hypothyroidism.
DOSAGE: ***Adults:*** Initially 25 mg/24h, then titration q1–2 wk according to clinical response and thyroid function tests to maintenance of 25–75 mg PO qd. ***Peds:*** Initially 5 mg/24h, then titration by 5 mg/24h increments at 1–2 wk intervals; maintenance 25–75 mg/24h PO qd.
NOTES: Reduce dose in elderly patients; monitor thyroid function test.

Lisinopril (Prinivil, Zestril)

COMMON USES: Treatment of hypertension, heart failure, and acute myocardial infarction.
DOSAGE: 5–40 mg/24h PO qd-bid. AMI: 5 mg within 24 h of MI, then 5 mg after 24 h, 10 mg after 48 h, then 10 mg qd.
NOTES: Dizziness, headache, and cough are common side effects; DO NOT use in pregnancy.

Lithium Carbonate (Eskalith, others)

COMMON USES: Manic episodes of manic-depressive illness; maintenance therapy in recurrent disease.
DOSAGE: Acute mania: 600 mg PO tid or 900 mg slow release bid. Maintenance: 300 mg PO tid–qid.
NOTES: Dosage must be titrated; follow serum levels (Table IX–3, page 457); common side effects are polyuria, tremor; contraindicated in patients with severe renal impairment; sodium retention or diuretic use may potentate toxicity.

Lodoxamide (Alomide Ophthalmic)

COMMON USES: Seasonal allergic conjunctivitis.
DOSAGE: ***Adults*** and ***Peds > 2 y:*** 1–2 drops in eye(s) qid up to 3 mo.

Lomefloxacin (Maxaquin)

COMMON USES: Treatment of UTI and lower respiratory tract infections caused by gram-negative bacteria; prophylaxis in transurethral procedures.
DOSAGE: 400 mg PO qd.
NOTES: May cause severe photosensitivity.

Loperamide (Imodium)

COMMON USES: Diarrhea.
DOSAGE: ***Adults:*** 4 mg PO initially, then 2 mg after each loose stool, up to 16 mg/d. ***Peds:*** 0.4–0.8 mg/kg/24h PO divided q6–12h until diarrhea resolves or for 7 d maximum.
NOTES: Do not use in acute diarrhea caused by *Salmonella, Shigella,* or *C difficile.*

Loracarbef (Lorabid)

COMMON USES: Treatment of infections caused by susceptible bacteria involving the upper and lower respiratory tract, skin, bone, urinary tract, abdomen and gynecologic system.
DOSAGE: ***Adults:*** 200–400 mg PO bid. ***Peds:*** 7.5–15 mg/kg/d PO divided bid.
NOTES: Has more gram-negative activity then first generation cephalosporins.

Loratadine (Claritin)

COMMON USES: Treatment of allergic rhinitis.
DOSAGE: 10 mg PO once daily.
NOTES: Take on empty stomach.

Lorazepam (Ativan, Alzapam) [C]

COMMON USES: Anxiety and anxiety mixed with depression; preop sedation; control of status epilepticus.
DOSAGE: ***Adults:*** Anxiety: 0.5–1.0 mg PO bid–tid. Preop: 0.05 mg/kg up to max of 4 mg IM 2 h before surgery. Insomnia: 2–4 mg PO qhs. Status epilepticus: 2.5–10 mg/dose IV repeated at 15–20 min interval prn. ***Peds:*** Status epilepticus: 0.05 mg/kg/dose IV repeated at 15–20 min interval prn.
NOTES: Decrease dose in elderly patients; may take up to 10 min to see effect when given IV.

Losartan (Cozaar)

COMMON USES: Treatment of hypertension.
DOSAGE: 25–50 mg PO qd-bid.
NOTES: Do not use in pregnancy; symptomatic hypotension may occur in patients on diuretics.

Lovastatin (Mevacor)

COMMON USES: Adjunct to diet for the reduction of elevated total and LDL cholesterol levels in patients with primary hypercholesterolemia (types IIa and IIb).
DOSAGE: 20 mg PO daily with evening meal; increase at 4– wk intervals to max 80 mg/d.
NOTES: Patient should be maintained on standard cholesterol-lowering diet throughout treatment; monitor LFTs every 6 wk during first year of therapy; headache and gastrointestinal intolerance common.

Magaldrate (Riopan, Lowsium)

COMMON USES: Hyperacidity associated with peptic ulcer; gastritis, and hiatal hernia.
DOSAGE: 1–2 tablets PO or 5–10 mL PO between meals and hs.
NOTES: Less than 0.3 mg sodium per tablet or teaspoon; do not use in renal insufficiency.

Magnesium Citrate

COMMON USES: Vigorous bowel prep; constipation.
DOSAGE: ***Adults:*** 120–240 mL PO prn. ***Peds:*** 0.5 mL/kg/dose, up to maximum 200 mL PO.
NOTES: Do not use in renal insufficiency, intestinal obstruction.

Magnesium Hydroxide (Milk of Magnesia)

COMMON USES: Constipation.
DOSAGE: ***Adults:*** 15–30 mL PO prn. ***Peds:*** 0.5 mL/kg/dose PO prn.
NOTES: Do not use in renal insufficiency or intestinal obstruction.

Magnesium Oxide (Uro-Mag, Mag-Ox 400, Maox)

COMMON USES: Replacement for low plasma magnesium levels.
DOSAGE: 400–800 mg/d divided qd–qid.
NOTES: May cause diarrhea.

Magnesium Sulfate

COMMON USES: Replacement for low plasma levels; refractory hypokalemia and hypocalcemia; preeclampsia and premature labor.
DOSAGE: ***Adults:*** Supplement: 1–2 g IM or IV; repeat dosing based on response and continued hypomagnesemia. Preeclampsia, premature labor: 1–4 g/h IV infusion. ***Peds:*** 25–50 mg/kg/dose IM or IV q4–6h for 3–4 doses; may repeat if hypomagnesemia persists.

NOTES: Reduce dose with low urine output or renal insufficiency.

Mannitol

COMMON USES: Osmotic diuresis (cerebral edema, oliguria, anuria, myoglobinuria, etc), bowel prep.
DOSAGE: ***Adults:*** Diuresis: 0.2 g/kg/dose IV over 3–5 min; if no diuresis within 2 h, discontinue. ***Peds:*** Diuresis: 0.75 g/kg/dose IV over 3–5 minutes; if no diuresis within 2 hours, discontinue. ***Adults*** and ***Peds:*** Cerebral edema: 0.25 g/kg/dose IV push repeated at 5-min intervals prn; increase incrementally to 1 g/kg per dose prn intracranial hypertension.
NOTES: Caution with CHF or volume overload.

Maprotiline (Ludiomil)

COMMON USES: Depressive neurosis; manic-depressive illness; major depressive disorder; anxiety associated with depression.
DOSAGE: 75–150 mg/d qhs, maximum of 300 mg/d.
NOTES: Contraindicated with MAO inhibitors or seizure history; for patients > 60 y, give only 50–75 mg/d; anticholinergic side effects.

Meclizine (Antivert)

COMMON USES: Motion sickness, vertigo associated with diseases of the vestibular system.
DOSAGE: ***Adults*** and ***Peds > 12 y:*** 25 mg PO tid–qid prn.
NOTES: Drowsiness, dry mouth, blurred vision commonly occur.

Medroxyprogesterone (Provera, Depo-Provera, others)

COMMON USES: Secondary amenorrhea and abnormal uterine bleeding owing to hormonal imbalance, endometrial cancer, contraceptive.
DOSAGE: Secondary amenorrhea: 5–10 mg PO qd for 5–10 d. Abnormal uterine bleeding: 5–10 mg PO qd for 5–10 days beginning on the 16th or 21st d of menstrual cycle. Endometrial Cancer: 400–1000 mg IM/wk.
NOTES: Contraindicated with past thromboembolic disorders or with hepatic disease.

Megestrol Acetate (Megace)

COMMON USES: Treatment of breast and endometrial cancer; appetite stimulation in cancer and HIV-related cachexia.
DOSAGE: Cancer: 40–320 mg/d PO in divided doses. Appetite: 80 mg PO qid.

Meloxicam (Mobic)

COMMON USES: Treatment of osteoarthritis.
DOSAGE: 7.5–15 mg PO once daily.

Melphalan (Alkeran)

COMMON USES: Treatment of breast and ovarian cancer, and multiple myeloma.
DOSAGE: 6 mg/d PO as single dose or 16 mg/m^2 IV every 2 wk for 4 doses.
NOTES: Monitor blood counts closely.

Meperidine (Demerol) [C]

COMMON USES: Relief of moderate-to-severe pain.
DOSAGE: ***Adults:*** 50–100 mg PO or IM q3–4h prn. ***Peds:*** 1–1.5 mg/kg/dose PO or IM q3–4h prn.
NOTES: 75 mg IM equivalent to 10-mg morphine IM; beware of respiratory depression. A useful preprocedure sedative, particularly in children, is a so-called cardiac cocktail, consisting of (per 30–lb body weight) 30 mg demerol, 6.25 mg thorazine, and 6.25 mg phenergan given IM.

Meprobamate (Equinil, Miltown) [C]

COMMON USES: Short-term relief of anxiety.
DOSAGE: 200–400 mg PO tid–qid; sustained release 400–800 mg PO bid.
NOTES: May cause drowsiness.

Mercaptopurine (Purinethol)

COMMON USES: Treatment of leukemia.
DOSAGE: ***Adults*** and ***Peds:*** 2.5 mg/kg/d PO.

Meropenem (Merrem)

COMMON USES: Serious infections caused by a wide variety of bacteria including intra-abdominal and polymicrobic; bacterial meningitis.
DOSAGE: ***Adults:*** 1 gm IV q8h. ***Peds:*** 20–40 mg/kg IV q8h.
NOTES: Adjust dose for renal function; less seizure potential than imipenem.

Mesalamine (Rowasa, Asacol, Pentasa)

COMMON USES: Treatment of mild-to-moderate distal ulcerative colitis, proctosigmoiditis, or proctitis.
DOSAGE: Retention enema at bedtime daily or insert 1 suppository bid. Oral: 800–1000 mg PO 3–4 times a day.

Mesna (Mesnex)

COMMON USES: Reduce the incidence of ifosfamide-induced hemorrhagic cystitis.
DOSAGE: 20% of the ifosfamide dose (w/w) IV at the time of ifosfamide infusion and 4 and 8 h after, for a total dose equal to 60% of the ifosfamide dose.

Mesoridazine (Serentil)

COMMON USES: Schizophrenia; acute and chronic alcoholism; chronic brain syndrome.
DOSAGE: 25–50 mg PO or IV tid initially; titrate to maximum of 300–400 mg/d.
NOTES: Low incidence of extrapyramidal side effects.

Metaproterenol (Alupent, Metaprel)

COMMON USES: Bronchodilator for asthma and reversible bronchospasm.
DOSAGE: ***Adults:*** Inhalation: 1–3 inhalations q3–4h to maximum of inhalations 12 per 24 h; allow at least 2 min between inhalations. Oral: 20 mg q6–8h. ***Peds:*** Inhalation: 0.5 mg/kg/dose up to max of 15 mg/dose inhaled q4–6h by nebulizer or 1–2 puffs q4–6h. Oral: 0.3–0.5 mg/kg/dose q6–8h.
NOTES: Fewer beta-1 effects than isoproterenol and longer acting.

Metaraminol (Aramine)

COMMON USES: Prevention and treatment of hypotension due to spinal anesthesia.
DOSAGE: ***Adults:*** Prevention: 2–10 mg IM q10–15min prn. Treatment: 0.5–5 mg IV bolus followed by IV infusion of 1–4 mg/kg/min titrated to effect. ***Peds:*** Prevention: 0.1 mg/kg/dose IM prn. Treatment: 0.01 mg/kg IV bolus followed by IV infusion of 5 mg/kg/min titrated to effect.
NOTES: Allow 10 min for maximal effect; employ other shock management techniques such as fluid resuscitation as needed; may cause cardiac arrhythmias.

Metaxalone (Skelaxin)

COMMON USES: Relief of painful musculoskeletal conditions.
DOSAGE: 800 mg PO 3–4 times a day.

Metformin (Glucophage)

COMMON USES: Treatment of non-insulin-dependent diabetes mellitus.
DOSAGE: Initial dose of 500 mg PO bid; may be increased to a maximum daily dose of 2500 mg.
NOTES: Administer with the morning and evening meals; may cause lactic acidosis; do not use if the creatinine is > 1.3 in females or > 1.4 in males.

Methadone (Dolophine) [C]

COMMON USES: Severe pain; detoxification and maintenance of narcotic addiction.
DOSAGE: ***Adults:*** 2.5–10 mg IM q8h or 5–15 mg PO q8h (titrate as needed). ***Peds:*** 0.7 mg/kg/24h PO or IM divided q8h.

NOTES: Equianalgesic with parenteral morphine; long half-life; increase dose slowly to avoid respiratory depression.

Methenamine (Hiprex, Urex, others)

COMMON USES: Suppression or elimination of bacteriuria associated with chronic and recurrent infections of the urinary tract.
DOSAGE: Initially: 2 tablets 4 times a day. Maintenance: 2–4 tablets daily in divided doses.
NOTES: Contraindicated in patients with renal insufficiency, sever hepatic disease, and severe dehydration

Methimazole (Tapazole)

COMMON USES: Hyperthyroidism; preparation for thyroid surgery or radiation.
DOSAGE: ***Adults:*** Initially, 15–60 mg/d PO divided tid; maintenance of 5–15 mg PO qd. ***Peds:*** Initially, 0.4–0.7 mg/kg/24h PO divided tid; maintenance of 0.2 mg/kg/d divided tid.
NOTES: Follow patient clinically and with thyroid function tests.

Methocarbamol (Robaxin)

COMMON USES: Relief of discomfort associated with painful musculoskeletal conditions.
DOSAGE: ***Adults:*** 1.5 g PO qid for 2–3 d, then 1 g PO qid maintenance therapy; IV form rarely indicated. ***Peds:*** 60 mg/kg/24h PO divided qid.
NOTES: Can discolor urine; may cause drowsiness or gastrointestinal upset; contraindicated with myasthenia gravis.

Methotrexate (Folex)

COMMON USES: ALL, AML, leukemic meningitis, trophoblastic tumors (chorioepithelioma, choriocarcinoma, chorioadenoma destruens, hydatidiform mole), breast cancer, Burkitt's lymphoma, mycosis fungoides, osteosarcoma, head and neck cancer, Hodgkin's and non-Hodgkin's lymphoma, lung cancer, psoriasis, and rheumatoid arthritis.
DOSAGE: Cancer: "conventional dose": 15–30 mg PO or IV 1–2 times a week every 1–3 wk; "intermediate dose": 50–240 mg or 0.5–1 g/m^2 IV once every 4 d to 3 wk, "high dose": 1–12 g/m^2 IV once every 1–3 wk; 12 mg/m^2 (maximum 15 mg) intrathecally, weekly until the CSF cell count returns to normal. Rheumatoid arthritis: 7.5 mg/wk PO as a single dose or 2.5 mg q12h PO for 3 doses each week.
NOTES: Toxicity includes myelosuppression, nausea and vomiting, anorexia, mucositis, diarrhea, hepatotoxicity (transient and reversible; may progress to atrophy, necrosis, fibrosis, cirrhosis), rashes, dizziness, malaise, blurred vision, renal failure, pneumonitis, and, rarely, pulmonary fibrosis. Chemical arachnoiditis and headache may occur with intrathecal delivery. "High-dose" therapy requires leucovorin rescue to prevent severe hematologic and mucosal toxicity (see page 500); monitor blood counts and methotrexate levels carefully.

Methoxamine (Vasoxyl)

COMMON USES: Support, restoration, or maintenance of blood pressure during anesthesia; for termination of some episodes of paroxysmal supraventricular tachycardia.
DOSAGE: ***Adults:*** Anesthesia: 10–15 mg IM; if emergency exists, 3–5 mg slow IV push. Paroxysmal SVT: 10 mg by slow IV push. ***Peds:*** 0.25 mg/kg/dose IM or 0.08 mg/kg/dose slow IV push.
NOTES: IM dose requires 15 min to act; use 5–10 mg phentolamine locally in case of extravasation; interaction with MAO inhibitors and tricyclic antidepressants to potentiate methoxamine effect.

Methyldopa (Aldomet)

COMMON USES: Essential hypertension.

DOSAGE: ***Adults:*** 250–500 mg PO bid–tid (max 2–3 g/d) or 250 mg to 1 g IV q4–8h. ***Peds:*** 10 mg/kg/24h PO in 2–3 divided doses (max 40 mg/kg/24h divided q6–12h) or 5–10 mg/kg/dose IV q6–8h to a total dose of 20–40 mg/kg/24h.
NOTES: Do not use in presence of patients with liver disease; can discolor urine; initial transient sedation or drowsiness occurs frequently.

Methylergonovine (Methergine)

COMMON USES: Prevention and treatment of postpartum hemorrhage caused by uterine atony.
DOSAGE: 0.2 mg IM after delivery of placenta, may repeat at 2–4-h intervals or 0.2–0.4 mg PO q6–12h for 2–7 d.
NOTES: IV doses should be given over a period of not less than 1 min with frequent BP monitoring.

Methylprednisolone (Solu-Medrol)

See "Steroids," page 529 and Table IX–4, page 475.

Metoclopramide (Reglan, Clopra, Octamide)

COMMON USES: Relief of diabetic gastroparesis; symptomatic gastroesophageal reflux; relief of cancer chemotherapy-induced nausea and vomiting.
DOSAGE: ***Adults:*** Diabetic gastroparesis: 10 mg PO 30 min ac and hs for 2–8 wk prn; or same dose given IV for 10 d, then switch to PO. Reflux: 10–15 mg PO 30 min ac and hs. Antiemetic: 1–3 mg/kg/dose IV 30 min before antineoplastic agent, then q2h for 2 doses, then q3h for 3 doses. ***Peds:*** Reflux: 0.1 mg/kg/dose PO qid. Antiemetic: 2 mg/kg/dose IV on same schedule as adults.
NOTES: Dystonic reactions common with high doses that can be treated with IV Benadryl; can also be used to facilitate small bowel intubation and radiologic evaluation of the upper gastrointestinal tract.

Metolazone (Diulo, Zaroxolyn)

COMMON USES: Mild to moderate essential hypertension; edema of renal disease or cardiac failure.
DOSAGE: ***Adults:*** Hypertension: 2.5–5 mg PO daily. Edema: 5–20 mg PO daily. ***Peds:*** 0.2–0.4 mg/kg/d PO divided q12h–qd.
NOTES: Monitor fluid and electrolyte status of patient during treatment.

Metoprolol (Lopressor, Toprol XL)

Used for emergency cardiac care.
COMMON USES: Treatment of hypertension, angina, and myocardial infarction.
DOSAGE: Angina: 50–100 mg PO bid. HTN: 100–450 mg PO qd. AMI: 5 mg IV x 3 doses, then 50 mg PO q6h x 48 h, then 100 mg PO bid.

Metronidazole (Flagyl)

COMMON USES: Amebiasis, trichomoniasis, *C difficile,* and anaerobic infections.
DOSAGE: ***Adults:*** Anaerobic infections: 500 mg IV q6–8h. Amebic dysentery: 750 mg PO qd for 5–10 d. Trichomoniasis: 250 mg PO tid for 7 d or 2 g PO in 1 dose. *C difficile:* 500 mg PO or IV q8h for 7–10 d. ***Peds:*** Anaerobic infections: 30 mg/kg/24h PO or IV divided q6h. Amebic dysentery: 35–50 mg/kg/24h PO in 3 divided doses for 5–10 d.
NOTES: For *Trichomonas* infections, also treat partner; reduce dose in hepatic failure; no activity against aerobic bacteria; use in combination in serious mixed infections; may cause disulfiram-like reaction.

Metyrapone (Metopirone)

COMMON USES: Diagnostic test for hypothalamic-pituitary ACTH function.
DOSAGE: Metapyrone test: Day 1: Control period: collect 24-h urine to measure 17-hydroxycorticosteroids (17-OHCS) or 17-ketogenic steroids (17-KSG). Day 2: acTH test: Infuse 50 units acTH over 8 h and measure 24-h urinary steroids. Days 3–4: Rest period. Day 5: Administer metapyrone with milk or snack.

Adults: 750 mg PO q4h for 6 doses. ***Peds:*** 15 mg/kg q4h for 6 doses (min 250-mg dose). Day 6: Determine 24–h urinary steroids.
NOTES: Normal 24-h urine 17-OHCS is 3–12 mg; following ACTH, it increases to 15–45 mg/24h; normal response to metapyrone is between a two- and fourfold increase in 17-OHCS excretion; drug interactions with phenytoin, cyproheptadine, and estrogens may lead to subnormal response.

Metyrosine (Demser)

COMMON USES: Pheochromocytoma; short-term preop and long term when surgery is contraindicated.
DOSAGE: ***Adults*** and **Peds:** > 12 y: 250 mg PO qid, increase by 250–500mg/d up to 4 g/d; maintenance dose 2–3 g/d divided qid.
NOTES: Administer at least 5–7 d preop.

Mexiletine (Mexitil)

COMMON USES: Suppression of symptomatic ventricular arrhythmias.
DOSAGE: Administer with food or antacids; 200–300 mg PO q8h, max 1200 mg/d.
NOTES: Not to be used in cardiogenic shock, second or third degree AV block if no pacemaker; may worsen severe arrhythmias; monitor liver function during therapy; drug interactions with hepatic enzyme inducers and suppressors requiring dosing changes.

Mezlocillin (Mezlin)

COMMON USES: Infections caused by susceptible strains of gram-negative bacteria including *Klebsiella, Proteus, E coli, Enterobacter, P aeruginosa, and Serratia)* involving the skin, bone, respiratory tract, urinary tract, abdomen, and septicemia.
DOSAGE: ***Adults:*** 3 mg IV q4–6h. ***Peds:*** 200–300 mg/kg/d divided q4–6h.
NOTES: Often used in combination with aminoglycosides

Miconazole (Monistat)

COMMON USES: Severe systemic fungal infections including coccidioidomycosis, candidiasis, *Cryptococcus,* and others; various tinea forms; cutaneous candidiasis; vulvovaginal candidiasis; tinea versicolor.
DOSAGE: ***Adults:*** Systemic: from 200–3600 mg/24h IV based on diagnosis divided into 3 doses. Topical: Apply to affected area twice daily for 2–4 wk. Intravaginally: Insert 1 full applicator or suppository at bedtime for 7 d. ***Peds:*** 20–40 mg/kg/24h IV divided q8h.
NOTES: Antagonistic to amphotericin-B in vivo; rapid IV infusion may cause tachycardia or arrhythmias; may potentiate warfarin drug activity.

Midazolam (Versed) [C]

COMMON USES: Preoperative sedation; conscious sedation for short procedures; induction of general anesthesia.
DOSAGE: ***Adults:*** 1–5 mg IV or IM, titrate dose to effect. ***Peds:*** Conscious sedation: 0.08 mg/kg IM 3 1. General anesthesia: 0.15 mg/kg IV followed by 0.05 mg/kg/dose q2min for 1–3 doses as needed to induce anesthesia.
NOTES: Monitor patient for respiratory depression; may produce hypotension in conscious sedation.

Miglitol (Glyset)

COMMON USES: Treatment of Type 2 diabetes mellitus.
DOSAGE: Initial 25 mg PO 3 times daily taken at the first bite of each meal; maintenance 50–100 mg 3 times daily with meals.
NOTES: May be used alone or in combination with sulfonylureas; can cause GI disturbances.

Milrinone (Primacor)

COMMON USES: Treatment of congestive heart failure.
DOSAGE: Loading dose of 50 mg/kg, followed by a continuous infusion of 0.375–0.75 mg/kg/min.
NOTES: Carefully monitor fluid and electrolyte status.

Mineral Oil

COMMON USES: Constipation.
DOSAGE: ***Adults:*** 15–45 mL PO prn. ***Peds:*** > 6 y: 10–20 mL PO bid.

Minoxidil (Loniten, Rogaine)

COMMON USES: Severe hypertension; treatment of male and female pattern baldness.
DOSAGE: ***Adults:*** Oral: 2.5–10 mg PO bid–qid. Topical Rogaine: Apply twice daily to affected area. ***Peds:*** 0.2–1 mg/kg/24h divided PO q12–24h.
NOTES: Pericardial effusion and volume overload may occur; hypertrichosis after chronic use.

Mirtazapine (Remeron)

COMMON USES: Treatment of depression.
DOSAGE: 15 mg PO qhs, up to 45 mg qhs.
NOTES: Do not increase dose at intervals of less than 1–2 wk.

Misoprostol (Cytotec)

COMMON USES: Prevention of NSAID-induced gastric ulcers.
DOSAGE: 200 mg PO qid.
NOTES: Do not take if pregnant; can cause miscarriage with potentially dangerous bleeding; gastrointestinal side effects are common.

Mitomycin (Mutamycin)

COMMON USES: Treatment of breast, cervical, ovarian cancer, and GI adenocarcinomas; intravesical for bladder cancer.
DOSAGE: 20 mg/m^2 IV as a single dose every 6–8 wk; bladder cancer 20–40 mg in 40 mL of NSS via a urethral catheter once a week for 8 wk, followed by monthly treatments for 1 y.
NOTES: May cause cumulative myelosuppression.

Mitoxantrone (Novantrone)

COMMON USES: Treatment of leukemia, lymphoma, prostate and breast cancer.
DOSAGE: 12 mg/m^2/d IV infusion for 2–3 d of each chemotherapy cycle.
NOTES: Causes severe myelosuppression.

Mivacurium (Mivacron)

COMMON USES: Adjunct to general anesthesia or mechanical ventilation.
DOSAGE: ***Adults:*** 0.15 mg/kg/dose IV, may need to repeat at 15-min intervals. ***Peds:*** 0.2 mg/kg/dose IV, may need to repeat at 10-min intervals.

Moexipril (Univasc)

COMMON USES: Treatment of hypertension.
DOSAGE: 7.5–30 mg in 1–2 divided doses administered 1 h before meals.

Molindone (Moban)

COMMON USES: Management of psychotic disorders.
DOSAGE: 5–100 mg PO tid–qid.

Montelukast (Singulair)

COMMON USES: Prophylaxis and treatment of chronic asthma.
DOSAGE: ***Adults:*** > 15 y: 10 mg PO daily taken in the evening. ***Peds:*** 6–14 y: 5 mg PO daily taken in the evening. ***Peds:*** 2–5 y: 4 mg PO daily taken in the evening.

NOTES: NOT for acute asthma attacks.

Moricizine (Ethmozine)

COMMON USES: Treatment of ventricular arrhythmias.
DOSAGE: 200–300 mg PO tid.

Morphine Sulfate [C]

COMMON USES: Relief of severe pain.
DOSAGE: ***Adults:*** Oral: 10–30 mg q4h prn; sustained release tablets 30–60 mg q8–12h. IV/IM: 2.5–15 mg q4h prn. ***Peds:*** 0.1–0.2 mg/kg/dose IM/IV q2–4h prn up to maximum 15 mg/dose.
NOTES: Large number of narcotic side effects; may require scheduled dosing to relieve severe chronic pain.

Moxifloxacin (Avelon)

COMMON USES: Treatment of acute sinusitis, acute bronchitis, and community-acquired pneumonia.
DOSAGE: 400 mg once daily.
NOTES: Active against gram-negative bacteria and *S pneumoniae;* interactions with Mg- , Ca- , Al- , and Fe-containing products and Class IA and III antiarrhythmic agents.

Mupirocin (Bactroban)

COMMON USES: Treatment of impetigo; eradication of MRSA nasal carrier state.
DOSAGE: Topical: apply small amount to affected area. Nasal: apply twice daily in the nostrils.
NOTES: Do not use concurrently with other nasal products.

Muromonab-CD3 (Orthoclone OKT3)

COMMON USES: Treatment of acute rejection following organ transplantation.
DOSAGE: 5 mg IV qd for 10–14 d.
NOTES: This is a murine antibody; may cause significant fever and chills after the first dose.

Mycophenolate Mofetil (Cellcept)

COMMON USES: Prevention of organ rejection following transplantation.
DOSAGE: 1 g PO bid.
NOTES: Used in conjunction with corticosteroids and cyclosporine.

Nabumetone (Relafen)

COMMON USES: Arthritis and pain.
DOSAGE: 1000–2000 mg/d divided qd–bid.

Nadolol (Corgard)

COMMON USES: Hypertension and angina, prevention of migraines.
DOSAGE: 40–80 mg qd; 160 mg/d max.

Nafcillin (Nallpen)

COMMON USES: Treatment of infections caused by susceptible strains of *S aureus* and *Streptococcus.*
DOSAGE: ***Adults:*** 250–500 mg (1 g max) PO q4–6h; 1–2 g IV q4–6h; 500 mg IM q4–6h. ***Peds:*** 50–200 mg/kg/d divided q4–6h(max 12 g/d); 50–100 mg/kg/d divided q6h.
NOTES: No adjustments for renal function.

Nalbuphine (Nubain)

COMMON USES: Moderate to severe pain.
DOSAGE: 10–20 mg IM, IV, SC q4–6h prn.
NOTES: Causes CNS depression and drowsiness; use with caution in patients receiving opiate drugs.

Nalidixic Acid (NegGram)

COMMON USES: Urinary tract infections caused by susceptible strains of *Proteus, Klebsiella, Enterobacter,* and *E coli* but not *Pseudomonas.*
DOSAGE: ***Adults:*** 1 g PO qid for 7–14 d. ***Peds:*** 55 mg/kg/24h in 4 divided doses.
NOTES: Resistance emerges within 48 h in significant percentage of trials; may enhance effect of oral anticoagulants; may cause CNS adverse effects which reverse on discontinuation of the drug.

Naloxone (Narcan)

COMMON USES: Reversal of narcotic effect.
DOSAGE: ***Adults:*** 0.4–2.0 mg IV, IM or SC every 5 min, max dose of 10 mg. ***Peds:*** 0.01 mg/kg/dose IV, IM, or SC; may repeat IV every 3 min for 3 doses prn.
NOTES: May precipitate acute withdrawal in addicts; if no response after 10 mg, suspect a non-narcotic cause.

Naltrexone (Revia)

COMMON USES: Treatment of alcoholism and narcotic addiction.
DOSAGE: 50 mg PO qd.
NOTES: May cause hepatotoxicity; do not give until opioid free for 7–10 d.

Naphazoline and Antazoline (Albalon-A Ophthalmic, others)

Naphazoline and Pheniramine (Naphcon-A Ophthalmic, others)

COMMON USES: Ocular congestion and itching.
DOSAGE: 1–2 drops in eye(s) every 3–4 h.

Naproxen (Naprosyn, Anaprox)

COMMON USES: Treatment of arthritis and pain.
DOSAGE: ***Adults*** and ***Peds:*** > 12 y: 200–500 mg bid–tid, to a maximum of 1500 mg per day.

Nedocromil (Tilade)

COMMON USES: Management of patients with mild-to-moderate asthma.
DOSAGE: 2 inhalations 4 times a day.

Nefazodone (Serzone)

COMMON USES: Treatment of depression.
DOSAGE: Initially, 100 mg PO bid; usual effective range is 300–600 mg/d in 2 divided doses.
NOTES: May cause postural hypotension and allergic reactions.

Neomycin

COMMON USES: Hepatic coma; preop bowel prep; minor skin infections.
DOSAGE: ***Adults:*** 3–12 g/24h PO in 3–4 divided doses. ***Peds:*** 50–100 mg/kg/24h PO in 3–4 divided doses.
NOTES: Part of Nichols-Condon bowel prep.

Neomycin, Polymyxin-B Bladder Irrigant Solution

COMMON USES: Continuous irrigant for prophylaxis against bacteriuria and gram-negative bacteremia associated with indwelling catheter use.
DOSAGE: 1-mL irrigant added to 1-L 0.9% NaCl; continuous irrigation of the bladder with 1–2 L of solution per 24 h.
NOTES: Potential for bacterial or fungal superinfection; possibility for neomycin-induced ototoxicity or nephrotoxicity.

Neomycin, Polymyxin-B and Dexamethasone, (Maxitrol)

COMMON USES: Steroid-responsive ocular conditions with bacterial infection.
DOSAGE: 1–2 drops in eye(s) q4–6h; apply ointment in eye 3–4 times/d.
NOTES: Should be used under supervision of ophthalmologist.

Neomycin, Polymyxin-B, and Hydrocortisone (Cortisporin Ophthalmic and Otic, others)

COMMON USES: Superficial bacterial infections of the eye or external auditory canal by organisms sensitive to neomycin or polymyxin and associated with inflammation; suspension used in the treatment of infections in mastoidectomy and fenestration cavities.
DOSAGE: ***Adults*** and ***Peds:*** Ophthalmic: ointment, apply every 3–4 h; suspension 1 drop q3–4h. Otic: 3–4 drops into external auditory canal tid–qid.
NOTES: Use suspension in cases of ruptured ear drum. Limit use to < 10 d; ocular use should be used under supervision of ophthalmologist

Neomycin, Polymyxin-B and Prednisolone (Poly-Pred)

COMMON USES: Steroid-responsive ocular conditions with bacterial infection.
DOSAGE: 1–2 drops in eye(s) q4–6h; apply ointment in eye 3–4 times/d.
NOTES: Should be used under supervision of ophthalmologist.

Niacin (Nicolar)

COMMON USES: Adjunctive therapy in patients with significant hyperlipidemia who do not respond adequately to diet and weight loss.
DOSAGE: 1–2 g PO tid with meals; up to 8 g/d.
NOTES: Upper body and facial flushing and warmth following dose; may cause gastrointestinal upset and pruritus.

Nicardipine (Cardene)

COMMON USES: Chronic stable angina, hypertension.
DOSAGE: Oral: 20–40 mg PO tid. Sustained release: 30–60 mg PO bid. Intravenous: 0.5–15 mg/h continuous IV infusion. Titrate to desired blood pressure.
NOTES: Oral to IV conversion: 20 mg tid = 0.5 mg/h; 30 mg tid = 1.2 mg/h; 40 mg tid = 2.2 mg/h.

Nicotine Gum (Nicorette, Nicorette DS)

COMMON USES: See Nicotine, Transdermal (below).
DOSAGE: 9–12 pieces/d prn. Maximum 30 pieces per day
NOTES: Patients must stop smoking and perform behavior modification for maximum effect.

Nicotine Nasal Spray (Nicotrol NS)

COMMON USES: Aid to smoking cessation for the relief of nicotine withdrawal.
DOSAGE: 0.5 mg/actuation.
NOTES: Patients must stop smoking and perform behavior modification for maximum effect

Nicotine, Transdermal (Habitrol, Nicoderm, Nicotrol, Prostep)

COMMON USES: Aid to smoking cessation for the relief of nicotine withdrawal.
DOSAGE: Individualized to the patient's needs; apply 1 patch (14–22 mg qd), and taper over 6 wk.
NOTES: Nicotrol to be worn for 16 h to mimic smoking patterns; others worn for 24 h; patients must stop smoking and perform behavior modification for maximum effect.

Nifedipine (Procardia, Procardia XL, Adalat, Adalat CC)

COMMON USES: Vasospastic or chronic stable angina; hypertension.
DOSAGE: ***Adults:*** 10–30 mg PO q8h, maximum 180 mg/d, or sustained release tablets 30–90 mg once daily. ***Peds:*** 0.6–0.9 mg/kg/24h divided tid–qid.
NOTES: Headaches common on initial treatment; reflex tachycardia may occur; Adalat CC and Procardia XL are not interchangeable dosing forms.

Nilutamide (Nilandron)

COMMON USES: Combination with surgical castration for the treatment of metastatic prostate cancer
DOSAGE: 300 mg/d in divided doses for the first 30 d, then 150 mg/d.
NOTES: Toxicity can include hot flashes, loss of libido, impotence, diarrhea, nausea, vomiting, gynecomastia, hepatic dysfunction (Follow LFT's), and interstitial pneumonitis.

Nimodipine (Nimotop)

COMMON USES: Prevention of vasospasms following subarachnoid hemorrhage.
DOSAGE: 60 mg PO q4h for 21 d.
NOTES: Contents of capsule may be extracted and administered through an NG tube if the capsule cannot be swallowed whole.

Nisoldipine (Sular)

COMMON USES: Treatment of hypertension.
DOSAGE: 10–60 mg PO once daily.
NOTES: Do not take with grapefruit juice or high-fat meal

Nitrofurantoin (Macrodantin, Furadantin)

COMMON USES: Urinary tract infections.
DOSAGE: ***Adults:*** Suppression: 50–100 mg PO qd. Treatment: 50–100 mg PO qid. ***Peds:*** 5–7 mg/kg/24h in 4 divided doses.
NOTES: Gastrointestinal side effects common; should be taken with food, milk, or antacid; macrocrystals (Macrodantin) cause less nausea than other forms of drug, may cause pulmonary fibrosis.

Nitroglycerin (Nitrostat, Nitrolingual, Nitro-Bid Ointment, Nitro-bid IV, Nitrodisc, Transderm-Nitro)

COMMON USES: Angina pectoris; acute and prophylactic therapy; congestive heart failure, blood pressure control, pulmonary hypertension in children.
DOSAGE: ***Adults:*** Sublingual: 1 tablet (0.3,0.4,0.6 mg) SL. q5min prn X 3 doses. Translingual: 1–2 doses sprayed under tongue q5 min prn X 3 doses. Oral: 2.5– , 6.5– , or 9-mg sustained-release capsule or tablet PO tid. Intravenous: 5–20 μg/min titrated to effect 200 μg/min max. Topical: 1–2 inches ointment to chest wall q6h, then wipe off at night. Transdermal: 0.2–0.4 mg/h, titrated to 0.4–0.8 mg/h; patches deliver in 24 h: 2.5, 5, 7.5, 10 or 15 mg; keep patch off 10–12 h each day. ***Peds:*** 1 μg/kg/min IV titrated to effect, max 5 μg/kg/min.
NOTES: Tolerance to nitrates develops with chronic use after 1–2 wk; this can be avoided by providing a nitrate-free period each day; shorter acting nitrates should be used on a tid basis, and long-acting patches and ointment should be removed before bedtime to prevent the development of tolerance.

Nitroprusside (Nipride, Nitropress)

COMMON USES: Hypertensive emergency, aortic dissection, pulmonary edema.
DOSAGE: ***Adults*** and ***Peds:*** 0.5–10 μg/kg/min IV infusion titrated to desired effect.
NOTES: Thiocyanate, the metabolite, is excreted by the kidney; thiocyanate toxicity occurs at plasma levels of 5–10 mg/dL; if used to treat aortic dissection, a beta-blocker must be used concomitantly.

Nizatidine (Axid)

COMMON USES: Treatment of duodenal ulcers.
DOSAGE: Active ulcer: 150 mg PO bid or 300 mg PO qhs. Maintenance: 150 mg PO qhs.

Norepinephrine (Levophed)

COMMON USES: Acute hypotensive states.

DOSAGE: ***Adults:*** 8–12 μg/kg/min IV titrated to desired effect. ***Peds:*** 0.1 μg/kg/min IV titrated to desired effect.
NOTES: Correct blood volume depletion as much as possible before initiation of vasopressor therapy; drug interaction with tricyclic antidepressants leading to severe profound hypertension; infuse into large vein to avoid extravasation; phentolamine 5–10 mg/10 mL normal saline injected locally is antidote to extravasation.

Norfloxacin (Noroxin, Chibroxin Ophthalmic)

COMMON USES: Complicated and uncomplicated urinary tract infections resulting from a wide variety of gram-negative bacteria, and prostatitis; topical for ocular infections.
DOSAGE: ***Adults:*** 400 mg PO bid; ophthalmic 1–2 drops qid; if severe use up to q2h. ***Peds:*** Not recommended for use in patients < 18 y.
NOTES: Not for use in pregnancy; drug interactions with antacids, theophylline, and caffeine.

Nortriptyline (Aventyl, Pamelor)

COMMON USES: Endogenous depression.
DOSAGE: 25 mg PO tid to qid; doses above 100 mg/d are not recommended.
NOTES: Many anticholinergic side effects including blurred vision, urinary retention, dry mouth.

Nystatin (Mycostatin, Nilstat)

COMMON USES: Treatment of mucocutaneous *Candida* infections (thrush, vaginitis).
DOSAGE: ***Adults:*** Oral: 400,000–600,000 U PO "swish and swallow" qid or troche 200,000 U 1–2 dissolved in mouth. Vaginal: 1 tablet inserted into vagina qhs. Topical: Apply 2–3 times daily to affected area (cream, ointment or powder). ***Peds:*** Infants: 200,000 U PO q6h. Children: See adult.
NOTES: Not absorbed orally, therefore not effective for systemic infections.

Octreotide Acetate (Sandostatin)

COMMON USES: Suppresses or inhibits severe diarrhea associated with carcinoid and vasoactive intestinal tumors.
DOSAGE: ***Adults:*** 100–600 mg/d SC in 2–4 divided doses. ***Peds:*** 1–10 mg/kg/24h SC in 2–4 divided doses.
NOTES: May cause nausea, vomiting, and abdominal discomfort.

Ofloxacin (Floxin, Ocuflox Ophthalmic)

COMMON USES: Infections of the lower respiratory tract, skin and skin structure, and urinary tract, prostatitis, uncomplicated gonorrhea, and chlamydia infections; topical for bacterial conjunctivitis and otitis externa.
DOSAGE: ***Adults:*** 200–400 mg PO bid or IV q12h. ***Adults*** and ***Peds > 1 y:*** Ophthalmic: 1–2 drops in eye(s) q2–4h for 2 d, then qid for 5 additional days. ***Peds:*** Systemic administration should not be used in children < 18 y. ***Peds 1–12 y:*** Otic: 5 drops in ear bid for 10 d. ***Peds > 12 y*** and ***Adults*** otic: 10 drops in ear bid for 10 d.
NOTES: May cause nausea, vomiting, diarrhea, insomnia and headache; drug interactions with antacids, sucralfate, and iron- and zinc-containing products that decrease the absorption of ofloxacin; may increase theophylline levels.

Olanzapine (Zyprexa)

COMMON USES: Treatment of psychotic disorders.
DOSAGE: Titrate up to maximum of 20 mg/d.
NOTES: May take many weeks to titrate to therapeutic dose; cigarette smoking will decease levels.

Olsalazine (Dipentum)

COMMON USES: Maintenance of remission of ulcerative colitis.
DOSAGE: 500 mg PO bid.
NOTES: Take with food; may cause diarrhea.

Omeprazole (Prilosec)

COMMON USES: Treatment of duodenal and gastric ulcers, Zollinger-Ellison syndrome, GERD, and *H pylori* infections.
DOSAGE: 20–40 mg PO qd-bid.
NOTES: Combination therapy necessary for *H pylori.*

Ondansetron (Zofran)

COMMON USES: Prevention of nausea and vomiting associated with cancer chemotherapy and postoperative nausea and vomiting.
DOSAGE: ***Adults*** and ***Peds:*** Chemotherapy: 0.15 mg/kg/dose IV before chemotherapy, then repeated 4 and 8 h after the first dose or 4–8 mg PO tid, administer first dose 30 min before chemotherapy. ***Adults:*** Postop: 4 mg IV immediately before induction or postop.
NOTES: May cause diarrhea and headache.

Orpernadrine (Norflex)

COMMON USES: Treatment of muscle spasms.
DOSAGE: 60–100 mg bid.
NOTES: Dose dependent on route of administration.

Oseltamivir (Tamiflu)

COMMON USES: Treatment of influenza A and B.
DOSAGE: 75 mg twice daily for 5 d.

Oxacillin (Bactocill, Prostaphlin)

COMMON USES: Treatment of infections caused by susceptible strains of *S aureus* and *Streptococcus.*
DOSAGE: ***Adults:*** 1–2 mg IV q4–6h. ***Peds:*** 150–200 mg/kg/d IV q4–6h.

Oxaprozin (Daypro)

COMMON USES: Treatment of arthritis and pain.
DOSAGE: 600–1200 mg qd.

Oxazepam (Serax) [C]

COMMON USES: Anxiety; acute alcohol withdrawal; anxiety with depressive symptoms.
DOSAGE: 10–15 mg PO tid–qid; severe anxiety and alcohol withdrawal may require up to 30 mg qid.
NOTES: Oxazepam is one of the metabolites of diazepam (Valium).

Oxcarbazepine (Trileptal)

COMMON USES: Treatment of partial seizures.
DOSAGE: ***Adults:*** 300 mg, increase dose weekly to a usual dose of 1200–2400 mg/d. ***Peds:*** 8–10 mg/kg PO bid, 600 mg/d max; increase dose weekly to target maintenance dose.
NOTES: May cause hyponatremia.

Oxybutynin (Ditropan, Ditropan XL)

COMMON USES: Symptomatic relief of urgency, nocturia, and incontinence associated with neurogenic or reflex neurogenic bladder.
DOSAGE: ***Adults*** and ***Peds > 5 y:*** 5 mg PO tid–qid. ***Adults:*** extended release 5 mg PO qd; can titrate up to 30 mg PO, qd (5 and 10 mg/tab). **Peds 1–5 y:** 0.02 mg/kg/dose 2–4 times a day (syrup 5 mg/5 mL).
NOTES: Anticholinergic side effects (dry mouth, constipation, dry eyes, somnolence, others).

Oxycodone (OxyContin, Roxicodone, others) [C]

COMMON USES: Moderate-to-severe pain usually in combination with other analgesics.

DOSAGE: ***Adults:*** 5 mg PO q4–6h prn; 10–40 mg PO q12h sustained release. ***Peds:*** 6–12 y: 1.25 mg PO q6h prn. >12 y :2.5 mg PO q6h prn
NOTES: Sustained release (OxyContin) 10, 20, 40, 80 mg; liquid 5 mg/5mL, solution 20 mg/mL

Oxycodone and Acetaminophen (Percocet, Tylox) [C]

COMMON USES: Moderate-to-severe pain.
DOSAGE: ***Adults:*** 1–2 tablets/capsules PO q4–6h prn (Specify oxycodone/acetaminophen dose). ***Peds:*** 0.05–0.15 mg/kg/dose q4–6h, max 5 mg/dose (based on oxycodone).
NOTES: Supplied as: (Percocet : oxycodone/acetaminophen, 2.5 mg/325 mg, 5 mg/325 mg, 7.5mg/500 mg, 10 mg/500 mg; Tylox: 5- mg oxycodone, 500-mg acetaminophen) solution 5-mg oxycodone/325-mg acetaminophen/5 mL.

Oxycodone and Aspirin (Percodan, Percodan-Demi) [C]

COMMON USES: Moderate to moderately severe pain.
DOSAGE: ***Adults:*** 1–2 tablets/capsules PO q4–6h prn. ***Peds:*** 0.05–0.15 mg/kg/dose q4–6h, max 5 mg/dose (based on oxycodone).
NOTES: (Percodan : 4.5-mg oxycodone hydrochloride 0.38-mg oxycodone terephthalate, 325-mg aspirin; Pedcodan-Demi: 2.25-mg oxycodone hydrochloride, 0.19-mg oxycodone terephthalate, 325-mg aspirin).

Oxymorphone (Numorphan) [C]

COMMON USES: Treatment of moderate-to-severe pain, sedative.
DOSAGE: 0.5 mg IM, SC, IV initially, 1–1.5 mg q4–6h prn. Rectal: 5 mg q4–6h prn
NOTES: Chemically related to hydromorphone.

Oxytocin (Pitocin, Syntocinon)

COMMON USES: Induction of labor; control of postpartum hemorrhage.
DOSAGE: 0.001–0.002 U/min IV titrate to effect, max 0.02 U/min.
NOTES: Can cause uterine rupture and fetal death; monitor vital signs closely.

Paclitaxel (Taxol)

COMMON USES: Treatment of ovarian cancer.
DOSAGE: 135 mg/m^2 IV every 3 wk.
NOTES: May cause severe neutropenia.

Pancreatin

Pancrelipase (Pancrease, Cotazym)

COMMON USES: For patients deficient in exocrine pancreatic secretions (cystic fibrosis, chronic pancreatitis, other pancreatic insufficiency), and for steatorrhea of malabsorption syndrome.
DOSAGE: ***Adults*** and ***Peds:*** 1–3 capsules (tablets) with meals and snacks may be increased up to 8 capsules (tablets).
NOTES: Avoid antacids; may cause nausea, abdominal cramps, or diarrhea; do not crush or chew enteric-coated products.

Pancuronium (Pavulon)

COMMON USES: Aids in the management of patients on mechanical ventilator, intraoperative muscle relaxation.
DOSAGE: ***Adults:*** 2–4 mg IV q2–4h prn. ***Peds:*** 0.02–0.10 mg/kg/dose q2–4h prn.
NOTES: Patient must be intubated and on controlled ventilation; use adequate amount of sedation or analgesia.

Paregoric [C]

COMMON USES: Diarrhea, pain and neonatal withdrawal syndrome.
DOSAGE: ***Adults:*** 5–10 mL qd–qid prn.
NOTES: Contains opium.

Paroxetine (Paxil)

COMMON USES: Depression.
DOSAGE: 20–50 mg PO as a single daily dose.

Pantoprazole (Protonix)

COMMON USES: GERD.
DOSAGE: 40 mg PO once daily.
NOTES: Delayed-release tablet, therefore do not crush or chew tablet

Penbutolol (Levatol)

COMMON USES: Hypertension
DOSAGE: 20–40 mg qd.

Penicillin G Aqueous, Potassium or Sodium (Pfizerpen, Pentids)

COMMON USES: Most gram-positive infections (except penicillin-resistant staphylococci) including streptococci, *N meningitidis,* syphilis, clostridia, corynebacteria, and some coliforms.
DOSAGE: ***Adults:*** 400,000–800,000 units PO qid; IV doses vary greatly depending on indications; range: 1.2–24 million U/d. ***Peds:*** Newborns < 1 wk: 25,000–50,000 U/kg/dose IV q12h. Infants 1 wk–1 mo: 25,000–50,000 U/kg/dose IV q8h. Children: 100,000–300,000 U/kg/24h IV divided q4h.
NOTES: Watch for hypersensitivity reactions; drug of choice for group A streptococcal infections and syphilis.

Penicillin G Benzathine (Bicillin)

COMMON USES: Useful as a single-dose treatment regimen for streptococcal pharyngitis, rheumatic fever and glomerulonephritis prophylaxis, and syphilis.
DOSAGE: ***Adults:*** 1.2–2.4 million U deep IM injection q2–4 wk. ***Peds:*** 50,000 U/kg/dose to a maximum of 2.4 million U/dose deep IM injection q2–4wk.
NOTES: Sustained action with detectable levels up to 4 wk; considered drug of choice for treatment of noncongenital syphilis; Bicillin L-A contains the benzathine salt only; Bicillin C-R contains a combination of the benzathine and procaine salts and is used for most acute strep infections (300,000 U procaine with 300,000 U benzathine/mL or 900,000 U benzathine with 300,000 U procaine/2 mL).

Penicillin G Procaine (Wycillin, others)

COMMON USES: Moderately severe infections caused by penicillin G-sensitive organisms that respond to low persistent serum levels (syphilis, uncomplicated pneumococcal pneumonia).
DOSAGE: ***Adults:*** 300,000–1.2 million U/d IM divided qd–bid. ***Peds:*** 25,000–50,000 U/kg/d IM divided qd–bid.
NOTES: A long-acting parenteral penicillin; blood levels up to 15 h; give probenecid at least 30 min before administration of penicillin to prolong action.

Penicillin V (Pen-Vee K, Veetids, others)

COMMON USES: Most gram-positive infections (except penicillin-resistant staphylococci) including streptococci, *N meningitidis,* syphilis, clostridia, corynebacteria, and some coliforms.
DOSAGE: ***Adults:*** 250–500 mg PO q6h. ***Peds:*** 25–50 mg/kg/24h PO in 4 divided doses.
NOTES: A well-tolerated oral penicillin; 250 mg = 400,000 U Penicillin G.

Pentamidine Isethionate (Pentam 300, NebuPent)

COMMON USES: Treatment and prevention of *P carinii* pneumonia.
DOSAGE: ***Adults*** and ***Peds:*** 4 mg/kg/24h IV daily for 14–21 d. ***Adults:*** Prevention: 300 mg once every 4 wk, administered via Respirgard II nebulizer.

NOTES: Monitor patient for severe hypotension following IV administration; associated with pancreatic islet-cell necrosis leading to hypoglycemia and hyperglycemia; monitor hematology labs for leukopenia and thrombocytopenia.

Pentazocine (Talwin) [C]

COMMON USES: Moderate-to-severe pain.
DOSAGE: 30 mg IM or IV; 50–100 mg PO q3–4h prn.
NOTES: 30–60 mg IM equianalgesic to 10-mg morphine IM; associated with considerable dysphoria.

Pentobarbital (Nembutal, others) [C]

COMMON USES: Insomnia, convulsions, induced coma following severe head injury.
DOSAGE: ***Adults:*** Sedative: 20–40 mg PO or PR q6–12h. Hypnotic: 100–200 mg PO or PR qhs prn. Induced coma: load 3–5 mg/kg IV 3 1, then maintenance 2–3.5 mg/kg/dose IV q1h prn to keep level between 25–40 mg/mL. ***Peds:*** Hypnotic: 2–6 mg/kg/dose PO qhs prn. Induced coma: See adult.
NOTES: Can cause respiratory depression; may produce hypotension when used IV for cerebral edema; tolerance to sedative-hypnotic effect acquired within 1–2 wk.

Pentosan Polysulfate Sodium (Elmiron)

COMMON USES: Bladder pain and discomfort associated with interstitial cystitis.
DOSAGE: 100 mg PO 3 times a day.
NOTES: Alopecia, diarrhea, nausea, and headaches have been reported.

Pentoxifylline (Trental)

COMMON USES: Intermittent claudication.
DOSAGE: 400 mg PO tid with meals.
NOTES: Treat for at least 8 wk to see full effect.

Pergolide (Permax)

COMMON USES: Parkinson's disease.
DOSAGE: Initially 0.05 mg PO tid, titrated every 2–3 d to desired effect.
NOTES: May cause hypotension during initiation of therapy.

Perindopril (Aceon)

COMMON USES: Treatment of hypertension and CHF.
DOSAGE: 4–8 mg daily.
NOTES: Avoid taking with food.

Permethin (Elimite, Nix)

COMMON USES: Eradication of lice.
DOSAGE: ***Adults*** and ***Peds:*** Lice: Saturate hair and scalp with cream rinse; allow to remain in hair for 10 min before rinsing out. Scabies: apply cream over entire body; rinse after 8–14 h.

Perphenazine (Trilafon)

COMMON USES: Psychotic disorders, intractable hiccups, severe nausea.
DOSAGE: Antipsychotic: 4–8 mg PO tid, maximum 64 mg/d. Hiccups: 5 mg IM q6h prn or 1 mg IV at not less than 1–2 mg/min intervals up to 5 mg.

Phenazopyridine (Pyridium)

COMMON USES: Symptomatic relief of discomfort from lower urinary tract irritation.
DOSAGE: ***Adults:*** 200 mg PO tid. ***Peds:*** 6–12 y: 12 mg/kg/24h PO in 3 divided doses.
NOTES: Gastrointestinal disturbances; causes red-orange urine color, which can stain clothing.

Phenobarbital [C]

COMMON USES: Seizure disorders, insomnia, anxiety.

DOSAGE: ***Adults:*** Sedative-hypnotic: 30–120 mg PO or IM qd prn. Anticonvulsant: Load 10–12 mg/kg in 3 divided doses, then 1–3 mg/kg/24h PO, IM, or IV. ***Peds:*** Sedative-hypnotic: 2–3 mg/kg/24h PO or IM qhs prn. Anticonvulsant: Load 15–20 mg/kg divided into 2 equal doses 4 h apart, then 3–5 mg/kg/24h PO divided in 2–3 doses.

NOTES: Tolerance develops to sedation; paradoxical hyperactivity seen in pediatric patients; long half-life allows single daily dosing. See levels page 457.

Phenylephrine (Neo-Synephrine)

COMMON USES: Treatment of vascular failure in shock, hypersensitivity, or drug-induced hypotension; nasal congestion; mydriatic.

DOSAGE: ***Adults:*** Mild to moderate hypotension: 2–5 mg IM or SC elevates BP for 2 h; 0.1–0.5 mg IV elevates BP for 15 min. Severe hypotension/shock: Infusion at 100–180 mg/min; after BP stabilized, maintenance rate of 40–60 mg/min. Nasal congestion: 1–2 sprays into each nostril prn. ***Adults*** and ***Peds:*** > 1: Mydriasis: 1 drop 2.5–10% solution in eye(s) 30 min before procedure; may repeat in 10–60 min if needed. ***Peds:*** Hypotension: 5–20 mg/kg/dose IV q10–15 min or 0.1–0.5 mg/kg/min IV infusion titrated to desired effect. Nasal congestion: 1 spray into each nostril q3–4h prn. ***Peds:*** < 1: Mydriasis: 1 drop 2.5% solution in eye(s) 30 min before procedure.

NOTES: Promptly restore blood volume if loss has occurred; use caution in patients with hyperthyroidism, bradycardia, partial heart block, myocardial disease, or severe arteriosclerosis; use large veins for infusion to avoid extravasation; phentolamine 10 mg in 10–15 mL saline for local injection as antidote for extravasation; activity potentiated by oxytocin, MAOIs, and tricyclic antidepressants.

Phenytoin (Dilantin)

COMMON USES: Tonic-clonic and partial seizures.

DOSAGE: ***Adults*** and ***Peds:*** Load: 15–20 mg/kg, IV at a max infusion rate of 25 mg/min or orally in 400-mg doses at 4-h intervals. ***Adults:*** Maintenance: 200 mg PO or IV bid or 300 mg qhs initially then follow serum level. ***Peds:*** Maintenance: 4–7 mg/kg/24h PO or IV divided qd–bid.

NOTES: Caution with cardiac depressant side effects, especially with IV administration; follow levels as needed (see Table IX–3, Page 457); nystagmus and ataxia are early signs of toxicity; gum hyperplasia occurs with long-term use; avoid use of oral suspension if possible because of erratic absorption; avoid use in pregnancy.

Physostigmine (Antilirium)

COMMON USES: Antidote for tricyclic antidepressant, atropine, and scopolamine overdose.

DOSAGE: ***Adults:*** 2 mg IV/IM q15min. ***Peds:*** 0.01–0.03 mg/kg/dose IV q15–30 min.

NOTES: Rapid IV administration associated with convulsions; cholinergic side effects; may cause asystole.

Phytonadione [Vitamin K] (AquaMEPHYTON, others)

COMMON USES: Coagulation disorders caused by faulty formation of factors II, VII, IX, and X, hyperalimentation.

DOSAGE: ***Adults*** and ***Peds:*** Anticoagulant-induced prothrombin deficiency: 2.5–10.0 mg PO or IV slowly. Hyperalimentation: 10 mg IM or IV every week. Infants: 0.5–1.0 mg/dose IM, SC, or PO.

NOTES: With parenteral treatment, usually see first change in prothrombin in 12–24 h; anaphylaxis can result from IV dosing; should be administered slowly IV.

Pilocarpine (Salagen Oral, Ocusert Pilo 20, Ocusert Pilo 40, others)

COMMON USES: Glaucoma and to reverse cycloplegia; radiation-induced xerostomia.

DOSAGE: Reversal mydriasis: 1 drop 1% solution to eye. Glaucoma: 1–2 drops hydrochloride solution up to 6 times a day; titrate based on pressures; 0.5″ ribbon into eye qhs; Ocusert: 1 in eye weekly.
NOTES: Ocusert implant system releases 20 or 40 μg/h over 1 wk.

Pindolol (Visken)

COMMON USES: Treatment of hypertension.
DOSAGE: 5–10 mg bid.

Pioglitazone (Actos)

COMMON USES: Management of Type 2 diabetes.
DOSAGE: 15–45 mg once daily.

Pipecuronium (Arduan)

COMMON USES: Adjunct to general anesthesia.
DOSAGE: ***Adults:*** 50–100 mg/kg IV. ***Peds:*** 40–57 mg/kg IV.

Piperacillin (Pipracil)

COMMON USES: Infections caused by susceptible strains of gram-negative bacteria including *Klebsiella, Proteus, E. coli, Enterobacter, P aeruginosa,* and *Serratia*) involving the skin, bone, respiratory tract, urinary tract, abdomen, and septicemia.
DOSAGE: ***Adults:*** 3 g IV q4–6h. ***Peds:*** 200–300 mg/kg/d IV divided q4–6h.
NOTES: Often used in combination with aminoglycosides

Piperacillin/Tazobactam (Zosyn)

COMMON USES: Treatment of infections caused by susceptible strains of gram-negative bacteria including *Klebsiella, Proteus, E coli, Enterobacter, P aeruginosa,* and *Serratia)* involving the skin, bone, respiratory tract, urinary tract, abdomen, and septicemia.
DOSAGE: ***Adults:*** 3.375–4.5 g IV q6h.
NOTES: Often used in combination with aminoglycosides

Pirbuterol (Maxair)

COMMON USES: Prevention and reversal of bronchospasm.
DOSAGE: ***Adults*** and ***Peds:*** > 12 y : 2 inhalations q4–6h, maximum of 12 inhalations per day.

Piroxicam (Feldene)

COMMON USES: Treatment of arthritis and pain.
DOSAGE: 10–20 mg qd.

Plasma Protein Fraction (Plasmanate, others)

COMMON USES: Shock and hypotension.
DOSAGE: ***Adults:*** 250–500 mL IV initially (not 0.10 mL/min); subsequent infusions should depend on clinical response. ***Peds:*** 10–15 mL/kg/dose IV; subsequent infusions should depend on clinical response.
NOTES: Hypotension associated with rapid infusion; 130–160 mEq sodium/L; not a substitute for red cells.

Plicamycin (Mithracin)

COMMON USES: Hypercalcemia of malignancy.
DOSAGE: 25 mg/kg/d IV for 3–4 d.

Pneumococcal Vaccine, Polyvalent (Pneumovax-23)

COMMON USES: Immunization against pneumococcal infections in patients predisposed to or at high risk of acquiring these infections (ie, before elective splenectomy).
DOSAGE: ***Adults*** and ***Peds:*** > 2 y: 0.5 mL IM.
NOTES: Do not vaccinate during immunosuppressive therapy.

Pneumococcal 7-Valent Conjugate Vaccine (Prevnar)

COMMON USES: Immunization against pneumococcal infections in infants and children.
DOSAGE: 0.5 mL IM per dose; series consists of 3 doses; first dose at 2 mo with subsequent doses every 2 mo.

Polyethylene Glycol-electrolyte Solution (Go-LYTLEY, CoLyte)

COMMON USES: Bowel cleansing before examination or surgery.
DOSAGE: ***Adults:*** Following 3–4 h fast, the patient must drink 240 mL of solution every 10 min until 4 L is consumed. ***Peds:*** 25–40 mL/kg/h over 4–10 h.
NOTES: First bowel movement should occur in approximately 1 h; may cause some cramping or nausea.

Porfimer (Photofrin)

COMMON USES: Photodynamic therapy of early endobronchial non-small cell cancer; palliation of esophageal cancer.
DOSAGE: 2 mg/kg IV over 3–5 min (follow up with photo dynamic therapy 40–50h later).

Potassium Citrate (Urocit-K)

COMMON USES: Alkalinize urine, prevention of urinary stones (uric acid, calcium stones if hypocitraturic; urinary alkalinizer.
DOSAGE: 10–20 mEq PO tid with meals, max 100 mEq/d.
NOTES: Tablets: 540 mg = 5 mEq, 1080 mg = 10 mEq.

Potassium Citrate and Citric Acid (Polycitra-K)

COMMON USES: Alkalinize urine, prevention of urinary stones (uric acid, calcium stones if hypocitraturic; urinary alkalinizer.
DOSAGE: 10–20 mEq PO tid with meals, max 100 mEq/d.
NOTES: Solution, 10 mEq/5 mL; powder, 30 mEq/packet.

Potassium Idodide [Lugol's solution] (SSKI, Thyro-Block)

COMMON USES: Thyroid crisis, reduction of vascularity before thyroid surgery, thin bronchial secretions.
DOSAGE: Preop thyroidectomy:***Adults*** and ***Peds:*** 50–250 mg PO tid 3 times/d (2–6 drops strong iodine solution); administer for 10 d before surgery. Thyroid crisis: ***Adults*** and ***Peds:*** > 1 y: 300 mg (6 drops SSKI q8h); Infants < 1 y: 1/2 dose.
NOTES: SSKI = 1 g/mL, Lugol's = 100 mg/mL.

Potassium Supplements

COMMON USES: Prevention or treatment of hypokalemia.
DOSAGE: ***Adults:*** 20–100 mEq/d PO divided qd–bid; IV 10–20 mEq/h, max 40 mEq/h and 150 mEq/d (monitor frequent potassium levels when using high-dose IV infusions). ***Peds:*** Calculate potassium deficit; 1–3 mEq/kg/d PO divided qd–qid; IV max dose 0.5–1 mEq/kg/h.
NOTES: Dosing ranges based on clinical conditions. See Table IX–6 on page 522 for oral agents. Can cause gastrointestinal irritation; powder and liquids must be mixed with beverage (unsalted tomato juice, etc); use cautiously in renal insufficiency, and along with NSAIDs and ACE inhibitors; chloride salt recommended in coexisting alkalosis; for coexisting acidosis, use acetate, bicarbonate, citrate or gluconate salt.

Pramipexole (Mirapex)

COMMON USES: Treatment of Parkinson's disease.
DOSAGE: 1.5–4.5 mg/d; titrated slowly.

Pramoxine (Anusol, ProctoFoam-NS, others)

TABLE IX–6. SOME COMMON ORAL POTASSIUM SUPPLEMENTS.

Brand Name	Salt	Form	mEq Potassium/ Dosing Unit
Glu-K	Gluconate	Tablet	2 mEq/tablet
Kaochlor 10%	KCl	Liquid	20 mEq/15 mL
Kaochlor S-F 10% (sugar-free)	KCl	Liquid	20 mEq/15 mL
Kaochlor Eff	Bicarbonate/KCl/ citrate	Effervescent tablet	20 mEq/tablet
Kaon Elixir	Gluconate	Liquid	20 mEq/15 mL
Kaon	Gluconate	Tablet	5 mEq/tablet
Kaon-Cl	KCl	Tablet, SR	6.67 mEq/tablet
Kaon-Cl 20%	KCl	Liquid	40 mEq/15 mL
KayCiel	KCl	Liquid	20 mEq/15 mL
K-Lor	KCl	Powder	15 or 20 mEq/packet
Klorvess	Bicarbonate/KCl	Liquid	20 mEq/15 mL
Klotrix	KCl	Tablet, SR	10 mEq/tablet
K-Lyte	Bicarbonate/citrate	Effervescent tablet	25 mEq/tablet
K-Tab	KCl	Tablet, SR	10 mEq/tablet
Micro-K	KCl	Capsule, SR	8 mEq/capsule
Slow-K	KCl	Tablet, SR	8 mEq/tablet
Tri-K	Acetate/bicarbonate and citrate	Liquid	45 mEq/15 mL
Twin-K	Citrate/gluconate	Liquid	20 mEq/5 mL

Pramoxine With Hydrocortisone (Proctofoam-HC, Anusol-HC, others)

COMMON USES: Relief of pain and itching from external and internal hemorrhoids and anorectal surgery.
DOSAGE: 1 suppository every morning and bedtime and following each bowel movement; apply cream, ointment, gel or spray, freely to anal area q6–12h.
NOTES: Anusol-HC/Proctofoam HC contains 1% hydrocortisone

Pravastatin (Pravachol)

COMMON USES: Reduction of elevated cholesterol levels.
DOSAGE: 10–40 mg PO qhs.

Prazepam (Centrax) [C]

COMMON USES: Anxiety disorders.
DOSAGE: 5–10 mg PO tid–qid, or 20–50 mg PO as single bedtime dose to minimize daytime drowsiness.

Prazosin (Minipres)

COMMON USES: Hypertension and CHF.
DOSAGE: ***Adults:*** 1 mg PO tid; to total daily dose of 20 mg/d prn. ***Peds:*** 5–25 mg/kg/dose q6h.

NOTES: Can cause orthostatic hypotension, so the patient should take the first dose at bedtime; tolerance develops to this effect; tachyphylaxis may result.

Prednisone

See "Steroids," page 529 and Table IX, page 475.

Prednisolone

See "Steroids," page 529 and Table IX, page 475.

Prednisolone, Ophthalmic (AK-Pred Ophthalmic, Pred-Forte Ophthalmic, others)

COMMON USES: Iritis, postoperative inflammation, palpebral and bulbar conjunctivitis, chemical, radiation or thermal injury, corneal abrasion.
DOSAGE: 1–2 drops in eye(s) every hour during day and q2h at night until inflammation subsides; then 1 drop q4h.
NOTES: Can increase intraocular pressure, cause cataracts, and worsen herpes keratitis.

Probenecid (Benemid)

COMMON USES: Gout, maintenance of serum levels of penicillins or cephalosporins.
DOSAGE: ***Adults:*** Gout: 0.25 g bid for 1 wk; then 0.5 g PO bid. Antibiotic effect: 1–2 g PO 30 min before dose of antibiotic. ***Peds:*** 25 mg/kg, then 40 mg/kg/d PO divided qid.

Procainamide (Pronestyl, Procan)

COMMON USES: Treatment of supraventricular and ventricular arrhythmias.
DOSAGE: ***Adults:*** Emergency cardiac care: 100–200 mg/dose IV q5min until dysrhythmia resolves, hypotension ensues, or dose totals 1 g; then maintenance of 1–4 mg/min IV infusion. Chronic dosing: 50 mg/kg/d PO in divided doses q4–6h. ***Peds:*** Emergency cardiac care: 3–6 mg/kg/dose IV over 5 min, then 20–80 mg/kg/min IV infusion. Maintenance: 15–50 mg/kg/24h PO divided q3–6h.
NOTES: Can cause hypotension and a lupus-like syndrome; dose adjustment renal impairment; see Table IX–3, page 457.

Prochlorperazine (Compazine)

COMMON USES: Nausea, vomiting, agitation, psychotic disorders.
DOSAGE: ***Adults:*** Antiemetic: 5–10 mg PO tid–qid or 25 mg PR bid or 5–10 mg IM q4–6h. Antipsychotic: 10–20 mg IM acutely or 5–10 mg PO tid–qid for maintenance. ***Peds:*** 0.1–0.15 mg/kg/dose IM q4–6h or 0.4 mg/kg/24h PO divided tid–qid.
NOTES: Much larger dose may be required for antipsychotic effect; extrapyramidal side effects common; treat acute extrapyramidal reactions with diphenhydramine.

Procyclidine (Kemadrin)

COMMON USES: Treatment of Parkinson's syndrome.
DOSAGE: 2.5 mg PO tid.
NOTES: Contraindicated for glaucoma patients.

Promethazine (Phenergan)

COMMON USES: Nausea, vomiting, motion sickness.
DOSAGE: ***Adults:*** 12.5–50 mg PO, PR, or IM bid–qid prn. ***Peds:*** 0.1–0.5 mg/kg/dose PO or IM q4–6h prn.
NOTES: High incidence of drowsiness.

Propafenone (Rythmol)

COMMON USES: Treatment of life-threatening ventricular arrhythmias.
DOSAGE: 150–300 mg PO q8h.
NOTES: May cause dizziness, unusual taste, and first- degree heart block.

Propantheline (Pro-Banthine)

COMMON USES: Symptomatic treatment of small intestine hypermotility, spastic colon, ureteral spasm, bladder spasm, and pylorospasm.

DOSAGE: ***Adults:*** 15 mg PO ac and 30 mg PO hs. ***Peds:*** 1.5–3.0 mg/kg/24h PO divided tid–qid.

NOTES: Anticholinergic side effects such as dry mouth, blurred vision are common.

Propofol (Diprivan)

COMMON USES: Induction or maintenance of anesthesia; continuous sedation in intubated patients.

DOSAGE: Anesthesia: 20–40 mg every 10 min until induction onset, then 50–200 mg/kg/min continuous infusion. ICU sedation: 5–50 mg/kg/min continuous infusion.

NOTES: 1 mL of propofol contains 0.1 g of fat; may increase serum triglycerides when administered for extended periods.

Propoxyphene (Darvon) [C]

Propoxyphene and Acetaminophen (Darvocet) [C]

Propoxyphene and Aspirin (Darvon Compound-65, Darvon-N With Aspirin) [C]

COMMON USES: Mild-to-moderate pain.

DOSAGE: 1–2 PO q4h prn.

NOTES: Darvon: propoxyphene HCl capsule 65 mg. Darvon-N: propoxyphene napsylate 100-mg tablet. Darvocet-N: Propoxyphene napsylate 50 mg/acetaminophen 325 mg. Darvocet-N 100: Propoxyphene napsylate 100 mg/acetaminophen 650 mg. Darvon Compound-65: Propoxyphene HCl 65-mg/aspirin 389-mg/caffeine 32-mg capsules. Darvon- N with Aspirin: Propoxyphene napsylate 100 mg/aspirin 325 mg.

Propranolol (Inderal)

COMMON USES: Treatment of hypertension, angina, myocardial infarction prophylaxis, arrhythmias (a-fib, a-flutter, others) essential tremor, pheochromocytoma, thyrotoxicosis, migraine prevention.

DOSAGE: ***Adults:*** Angina: 80–320 mg PO qd divided bid–qid or 80–160 mg SR qd. Arrhythmia: 10–80 mg PO tid–qid or 1 mg IV slowly, repeat q5min up to 5 mg. HTN: 40 mg PO bid or 60–80 mg SR qd, increase weekly to max 640 mg/d. Hypertrophic Subaortic Stenosis: 20–40 mg PO tid–qid. MI: 180–240 mg PO divided tid–qid. Migraine Prophylaxis: 80 mg/d divided qid–tid, increase weekly to max 160–240 mg/d divided tid–qid; wean off if no response in 6 wk. Pheochromocytoma: 30–60 mg/d divided tid–qid. Thyrotoxicosis: 1–3 mg IV single dose; 10–40 mg PO q6h. Tremor: 40 mg PO bid, increase as needed to max 320 mg/d. ***Peds:*** Arrhythmia 0.5–1.0 mg/kg/d divided tid–qid, increase as needed q3–7d to max 60 mg/d; 0.01–0.1 mg/kg IV over 10 min, max dose 1 mg. Hypertension: 0.5–1.0 mg/kg divided bid–qid, increase as needed q3–7d to 2 mg/kg/d max.

Propylthiouracil [PTU]

COMMON USES: Hyperthyroidism.

DOSAGE: ***Adults:*** 100 mg PO q8h increase up to 1200 mg/d); after euthyroid (6–8 wk), taper dose by 1/3 every 4–6 wk to a maintenance dose of 50–150 mg/24h; treatment is often discontinued in 2–3 y. ***Peds:*** Initial 5–7 mg/kg/24h PO divided q8h, then maintenance of 1/3–2/3 of initial dose.

NOTES: Follow patient clinically; monitor thyroid function tests.

Protamine Sulfate

COMMON USES: Reversal of heparin effect.

DOSAGE: ***Adults*** and ***Peds:*** Based on amount of heparin reversal desired; given slow IV, 1 mg will reverse approximately 100 U of heparin given in the preceding 3–4h to max dose of 50 mg.

NOTES: Follow coagulation studies; may have anticoagulant effect if given without heparin.

Pseudoephedrine (Sudafed, Novafed, Afrinol)

COMMON USES: Decongestant.
DOSAGE: ***Adults:*** 30–60 mg PO q6–8h; sustained release capsules 120 mg PO q12h. ***Peds:*** 4 mg/kg/24h PO divided qid.
NOTES: Contraindicated in patients with hypertension or coronary artery disease and in patients taking MAO inhibitors; an ingredient in many cough and cold preparations.

Psyllium (Metamucil, Serutan, Effer-Syllium)

COMMON USES: Constipation, diverticular disease of the colon.
DOSAGE: 1 teaspoon (7 g) in a glass of water qd–tid.
NOTES: Do not use if bowel obstruction is suspect; one of the safest laxatives; psyllium in effervescent (Effer-syllium) form usually contains potassium and should be used with caution in patients with renal failure.

Pyrazinamide

COMMON USES: Treatment of active tuberculosis.
DOSAGE: ***Adults:*** 20–35 mg/kg/24h PO divided tid–qid, maximum dose is 3 g/d. ***Peds:*** 15–30 mg/kg/d PO divided bid or qd.
NOTES: May cause hepatotoxicity; use in combination with other antituberculosis drugs.

Pyridoxine (Vitamin B6)

COMMON USES: Treatment and prevention of vitamin B6 deficiency.
DOSAGE: Deficiency: 2.5–10.0 mg PO qd. Drug-induced neuritis: 50 mg PO qd.

Quazepam (Doral) [C]

COMMON USES: Insomnia.
DOSAGE: 7.5–15 mg PO qhs prn.
NOTES: Reduce dose in elderly patients.

Quinapril (Accupril)

COMMON USES: Treatment of hypertension.
DOSAGE: 10–80 mg PO qd in single dose.

Quinidine (Quinidex, Quinaglute)

COMMON USES: Prevention of tachydysrhythmias.
DOSAGE: ***Adults:*** PACs, PVCs: 200–300 mg PO tid–qid. Conversion of atrial fibrillation or flutter: Use after digitalization, 200 mg q2–3h for 8 doses; then increase daily dose to maximum of 3–4 g or until normal rhythm. ***Peds:*** 30 mg/kg/24h PO in 4–5 divided doses.
NOTES: Contraindicated in digitalis toxicity, AV block; follow serum levels if available (see Table IX–3, page 457); extreme hypotension seen with IV administration. Sulfate salt contains 83% quinidine, gluconate salt is 62% quinidine.

Quinupristin/Dalfopristin (Synercid)

COMMON USES: Infections caused by vancomycin-resistant *Enterococcus faecium,* and other gram-positive organisms.
DOSAGE: ***Adults*** and ***Peds:*** 7.5 mg/kg IV q8–12h.
NOTES: Administer through central line if possible; NOT compatible with saline or heparin, therefore flush IV lines with dextrose.

Rabeprazole (Aciphex)

COMMON USES: Peptic ulcers, GERD, and hypersecretory conditions.
DOSAGE: 20 mg once daily; may be increased to 60 mg daily.
NOTES: Do not crush tablets.

Raloxifene (Evista)

COMMON USES: Prevention of osteoporosis.
DOSAGE: 60 mg/d.

Ramipril (Altace)

COMMON USES: Hypertension and heart failure.
DOSAGE: 2.5–20 mg/d PO divided qd-bid.
NOTES: May use in combination with diuretics; may cause a nonproductive cough.

Ranitidine (Zantac)

COMMON USES: Duodenal ulcer, active benign ulcers, hypersecretory conditions, gastroesophageal reflux.
DOSAGE: ***Adults:*** Ulcer: 150 mg PO bid, 300 mg PO qhs, or 50 mg IV q6–8h; or 400 mg IV/d continuous infusion. Maintenance: 150 mg PO qhs. Hypersecretion: 150 mg PO bid. ***Peds:*** 0.1–0.8 mg/kg/dose IV q6–8h or 1.25–2.0 mg/kg/dose PO q12h.
NOTES: Reduce dose with renal failure; note oral and parenteral doses are different.

Rimexolone (Vexol Ophthalmic)

COMMON USES: Postoperative inflammation and uveitis
DOSAGE: ***Adults*** and ***Peds > 2 y:*** Uveitis: 1–2 drops q1h daytime and q2h at night, can taper to 1 drop q4h; postoperative 1–2 drops qid for up to 2 wk.
NOTES: Should taper dose to zero.

Repaglinide (Prandin)

COMMON USES: Management of Type 2 diabetes.
DOSAGE: 0.5–4 mg ac.

Reteplase (Retavase)

COMMON USES: Thrombolytic after acute myocardial infarction.
DOSAGE: 10 U IV over 2 min, 2nd dose 30 min later of 10 U IV over 2 min.

Ribavirin (Virazole, Rebetron)

COMMON USES: Treatment of infants and children with respiratory syncytial virus infection; treatment of Hepatitis C.
DOSAGE: RSV: 6 g in 300 mL of sterile water inhaled over 12–18 h. Hep C: 600 mg PO bid in combination with interferon alfa-2b.
NOTES: Aerosolized by a SPAG generator; may accumulate on soft contact lenses; monitor Hgb and Hct frequently; pregnancy test every month.

Rifampin (Rifadin)

COMMON USES: Tuberculosis, treatment, and prophylaxis of *N meningitidis, H influenzae,* or *S aureus* carriers.
DOSAGE: ***Adults:*** *N meningitidis* and *H influenzae* carrier: 600 mg PO qd 3–4 d. Tuberculosis: 600 mg PO or IV qd or twice weekly with combination therapy regimen. ***Peds:*** 10–20 mg/kg/dose PO or IV qd–bid.
NOTES: Multiple side effects; causes orange-red discoloration of bodily secretions including tears; never used as a single agent to treat active tuberculosis infections.

Rifapentine (Priftin)

COMMON USES: Treatment of tuberculosis.
DOSAGE: Intensive phase: 600 mg PO twice weekly for 2 mo; separate doses by 3 or more days. Continuation phase: 600 mg once weekly.
NOTES: Has similar adverse effects and drug interactions as rifampin.

Rimantadine (Flumadine)

COMMON USES: Prophylaxis and treatment of influenza A virus infections.

DOSAGE: *Adults:* 100 mg PO bid. *Peds:* 5 mg/kg PO qd, not to exceed 150 mg/d.

Risedronate (Actonel)

COMMON USES: Prevention and treatment of postmenopausal osteoporosis.
DOSAGE: 5 mg PO once daily with 6–8 oz of water.
NOTES: Take 30 min before first food or drink of the day; interaction with calcium supplements; may cause GI distress and arthralgia.

Risperidone (Risperdal)

COMMON USES: Management of psychotic disorders.
DOSAGE: 1–8 mg PO bid.

Ritonavir (Norvir)

COMMON USES: HIV in combination with two or three other agents.
DOSAGE: 600 mg PO bid with food.

Rofecoxib (Vioxx)

COMMON USES: Osteoarthritis, acute pain, and primary dysmenorrhea.
DOSAGE: 12.5–50 mg/d.
NOTES: Alert patients to be aware of GI ulceration or bleeding.

Rosiglitazone (Avandia)

COMMON USES: Treatment of type 2 diabetes mellitus.
DOSAGE: 4–8 mg PO once daily or in 2 divided doses.
NOTES: May be taken with or without meals.

Salmeterol (Serevent)

COMMON USES: Treatment of asthma and exercise-induced bronchospasm.
DOSAGE: 2 inhalations twice daily.

Saquinavir (Fortovase,Invirase)

COMMON USES: HIV in combination with two or three other agents.
DOSAGE: Fortovase: 1200 mg tid after meals; Invirase: 600 mg PO tid after meals.

Sargramostim [GM-CSF] (Prokine, Leukine)

COMMON USES: Treatment of myeloid recovery following bone marrow transplantation.
DOSAGE: *Adults* and *Peds:* 250 mg/m^2/d IV for 21 d.
NOTES: May cause bone pain.

Scopolamine

Scopolamine, Transdermal (Transderm-Scop)

COMMON USES: Prevention of nausea and vomiting associated with motion sickness; preop control of secretions.
DOSAGE: Transderm-Scop: Apply 1 patch behind the ear every 3 d; 0.3–0.65 IM/IV/SC repeat prn q4–6h.
NOTES: May cause dry mouth, drowsiness, and blurred vision.

Secobarbital (Seconal) [C]

COMMON USES: Insomnia.
DOSAGE: *Adults:* 100 mg PO, or IM qhs prn. *Peds:* 3–5 mg/kg/dose PO or IM qhs prn.
NOTES: Beware of respiratory depression; tolerance acquired within 1–2 wk.

Selegiline (Eldepryl)

COMMON USES: Parkinson's disease.
DOSAGE: 5 mg PO bid.
NOTES: May cause nausea and dizziness.

Sertraline (Zoloft)

COMMON USES: Treatment of depression.
DOSAGE: 50–200 mg PO qd.
NOTES: Can activate manic/hypomanic state; has caused weight loss in clinical trials.

Sibutramine (Meridia)

COMMON USES: Management of obesity.
DOSAGE: 10–15 mg/d.
NOTES: Use with low-calorie diet, monitor blood pressure.

Sildenafil (Viagra)

COMMON USES: Erectile dysfunction.
DOSAGE: 25–100 mg 1 hour prior to sexual activity, maximum dosing is once daily.
NOTES: Do not take with nitrates in any form; adjust dose in persons > 65 y.

Silver Nitrate

COMMON USES: Prevention of ophthalmia neonatorium due to GC; removal of granulation tissue cauterization of wounds.
DOSAGE: ***Adults*** and ***Peds:*** Apply to moist surface 2–3 times a week for several weeks or until desired effect. ***Peds:*** newborns apply 2 drops into conjunctival sac immediately after birth.

Silver Sulfadiazine (Silvadene)

COMMON USES: Prevention of sepsis in second-degree and third-degree burns.
DOSAGE: ***Adults*** and ***Peds:*** Aseptically cover affected area with thin coating bid.
NOTES: Can have systemic absorption with extensive application; must be aggressively debrided daily.

Simethicone (Mylicon)

COMMON USES: Symptomatic treatment of flatulence.
DOSAGE: ***Adults*** and ***Peds:*** 40–125 mg PO pc and hs prn.

Simvastatin (Zocor)

COMMON USES: Reduction of elevated cholesterol levels.
DOSAGE: 5–40 mg PO qhs.

Sirolimus (Rapamune)

COMMON USES: Prophylaxis of organ rejection.
DOSAGE: 2 mg PO per day.
NOTES: Dilute in water or orange juice; do NOT drink grapefruit juice while on sirolimus; take 4 h after cyclosporin.

Sodium Bicarbonate

COMMON USES: Alkalinization of urine, renal tubular acidosis (RTA), treatment of metabolic acidosis.
DOSAGE: ***Adults:*** Emergency cardiac care: initiate adequate ventilation, 1 mEq/kg/dose IV ; can repeat 0.5 mEq/kg in 10 min one time or based on acid/ base status. Metabolic acidosis: 2–5 mEq/kg IV over 8 h and prn based on acid/ base status. Alkalinize urine: 4 g (48 mEq) PO, then 1–2 g q4h; adjust based on urine pH. Chronic renal failure: 1–3 mEq/kg/d. Distal RTA: 1 mEq/kg/d PO. ***Peds:*** > 1 y: Emergency cardiac care: see Adult. < 1 y: Emergency cardiac care: initiate adequate ventilation, 1:1 dilution 1 mEq/mL dosed 1 mEq/kg IV; can repeat with 0.5 mEq/kg in 10 min one time or based on acid/base status. Chronic renal failure: see Adult. Distal RTA: 2–3 mEq/kg/d PO. Proximal RTA: 5–10 mEq/kg/d titrate based on serum bicarbonate levels. Urine alkalinization: 84–840 mg/kg/d (1–10 mEq/kg/d) divided doses; adjust based on urine pH.

NOTES: 1 g neutralizes 12 mEq of acid; in infants, do not exceed 10 mEq/min infusion; supplied as IV infusion, powder and tablets: 300 mg = 3.6 mEq; 325 mg = 3.8 mEq; 520 mg = 6.3 mEq; 600 mg = 7.3 mEq; 650 mg = 7.6 mEq.

Sodium Citrate (Bicitra)

COMMON USES: Alkalinization of urine; dissolve uric acid and cysteine stones.
DOSAGE: ***Adults:*** 2–6 teaspoonfuls (10–30 mL) diluted in 1–3 ounces of water pc and hs. ***Peds:*** 1–3 teaspoonfuls (5–15 mL) diluted in 1–3 ounces of water pc and hs. Supplied: 15– or 30-mL unit dose: 16 (473 mL) or 4 (118 mL) fluid ounces.
NOTES: Should not be given to patients on aluminum-based antacids. Contraindicated in patients with severe renal impairment of sodium-restricted diets.

Sodium Polystyrene Sulfonate (Kayexalate)

COMMON USES: Treatment of hyperkalemia.
DOSAGE: ***Adults:*** 15–60 g PO or 30–60 g PR q6h based on serum K. ***Peds:*** 1 g/kg/dose PO or PR q6h based on serum K.
NOTES: Can cause hypernatremia; given with agent such as sorbitol (mixed in 20–100 mL of 70% solution) to promote movement through bowel.

Sorbitol

COMMON USES: Constipation.
DOSAGE: ***Adults*** and ***Peds > 12 y:*** 30–150 mL of a 20–70% solution prn.

Sotalol (Betapace)

COMMON USES: Treatment of ventricular arrhythmias.
DOSAGE: 80 mg PO bid; may be increased to 240–320 mg/d.
NOTES: Dose should be adjusted for renal insufficiency.

Spironolactone (Aldactone)

COMMON USES: Treatment of hyperaldosteronism, essential hypertension, edematous states (CHF, cirrhosis), polycystic ovary.
DOSAGE: ***Adults:*** 25–100 mg PO qid. ***Peds:*** 1–3.3 mg/kg/24h PO divided bid–qid.
NOTES: Can cause hyperkalemia and gynecomastia; avoid prolonged use; diuretic of choice for cirrhotic edema and ascites.

Steroids, Systemic

(See also Table IX–4, page 475)

The following relates only to the commonly used systemic glucocorticoids:
COMMON USES: Endocrine disorders (adrenal insufficiency), rheumatoid disorders, collagen-vascular diseases, dermatologic diseases, allergic states, edematous states (cerebral, nephrotic syndrome), immunosuppression for transplantation, hypercalcemia, malignancies (breast, lymphomas), preoperatively (in any patient who has been on steroids in the previous year, known hypoadrenalism, preop for adrenalectomy); injection into joints/tissue.
DOSAGE: Varies with use and institutional protocols. Some commonly used doses are: Adrenal insufficiency, Acute (Addisonian crisis): ***Adults:*** hydrocortisone 100 mg IV q8h; then 300 mg/d divided q8h; convert to 50 mg PO q8h X 6 doses, taper to 30–50 mg/d divided bid. ***Peds:*** hydrocortisone: 1–2 mg/kg IV; then 150–250 mg/d divided tid. Adrenal insufficiency, chronic (physiologic replacement: may also need mineralocorticoid supplementation such as DOCA. ***Adults:*** hydrocortisone 20 mg PO QAM, 10 mg PO QPM; cortisone 0.5–0.75 mg/kg/d divided bid; cortisone 0.25–0.35 mg/kg IM qd; dexamethasone: 0.03–0.15 mg/kg/d or 0.6–0.75 mg/m^2/d in divided q6–12h PO, IM, IV. ***Peds:*** hydrocortisone 0.5–0.75 mg/kg/d PO tid; hydrocortisone succinate 0.25–0.35 mg/kg/d IM. Asthma, Acute: ***Peds:*** prednisolone 1–2 mg/kg/d or prednisone 1–2 mg/kg/d divided qd–bid for up to 5 d; prednisolone 2–4 mg/kg/d IV divided tid. Congenital Adrenal Hyperplasia: ***Peds:*** Initially hydrocortisone 30–36 mg/m^2/d PO divided 1/3 dose QAM, 2/3 dose QPM; maintenance: 20–25 mg/m^2/d divided

bid. Extubation/airway edema: Dexamethasone 0.5–1 mg/kg/d IM/IV divided 6h, start beginning 24 h before extubation; continue 4 additional doses. Immunosuppressive/anti-inflammatory: ***Adults*** and older ***Peds:*** Hydrocortisone: 15–240 mg PO, IM, IV q12h; methylprednisolone: 4–48 mg/d PO; taper to lowest effective dose; methylprednisolone sodium succinate 10–80 mg IM qd. ***Adults:*** prednisone or prednisolone 5–60 mg/d PO, divided qd-qid. ***Infants and Younger Children:*** 2.5–10 mg/kg/d hydrocortisone PO divided q6–8h; 1–5 mg/kg/d IM/IV divided bid/qd. Nephrotic Syndrome: ***Children:*** prednisolone or prednisone 2 mg/kg/d PO divided tid–qid until urine is protein free for 5 d, use up to 28 d; for persistent proteinuria, 4 mg/kg/dose PO qod max 120 mg/d for an additional 28 d; maintenance: 2 mg/kg/dose qod for 28 d; taper over 4–6 wk (max 80 mg/d). Septic Shock: ***Adults:*** hydrocortisone 500 mg–1 g IM/IV q2–6h. ***Peds:*** hydrocortisone 50 mg/kg IM/IV, repeat q4–24h prn. Status Asthmaticus: ***Adults*** and ***Peds:*** hydrocortisone 1–2 mg/kg/dose IV q6h; then by 0.5–1 mg/kg q6h. Rheumatic disease **(Adults):** Intra-articular: hydrocortisone acetate 25–37.5 mg large joint; 10–25 mg small joint; methylprednisolone acetate 20–80 mg large joint, 4–10 mg small joint. Intra-bursal: hydrocortisone acetate 25–37.5 mg. Intra-ganglia: hydrocortisone acetate 25–37.5 mg. Tendon sheath: hydrocortisone acetate 5–12.5 mg. Perioperative steroid coverage: Hydrocortisone 100 mg IV night before surgery, 1 h preop, intraoperatively, and 4, 8, and 12 h postoperatively; POD No. 1: 100 mg IV q6h; POD No. 2: 100 mg IV q8h; POD No. 3: 100 mg IV q12h; POD No. 4: 50 mg IV q12h; POD No. 5: 25 mg IV q12h; then, resume prior oral dosing if chronic use or discontinue if only perioperative coverage is required. Cerebral edema: Dexamethasone 10 mg IV; then 4 mg IV q4–6h.

NOTES: See Table IX–4, page 475. All can cause hyperglycemia, "steroid psychosis", adrenal suppression; never acutely stop steroids, especially if chronic treatment; taper dose. Hydrocortisone succinate administered systemically, acetate form intra-articular.

Steroids, Topical

COMMON USES: Topical therapy of a variety of inflammatory and pruritic dermatologic conditions that respond to corticosteroid therapy.

DOSAGE: Application based on individual agent (see Table IX–7 below).

TABLE IX–7. TOPICAL STEROID PREPARATIONS.

Agent	Common Trade Names	Potency	Apply
Alclometasone dipropionate	Aclovate, cream, ointment 0.05%	Low	bid/tid
Betamethasone valerate	Valisone cream, lotion 0.01%	Low	qd/bid
	Valisone cream 0.01, 0.1%, ointment, lotion 0.1%	Intermediate	qd/bid
Betamethasone dipropionate	Diprosone cream, lotion, ointment 0.05%	High	qd/bid
	Diprosone aerosol (0.1%)		
Betamethasone dipropionate, augmented	Diprolene ointment, gel 0.05%	Ultrahigh	qd/bid

TABLE IX–7. TOPICAL STEROID PREPARATIONS. (*continued*)

Agent	Common Trade Names	Potency	Apply
Clobetasol propionate	Temovate cream, gel, ointment, solution 0.05%,	Ultrahigh	Scalp, bid (2 weeks max)
Clocortolone pivalate	Cloderm cream 0.1%	Intermediate	qd/qid
Desonide	DesOwen, cream, ointment, lotion 0.05%	Low	bid/qid
Desoximetasone	Topicort LP cream, gel 0.05%	Intermediate	bid/tid
	Topicort cream, ointment 0.25%	High	
Dexamethasone base	Aeroseb-Dex aerosol 0.01%	Low	bid/qid
	Decadron cream 0.1%		
Diflorasone diacetate	Psorcon cream, ointment 0.05%	Ultrahigh	bid/qid
Fluocinolone	Fluocinolone acetonide 0.01%		
	Synalar cream, solution 0.01%	Low	bid/tid
	Synalar ointment, cream 0.025%	Intermediate	bid/tid
	Synalar-HP cream 0.2%	High	bid/tid
Fluocinonide 0.05%	Lidex, anhydrous cream, gel, ointment, solution 0.05%	High	bid/tid
	Lidex-E aqeous cream 0.05%		
Flurandrenolide	Cordran cream, ointment 0.025%	Intermediate	bid/tid
	cream, lotion, ointment 0.05%	Intermediate	bid/tid
	tape, 4 μg/cm^2	Intermediate	qd
Fluticasone propionate	Cutivate cream 0.05%, ointment 0.005%	Intermediate	bid
Halobetasol	Ultravate cream, ointment 0.05%	Very HIgh	bid
Halcinonide	Halog cream 0.025%, emollient base 0.1%	High	qd/tid
	Cream, ointment, solution 0.1%		
Hydrocortisone	Hydrocortisone Cortizone, Caldecort, Hycort, Hytone, others	Low	tid/qid
	Aerosol: 1%; Cream: 0.5, 1, 2.5%; Gel 0.5%; Ointment 0.5, 1, 2.5% Lotion 0.5, 1.25%; Paste 0.5%; Solution 1%		

(*continued*)

TABLE IX–7. TOPICAL STEROID PREPARATIONS. (*continued*)

Agent	Common Trade Names	Potency	Apply
Hydrocortisone acetate	Corticaine cream, ointment 0.5, 1%	Low	tid/qid
Hydrocortisone butyrate	Locoid ointment, solution 0.1%	Intermediate	bid/tid
Hydrocortisone valerate	Westcort cream, ointment 0.2%	Intermediate	bid/tid
Mometasone furoate	Elocon 0.1% cream, ointment, lotion	Intermediate	qd
Prednicarbate	Dermatop 0.1% cream	Intermediate	bid
Triamcinolone acetonide	Aristocort, Kenalog cream, ointment, lotion 0.025%	Low	tid/qid
	Aristocort, Kenalog cream, ointment, lotion 0.1%	Intermediate	tid/qid
	Aerosol 0.2 mg/2s spray		
Triamcinolone acetonide	Aristocort, Kenalog cream, ointment 0.5%	High	tid/qid

Streptokinase (Streptase, Kabikinase)

COMMON USES: Coronary artery thrombosis; acute massive pulmonary embolism; deep vein thrombosis; some occluded vascular grafts.

DOSAGE: Pulmonary embolus: Loading dose of 250,000 IU IV through a peripheral vein over 30 min, then 100,000 IU/h IV for 24–72 h. Deep vein thrombosis or arterial embolism: Load as with pulmonary embolus, then 100,000 IU/h for 72 h.

NOTES: If maintenance infusion is not adequate to maintain thrombin clotting time 2–5 times control, refer to package insert, PDR, or Hospital Formulary Service for adjustments.

Succinylcholine (Anectine, Quelicin, Sucostrin)

COMMON USES: Adjunct to general anesthesia to facilitate endotracheal intubation and to induce skeletal muscle relaxation during surgery or mechanically supported ventilation.

DOSAGE: ***Adults:*** 0.6 mg/kg IV over 10–30 s followed by 0.04–0.07 mg/kg as needed to maintain muscle relaxation. ***Peds:*** 1–2 mg/kg/dose IV followed by 0.03–0.06 mg/kg/dose at intervals of 10–20 min.

NOTES: May precipitate malignant hyperthermia; respiratory depression or prolonged apnea may occur; many drug interactions potentiating activity of succinylcholine; observe for cardiovascular effects; use only freshly prepared solutions.

Sucralfate (Carafate)

COMMON USES: Treatment of duodenal ulcers, gastric ulcers.

DOSAGE: ***Adults:*** 1 g PO qid, 1 h before meals and hs. ***Peds:*** 40–80 mg/kg/d divided q6h.

NOTES: Treatment should be continued for 4–8 wk unless healing is demonstrated by radiograph or endoscopy; constipation is the most frequent side effect.

Sufentanil (Sufenta) [C]

COMMON USES: Analgesic adjunct to maintain balanced general anesthesia.
DOSAGE: Adjunctive: 1–8 mg/kg with nitrous oxide/oxygen; maintenance of 10–50 mg prn. General anesthesia: 8–30 mg/kg with oxygen and a skeletal muscle relaxant; maintenance of 25–50 mg prn.
NOTES: Respiratory depressant effects persisting longer than the analgesic effects; 80 times more potent than morphine.

Sulfacetamide

COMMON USES: Conjunctival infections.
DOSAGE: 10% ointment apply qid and qhs; 10–, 15–, 30–% solution for keratitis apply q2–3h depending on severity.

Sulfasalazine (Azulfidine)

COMMON USES: Ulcerative colitis.
DOSAGE: ***Adults:*** 1–2 g PO initially, increase to maximum of 8 g/d in 3–4 divided doses; maintenance 500 mg PO qid. ***Peds:*** 40–60 mg/kg/24h PO divided q4–6h initially; maintenance 20–30 mg/kg/24h PO divided q6h.
NOTES: Can cause severe gastrointestinal upset; discolors urine.

Sulfinpyrazone (Anturane)

COMMON USES: Acute and chronic gout.
DOSAGE: 100–200 mg PO bid for 1 wk, then increase as needed to maintenance of 200–400 mg bid.

Sulindac (Clinoril)

COMMON USES: Treatment of arthritis and pain.
DOSAGE: 150–200 mg bid.

Sulfisoxazole (Gantrisin, others)

COMMON USES: Acute uncomplicated urinary tract infections.
DOSAGE: ***Adults:*** Between 500 mg and 1 g PO qid. ***Peds > 2 mo:*** 120–150 mg/kg/24h PO divided q4–6h.
NOTES: Avoid use in last half of pregnancy (causes fetal hyperbilirubinemia).

Tacrine (Cognex)

COMMON USES: Treatment of mild-to-moderate dementia.
DOSAGE: 10–40 mg PO qid.
NOTES: May cause elevations in transaminases; LFTs should be monitored regularly.

Tacrolimus [FK 506] (Prograf)

COMMON USES: Prophylaxis of organ rejection.
DOSAGE: IV: 0.05–0.1 mg/kg/d as continuous infusion. PO: 0.15–0.3 mg/kg/d divided into 2 doses.
NOTES: May cause neurotoxicity and nephrotoxicity.

Tamoxifen (Nolvadex)

COMMON USES: Adjuvant treatment of breast cancer.
DOSAGE: 10–20 mg PO bid.
NOTES: May increase the risk of secondary uterine cancer.

Tamsulosin (Flomax)

COMMON USES: Treatment of benign prostatic hyperplasia.
DOSAGE: 0.4–0.8 mg qd

Telmisartan (Micardis)

COMMON USES: Treatment of hypertension.

DOSAGE: 40–80 mg once daily.
NOTES: Avoid use during pregnancy.

Temazepam (Restoril) [C]

COMMON USES: Insomnia.
DOSAGE: 15–30 mg PO qhs prn.
NOTES: Reduce dose in elderly patients.

Tenecteplase (TNKase)

COMMON USES: Reduction of mortality associated with acute myocardial infarction.
DOSAGE: 30–50 mg IV; see product information for weight- based dosing.

Teniposide (Vumon)

COMMON USES: Treatment of leukemia.
DOSAGE: 165 mg/m^2 IV twice weekly for 8–9 doses.

Terazosin (Hytrin)

COMMON USES: Treatment of hypertension and benign prostatic hyperplasia.
DOSAGE: Initially 1 mg PO hs; titrate up to maximum of 20 mg PO qhs.
NOTES: Hypotension and syncope following first dose; dizziness, weakness, nasal congestion, peripheral edema common; often used with thiazide diuretic.

Terbutaline (Brethine, Bricanyl)

COMMON USES: Reversible bronchospasm (asthma, COPD); inhibition of labor.
DOSAGE: ***Adults:*** Bronchodilator: 2.5–5 mg PO qid or 0.25 mg SC, may repeat in 15 min (maximum 0.5 mg in 4 h). Metered dose inhaler: 2 inhalations q4–6h. Premature labor: 10–80 mg/min IV infusion for 4h, then 2.5 mg PO q4–6h until term. ***Peds:*** Oral: 0.05–0.15 mg/kg/dose PO tid; max 5 mg/24h.
NOTES: Caution with diabetes, hypertension, hyperthyroidism; high doses may precipitate β-1-adrenergic effects.

Terconazole (Terazol 7)

COMMON USES: Vaginal fungal infections.
DOSAGE: 1 applicator intravaginally qhs for 7 d.

Tetanus Immune Globulin

COMMON USES: Passive immunization against tetanus for any person with a suspect contaminated wound and unknown immunization status (see Appendix).
DOSAGE: ***Adults*** and ***Peds:*** 250–500 U IM (higher doses if delay in initiation of therapy).
NOTES: May begin active immunization series at different injection site if required.

Tetanus Toxoid

COMMON USES: Protection against tetanus.
DOSAGE: See Appendix for tetanus prophylaxis.

Tetracycline (Achromycin V, Sumycin)

COMMON USES: Broad-spectrum antibiotic treatment against *Staphylococcus, Streptococcus, Chlamydia, Rickettsia,* and *Mycoplasma.*
DOSAGE: ***Adults:*** 250–500 mg PO bid–qid. ***Peds > 8 y:*** 25–50 mg/kg/24h PO q6–12h. Do not use in children < 8 y.
NOTES: Can stain enamel and depress bone formation in children; caution with use in pregnancy; do not use in presence of impaired renal function (see Doxycycline, page 482).

Theophylline (Theolair, Theo-Dur, Somophyllin, others)

COMMON USES: Asthma, bronchospasm.
DOSAGE: ***Adults:*** 24 mg/kg/24h PO divided q6h; sustained release products may be divided q8–12h. ***Peds:*** 16 mg/kg/24h PO divided q6h; SR products may be divided q8–12h.

NOTES: See drug levels in Table IX–3 on page 457; many drug interactions; side effects include nausea, vomiting, tachycardia, and seizures.

Thiamine (Vitamin B1)

COMMON USES: Thiamine deficiency (beriberi); alcoholic neuritis; Wernicke's encephalopathy.
DOSAGE: ***Adults:*** Deficiency: 100 mg IM qd for 2 wk, then 5–10 mg PO qd for 1 mo. Wernicke's encephalopathy: 100 mg IV 3 1 dose, then 100 mg IM qd for 2 wk. ***Peds:***10–25 mg IM qd for 2 wk, then 5–10 mg/24h PO qd for 1 mo.
NOTES: IV thiamine administration associated with anaphylactic reaction; must be given slowly IV.

Thiethylperazine (Torecan)

COMMON USES: Nausea and vomiting.
DOSAGE: 10 mg PO, PR or IM qd–tid.
NOTES: Extrapyramidal reactions may occur.

Thioridazine (Mellaril)

COMMON USES: Psychotic disorders; short-term treatment of depression, agitation, organic brain syndrome.
DOSAGE: ***Adults:*** Initially 50–100 mg PO tid; maintenance 200–800 mg/24h PO in 2–4 divided doses. ***Peds:*** > 2 y: 1–2.5 mg/kg/24h PO divided bid–tid.
NOTES: Low incidence of extrapyramidal effects.

Thiotepa /Triethylene-thiophosphoramide (Thio-TEPA, TESPA, TSPA, Thioplex)

COMMON USES: Breast, ovarian cancer; intracavitary for serosal malignant implants; intravesical for superficial papillary bladder cancer.
DOSAGE: 0.3–0.4 mg/kg IV at 1–4-wk intervals. Intravesical: 60 mg in 30–60-mL saline, held for 2 h if possible; treat weekly for 4 wk. Additional 4-wk course should be given with caution since myelosuppression can occur.
NOTES: Toxicity includes myelosuppression, nausea, vomiting, dizziness, headache, allergy, paresthesias.

Thiothixene (Navane)

COMMON USES: Psychotic disorders.
DOSAGE: ***Adults*** and ***Peds:*** > 12 y: Mild-to-moderate psychosis: 2 mg PO tid. Severe psychosis: 5 mg PO bid; increase to maximum dose of 60 mg/24h prn. Intramuscular use: 16–20 mg/24h divided bid–qid; maximum 30 mg/d. < 12 y: 0.25 mg/kg/24h PO divided q6–12h.
NOTES: Drowsiness and extrapyramidal side effects most common.

Thyroid (Dessicated extract)

COMMON USES: Replacement in hypothyroidism
DOSAGE: 30 mg/d PO, titrate 30 mg/d over several weeks; maintenance 60–120 mg/d.

Tiagabine (Gagitril)

COMMON USES: Adjunctive therapy in treatment of partial seizures.
DOSAGE: Initially 4 mg once daily, increase by 4 mg during 2nd week; increase by 4–8 mg/d until clinical response is achieved; maximum dose 32 mg/d.
NOTES: Withdraw gradually; used in combination with other anticonvulsants.

Ticarcillin (Ticar)

COMMON USES: Infections caused by susceptible strains of gram-negative bacteria including *Klebsiella, Proteus, E coli, Enterobacter, P aeruginosa,* and *Serratia* involving the skin, bone, respiratory tract, urinary tract, abdomen, and septicemia.
DOSAGE: ***Adults:*** 3 g IV q4–6h. ***Peds:*** 200–300 mg/kg/d IV divided q4–6h.
NOTES: Often used in combination with aminoglycosides

Ticarcillin/Potassium Clavulanate (Timentin)

COMMON USES: Infections caused by susceptible strains of gram-negative bacteria (*Klebsiella, Proteus, E coli, Enterobacter, P aeruginosa,* and *Serratia*) involving the skin, bone, respiratory tract, urinary tract, abdomen, and septicemia.
DOSAGE: ***Adults:*** 3.1 g IV q4–6h. ***Peds:*** 200–300 mg/kg/d IV divided q4–6h.
NOTES: Often used in combination with aminoglycosides.

Ticlopidine (Ticlid)

COMMON USES: Reduce the risk of thrombotic stroke.
DOSAGE: 250 mg PO bid.
NOTES: Should be administered with food.

Timolol (Blocadren, Timoptic)

COMMON USES: Treatment of hypertension and myocardial infarction; glaucoma.
DOSAGE: HTN: 10–20 mg bid. MI: 10 mg bid. Ophthalmic: 0.25% 1 drop bid; decrease to qd when controlled; use 0.5% if needed; 1 drop gel qd.
NOTES: Timoptic XE (0.25, 0.5%) is a gel-forming solution.

Tioconazole (Vagistat)

COMMON USES: Vaginal fungal infections.
DOSAGE: 1 applicator intravaginally at bedtime (single dose).

Tirofiban (Aggrastat)

COMMON USES: Management of acute coronary syndrome
DOSAGE: Initial 0.4 μg/kg/min for 30 min, followed by 0.1 μg/kg/min.
NOTES: Adjust dose in renal insufficiency; use in combination with heparin.

Tobramycin (Nebcin)

COMMON USES: Serious gram-negative infections, especially *Pseudomonas.*
DOSAGE: Based on renal function 2 mg/kg IV load followed 1.5 mg/kg IV q8h; refer to Aminoglycoside Dosing on page 455.
NOTES: Nephrotoxic and ototoxic; decrease dose with renal insufficiency; monitor creatinine clearance and serum concentrations for dosing adjustments; see Table IX–3, page 457.

Tobramycin Ophthalmic (Tobrex)

COMMON USES: Ocular bacterial infections.
DOSE: 0.3% ointment apply q3–8h or 0.3% solution apply 1–2 drops q1–4h based on severity of infection.

Tobramycin and Dexamethasone Ophthalmic (Tobradex)

COMMON USES: Ocular bacterial infections associated with significant inflammation.
DOSE: 0.3% ointment apply Q3–8 H or solution 0.3% apply 1–2 drops Q 1–4 H;

Tocainide (Tonocard)

COMMON USES: Suppression of ventricular arrhythmias including PVCs, and ventricular tachycardia.
DOSAGE: 400–600 mg PO q8h.
NOTES: Properties similar to lidocaine; reduce dose in renal failure; CNS and gastrointestinal side effects are common.

Tolazamide (Tolinase)

COMMON USES: Management of non-insulin-dependent diabetes mellitus.
DOSAGE: 100–500 mg qd.

Tolazoline (Priscoline)

COMMON USES: Persistent pulmonary vasoconstriction and hypertension of the newborn, peripheral vasospastic disorders.

DOSAGE: ***Adults:*** 10–50 mg IM/IV/SC qid. ***Neonates:*** 1–2 mg/kg IV over 10–15 min, followed by 1–2 mg/kg/h.

Tolbutamide (Orinase)

COMMON USES: Management of non-insulin-dependent diabetes mellitus.
DOSAGE: 500–1000 mg bid.

Tolmetin (Tolectin)

COMMON USES: Treatment of arthritis and pain.
DOSAGE: 200–600 mg tid, to a maximum of 2000 mg/d.

Topiramate (Topamax)

COMMON USES: Treatment of partial onset seizures.
DOSAGE: Total dose 400 mg/d. See product information of 8-wk titration schedule.
NOTES: May precipitate kidney stones.

Torsemide (Demadex)

COMMON USES: Edema, hypertension, congestive heart failure, and hepatic cirrhosis.
DOSAGE: 5–20 mg PO or IV once daily.

Tramadol (Ultram)

COMMON USES: Management of moderate-to-severe pain.
DOSAGE: 50–100 mg PO q4–6h prn, not to exceed 400 mg/d.

Trandolapril (Mavik)

COMMON USES: Treatment of hypertension, CHF, left-ventricular systolic dysfunction, post acute MI.
DOSAGE: HTN: 2–4 mg/d. CHF/LV dysfunction: 4 mg/d.

Trazodone (Desyrel)

COMMON USES: Major depression.
DOSAGE: 50–150 mg PO qd–qid; maximum 600 mg/d.
NOTES: May take 1–2 wk for symptomatic improvement; anticholinergic side effects.

Triamterene (Dyrenium)

COMMON USES: Edema associated with CHF, cirrhosis.
DOSAGE: 100–300 mg/24h PO divided qd–bid.
NOTES: Can cause hyperkalemia; blood dyscrasias, liver damage, and other reactions.

Triazolam (Halcion) [C]

COMMON USES: Insomnia.
DOSAGE: 0.125–0.5 mg PO qhs prn.
NOTES: Additive CNS depression with alcohol and other CNS depressants.

Triethanolamine Polypeptide Oleate (Cerumenex Otic)

COMMON USES: Removal of symptomatic ear wax, ceruminolytic.
DOSAGE: ***Adults*** and ***Peds:*** Fill ear canal and insert cotton plug; allow to remain 15–30 min, then flush ear with water.

Trifluoperazine (Stelazine)

COMMON USES: Psychotic disorders.
DOSAGE: ***Adults:*** 2–10 mg PO bid. ***Peds 6–12 y:*** 1 mg PO qd–bid, gradually increase up to 15 mg/d.
NOTES: Decrease dose in elderly and debilitated patients; oral concentrate must be diluted to 60 mL or more before administration.

Trifluridine (Viroptic)

COMMON USES: Herpes simplex keratitis and conjunctivitis.

DOSAGE: 1 drop q2h (max 9 drops/d); decrease to 1 drop q4h after healing begins; treat up to 14 d.

Trihexyphenidyl (Artane)

COMMON USES: Parkinson's disease.
DOSAGE: 2–5 mg PO qd–qid.
NOTES: Contraindicated in narrow angle glaucoma.

Trimethaphan (Arfonad)

COMMON USES: Controlled hypotension during surgery; treatment of hypertensive crisis; treatment of pulmonary edema with pulmonary hypertension and systemic hypertension; dissecting aortic aneurysm.
DOSAGE: ***Adults:*** 0.3–6 mg/min IV infusion titrated to effect. ***Peds:*** 50–150 mg/kg/min IV infusion.
NOTES: Additive effect with other antihypertensive agents; vasopressors may be used to reverse hypotension if required; phenylephrine is vasopressor of choice for reversal of effects.

Trimethobenzamide (Tigan)

COMMON USES: Nausea and vomiting.
DOSAGE: ***Adults:*** 250 mg PO or 200 mg PR or IM tid–qid prn. ***Peds:*** 20 mg/kg/24h PO or 15 mg/kg/24h PR or IM in 3–4 divided doses (not recommended for infants).
NOTES: In the presence of viral infections, may contribute to Reye's syndrome; may cause parkinsonian-like syndrome.

Trimethoprim (Trimpex, Proloprim)

COMMON USES: Urinary tract infections caused by susceptible gram-positive and gram-negative organisms.
DOSAGE: 100 mg PO bid or 200 mg PO qd.
NOTES: Reduce dose in renal failure.

Trimethoprim-Sulfamethoxazole [Co-trimoxazole] (Bactrim, Septra)

COMMON USES: Urinary tract infections, otitis media, sinusitis, bronchitis, Shigella, Pneumocystis carinii, Nocardia.
DOSAGE: ***Adults:*** 1 double strength (DS) tablet PO bid or 5–10 mg/kg/24h (based on trimethoprim component) IV in 3–4 divided doses. *P carinii:* 15–20 mg/kg/d IV or PO (trimethoprim component) in 4 divided doses. ***Peds:*** 8–10 mg/kg/24h (trimethoprim) PO divided into 2 doses or 3–4 doses IV; do not use in newborn.
NOTES: Synergistic combination; reduce dosage in renal failure.

Trimipramine (Surmontil)

COMMON USES: Treatment of depression.
DOSAGE: 75–300 mg PO qhs.

Tropicamide (Mydriacyl)

COMMON USES: Ocular exam; mydriatic and cycloplegic.
DOSAGE: 1–2 drops of 0.5–1% solution 30 min before exam; repeat q30min prn
NOTES: Effects last 4–6 h.

Urokinase (Abbokinase)

COMMON USES: Pulmonary embolism, deep venous thrombosis, restore patency to IV catheters, coronary artery thrombosis.
DOSAGE: ***Adults*** and ***Peds:*** Systemic effect: 4400 IU/kg IV over 10 min, followed by 4400 IU/kg/h for 12 h. Restore catheter patency: Inject 5000 IU into catheter and gently aspirate.
NOTES: Do not use systemically within 10 d of surgery, delivery, or organ biopsy.

Valacyclovir (Valtrex)

COMMON USES: Treatment of herpes zoster.
DOSAGE: 1 g PO tid.

Valproic Acid and Divalproex (Depakene and Depakote)

COMMON USES: Epilepsy, mania, and prophylaxis of migraines.
DOSAGE: ***Adults*** and ***Peds:*** Seizures: 30–60 mg/kg/24h PO divided tid. Mania: 750 mg in three divided doses, increased to a maximum of 60 mg/kg/d. Migraines: 250 mg bid, increased to 1000 mg/d
NOTES: Monitor liver functions and follow serum levels; concurrent use of phenobarbital and phenytoin may alter serum levels of these agents.

Valsartan (Diovan)

COMMON USES: Hypertension.
DOSAGE: 80 mg once daily.
NOTES: Use with caution with potassium-sparing diuretics or potassium supplements.

Vancomycin (Vancocin, Vancoled)

COMMON USES: Serious infections resulting from methicillin-resistant staphylococci and in enterococcal endocarditis in combination with aminoglycosides in penicillin-allergic patients; oral treatment of *C difficile* pseudomembranous colitis.
DOSAGE: ***Adults:*** 1 g IV q12h; for colitis 250–500 mg PO q6h. ***Peds (not neonates):*** 40 mg/kg/24h IV in divided doses q12–6h.
NOTES: Ototoxic and nephrotoxic; not absorbed orally, provides local effect in gut only; IV dose must be given slowly over 1 h to prevent "red-man syndrome"; adjust dose in renal failure; see Table IX–3 and page 457.

Vasopressin (Antidiuretic Hormone) (Pitressin)

COMMON USES: Treatment of diabetes insipidus; gaseous gastrointestinal tract distention; severe gastrointestinal bleeding.
DOSAGE: ***Adults*** and ***Peds:*** Diabetes insipidus: 2.5–10 U SC or IM tid–qid or 1.5–5.0 U IM q1–3d of the tannate. Gastrointestinal hemorrhage: 20 U in 50–100-mL D5W or NS given IV over 15–30 min.
NOTES: Should be used with caution with any vascular disease.

Vecuronium (Norcuron)

COMMON USES: Skeletal muscle relaxation during surgery or mechanical ventilation.
DOSAGE: ***Adults*** and ***Peds:*** 0.08–0.1 mg/kg IV bolus; maintenance of 0.010–0.015 mg/kg after 25–40 min followed with additional doses every 12–15 min.
NOTES: Drug interactions leading to increased effect of vecuronium include aminoglycosides, tetracycline, and succinylcholine; less cardiac effects then pancuronium.

Venlafaxine (Effexor)

COMMON USES: Treatment of depression.
DOSAGE: 75–225 mg/d divided into 2–3 equal doses.

Verapamil (Calan, Isoptin)

COMMON USES: Supraventricular tachyarrhythmias (PAT, Wolff-Parkinson-White syndrome, atrial flutter or fibrillation); vasospastic (Prinzmetal's) and unstable (crescendo, preinfarction) angina; chronic stable angina (classical effort-associated); hypertension.
DOSAGE: ***Adults:*** Tachyarrhythmias: 5–10 mg IV over 2 min (may repeat in 30 min). Angina: 240–480 mg/24h divided in 3–4 doses. Hypertension: 80–180 mg PO tid or SR tablet 240 mg PO qd. ***Peds:*** <1 y: 0.1–0.2 mg/kg IV over 2 min (may

repeat in 30 min). 1–15 y: 0.1–0.3 mg/kg IV over 2 min (may repeat in 30 min); Do not exceed 5 mg.

NOTES: Use caution with elderly patients; reduce dose in renal failure; constipation is a common side effect.

Vidarabine (Vira-A)

COMMON USES: Herpes simplex keratitis and conjunctivitis

DOSAGE: Apply ointment 5 times a day divided q3–4h; after healing begins, decrease to bid for up to 7 d.

Vinblastine (Velban)

COMMON USES: Hodgkin's disease, lymphoma, and testicular and ovarian cancer.

DOSAGE: On the basis of protocol; typical dosing 4–12 mg/m^2 q7–10d or 5–d continuous infusion 1.4–1.8 mg/m^2/d.

NOTES: May cause neutropenia; reduce dose after radiation exposure.

Vincristine (Oncovin)

COMMON USES: Cervical and ovarian cancer, sarcoma, leukemia, and Hodgkin's disease.

DOSAGE: Varies with protocol 1.4–2 mg/m^2 IV once a week.

NOTES: May cause severe extravasation.

Vitamin B12

See "Cyanocobalamin," page 475.

Vitamin K

See "Phytonadione," page 519.

Warfarin Sodium (Coumadin)

COMMON USES: Prophylaxis and treatment of pulmonary embolism and venous thrombosis, atrial fibrillation with embolization, other postop uses.

DOSAGE: ***Adults:*** Need to individualize dose to keep INR level at 2–3; some mechanical heart valves require INR to be 2.5–3.5; initially, 10–15 mg PO, IM, or IV qd for 1–3 d; then maintenance, 2–10 mg PO, IV, or IM qd; follow INR levels during initial phase to guide dosing. ***Peds:*** 0.05–0.34 mg/kg/24h PO, IM, or IV qd. Follow PT closely to adjust dose.

NOTES: Follow INR while on maintenance dose; beware of bleeding caused by over anticoagulation (PT > 3 times control); caution patient on effects of taking Coumadin with other medications, especially aspirin; to rapidly correct over coumadinization, use vitamin K or fresh frozen plasma or both; highly teratogenic, do not use in pregnancy.

Witch Hazel (Tucks Pads)

COMMON USES: After bowel movement cleansing to decrease local irritation or relieve hemorrhoids; after anorectal surgery and episiotomy.

DOSAGE: Apply as needed.

Zafirlukast (Accolate)

COMMON USES: Prophylaxis and chronic treatment of asthma.

DOSAGE: 20 mg bid.

NOTES: Not for acute exacerbations of asthma, contraindicated in nursing women.

Zalcitabine (Hivid)

COMMON USES: HIV infection in patients intolerant to zidovudine and didanosine.

DOSAGE: 0.75 mg PO tid.

NOTES: May be used in combination with zidovudine; may cause peripheral neuropathy.

Zaleplon (Sonata)

COMMON USES: Insomnia.
DOSAGE: 5–20 mg qhs prn.

Zanamivir (Relenza)

COMMON USES: Treatment of influenza.
DOSAGE: 2 inhalations (10 mg) twice daily.
NOTES: Uses a diskhaler for administration.

Zidovudine (Retrovir)

COMMON USES: Management of patients with HIV infections.
DOSAGE: ***Adults:*** 200 mg PO tid or 300 mg PO bid or 1–2 mg/kg/dose IV q4h. Pregnancy: 100 mg PO 5 times/d until labor; during labor 2 mg/kg over 1 h followed by 1 mg/kg/h until clamping of the umbilical cord. ***Peds:*** 720 mg/m^2/24h PO divided 5 times/d.
NOTES: Not a cure for HIV infections.

Zidovudine and Lamivudine (Combivir)

COMMON USES: Management of patients with HIV infections.
DOSAGE: ***Adults*** and **Peds:** > 12 y: 1 tablet bid.

Zileution (Zyflo)

COMMON USES: Prophylaxis and chronic treatment of asthma.
DOSAGE: 600 mg qid.
NOTES: MUST take on a regular basis; does not treat acute exacerbation.

Zolpidem (Ambien) [C]

COMMON USES: Short-term treatment of insomnia.
DOSAGE: 5–10 mg PO qhs prn.

Zonisamide (Zonegran)

COMMON USES: Partial seizures.
DOSAGE: Initial 100 mg once daily; may be increased to 400 mg/d.
NOTES: Contraindicated in persons with hypersensitivity to sulfonamides.

Appendix

BODY SURFACE AREA: ADULT (See Figure A–1)

BODY SURFACE AREA: ADULT

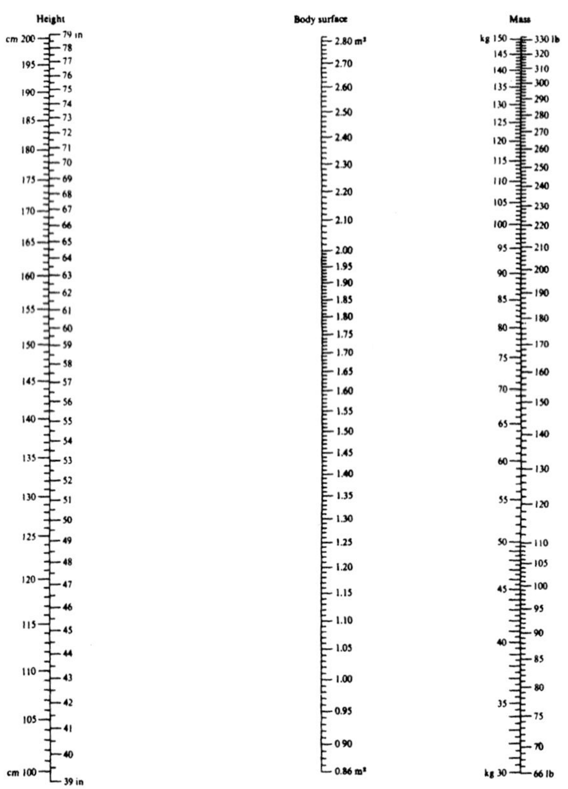

Figure A-1. To determine the body surface area in an adult, use a straight edge to connect the height and mass. The point of intersection on the body surface line gives the area in m^2. (From Lentner C (editor): *Geigy Scientific Tables,* 8th ed. CIBA-GEIGY 1981;1:226.)

BODY SURFACE AREA: CHILDREN (See Figure A–2)

BODY SURFACE AREA: CHILDREN

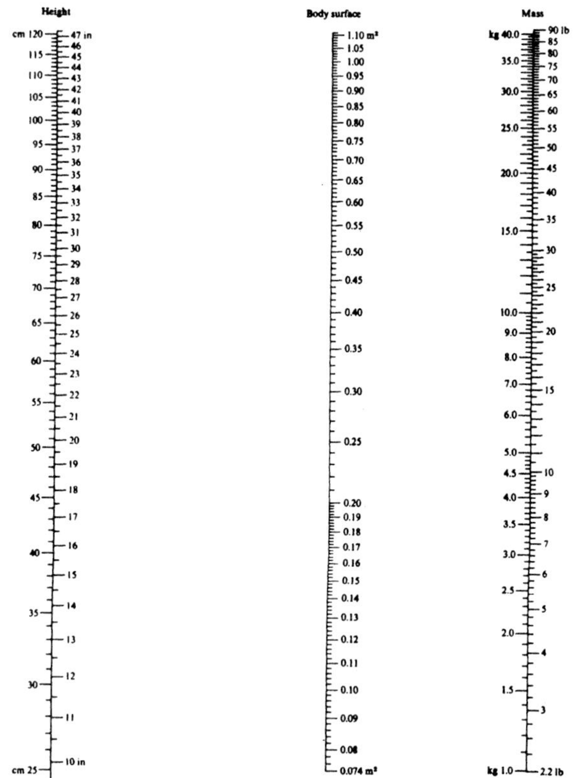

Figure A-2. To determine the body surface area in a child, use a straight edge to connect the height and mass. The point of intersection on the body surface line gives the area in m². (From Lentner C (editor): *Geigy Scientific Tables,* 8th ed. CIBA-GEIGY 1981;1:227.)

BOWEL PREPS

The purpose of a bowel preparation is the removal of all solid material from the bowel and the reduction of the bacterial population to decrease the incidence of complications of surgical procedures and to provide a clean bowel for endoscopic procedures.

A. Noncolonic surgery.

1. The patient should remain NPO after midnight before surgery.
2. Bowel preparation may be indicated for upper gastrointestinal surgical procedures.
    a. Surgery may involve the colon (eg, extensive surgery for gynecologic malignancy or large gastric tumors).
    b. Achlorhydria, gastric carcinoma, prolonged H_2-receptor blocker use, and obstructive peptic ulcer disease will allow bacterial growth in the stomach. Consider using an oral antibiotic prep (eg, neomycin) for gastric surgery in these patients (see below).

B. Colonic surgery mechanical or whole gut lavage prep with or without oral antibiotic prep. Many variations exist.

1. Mechanical prep.
    a. Day 1—diet should be clear liquids; give a laxative of choice (castor oil 60 mL, Milk of Magnesia (MOM) 30 mL, magnesium citrate 250 mL), and a tap water or a soap-suds enema until bowel is clear.
    b. Day 2—diet should be clear liquids, give IV fluids, a laxative of choice, and an enema (both AM and PM).
    c. Day 3—operation.

OR

    d. Day 1—diet should be clear liquids; give IV fluids, Fleets, Phospho-soda 1–2 oz with water (repeat × 1), a Dulcolax suppository in the evening and an enema × 1.
    e. Day 2—operation.
2. Whole gut lavage (GoLYTELY, a polyethylene glycol electrolyte-balanced solution).
    a. Day 1—GoLYTELY 4 L PO or per NG tube over 4 h.
    b. Give metoclopramide 10 mg PO to reduce bloating and nausea.
    c. Day 2—operation.
3. Oral antibiotic prep, mechanical prep, or whole gut lavage should be completed before the administration of the oral antibiotic prep.
    a. Nichols-Condon prep—on day before surgery, give neomycin 1 g and erythromycin base 1 g of each

PO at 1 PM, 2 PM, and 11 PM for a patient scheduled at 8 AM.

   b. Metronidazole (500 mg) PO—This may be substituted for erythromycin base in the Nichols-Condon prep (causes less nausea than with erythromycin base).

4. Perioperative IV antibiotics may be used in conjunction with, or instead of, the oral antibiotic prep, depending on the preference of the attending surgeon.

   a. These antibiotics should be administered immediately preoperatively (see above) and intraoperatively for prolonged operations. Any further postoperative doses reportedly are not effective in preventing wound infection; however, most surgeons still administer at least one dose of antibiotic postoperatively, and it is common to continue the antibiotic for 24 h postoperatively.

   b. Choice of antibiotic (See Table A–1)—The key here is to obtain broad coverage of enteric organisms (gram-negatives, anaerobes, eg, gentamicin and clindamycin, cefazolin and metronidazole, or cefotetan).

(From Preoperative Preparation. In Koutlas TC (editor): *The Mont Reid Surgical Handbook,* Mosby, 1994, with permission.)

CHARTWORK

Preoperative Note

The specific items in the preoperative note are dependent on institutional guidelines, the nature of the procedure, and the age and health of the patient. For example, an ECG and blood set-up may not be necessary for a 2-year-old child for a herniorrhaphy, but it is essential for a 70-year-old scheduled for vascular surgery.

Preop diagnosis: State the preop diagnosis, such as "Acute appendicitis."

Procedure: Indicate what the planned procedure is, such as "Exploratory laparotomy."

Labs: Note results of the complete blood count (CBC), electrolytes, urinalysis, and so forth.

Chest Radiograph (CXR): Note the results.

ECG: Note the results.

Blood: Type and cross (T&C) 2 units packed red cells, blood not needed, and so forth.

History and physical: Data should be "on chart."

Orders: Note special preop orders written, such as preoperative colon preps, vaginal douches, and prophylactic antibiotics.

Permit: If this has been completed, write "Signed and on chart."

TABLE A–1. PREVENTION OF WOUND INFECTION AND SEPSIS IN SURGICAL PATIENTS

Nature of operation	Likely pathogens	Recommended drugs	Adult dosage before surgery[1]
Cardiac			
Prosthetic valve, coronary artery bypass, other open-heart surgery, pacemaker or defibrillator implant	*Staphylococcus epidermidis, S. aureus, Corynebacterium,* enteric gram-negative bacilli	cefazolin or cefuroxime *or* vancomycin[3]	1–2 grams IV[2] 1–2 grams IV[2] 1 gram IV
Gastrointestinal			
Esophageal, gastroduodenal	Enteric gram-negative bacilli, gram-positive cocci	*High risk*[4] only: cefazolin[5]	1–2 grams IV
Biliary tract	Enteric gram-negative bacilli, enterococci, clostridia	*High risk*[6] *only:* cefazolin[5]	1–2 grams IV
Colorectal	Enteric gram-negative bacilli, anaerobes, enterococci	*Oral:* neomycin+ erythromycin base[7] *Parenteral:* cefoxitin or cefatetan or cefazolin + metronidazole	 1–2 grams IV 1–2 grams IV 1–2 grams IV 0.5 grams IV
Appendectomy, non-perforated	Enteric gram-negative bacilli, anaerobes, enterococci	cefoxitin or cefotetan	1–2 gramsIV 1–2 grams IV
Genitourinary	Enteric gram-negative bacilli, enterococci	*High risk*[8] *only:* ciprofloxacin	500 mg PO or 400 mg IV
Gynecologic and Obstetric			
Vaginal or abdominal hysterectomy	Enteric gram-negatives, anaerobes, Gp B strep, enterococci	cefazolin or cefotetan or cefoxitin	1–2 grams IV 1–2 grams IV 1 gram IV
Cesarean section	same as for hysterectomy	*High risk*[9] *only:* cefazolin	1 gram IV after cord clamping

Abortion	same as for hysterectomy	*First trimester, high risk*[10]: aqueous penicillin G or doxycycline	 2 mill units IV 300 mg PO[11]
		Second trimester: cefazolin	1 gram IV
Head and Neck Surgery			
Incisions through oral or pharyngeal mucosa	Anaerobes, enteric gram-negative bacilli, *S. aureus*	clindamycin + gentamicin	600–900 mg IV 1.5 mg/kg IV
Neurosurgery			
Craniotomy	*S. aureus, S. epideridis*	cefazolin *or* vancomycin[3]	1–2 grams IV 1 gram IV
Opthalmic	*S. epidermidis, S. aureus,* streptococci, enteric gram-negative bacilli, Pseudomonas	gentamicin, tobramycin, ciprofloxacin, ofloxacin or neomycin-gramicidin-polymyxin B cefazolin	multiple drops topically over 2 to 24 hours 100 mg subconjunctivally
Orthopedic			
Total joint replacement, internal fixation of fractures	*S. aureus, S. epidermidis*	cefazolin *or* vancomycin[3]	1–2 grams IV 1 gram IV
Throracic (Non-Cardiac)	*S.aureus, S epidermidis,* streptococci, enteric gram-negative bacilli	cefazolin or cefuroxime *or* vancomycin[3]	1–2 grams IV 1–2 grams IV 1 gram IV
Vascular			
Arterial surgery involving a prosthesis, the abdominal aorta, or a groin incision	*S. aureus, S. epidermidis,* enteric gram-negative bacilli	cefazolin *or* vancomycin[3]	1–2 grams IV 1 gram IV
Lower extremity amputation for ischemia	*S. aureus, S. epidermidis,* enteric gram-negative bacilli, clostridia	cefazolin[5] *or* vancomycin[3]	1–2 grams IV 1 gram IV

(*continued*)

TABLE A–1. PREVENTION OF WOUND INFECTION AND SEPSIS IN SURGICAL PATIENTS (*continued*)

Nature of operation	Likely pathogens	Recommended drugs	Adult dosage before surgery[1]
CONTAMINATED SURGERY[12]			
Ruptured viscus	Enteric gram-negative bacilli, anaerobes, enterococci	cefoxitin or cefotetan ± gentamicin *or* clindamycin + gentamicin	1–2 g IV q6h 1–2 IV q12h 1.5 mg/kg IV q8h 600 mg IV q6h 1.5 mg/kg IV q8h
Traumatic wound	*S. aureus,* Gp A strep, clostridia	cefazolin[13]	1–2 grams IV q8h

[1]Parenteral prophylactic antimicrobials can be given as a single intravenous dose just before the operation. For prolonged operations, additional intraoperative doses should be given q4–8h for the duration of the procedure.
[2]Some consultants recommend an additional dose when patients are removed from bypass during open-heart surgery.
[3]For hospitals in which methicillin-resistant *S. aureus* and *S. epidermidis* are a frequent cause of postoperative wound infection, or for patients allergic to penicillins or cephalosporins. Rapid IV administration may cause hypotension, which could be especially dangerous during induction of anesthesia. Even if the drug is given over 60 minutes, hypotension may occur; treatment with diphenhydramine (*Benadryl,* and others) and further slowing of the infusion rate may be helpful (DG Maki et al, *J Thorac Cardiovasc Surg,* 104:1423, 1992). For procedures in which enteric gram-negative bacilli are likely pathogens, such as vascular surgery involving a groin incision, cefazolin should be included in the prophylaxis regimen for patients not allergic to cephalosporins.
[4]Morbid obesity, esophageal obstruction, decreased gastric acidity or gastrointestinal motility.
[5]Some Medical Letter consultants favor cefoxitin for better anaerobic coverage in this setting.
[6]Age > 70 years, acute cholecystitis, non-functioning gall bladder, obstructive jaundice or common duct stones.
[7]After appropriate diet and catharsis, one gram of each at 1 PM, 2 PM and 11 PM the day before an 8 AM operation.
[8]Urine culture positive or unavailable, preoperative catheter, transrectal prostatic biopsy.
[9]Active labor or premature rupture of membranes.
[10]Patients with previous pelvic inflammatory disease, previous gonorrhea or multiple sex partners.
[11]Divided into 100 mg one hour before the abortion and 200 mg one half hour after.
[12]For contaminated or "dirty" surgery, therapy should usually be continued for about five days. Ruptured viscus in postoperative setting (dehiscence) requires antibaterials to include coverage of nosocomial pathogens.
[13]For bite wounds, in which likely pathogens may also include oral anaerobes, *Eikenella corrodens* (human), or *Pasteurella multocida* (dog and cat), some Medical Letter consultants recommend use of amoxicillin/clavulanic acid (*Augmentin*) or ampicillin/sulbactam (*Unasyn*).
(Reproduced with permission from The Medical Letter *1999;41:76.)*

Operative Note

The operative note is written immediately after surgery to summarize the operation for those who were not present and is meant to complement the formal operative summary that is dictated by the surgeon.

Preop diagnosis: Indicate why the patient was taken to surgery such as "Acute appendicitis."

Postop diagnosis: This should be based on the operative findings, such as "Mesenteric lymphadenitis."

Procedure: Indicate what procedure was actually performed, such as "Exploratory laparotomy."

Surgeons: List the attending, residents, and students who scrubbed on the case along with titles (eg, MD, CCIV, MSII). It is often helpful to identify the dictating surgeon.

Findings: Briefly note operative findings, such as "Normal appendix with marked lymphadenopathy."

Anesthesia: State type of anesthesia used (Local, spinal, general, endotracheal, etc).

Fluids: Indicate amount and type used during case (eg, normal saline, blood, albumin). This is usually obtained for the anesthesia records.

Estimated Blood Loss (EBL): This is usually obtained from the anesthesia or nursing records.

Drains: State location and type of drain, such as "Jackson-Pratt drain in left upper quadrant," "T-tube in midline," and so forth.

Specimens: State whether any specimens were sent to the pathology lab, and indicate the test results of any intraoperative frozen sections.

Complications: Hopefully, you would write "None."

Condition: Note where the patient is taken immediately after surgery and indicate the patient's condition (eg, "transferred to the recovery room in stable condition").

Night of Surgery Note (Postoperative Note)

This is a specific type of progress note written several hours after surgery or on the same night.

Procedure: Indicate the operation performed.

Level of consciousness: Note whether the patient is alert, drowsy, and so forth.

Vital signs: Indicate blood pressure, pulse, respiration.

Intake and output (I&O): Calculate IV fluids, urine output, and other drainage, and attempt to assess fluid balance.

Labs: Review results, if any were obtained since surgery.

Physical exam: Examine and note the findings for the chest, heart, abdomen, extremities, and any other part as needed; examine the dressing for bleeding.

Assessment: Evaluate the postop course thus far (stable, etc).

Plan: Note any changes in orders.

Glasgow Coma Scale (Table A–2)

The Glasgow Coma Scale (EMV Scale) is a fairly reliable, objective method of monitoring changes in levels of consciousness. It is based on eye opening, motor responses, and verbal responses (EMV). A person's EMV score is based on the total of the three different responses. The score ranges from 3 (lowest) to 15 (highest).

TABLE A–2. GLASGOW COMA SCALE.

Parameter	Response		Score
Eyes	Open: spontaneously		4
	To verbal command		3
	To pain		2
	No response		1
Best motor response	To verbal command	Obeys	6
	To painful stimulus	Localizes pain	5
		Flexion-withdrawal	4
		Decorticate (flex)	3
		Decerebrate (extend)	2
		No response	1
Best verbal response	Oriented, converses		5
	Disoriented, converses		4
	Inappropriate responses		3
	Incomprehensible sounds		2
	No response		1

SBE Prophylaxis

The following recommendations (Tables A–3, 4, 5) are based on guidelines published by the American Heart Association. (JAMA. 1997;277:1794). These updated guidelines now specify those patients who are at high, moderate, and low risk of bacteremia, and they provide general guidelines for procedures that are more likely to be associated with bacterial endocarditis. SBE prophylaxis is recommended for patients with high or moderate risk conditions.

High-risk: Prosthetic cardiac valves, history of bacterial endocarditis; complex cyanotic congenital heart disease, surgically constructed systemic pulmonary shunts.

Moderate-risk: Most other congenital cardiac malformations (other than above and below), acquired valvar disease (eg, rheumatic heart disease), hypertrophic cardiomyopathy, mitral valve prolapse with regurgitation and/or thickened leaflets.

Low-risk: Isolated ASD secundum; repair of atrial/ventricular septal defect, or PDA; prior CABG; mitral valve prolapse without regurgitation; innocent heart murmurs; previous Kawasaki disease or rheumatic fever without valve dysfunction; pacemakers or implanted defibrillator.

TABLE A–3. SBE PROPHYLAXIS BASED ON PROCEDURE.

Dental: Dental extractions, periodontal procedures, dental implants; reimplantation of avulsed teeth; endodontic instrumentation only beyond the apex; subgingival placement of antibiotic fibers or strips; placement of orthodontic bands (not brackets); intraligamentary anesthetic injections; cleaning of teeth or implants where bleeding likely

Respiratory: Tonsillectomy and/or adenoidectomy; surgery on the respiratory mucosa; rigid bronchoscopy

Gastrointestinal tract: Sclerotherapy for esophageal varices; esophageal stricture dilation; ERCP with biliary obstruction; biliary tract surgery; operations involoving intestinal mucosa

Genitourinary: Prostate surgery, cystoscopy, urethral dilation

TABLE A–4. SBE PROPHYLAXIS FOR ORAL, RESPIRATORY OR ESOPHAGEAL PROCEDURES.

	Agent	Regimen*
Standard prophylaxis	Amoxicillin	Adults: 2.0 g; children: 50 mg/kg PO 1 h before procedure
Unable to take oral medications	Ampicillin	Adults: 2.0 g IM or IV; children: 50 mg/kg IM or IV 30 min before procedure
Allergic to penicillin	Clindamycin **or**	Adults: 600 mg; children 20 mg/kg PO 1 h before procedure
	Cephalexin **or** Cefadroxil	Adults: 2.0 g; children: 50 mg/kg PO 1 h before procedure
	Azithromycin **or** Clarithromycin	Adults: 500 mg; children: 15 mg/kg PO 1 h before procedure
Penicillin allergic and unable to take oral medications	Clindamycin **or** Cefazolin	Adults: 600 mg; children: 20 mg/kg IV 30 min before procedure Adults: 1.0 g; children: 25 mg/kg IM or IV 30 min before procedure

*Total children's dose should not exceed adult dose.

TABLE A–5. SBE PROPHYLAXIS FOR GU/GI (EXCLUDING ESOPHAGEAL) PROCEDURES.

	Agents	Regimen*
High-risk patients	Ampicillin + gentamicin	Adults: ampicillin 2.0 g IM/IV + gentamicin 1.5 mg/kg (max 120 mg) within 30 min of procedure; 6 h later, ampicillin 1 g IM/IV or amoxicillin 1 g PO
		Children: ampicillin 50 mg/kg IM or IV (2.0 g max) + gentamicin 1.5 mg/kg within 30 min of procedure; 6 h later, ampicillin 25 mg/kg IM/IV or amoxicillin 25 mg/kg PO
High-risk patients allergic to ampicillin/ amoxicillin	Vancomycin + gentamicin	Adults: vancomycin 1.0 g IV over 1–2 h + gentamicin 1.5 mg/kg IV/IM (120 mg max); dose within 30 min of starting procedure
		Children: vancomycin 20 mg/kg IV over 1–2 h + gentamicin 1.5 mg/kg IV/IM; complete dose within 30 min of starting procedure
Moderate-risk patients	Amoxicillin or ampicillin	Adults: amoxicillin 2.0 g PO 1 h before procedure, or ampicillin 2.0 g IM/IV within 30 min of starting procedure
		Children: amoxicillin 50 mg/kg PO 1 h before procedure, or ampicillin 50 mg/kg IM/IV within 30 min of starting procedure
Moderate-risk patients allergic to ampicillin/ amoxicillin	Vancomycin	Adults: vancomycin 1.0 g IV over 1–2 h complete infusion within 30 min of starting procedure
		Children: vancomycin 20 mg/kg IV over 1–2 h; complete infusion within 30 min of starting procedure

*Total children's dose should not exceed adult dose.

SPECIMEN TUBES FOR VENIPUNCTURE

TABLE A–6. SPECIMEN TUBES FOR VENIPUNCTURE.[1]

Tube Color	Additives	General Use
Red	None	Clot tube to collect serum for chemisty, crossmatching, serology
Red and black (hot pink)	Silicone gel for rapid clot	As above, but not for osmolality or blood bank work
Blue	Sodium citrate (binds calcium)	Coagulation studies (best kept on ice, not for fibrin split products)
Blue/yellow label		Fibrin split products
Royal blue		Heavy metals, arsenic
Purple	Disodium EDTA (binds calcium)	Hematology, not for lipid profiles
Green	Sodium heparin	Ammonia, cortisol, ionized calcium (best kept on ice)
Green/glass beads		LE prep
Grey	Sodium fluoride	Lactic acid
Yellow	Transport media	Blood cultures

[1]Individual labs may vary slightly from these listings.

TETANUS PROPHYLAXIS

TABLE A–7. TENTANUS PROPHYLAXIS, BASED ON GUIDELINES FROM THE CENTERS FOR DISEASE CONTROL AND PREVENTION AND REPORTED IN MMWR 1990:39. [NO. 3].

History Tetanus Toxoid Immunization	Clean, Minor Wounds		All Other Wounds	
	Td[2]	TIG[3]	Td[2]	TIG[3]
Unknown or <3 doses	Yes	No	Yes	Yes
> or = 3 doses[4]	No[5]	No	No[6]	No

Such as, but not limited to, wounds contaminated with dirt, feces, soil, saliva, etc; puncture wounds; avulsions; and wounds resulting from missiles, crushing, burns, and frostbite.
[2]Td = tetanus-diphtheria toxoid, (Adult type) dose: 0.5 mL IM. For children younger than 7 years DPT (DT, if pertussis vaccine cantraindiacted) is preferred to tetanus toxoid alone. For persons 7 years of age or older, Td is preferred to tetanus toxoid alone. DT = diptheria-tetanus toxoid (Pediatric) used for those who cannot receive pertussis.
[3]TIG = tetanus immune globulin, 250 units IM.
[4]If only three doses of fluid toxoid have been received, then a fourth dose of toxoid, preferably an absorbed toxoid, should be given.
[5]Yes, if more than 10 years since last dose.
[6]Yes, if more than 5 years since last dose.

TEMPERATURE CONVERSION CHART.

TABLE A–8. TEMPERATURE CONVERSION TABLE[1]

F	C	C	F
0	–17.7	0	32.0
95.0	35.0	35.0	95.0
96.0	35.5	35.5	95.9
97.0	36.1	36.0	96.8
98.0	36.6	36.5	97.7
98.6	**37.0**	**37.0**	**98.6**
99.0	37.2	37.5	99.5
100.0	37.7	38.0	100.4
101.0	38.3	38.5	101.3
102.0	38.8	39.0	102.2
103.0	39.4	39.5	103.1
104.0	40.0	40.0	104.0
105.0	40.5	40.5	104.9
106.0	41.1	41.0	105.8

$C = (F - 32) \times 5/9$ $F = (C \times 9/5) + 32$

[1]F = degrees Fahreheit; C = degrees Celsius.

Index

Page numbers followed by italicized *f* and *t* refer to figures and tables, respectively

C

O